चरक संहिता III

ENGLISH TRANSLATION

डा. जनार्धन वि हेब्बार

Made with ♥ on the Notion Press Platform
www.notionpress.com

|| Jai Guruji ||

I, Dr. Janardhana V. Hebbar, dedicate this book at the holy feet of Sri Guruji – Swami Vivekananda and my spiritual Guru, Dr. A. Chandrashekhara Udupa MBBS, F.A.G.E., Managing Director, Divine Park Trust (R), Saligrama, Udupi. (www.divinepark.org)

He guides, He energizes, He shows the path,
He holds my hand and makes me walk!

क्रम-सूची

भूमिका

This book covers the 23 chapters of Chikitsasthana of Charaka Samhita.

Charaka Samhita is a popular Ayurvedic treatise. As the name indicates, it is a compilation of Ayurveda lessons comprising of various aspects including basic concepts (Sutra sthana), diagnosis of diseases (Nidana sthana), treatment concepts (Chikitsa sthana) etc. and is written by Charaka. (Charaka Samhita means 'treatise written by Charaka).

Acharya Charaka redacted the treatise 'Agnivesha Tantra' which has become popular in the name of 'Charaka Samhita'. This means to tell that the text 'Agnivesha Tantra' written by Agnivesha was re-modulated by Charaka, which later came to be called as 'Charaka Samhita'.

Charaka Samhita is the first and foremost authentic treatise of Ayurveda and is one of the 'greatest trio' (Brihat-Trayee).

Master Charaka was so keen to help people with Ayurveda that he used to roam from one place to the other continuously. Hence he got the name Charaka.

Charati iti Charakaha – One who moves continuously.

Charaka Samhita

Charaka Samhita, a part of Brihat Trayi or greater trio of Ayurveda occupies a significant place in the history of world's medical science.

Atreya Punarvasu has many intelligent students. Punarvasu was the most respected, learned Guru (teacher) and preacher of Ayurveda. Among the clan of his elite students Agnivesha was the best.

According to the directions and teachings of his teacher Punarvasu Atreya, Agnivesha recorded, documented and composed his work on Ayurveda.

It was called as Agnivesha Tantra. It was subsequently redacted by Charaka which in due course of time got popular in the name 'Charaka Samhita'. This Charaka Samhita was further redacted by Dridhabala.

In Charaka Samhita, we can find that the justice has been done in covering all the aspects and 8 branches of Ayurveda. But the emphasis has been given in covering the concepts of Kaya Chikitsa (General medicine) in detail. That is why, Charaka Samhita is considered to be the best reference and authentic text of Kaya Chikitsa.

More than 40 commentaries are written on Charaka Samhita. It is translated into all the Indian languages. It is also translated into many foreign languages including Persian, Simhali, Nepali, Arabic etc.

Sections and Chapters of Charaka Samhita:

Charaka Samhita has been dealt with in 8 sections and 120 chapters.

Sutrasthana – Basic Principles – 30 chapters, 1952 Verses.

Nidana Sthana – Pathology – 8 chapters, 247 verses

Vimana Sthana – Specific determination – 8 chapters, 354 verses

Shareera Sthana – Anatomy – 8 chapters , 382 verses

Indriya Sthana – Sensory organ based prognosis – 12 chapters, 378 verses

Chikitsa Sthana – Therapeutics – 30 chapters, 4904 verses

Kalpasthana – Pharmaceutics and toxicology – 12 chapters – 378 verses

Siddhi Sthana – Success in treatment – 12 chapters – 700 verses

Total – 9295 verses (Sutras)

Sutra sthana

Deals with fundamental principles of Ayurveda covered in 30 chapters

Sutra Sthana is sub-divided into Sapta Chatushkas (7 quadrates), having 4 chapters each.

They are:

Bheshaja Chatushka – quadrate on drugs

Swasta Chatushka – quadrate on regimen for the maintenance of health

Nirdesha Chatushka – quadrate on various instructions

Kalpana Chatushka – quadrate on description of therapeutic procedures
Roga Chatushka – quadrate on description of diseases
Yojana Chatushka – quadrate on administration of various therapies
Annapana Chatushka – quadrate on description of diet and drinks
Sangraha adhyaya – 2 chapters at the end of Sutra Sthana are known by the name Sangraha Adhyaya, the concluding chapters

Vimana Sthana

Deals with the principles governing the bodily factors that cause diseases – drugs and medicaments covered in 8 chapters

a. In Rasa Vimana chapter, sweet, sour etc tastes, qualities, functions, effect on Dosha, oils, ghee, honey etc, their effect on health and asta vidha vishesha Ayatana are explained.

b. In Trividha Kuksheeya Vimana, GI tract, quantity of food to be taken, what happens if the food is taken excessively or in low quantities, Visuchika, Alasaka etc digestive tract disorders are mentioned.

c. In Janapadodhvamsaneeya chapter – communicable disorders, endemic diseases, reasons, preventive measures are mentioned.

d. In Trividha Roga VIshesha Vijnaneeya chapter, Pratyaksha – direct observation, Anumana, Aptaopadesha – means of knowledge, etc are explained.

e. In Sroto Vimana chapter, all the body channels, causes, symptoms and treatment of vitiation of body channels are mentioned.

f. In Roganeeka Vimana – types of diseases – mental, physical, types of Agni, Prakriti – body types etc are mentioned.

g. In Vyadhita Rupeeya Vimana – Guru, Laghu etc patient features, Krumi causes and treatment are mentioned.

h. In Roga Bhishag Jiteeya chapter, causes for diseases, sambhasha – discussion, 10 types of patient examination etc are explained.

Nidana Sthana

Deals with aetiology, pathogenesis and diagnosis of diseases covered in 8 chapters.
For each disease, causative factors, prodromal symptoms, signs and symptoms, pathogenesis, prognosis are explained in detail.

Jwara, Rakthapitha, Gulma, Prameha, Kushta etc diseases are explained in detail.

Shareera Sthana

Deals with embryology, anatomy and physiology covered in 8 chapters. This section gives detail discription about Human Anatomy and its application in treatment, panchamahabhutha (Basic 5 elements of earth), conception, embryology, signs of pregnancy, monthwise fetal development, manas prakruti (constitution of mind), determination of prakruti in the fetus, procedure of labour, diseases of children, bala samskara (Agewise ceremony), child nutrition and treatment of child disease.

Indriya Sthana

Deals with prognostic signs and symptoms covered in 12 chapters
In this section signs and symptoms of bad prognosis, inauspicious symptoms pertaining to skin complexion, voice, odour, taste, touch, sight, sound, mind, tongue, nose, fire, hygiene, behavioural activities, memory, tolerance capacity of patient, strength, structure of body, dryness, unctuousness, heaviness, digestion of food etc

Importance of inauspicious symptoms in the origin of disease, pain, advice, shadow, dreams, to see inauspicious signs on the road, auspicious and inauspicious signs related to sense organs and its perceived senses, curable and incurable signs of disease and patients life span are mentioned.

Chikitsa Sthana

Deals with treatment of various diseases covered in 30 chapters
This section explains in detail under Rasayana chapters – Rasayana medicines, intake procedure of rasayana, types of rasayana, rasayana properties of hareethaki and amalaki, procedure of its preparation, intake and its doses. It also deals with acharya rasayana.

Vachikarana chapters deals with – causes, types and treatment of infertility, use of vajikaran medicines, its method of preparation and intake.

Causes, signs and symptoms, types and treatment of various disease beginning from jwara, rakthapitha, gulma, prameha, doshagatha diseases, mental disorders, alcoholism,poisoning etc are mentioned here.

Kalpa Sthana

Deals with formulations for vamana (emesis), virechana (purgation) etc covered in 12 chapters.

This section deals with various medicinal formulations of madanaphala, jeemuthaka, dhamargava, krethavedhana, trivruth, aaragvadha, bilva, sapthala, danthi, dravathi etc, its origin, collection, types and properties are also mentioned here.

Siddhi Sthana

Deals with principles governing the administration of elimination therapies covered in 12 chapters

This section explains in detail – procedure of administration of elimination therapies(panchakarma), its indication and contraindications, complications developed due to improper administration of elimination therapy and its treatment. It also explains signs and symptoms produced due to excess, improper and proper administration of elimination therapy.

The three stages of Panchakarma – priliminary therapy (purvakarma), main therapy (pradhanakarma), post therapy procedures (paschathkarma) are explained orderly.

Persons indicated and contraindicated for elimination therapy and purificatory procedure for contraindicated person is also explained here.

Salient features of Charaka Samhita –

The titles of some chapters are based on the first word occurring in the chapter and others are based on the subject matter discussed in that particular chapter

4 types of Sutras are found in Charaka Samhita such as:

Guru Sutra – statements made by the teacher

Shishya Sutra – statements / enquires made by the disciple

Pratisamskarta Sutra – Statement of the redactor

Ekiya Sutra – statements made by individual scholars

Subject matter of each chapter is described as Uddeshya (brief statement and intention of chapter) followed by Nirdesha (detailed expansion of the above statement) and Lakshana (definition)

The colophons give the information of the author's name, name of redactor, title of the section and chapter and also the serial number of the chapter

The explanation of topics like Swabhavoparama vada highlights the influence of Buddhism on Charaka Samhita

Scientific explanation of the Ayurvedic fundamental principles like Tridoshas, Pancha Mahabhutas and Rasa Panchakas etc can be seen

Importance of Roga and Rogi Pareeksha (examination of disease and the diseased) has been emphasised

At the end of each chapter, the complete contents of the chapter are enlisted

Commentaries

More than 40 Sanskrit Commentaries were written on Charaka Samhita. Out of them the following are available partly or in full form.

Charakanyasa – By Bhattara Harishchandra in 4th century AD

Charaka Panjika – By Swami Kumara after 4th century AD

Nirantarapada Vyakhya – By Jejjata in 6th century AD

Ayurveda Deepika – By Chakrapani in 11th century AD

Tatwa Chandrika – By Shivadas Sen in 15th century AD

Jalpakalpataru – By Gangadhar Sen in 19th century AD

Charakopaskara – By Yogendranath Sen in 20th century AD

Charaka Pradipika – By Jyotishchandra Saraswati in 20th century AD

Charaka, the highly valued

Since 4th century A.D. onwards great scholars of Ayurveda, authors, scientists, commentators etc gave utmost respect to the sage 'Charaka'.

Famous commentators like Bhattara Harischandra, Swami Kumara, Yogendranatha Sen etc, paid their tributes to Acharya Charaka by naming their works as Charakanyasa, Charaka Panjika and Charakopaskara respectively. There are as many as 43 Sanskrit commentaries on this work.

In the beginning of 8th century AD Charaka Samhita was translated into Arabic language.

According to the Colophon, Agnivesha, on the advice of his preceptor Punarvasu Atreya, composed this work which was subsequently redacted by Charaka and Dridhabala

Charaka's Club – It is a medical organization which was established in New York in November 1898. It was founded by a group of 4 doctors Charles. L. Dana, Joseph Colliers, Fredrick Peterson and Barnad Sachs. This club discussed a wide array of subjects involving fields like medical, medical history, literature, poetry etc.

पावती (स्वीकृति)

Special thanks to Dr Raghuram YS for painstakingly editing the entire book.
Special thanks to my family members who have been supporting me unconditionally throughout this journey of Easy Ayurveda. Thank you for tolerating all the pains.
Smt. Padmakshamma (mother), Karthyayini (wife and staff), Smt. Vanamala (mother-in-law).
Daughters – Sadhvi & Chinmayi
Sister Sharada, brother-in-law Mr ShashiKumar, Tushar, Ms Sharada.
All my staff who make Easy Ayurveda possible, everyday.
Dr Sudarshan CH, Dr Shilpa Ramdas, Dr Renita D'Souza,
Mr Sachidananda Bhat, Smt. Nayana, Mr Nikhil and Smt. Sumangala.
My mentors - Dr MB Gururaja, Dr MS Krishnamurthy and Dr Prashanth BK

1

Chikitsasthana Chapter 1.1 Abhaya Amalakeeya Rasayanam

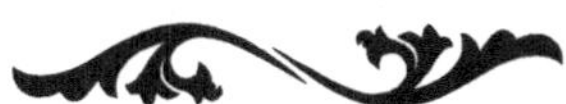

CharakaChikitsasthana 1.1

AbhayaAmalakeeyaRasayana

We are starting with Chikitsa Sthana section of Charaka Samhita. It has 30 chapters. Chikitsa refers to treatment. Hence, this section deals with the treatment and medicines for diseases.

The first chapter of Charaka Samhita Chikitsa Sthana is Rasayana Chikitsa. Rasayana means – anti ageing treatment. This chapter has four sub-sections.

1.1 AbhayaAmalakeeyaRasayana Pada

1.2 PraanaKameeyaRasayana Pada

1.3 Kara PrachiteeyaRasayana Pada

1.4 Ayurveda SamutthaniyaRasayana Pada

First Quarter of the Chapter on Rejuvenation:

अथातोऽभयामलकीयं रसायनपादं व्याख्यास्यामः||१||

इति ह स्माह भगवानात्रेयः||२||

    We shall now explore AbhayaAmalakeeyaRasayana Pada – the first sub section of the first Chapter of Charak Samhita Chikitsa Sthana. Thus said Lord Atreya:[1-2]

Synonyms of Medicine:

चिकित्सितं व्याधिहरं पथ्यं साधनमौषधम्|

प्रायश्चित्तं प्रशमनं प्रकृतिस्थापनं हितम्||३||

विद्यादभेषजनामानि, ...|४|

The synonyms of the term Bheshaja (medicine) are as below. Some refer it to as synonym for treatment:

- Chikitsa – Tool for treatment
- Vyadhihara – Tool to get rid of disease
- Pathya – the wholesome regime (dietary & behavioural) which is beneficial to maintain health or to treat illness
- Sadhana – means or tools of treatment
- Aushadha – drug / medicine
- Prayashchitta – corrective, reconciliation
- Prashamana – pacifier, balancing
- Prakriti-sthapana — Restoration of health.
- Hita – one which is beneficial, wholesome [3-4]

Categories of Medicines:
... भेषजं द्विविधम्च तत् I
स्वस्थस्योर्जस्करं किञ्चित् किञ्चिदार्तस्य रोगनुत् ||४||
Medicines are of two types:
Swasthasya Urjaskara – To maintain health of the healthy individuals, to improve immunity and quality of health etc.
Arthasya Roganut – To relieve the disease in the patient. [4]

Types of Abheshaja – Side Effects Of Medicines:
अभेषजं च द्विविधम्बाधनं सानुबाधनम्||५|
Abhesaja (medicines with adverse effects) are of two types viz.,
Badhana – those which cause miseries immediately after their use, which cause quick side effects
Sanubadhana – those which produce disease after they are used constantly for a long time [5]

Distinctive features of medicines:
स्वस्थस्योर्जस्करं यत्तु तद्वृष्यं तद्रसायनम्||५||
प्रायः, प्रायेण रोगाणां द्वितीयं प्रशमे मतम्|
प्रायःशब्दो विशेषार्थो ह्युभयं ह्युभयार्थकृत्||६||
The treatment / medicines that enhance quality of health in a healthy person are –
Vrushya – aphrodisiacs
Rasayana – anti ageing treatments
The other types of medicines are useful in the alleviation of diseases. However, both these types (health maintaining and disease alleviating) are considered medicines as they help to keep diseases at bay.
Sometimes Vrushya (aphrodisiac) and Rasayana medicines are used in treating diseases. Similarly, some medicines meant for treating diseases also act as Vrushya / Rasayana. For example: Agasthya Hareetaki Rasayana – medicine explained for Kasa (cough treatment) is also useful for anti-ageing purpose. [5-6]

Benefits of Anti-aging treatment (Rasayana – Rejuvenation therapy):
दीर्घमायुः स्मृतिं मेधामारोग्यं तरुणं वयः |
प्रभावर्णस्वरौदार्यं देहेन्द्रियबलं परम् ||७||
वाक्सिद्धिं प्रणतिंकान्तिं लभते ना रसायनात् |
लाभोपायो हि शस्तानां रसादीनां रसायनम्||८||
A person undergoing rejuvenation therapy gains
Deergham Aayu – Longevity
Smruti – good Memory
Medha – Intelligence
Arogya – Good health, free from diseases
Taruna – Youth
Vayaha – Long life
Prabha – Excellent aura, lustre
Varna – Good skin complexion
Swara – good voice
Dehabala – physical strength
IndriyaBala – Strong sense organs
Vak Siddhi – good oration skills
Pranati, Kanti – respect and brilliance.

The means by which one gets the maximum utilization of the end product of digestion (Rasa) is known as Rasayana or anti-ageing / rejuvenation therapy. [7-8]

Effects of Aphrodisiac therapy:
अपत्यसन्तानकरं यत् सद्यः सम्प्रहर्षणम्|
वाजीवातिबलो येन यात्यप्रतिहतः स्त्रियः ||९||
भवत्यतिप्रियः स्त्रीणां येन येनोपचीयते |
जीर्यतोऽप्यक्षयं शुक्रं फलवद्येन दृश्यते||१०||
प्रभूतशाखः शाखीव येन चैत्यो यथा महान् |
भवत्यच्र्याबहुमतः प्रजानां सुबहुप्रजः ||११||
सन्तानमूलं येनेह प्रेत्य चानन्त्यमश्नुते |
यशः श्रियं बलं पुष्टिं वाजीकरणमेव तत्||१२||
Vrushya – Aphrodisiac therapy yields following benefits :
Apatya, Santaanakara – potentiality for getting offspring's for the maintenance of the continuity of the lineage,
Sadya Sampraharshana – instantaneous sexual excitation,
Vaajivatibala – sexual strength of a horse
Apratihata Striyaha – does not get exhausted by sexual act
Atipriyaha streenaam – being liked by women

Aphrodisiac therapy nourishes Dhatu – tissue elements, by which even in old age, one does not get seminal debility or deficiency. It enables one to remain firm like a Chaitya (a big tree) with many branches. It enables the person to earn respect from people by virtue of him having procreated several children, which is conducive to his enjoying happiness and eternity in this world and beyond. Children bring about success, auspiciousness, strength and immunity. Vajikarana treatment is the reason for all these. [9-13]

Two categories of Medicines:
स्वस्थस्योर्जस्करं त्वेतद्दि्द्वविधं प्रोक्तमौषधम् |
यद्व्याधिनिर्घातकरं वक्ष्यते तच्चिकित्सिते ||१३||
चिकित्सितार्थ एतावान् विकाराणां यदौषधम् |
रसायनविधिश्चाग्रे वाजीकरणमेव च ||१४||
Swasthasya Urjaskara – The treatment that improves quality of a healthy person is described in this chapter. Those which help in the cure of diseases will be described later, from 3rd chapter onward. the primary aim of medicines is to cure diseases. The method of administration of rejuvenation and aphrodisiac therapies are described first. [13-14]

Abheshaja – Anti-medicine :
अभेषजमिति ज्ञेयं विपरीतं यदौषधात् |
तदसेव्यं निषेव्यं तु प्रवक्ष्यामि यदौषधम्||१५||
Things which are opposite in action to those of medicines are known as Abhesaja. These should not be used. Only medicines which are required to be used will be described here. [15]

Types of Rejuvenation Therapy:
रसायनानां द्विविधं प्रयोगमृषयो विदुः |
कुटीप्रावेशिकं चैव वातातपिकमेव च||१६||
कुटीप्रावेशिकस्यादौ विधिः समुपदेक्ष्यते |
नृपवैद्यद्विजातीनां साधूनां पुण्यकर्मणाम् ||१७||
निवासे निर्भये शस्ते प्राप्योपकरणे पुरे |

दिशि पूर्वोतरस्यां च सुभूमौ कारयेत् कुटीम्||१८||
विस्तारोत्सेधसम्पन्नां त्रिगर्भां सूक्ष्मलोचनाम् |
घनभित्तिमृतुसुखां सुस्पष्टां मनसः प्रियाम् ||१९||
शब्दादीनामशस्तानामगम्यं स्त्रीविवर्जिताम् |
इष्टोपकरणोपेतां सज्जवैद्यौषधद्विजाम्||२०||
अथोदगयने शुक्ले तिथिनक्षत्रपूजिते |
मुहूर्तकरणोपेते प्रशस्ते कृतवापनः ||२१||
धृतिस्मृतिबलं कृत्वा श्रद्दधानः समाहितः |
विधूय मानसान् दोषान् मैत्रीं भूतेषु चिन्तयन् ||२२||
देवताः पूजयित्वाऽग्रे द्विजातींश्च प्रदक्षिणम् |
देवगोब्राह्मणान् कृत्वा ततस्तां प्रविशेत् कुटीम् ||२३||
तस्यां संशोधनैः शुद्धः सुखी जातबलः पुनः |
रसायनं प्रयुञ्जीत तत्प्रवक्ष्यामिशोधनम् ||२४||

According to the sages, Rasayana (Rejuvenation / anti ageing) therapy is of two types:

Kutipraveshika – The patient is confined to a cottage throughout the treatment)

Vatatapika - It is administered even if the individual is exposed to the wind and the sun. He is not confined to a room.

Description of KutipraveshikaRasayana:

- One should get a cottage constructed in a good site inhabited by the king, physician, Brahmins, saints and those who perform virtuous acts,
- The place should be free from alarm, auspicious and where the required appliances can easily be procured.
- This cottage should face towards the east or the north. It should have three concentric courts and should be furnished with narrow ventilators.
- Its walls should be thick and it should be pleasant to reside in all seasons.
- It should be well-lit, and pleasant to the mind and be free from undesirable noise etc.
- It should not be accessible to women. This is because, the person undergoing Rasayana treatment is prohibited from having sex.
- It should be equipped with all the required appliances.
- Physicians, medicines and Brahmanas should be readily available there.

The time and duration:

- During the sun's northern course, in the light half of the month (Shukla Paksha), on an auspicious day (Tithi) with an auspicious constellation (Nakshatra), and favourable Muhurta (moment) and Karana.
- A person desirous of undergoing rejuvenation therapy should enter into the cottage after shaving, endowed with the perseverance and memory, full of faith, single minded, having removed all mental afflictions, cherishing good will for all living and performed the Pradakshina (going round) of the Gods, Cows and the Brahmanas.

That individual should then be cleansed by Panchakarma – elimination therapy. Thereafter, when he is happy and has regained his strength, the rejuvenation therapy should be administered. [16-24]

Preparation Elimination therapy:

हरीतकीनां चूर्णानि सैन्धवामलके गुडम् |
वचां विडङ्गं रजनीं पिप्पलीं विश्वभेषजम् ||२५||

पिबेदुष्णाम्बुना जन्तुः स्नेहस्वेदोपपादितः |
तेन शुद्धशरीराय कृतसंसर्जनाय च ||२६||
त्रिरात्रं यावकं दद्यात् पञ्चाहं वाऽपि सर्पिषा |
सप्ताहं वा पुराणस्य यावच्छुद्धेस्तु वर्चसः | |२७||
शुद्धकोष्ठं तु तं ज्ञात्वा रसायनमुपाचरेत् |
वयःप्रकृतिसात्म्यज्ञो यौगिकं यस्य यद्भवेत् ||२८||

The person after oleation (Snehana) and sweating (Swedana) therapies , should take the following combination of herbal powders with a cup of hot water.

The herbal powder is prepared with equal amounts of each of :

Haritaki – Terminalia chebula with

Saindhava – Rock-salt,

Amalaki (Emblica officinalis)

Guda – Jaggery

Vacha - Acorus calamus

Vidanga (Embelia ribes)

Rajani - Turmeric

Pippali (long pepper)

Vishwa Bheshaja – ginger

After administering the above combination with hot water, the person's body undergoes natural cleansing. For next 3, 5 or 7 days, the patient is administered with

Yaavaka – barley-gruel with Purana ghrita (old ghee)

Having ascertained that the Koshta (internal organs) is purged of all the impurities, he should be administered anti-ageing therapy, suitable for him by a physician who is well versed with

Vaya – age

Prakruti – Tridosha body constitution

Satmya – what is congenial and what is not, of the individual. [24-28]

Qualities and functions of Haritaki:

हरीतकीं पञ्चरसामुष्णामलवणां शिवाम् |
दोषानुलोमनीं लघ्वीं विद्याद्दीपनपाचनीम् ||२९||
आयुष्यां पौष्टिकीं धन्यां वयसः स्थापनीं पराम् |
सर्वरोगप्रशमनीं बुद्धीन्द्रियबलप्रदाम् ||३०||
कुष्ठं गुल्ममुदावर्तं शोषं पाण्डवामयं मदम् |
अर्शांसि ग्रहणीदोषं पुराणं विषमज्वरम् ||३१||
हृद्रोगं सशिरोरोगमतीसारमरोचकम् |
कासं प्रमेहमानाहं प्लीहानमुदरं नवम् ||३२||
कफप्रसेकं वैस्वर्यं वैवर्ण्यं कामलां क्रिमीन् |
श्वयथुं तमकं छर्दिं क्लैब्यमङ्गावसादनम् ||३३||
स्रोतोविबन्धान् विविधान् प्रलेपं हृदयोरसोः |
स्मृतिबुद्धिप्रमोहं च जयेच्छीघ्रं हरीतकी ||३४||
(अजीर्णिनोरूक्षभुजः स्त्रीमद्यविषकर्शिताः |
सेवेरन्नाभयामेते क्षुत्तृष्णोष्णादिताश्च ये)| |३५||
तान् गुणांस्तानि कर्माणि विद्यादामलकीष्वपि |
यान्युक्तानि हरीतक्या वीर्यस्य तु विपर्ययः ||३६||
अतश्चामृतकल्पानि विद्यात् कर्मभिरीदृशैः |

हरीतकीनां शस्यानि भिषगामलकस्य च ||३७||

Qualities of Haritaki – Terminalia chebula:
Has five tastes viz, sweet, sour, pungent, bitter and astringent
Ushna – It is hot in potency
Alavanam – It is free from saline taste
Shiva – It is good for general health
Dosha Anulomi – It eliminates the Doshas through intestines
Laghvi – light to digest
Deepana – improves digestion strength
Pachana – digestive
VayasaSthapani, Ayushya – anti aging, rejuvenating
Paushtiki – nourishing
SarvaRogaPrashamani – eradicates all diseases and
Buddhi IndriyaBalaprada – promotes intellect, sense perception and vitality.

Haritaki is indicated in:
Kustha (skin disease)
Gulma (phantom Tumor)
Udavarta (upward movement of the wind in abdomen)
Shosha (consumption)
Pandu (anemia)
Mada (intoxication)
Arshas (piles)
Grahani-dosa (sprue syndrome)
Purana Vishama Jwara – chronic and irregular fever
Hrudroga (heart diseases)
Shiroroga – diseases of the head
Atisara – Diarrhea
Arochaka (anorexia)
Kasa (cough)
Prameha (urinary diseases, including diabetes mellitus)
Anaha (abdominal distension, bloating)
recently occurred udara (obstinate diseases of abdomen, including ascites)
KaphaPraseka – excessive salivation
Vaiswaryam (hoarseness of voice)
Vaivarnayam (impairment of complexion)
Kamala (jaundice)
Krimi (intestinal worms)
Shvayathu – oedema, inflammation
Tamaka Swasa (bronchial Asthma)
Chardi (vomiting)
Klaibya (impotency)
Angasaada (lassitude in the body)
Sroto Vibandha – various types of obstructions in the channels of circulations
Pralepa HrudayoRaso – collection of adhesive material (like fat) around the heart and chest
Smruti, Buddhi Pramoha – affliction of memory and intellect

Contraindications of Haritaki :

Ajeerni – Those suffering from indigestion

Rookshabhuja – Taking dry food

Stri Karshita – those who are weak due to sexual indulgence

Madya Karshita – emaciated due to excess of alcohol

Visha Karshita – emaciated due to poisons

Kshut – afflicted with excess hunger

Trushna – afflicted with excess thirst

Ushnardita – afflicted with excess heat (such as Sun stroke)

Qualities of Amalki:

Amalaki (Emblica officinalis) – Amla possesses similar qualities to that of Haritaki, except in potency, (Amalaki is cold, Haritaki is hot). In view of these actions, the physician should consider the fruit pulp of Haritaki and Amalaki, like nectar. [29-37]

Method of Herb collection – Dravya Sangraha Vidhi:

ओषधीनां परा भूमिर्हिमवाञ् शैलसत्तमः |
तस्मात्फलानि तज्जानि ग्राह्येत्कालजानि तु ||३८||
आपूर्णरसवीर्याणि काले काले यथाविधि |
आदित्यपवनच्छायासलिलप्रीणितानि च ||३९||
यान्यजग्धान्यपूतीनि निर्व्रणान्यगदानि च |
तेषां प्रयोगं वक्ष्यामि फलानां कर्म चोत्तमम् ||४०||

Method of Herb collection:

Medicinal herbs should be collected from Himalayas. Collection should be done in proper season, when they are rich with fully manifested taste and potency (Aapoorna rasaveerya) collected in proper season.

The medicinal herbs should be:

- mellowed by sun rays, wind, shade and water
- not eaten by birds and insects
- unspoiled, not rotten
- without any cuts and wounds,
- not afflicted with any disease

The method of administration of these herbs and their excellent effects will now be described. [38-40]

Brahma Rasayana (First Type) :

पञ्चानां पञ्चमूलानां भागान् दशपलोन्मितान् |
हरीतकीसहस्रं च त्रिगुणामलकं नवम्||४१||
विदारिगन्धां बृहतीं पृश्निपर्णीं निदिग्धिकाम् |
विद्यादिविदारिगन्धाद्यं श्वदंष्ट्रापञ्चमं गणम् ||४२||
बिल्वाग्निमन्थश्योनाकं काश्मर्यमथ पाटलाम् |
पुनर्नवां शूर्पपर्ण्यौ बलामेरण्डमेव च ||४३||
जीवकर्षभकौ मेदां जीवन्तीं सशतावरीम् |
शरेक्षुदर्भकाशानां शालीनां मूलमेव च ||४४||
इत्येषां पञ्चमूलानां पञ्चानामुपकल्पयेत् |

भागान् यथोक्तांस्तत्सर्वं साध्यं दशगुणेऽम्भसि ||४५||
दशभागावशेषं तु पूतं तं ग्राहयेद्रसम् |
हरीतकीश्च ताः सर्वाः सर्वाण्यामलकानि च ||४६||
तानि सर्वाण्यनस्थीनि फलान्यापोथ्य कूर्चनैः |
विनीय तस्मिन्निर्यूहे चूर्णानीमानि दापयेत् ||४७||
मण्डूकपर्ण्याः पिप्पल्याः शङ्खपुष्प्याः प्लवस्य च |
मुस्तानां सविडङ्गानां चन्दनागुरुणोस्तथा ||४८||
मधुकस्य हरिद्राया वचायाः कनकस्य च |
भागांश्चतुष्पलान् कृत्वा सूक्ष्मैलायास्त्वचस्तथा ||४९||
सितोपलासहस्रं च चूर्णितं तुलयाऽधिकम् |
तैलस्य द्व्याढकं तत्र दद्यात्रीणि च सर्पिषः ||५०||
साध्यमौदुम्बरे पात्रे तत् सर्वं मृदुनाऽग्निना |
ज्ञात्वा लेह्यमदग्धंच शीतं क्षौद्रेण संसृजेत् ||५१||
क्षौद्रप्रमाणं स्नेहार्धं तत् सर्वं घृतभाजने |
तिष्ठेत्सम्मूर्च्छितं तस्य मात्रां काले प्रयोजयेत् ||५२||
या नोपरुन्ध्यादाहारमेकंमात्रा जरां प्रति |
षष्टिकः पयसा चात्र जीर्णे भोजनमिष्यते ||५३||
वैखानसा वालखिल्यास्तथा चान्ये तपोधनाः |
रसायनमिदं प्राश्यबभूवुरमितायुषः ||५४||
मुक्त्वा जीर्णं वपुश्चाब्यमवापुस्तरुणं वयः |
वीततन्द्राक्लमश्वासा निरातङ्काः समाहिताः ||५५||
मेधास्मृतिबलोपेताश्चिररात्रं तपोधनाः |
ब्राह्मं तपो ब्रह्मचर्यं चेरुश्चात्यन्तनिष्ठया ||५६||
रसायनमिदं ब्राह्ममायुष्कामः प्रयोजयेत् |
दीर्घमायुर्वयश्चाब्यं कामांश्चेष्टान् समश्नुते ||५७||
(इति ब्राह्मरसायनम्) |

Ingredients used :
PanchaPanchamoola – 25 roots – are taken in 10 Pala each – 480 grams each.

a. Vidarigandhi-panchamoola :

1. Vidarigandha(Pueraria tuberosa)
2. Brihati - Solanum indicum
3. Prishniparni - Uraria picta
4. Nidigdhika
5. Shwadamshtra - Tribulus terrestris

b. Brihat -panchamoola :

1. Bilva – Aegle marmelos
2. Shyonaka – Oroxylum indicum
3. Gambhari – Coomb Teak (root) – Gmelina arborea
4. Patala – Trumpet (root) – Stereospermum suaveolens

5.   Agnimantha – Premna corymbosa (Burm.f) Merr

c. Punarnavadi-panchamoola:
Punarnava - Boerhaavia diffusa
Mudgaparni – Phaseolus trilobus
Mashaparni – Teramnus labialis
Bala - Sida cordifolia
Eranda - Castor root

d. Jivaneeya-Panchamoola :
Jeevaka – Malaxis acuminata
Rishabhaka – Manilkara hexandra
Meda – Polygonatum cirrhifolium
Jeevanti – Leptadenia reticulata
Shatavari – Asparagus racemosus

e. Truna Panchamoola
Kusha – Desmostachya bipinnata
Kasha – Saccharum spontaneum
Shara – Saccharum munja
Darbha –Imperata cylindrica
Ikshu – Sugarcanne – Saccharum officinarum
To this, 1000 freshly collected fruits of Haritaki and 3000 freshly collected fruits of Amalaki are added.

Procedure:
The first 25 root powders of the above herbs should be boiled with ten times of water, and when the water is reduced to one tenth, it is filtered and the decoction should be collected. The fruits of Haritaki and Amlaki should be removed of their seeds and made to a paste with a pestle and mortar.
To this decoction:
1. Add the paste of Haritaki and Amalaki
2. Add 192 gm of each of the powder of:
Mandukaparni – Gotu kola
Pippali – long pepper
Shankhapushpi - Convolvulus pluricaulis
Plava – Nyctanthes arbor-tristis
Musta - Cyperus rotundus
Vidanga – False black pepper
Chandana – Sandalwood
Aguru - Aquilaria agallocha
Madhuka – Madhuca longifolia
Haridra – Turmeric
Vacha – Acorus calamus
Kanaka - Datura metel
Sukshma Ela – Lesser cardamom
Twak – Cinnamon

52,800 g of sugar (in powder form) + 6,144 ml of Til oil (sesame oil) + 9,216 ml of ghee. This whole mixture is boiled in a copper vessel on a low fire till it takes the consistency of a linctus, but not burnt. When it is cooled, honey should be mixed. The quantity of honey should be half of the quantity of oil and ghee taken together. This whole mixture should be mixed well and kept in an earthen jar smeared with ghee.

Pathya Apathya : After the medicine is digested the patient should be given shashtika type of rice with milk to eat.

Benefits of this therapy:

Vaikhanasas, Valakhilyas and such of the types of the hermits, by the intake of this rejuvenation therapy, attained immense longevity;

- they were free from the aging effects of the body and became youthful
- they were free from drowsiness, weariness, breathlessness and fear and they became single minded and were endowed with intellect, memory and strength.
- these ascetics became worthy of severe spiritual practices and Vedic recitation and celibacy (Brahmacharya) with exceeding devotion for a long time

Therefore, this therapy which has spiritual value should be taken by a person who desires longevity. After having undergone this therapy, he is sure to enjoy a long span of life, youthfulness and to attain all his ambitions. [41-57].

Brahma Rasayana (SecondType) :

यथोक्तगुणानामामलकानां सहस्रं पिष्टस्वेदनविधिना पयस ऊष्मणा सुस्विन्नमनातपशुष्कमनस्थि चूर्णयेत्‌|
तदामलकसहस्रस्वरसपरिपीतं
स्थिरापुनर्नवाजीवन्तीनागबलाब्रह्मसुवर्चलामण्डूकपर्णीशतावरीशङ्खपुष्पीपिप्पलीवचाविडङ्गस्वयङ्गुप्तामृता-
चन्दनागुरुमधुकमधूकपुष्पोत्पलपद्ममालतीयुवतीयूथिकाचूर्णाष्टभागसंयुक्तं   पुनर्नागबलासहस्रपलस्वरसपरिपीतमनातपशुष्कं
द्विगुणितसर्पिषा क्षौद्रसर्पिषा वा क्षुद्रगुडाकृतिं कृत्वा शुचौ दृढे घृतभाविते कुम्भे भस्मराशेरधः स्थापयेदन्तर्भूमेः पक्षं
कृतरक्षाविधानमथर्ववेदविदा, पक्षात्यये चोद्धृत्य कनकरजतताम्रप्रवालकालायसचूर्णाष्टभागसंयुक्तमर्धकर्षवृद्ध्या यथोक्तेन विधिना प्रातः
प्रातः प्रयुञ्जानोऽग्निबलमभिसमीक्ष्य, जीर्णे च षष्टिकं पयसा ससर्पिष्कमुपसेवमानो यथोक्तान्‌ गुणान्‌ समश्नुत इति||५८||
भवन्ति चात्र-
इदं रसायनं ब्राह्मं महर्षिगणसेवितम्‌|
भवत्यरोगो दीर्घायुः प्रयुञ्जानो महाबलः||५९||
कान्तः प्रजानां सिद्धार्थश्चन्द्रादित्यसमद्युतिः|
श्रुतं धारयते सत्त्वमार्षं चास्य प्रवर्तते||६०||
धरणीधरसारश्च वायुना समविक्रमः|
स भवत्यविषं चास्य गात्रे सम्पद्यते विषम्‌||६१||
(इति द्वितीयं ब्राह्मरसायनम्‌)|

PROCEDURE:

1. 1000 fruits of Amla is steam-boiled with water and made to a paste
2. After they are well-cooked it is dried without exposing it to sun and made to a powder by removing the seeds.
3. This powder should be impregnated (triturated) with the juice of another 1000 fruits of Amalaki and added with the powder of

Sthira – Desmodium gangeticum
Punarnava – Boerhavia diffusa
Jivanti – Leptadenia reticulata
Nagabala – Grewia populifolia

Bramha- suvarchala,

Mandaukaparni – Gotu kola

Shatavari – Indian Asparagus

Shankhapushpi – Convolvulus pluricaulis

Pippali – Long pepper

Vacha – Acorus calamus

Vidanga – Embelia ribes

Swayamgupta – Mucuna pruriens

Amruta - Tinospora cordifolia

Chandana – Sandalwood

Aguru – Aquilaria agallocha

Madhuka – Liquorice

Madhuka Pushpa – Madhuca longifolia

Utpala - Water lily

Padma - Lotus

Malati – Jasminum grandiflorum

Yuvati – Turmeric

Yuthika -Jasminum auriculatum

All the above mentioned should measure one-eighth of the powder of Amalaki. This compound should then be impregnated (ground) with the juice of 48,000 g of Nagabala (Grewia populifolia) and dried in shade. To this add double the quantity of ghee or both honey and ghee so as to make it Kshudraguda (a thick syrup like consistency). It is kept in a clean and strong earthen jar and is placed underground below a heap of ash for a fortnight. During this period, scholars who are well versed in the Atharva Veda should perform rituals for its protection. After a fortnight, this jar is removed, and the powder of gold, silver, copper, coral, black iron- all one-eighth in quantity is added with the prescribed procedure in a dose of 6 grams and then be gradually increased every day. When the medicine is digested, the patient is given shashtika type of rice with milk and ghee to take. By doing so, one attains all the benefits already described.

Thus, it is said:

Ancient great sages were using this rejuvenation therapy, called Brahma-rasayana. By its use, one becomes free from diseases and gains longevity and vigour. He bears a lovable complexion and is liked by everybody. His ambitions are fulfilled and he wears a lustre like that of the moon and the sun and is capable of retaining memory, all that he hears (Shrutamdharayate), and he possesses the mental faculty like that of seers. His body becomes compact like steel and in strength; he can be compared to wind. Even the poison becomes non-poisonous in his body. [58-61]

ChyavanaPrasha:

बिल्वोऽग्निमन्थः श्योनाकः काश्मर्यः पाटलिर्बला|
पर्ण्यश्चतस्रः पिप्पल्यः श्वदंष्ट्रा बृहतीद्वयम्||६२||
शृङ्गी तामलकी द्राक्षा जीवन्ती पुष्करागुरु|
अभया चामृता ऋद्धिर्जीवकर्षभकौ शटी||६३||
मुस्तं पुनर्नवा मेदा सैला चन्दनमुत्पलम्|
विदारी वृषमूलानि काकोली काकनासिका||६४||
एषां पलोन्मितान् भागाञ्छतान्यामलकस्य च|
पञ्च दद्यादतदैकध्यं जलद्रोणे विपाचयेत्||६५||
ज्ञात्वा गतरसान्येतान्योषधान्यथ तं रसम्|

तच्चामलकमुद्धृत्य निष्कुलं तैलसर्पिषोः||६६||
पलद्वादशके भृष्ट्वा दत्त्वा चार्धतुलां भिषक्|
मत्स्यण्डिकायाः पूताया लेहवत्साधु साधयेत्||६७||
षट्पलं मधुनश्चात्र सिद्धशीते प्रदापयेत्|
चतुष्पलं तुगाक्षीर्याः पिप्पलीद्विपलं तथा||६८||
पलमेकं निदध्याच्च त्वगेलापत्रकेशरात्|
इत्ययं च्यवनप्राशः परमुक्तो रसायनः||६९||
कासश्वासहरश्चैव विशेषेणोपदिश्यते|
क्षीणक्षतानां वृद्धानां बालानां चाङ्गवर्धनः||७०||
स्वरक्षयमुरोरोगं हृद्रोगं वातशोणितम्|
पिपासां मूत्रशुक्रस्थान् दोषांश्चाप्यपकर्षति||७१||
अस्य मात्रां प्रयुञ्जीत योपरुन्ध्यान्न भोजनम्|
अस्य प्रयोगाच्च्यवनः सुवृद्धोऽभूत् पुनर्युवा||७२||
मेधां स्मृतिं कान्तिमनामयत्वमायुःप्रकर्षं बलमिन्द्रियाणाम्|
स्त्रीषु प्रहर्षं परमग्निवृद्धिं वर्णप्रसादं पवनानुलोम्यम्||७३||
रसायनस्यास्य नरः प्रयोगाल्लभेत जीर्णोऽपि कुटीप्रवेशात्|
जराकृतं रूपमपास्य सर्वं बिभर्ति रूपं नवयौवनस्य||७४||
(इति च्यवनप्राशः)|

INGREDIENTS AND PROCEDURE :

Bilva – Aegle marmelos
Agnimantha – Premna mucronata
Shyonaka – Oroxylum indicum
Kashmarya – Gmelina arborea
Patali – Stereospermum suaveolens
Bala – Country mallow – Sida cordifolia
Shalaparni – Desmodium gangeticum
Prishniparni – Uraria picta
Mashaparni – Teramnus labialis
Mudgaparni – Phaseolus trilobus
Pippali – Long pepper
Shvadamstra – Tribulus terrestris
Brihati – Solanum indicum
Kantakari – Solanum xantocarpum
Shringi – Pistacia chinensis
Tamalaki – Phyllanthus niruri
Draksha – Grapes
Jivanti – Leptadenia reticulata
Pushkara – Inula racemosa
Aguru – Aquilaria agallocha
Abhaya – Harad – Terminalia chebula
Riddhi
Jivaka – Malaxis acuminata
Rishabhaka – Manilkara hexandra
Shati – Zadoary (root) – Hedychium spicatum / Curcuma zedoaria
Musta – Cyperus rotundus

Punarnava – Boerhavia diffusa
Meda – Polygonatum cirrhifolium
Ela – Cardamom
Chandana – Sandalwood
Utpala – Water Lily
Vidari – Pueraria tuberosa
Vrusha – Adhatoda vasica
Kakoli – Fritillaria roylei
Kakanasika – Martynia annua
1 pala – 48 g of each of the above herbs is taken in coarse powder form. It is added with 500 fruits of Amalaki.

All these are boiled together in 1 Drona – 12.288 litres of water. When it is fully boiled, the decoction and the fruits of Amalaki should be taken out. The fruits of Amalaki, after the removal of seeds, be fried in 12 Pala – 567 g, of each of ghee and sesame oil. This should be added to the decoction. This paste along with 2.400 kg of (half Tula) of sugar (Matsyandika), boiled with the decoction earlier obtained, until it takes the consistency of a linctus (semi solid).

When it has cooled down, the below ingredients are added and stirred well.
6 Pala – 288 g of honey;
4 Pala – 192 g of Tugaksiri;
2 Pala – 96 g of Pippali – Long pepper
1 pala – 48 g each of –
Twak – Cinnamon
Ela – Cardamom
Patra – Cinnamon leaves
Keshara – Nagakeshara – Mesua ferrea
This is called ChyavanaPrasha.

Benefits:
Parammukto Rasayana – best rejuvenators and anti-ageing medicine.
Indicated in :
Kasa – cold, cough
Shwasa – asthma, respiratory disorders involving difficulty in breathing
Kshataksheena – chest injury
Svarakshaya – voice problems
Uroroga – Chest disorders
Hrudroga – Cardiac disorders
Vatashonita – Gout
Pipasa – excessive thirst
Mutradosha – Urinary tract disorders
Shukra Dosha – semen, sperm anomalies
It is good for tissue growth and development of elderly and children. The dose should be such that it does not disturb the quantity of meals. By the use of this medicine, Sage Chyavana, who had become very old, became young once again.

Administration of this rejuvenation medicine promotes :
Medha – intelligence
Smruti – memory
Kanti – lustre

Anamayatva – freedom from diseases
Ayu – age, life expectancy
Indriyabala – strength of sense organs
Agni – digestion strength
Varna – skin complexion
Pavana Anuloma – Movement of Vata Dosha in its normal direction, easy bowel movement.

By using this therapy according to Kuti-Praveshika method (while residing in a cottage), even an old man can shed all his problems related to aging and emerge with fresh youthful complexion. [62-74]

Amalaka Rasayana:

अथामलक हरीतकीनामामलक बिभीतकानां हरीतकी बिभीतकानामामलक हरीतकी बिभीतकानां वा पलाशत्वगवनद्धानां मृदाऽवलिप्तानां कुकूलस्विन्नानामकुलकानां पलसहस्रमुलूखले सम्पोथ्य दधिघृतमधुपललतैलशर्करासंयुक्तं भक्षयेदनन्नभुग्यथोक्तेन विधिना; तस्यान्ते यवाग्वादिभिः प्रत्यवस्थापनम्, अभ्यङ्गोत्सादनं सर्पिषा यवचूर्णैश्च, अयं च रसायनप्रयोगप्रकर्षो द्विस्तावदग्निबलमभिसमीक्ष्य, प्रतिभोजनं यूषेण पयसा वा षष्टिकः ससर्पिष्कः, अतः परं यथासुखविहारः कामभक्ष्यः स्यात् |
अनेन प्रयोगेणर्षयः पुनर्युवत्वमवापुर्बभूवुश्चानेकवर्षशतजीविनो निर्विकाराः परं शरीर बुद्धीन्द्रियबलसमुदिताश्चेरुश्चात्यन्तनिष्ठया तपः ||७५|| (इति चतुर्थामलकरसायनम्)|

Method of preparation:

Amalaki, Haritaki and Bhibhitaki or combination of these, is tied to the bark of Palasha (Butea monosperma). This is covered with a layer of wet mud. This big ball is fried using cow dung cake fire. Then the mud and Palasha layers are scraped, pulp is taken in a dose of 48 Kg (1000 Pala = 1 Tula) and crushed properly, in pestle and mortar. This paste is administered by adding equal quantities of curd, ghee, honey, till paste (sesame), oil and sugar. It is administered according to the procedure laid down and during this period, the patient should be restrained from food. The patient should return to the normal diet gradually and he must be given massage and unction with ghee and the powder of barley. Two such courses of rejuvenation therapy should be administered, keeping in view the power of digestion of the individual. He should thereafter resort to meals containing Sastika type of rice and ghee with soup or milk. Thereafter, he should be left free to resort to regimens liked by him and take food desired by him.

By the administration of this rejuvenation therapy, the sages regained their youth and lived for many hundreds of years free from diseases, and with great devotion, practiced penance, endowed with the excellence of the body, the intellect, and normal functioning of the senses. [75]

Recipe of Haritaki:

हरीतक्यामलक बिभीतक पञ्चपञ्चमूलनिर्यूहे पिप्पली मधूक मधूक काकोली क्षीरकाकोल्यात्मगुप्ता जीवकर्षभक क्षीरशुक्ला कल्कसम्प्रयुक्तेन विदारीस्वरसेन क्षीराष्टगुण सम्प्रयुक्तेन च सर्पिषः कुम्भं साधयित्वा प्रयुञ्जानोऽग्निबलसमां मात्रां जीर्णे च क्षीरसर्पिभ्यां शालिषष्टिकमुष्णोदकानुपानमश्नञ्जरा व्याधि पापाभिचारव्यपगतभयः शरीरेन्द्रिय बुद्धि बलमतुलमुपलभ्याप्रतिहत सर्वारम्भः परमायुरनवाप्नुयात् ||७६|| (इति पञ्चमो हरीतकीयोगः)|

Method of preparation:

A decoction should be prepared of Haritaki, Amalaki, Bibhitaka and five groups of Pancamulas – PanchaPanchamoola - PanchaPanchamoola – 25 roots – are taken in 10 Pala each – 480 grams each.

a. Vidarigandhi-pancha :
Vidarigandha (Pueraria tuberosa)
Brihati – Solanum indicum
Prishniparni – Uraria picta

Nidigdhika
Shwadamshtra – Tribulus terrestris

b. Brihat -panchamoola :
Bilva – Aegle marmelos
Shyonaka – Oroxylum indicum
Gambhari – Coomb Teak (root) – Gmelina arborea
Patala – Trumpet (root) – Stereospermum suaveolens
Agnimantha – Premna corymbosa (Burm.f) Merr

c. Punarnavadi-panchamoola:
Punarnava – Boerhaavia diffusa
Mudgaparni – Phaseolus trilobus
Mashaparni – Teramnus labialis
Bala – Sida cordifolia
Eranda - castor root

d. Jivaneeya-Panchamoola :
Jeevaka – Malaxis acuminata
Rishabhaka – Manilkara hexandra
Meda – Polygonatum cirrhifolium
Jeevanti – Leptadenia reticulata
Shatavari – Asparagus racemosus

e. Truna-Panchamoola
Kusha – Desmostachya bipinnata
Kasha – Saccharum spontaneum
Shara – Saccharum munja
Darbha –Imperata cylindrica
Ikshu – Sugarcane – Saccharum officinarum

To this decoction the paste of the below mentioned are added :
Pippali – Long pepper
Madhuka (Licorice – Glycyrrhiza glabra),
Kakoli (Fritillaria roylei),
Ksheerakakoli (Lilium polyphyllum),
Atmagupta (Mucuna pruriens)
Jivaka (Malaxis acuminata),
Rishabhaka (Manilkara hexandra) and
Ksheerashukla are added.

The juice of Vidari (Ipomoea paniculata / Pueraria tuberosa), eight times of milk and 24, 576 g of ghee is added and boiled. This recipe is administered in a dose based on the power of digestion, and after it is digested, the individual should be advised to take Sali and Sastika type of rice along with milk and ghee. Hot water should be given to him as post-prandial potion.

By this therapy one becomes free from the consequences of old age, disease, sins and effects of black magic, and he becomes endowed with unrivalled strength of body, senses as well as intelligence. He develops powers to see through the completion of all projects in hand and leads a long life. [76]

Another Rasayana medicine with Haritaki:
हरीतक्यामलक बिभीतक हरिद्रा स्थिरा बला विडङ्गामृतवल्ली विश्वभेषज मधुक पिप्पली सोमवल्क सिद्धेन क्षीरसर्पिषा मधु शर्कराभ्यामपि च सन्नीयामलक स्वरस शतपरिपीतमामलक चूर्णमयश्चूर्ण चतुर्भागसम्प्रयुक्तं पाणितलमात्रं प्रातः प्रातः प्राश्य यथोक्तेन विधिना सायं मुद्गयूषेण पयसा वा ससर्पिष्कं शालिषष्टिकान्नमश्नीयात्, त्रिवर्षप्रयोगादस्य वर्षशतमजरं वयस्तिष्ठति, श्रुतमवतिष्ठते, सर्वामयाः प्रशाम्यन्ति, विषमविषं भवति गात्रे, गात्रमश्मवत् स्थिरीभवति, अधृष्यो भूतानां भवति॥७७॥

भवन्ति चात्र-
यथाऽमराणाममृतं यथा भोगवतां सुधा ।
तथाऽभवन्महर्षीणां रसायनविधिः पुरा ॥७८॥
न जरां न च दौर्बल्यं नातुर्यं निधनं न च ।
जग्मुर्वर्षसहस्राणि रसायनपराः पुरा । ॥७९॥
न केवलं दीर्घमिहायुरश्नुते रसायनं यो विधिवन्निषेवते ।
गतिं स देवर्षि निषेवितां शुभां प्रपद्यते ब्रह्म तथेति चाक्षयम् ॥८०॥

Method of preparation
Haritaki, Amalaki, Bibhitaka,
Haridra (turmeric – Curcuma longa),
Sthira (Desmodium gangeticum),
Bala(Country mallow (root) – Sida cordifolia),
Vidanga (Embelia ribes),
Amrutavalli,
Vishvabhesaja – ginger
Madhuka (Licorice – Glycyrrhiza glabra),
Pippali (Long pepper fruit – Piper longum),
Somavalka- these drugs should be cooked with ghee extracted from milk and added with honey and sugar.

To this, Amalaki which is impregnated with 100 times juice of the same fruit (Amalaka) and the powder of iron one-fourth in quantity, should be added. Following the prescribed procedure, this recipe should be taken every morning in a dose of 12 g. In the evening, Shali or Sastika type of rice, mixed with ghee or milk, or the soup of Mudga should be taken.

BENEFITS:
By the administration of this therapy for three years, the individual becomes free from old age for 100 years. He develops the power to recollect anything he hears. All these diseases are eradicated and even poisons become non-poisonous in his body. His body becomes compact like a stone and he attains invincibility.

As the nectar is to the Gods and the nectar is for serpents, so in ancient times, this rejuvenation therapy became useful to the great sages. It kept them free from old age, weakness, diseases and death and they lived for thousands of years by the intake of this rejuvenating drug.

He who makes use of this rejuvenation therapy, according to the prescribed procedure, not merely enjoys long life in this world, but also enjoys the auspicious life of the Devas and Rishis after death and gets submerged in immutable Brahman. [77-80]

तत्र श्लोकः-
अभयामलकीयेऽस्मिन् षड्योगाः परिकीर्तिताः ।

रसायनानां सिद्धानामायुर्यैरनुवर्तते ||८१||

Summary:

In this quarter, dealing with Abhaya and Amalaki, six recipes for rejuvenation therapy are described. By the administration of these recipes the life of the great Siddhas (those who have attained perfection) was prolonged. [81]

इत्यग्निवेशकृते तन्त्रे चरकप्रतिसंस्कृते चिकित्सास्थाने रसायनाध्यायेऽभयामलकीयो नाम रसायनपादः प्रथमः||१||

Thus, ends the first quarter dealing with Abhaya and Amalaki of the Chapter on Rejuvenation Therapy of the Section on Therapeutics of the work of Agnivesha redacted by Charaka.

2

Chikitsasthana Chapter 1.2 Prana Kameeya Rasayanam

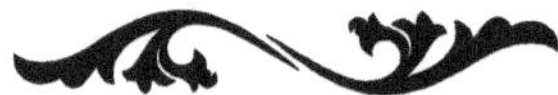

The second quarter of Charaka Chikitsa Sthana 1st chapter deals with Rasayana – rejuvenation, anti ageing. This sub-chapter is called Prana KameeyaRasayana Pada.Prana means life. Kameeya means desirous. So, it deals with 37 Ayurvedic medicines designed to improve life expectancy and quality.

अथातः प्राणकामीयं रसायनपादं व्याख्यास्यामः||१||

इति ह स्माह भगवानात्रेयः||२||

We shall now explore the second quarter of the Chapter on rejuvenation therapy (Rasayana) beginning with the term Pranakama (desirous for vitality).

Thus said lord Atreya.[1-2]

The importance of Rejuvenation Therapy:

प्राणकामाः शुश्रूषध्वमिदमुच्यमानममृतमिवापरमदितिसुत हितकरमचिन्त्याद्भुत प्रभावमायुष्यमारोग्यकरं वयसः स्थापनं निद्रा तन्द्रा श्रम क्लमालस्य दौर्बल्यापहरमनिल कफ पित्त साम्यकरं स्थैर्यकरमबद्ध मांसहरमन्तराग्नि सन्धुक्षणं प्रभा वर्ण स्वरोत्मकरं रसायन विधानम् | अनेन च्यवनादयो महर्षयः पुनर्युवत्वमापुर्नरीणां चेष्टतमा बभूवुः, स्थिर समसुविभक्तमांसाः, सुसंहत स्थिरशरीराः, सुप्रसन्न बल वर्णेन्द्रियाः, सर्वत्राप्रतिहत पराक्रमाः, क्लेश सहाश्च|

Lord Punarvasu Atreya said, "Listen to me, O! Persons desirous for vitality: the revitalization therapy is like ambrosia and is beneficial to the Gods, the sons of Aditi.

Effects of Rasayana treatment (anti ageing Therapy):

It has unimaginable and wonderful effects.

Ayushya – It promotes life

Arogyakara – Maintains positive health

VayasaSthapanam – anti ageing

And cures

Nidra – morbid sleep,

Tandra – Drowsiness

Shrama, Klama – Physical as well as mental fatigue

Alasya - Laziness and

Dourbalya – weakness

It maintains proper balance among Vata, Pitta and Kapha;

Sthairyakara – It produces stability,

Cures slothness, wasting of muscles

Agni Sandhukshana – Stimulates digestive fire (enzymes responsible for digestion and metabolism)
Prabha Varna Swarottamakara – Brings about excellence in lustre, complexion as well as voice

Benefits:
The great sages like Chyavana etc., regained their youth and were liked most by women. Their muscles and bodies became compact, even and well proportioned.

They were endowed with:

- Excellence of strength, complexion and senses.
- Unchallengeable prowess everywhere.
- And developed powers of resistance to hardships

सर्वे शरीरदोषा भवन्ति ग्राम्याहारादम्ल लवण कटुक क्षार शुष्क शाक मांस तिल पलल पिष्टान्न भोजिनां विरूढ नव शूक शमी धान्य विरुद्धासात्म्य रूक्ष क्षाराभिष्यन्दि भोजिनां क्लिन्न गुरु पूति पर्युषित भोजिनां विषमाध्यशन प्रायाणां दिवास्वप्न स्त्री मद्य नित्यानां विषमाति मात्र व्यायाम सङ्क्षोभित शरीराणां भय क्रोध शोक लोभ मोहायास बहुलानाम्;

Causes for body defects (Shareera Dosha):
Intake of
Gramya Ahara – substandard diet
Amla, Lavana, Katuka, Kshara, Shushka Shaka – green vegetables with sour, saline, pungent and alkaline tastes, dry vegetables, meat, sesame seeds, paste of sesame seeds and pastries
Viruda Nava Shooka Shami Dhanya – Germinated cereals and pulses, freshly harvested corns with bristles and pulses
Viruddha – intake of wrong food combinations
Asathmya – uncongenial foods
Klinna, Guru, PootiParyushitaBhojana – softened, moist, heavy, putrid and stale food
Vishamashana – eating at random times
Adhyashana – eating before previously food getting digested

Bad habits that cause illness :
Divasvapna, Stree Madya Nitya – daily indulgence in day-sleep,sex and alcohol
Vishama, Ati Vyayama – irregular, excessive exercise,
Bhaya, Krodha, Shoka, Lobha, Moha, AyasaBahula – excessive fear, anger, grief, greed, infatuation and over-work.

अतोनिमित्तं हि शिथिलीभवन्ति मांसानि, विमुच्यन्ते सन्धयः, विदह्यते रक्तं, विष्यन्दते चानल्पं मेदः, न सन्धीयतेऽस्थिषु मज्जा, शुक्रं न प्रवर्तते, क्षयमुपैत्योजः; स एवम्भूतो ग्लायति, सीदति, निद्रा तन्द्रालस्य समन्वितो निरुत्साहः श्वसिति, असमर्थश्चेष्टानां शारीरमानसीनां, नष्ट स्मृति बुद्धिच्छायो रोगाणामधिष्ठानभूतो न सर्वमायुरवाप्नोति | तस्मादेतान् दोषानवेक्षमाणः सर्वान् यथोक्तानहितानपास्याहार विहारान् रसायनानि प्रयोक्तुमर्हतीत्युक्त्वा भगवान् पुनर्वसुरात्रेय उवाच-||३||

Effect of bad food, physical and mental habits:

- Shithileebhavati Mamsani – muscles become flabby, fragile
- Vimuchyante Sandhayaha – Joints become loosened, weak
- Vidahyate Raktam – blood becomes vitiated, burnt out
- Vishyandate cha analpam medaha – The fat which is accumulated in excess gets liquefied, vitiated
- Na sandheeyate asthishu majja – The marrow does not remain intact inside the (hollow part) bones,

- Shukram na pravartate – Impairment in the ejaculation of semen and
- Kshayamupaiti Ojaha – The Ojas (vital fluid, responsible for immunity) undergoes diminution.

Such a person suffers from

- Glayati, Seedati, Nidra, Tandra, Alasya, Nirutsaha – Feels exhausted, languid, sleepy, drowsy and lazy, lack of enthusiasm
- Shwasa – dyspnea
- Becomes incapable of physical and mental work,
- Loses his memory, intellect and complexion and
- Becomes an abode of diseases.
- Thus he fails to enjoy the full span of his life.

In view of all these miseries, one should give up all types of unwholesome diet and regimens and should undergo revitalization treatment. Lord Punarvasu Atreya continued his discourse as follows [3]

Amalaka ghrita – Ghee prepared with Amla:
आमलकानां सुभूमिजानां कालजानामनुपहत गन्ध वर्ण रसानामापूर्णरस प्रमाणवीर्याणां स्वरसेन पुनर्नवा कल्क पाद सम्प्रयुक्तेन सर्पिषः साधयेदाढकम्, अतः परं विदारी स्वरसेन जीवन्ती कल्क सम्प्रयुक्तेन, अतः परं चतुर्गुणेन पयसा बलातिबला कषायेण शतावरी कल्क संयुक्तेन; अनेन क्रमेणैकैकं शतपाकं सहस्रपाकं वा शर्करा क्षौद्र चतुर्भाग सम्प्रयुक्तं सौवर्णे राजते मार्तिके वा शुचौ दृढे घृतभाविते कुम्भे स्थापयेत्; तद्यथोक्तेन विधिना यथाग्नि प्रातः प्रातः प्रयोजयेत्, जीर्णे च क्षीरसर्पिभ्र्या शालिषष्टिकमश्नीयात् |
अस्य प्रयोगाद्वर्षशतं वयोऽजरं तिष्ठति, श्रुतमवतिष्ठते, सर्वामयाः प्रशाम्यन्ति, अप्रतिहतगतिः स्त्रीषु, अपत्यवान् भवतीति ||४||
भवतश्चात्र-
बृहच्छरीरं गिरिसारसारं स्थिरेन्द्रियं चातिबलेन्द्रियं च |
अधृष्यमन्यैरतिकान्तरूपं प्रशस्ति पूजा सुखचित्तभाक् च ||५||
बलं महद्वर्ण विशुद्धिधरग्या स्वरो घनौघस्तनितानुकारी |
भवत्यपत्यं विपुलं स्थिरं च समशनतो योगमिमं नरस्य ||६||
(इत्यामलक घृतम्) |

Method of preparation of Amalaka Ghritam:
One Adhaka (3.072 liters) of ghee is boiled with
- The paste of Punarnava (Spreading Hogweed – Boerhaavia diffusa)
- Juice of Amalaki (Indian gooseberry fruit – Emblica officinalis Gaertn).

The Amalaki fruits should be :
Subhoomija– collected from trees which are grown in good soil, good place.
Kaalaja – seasonal
Anupahata Gandha Varna – Their smell, colour and taste should not have been impaired and heavy
Aapoorna Rasa PramanaVeerya – Should be full in juice, size and potency.
The ghee thus obtained is filtered.

Thereafter, this ghee is again boiled with the:
- juice of Vidari (Pueraria tuberosa)
- the paste of Jivanti(Leptadenia reticulata).
Then the obtained herbal ghee is filtered.

Thereafter, the obtained herbal ghee is boiled with 4 parts of milk and Decoction of:

- Bala – Country mallow (root) – Sida cordifolia
- Atibala (Abutilon indicum)
- The paste of Shatavari (Asparagus racemosus)
In this manner, this ghee should be boiled consecutively for 100 times or 1000 times.

Thereafter,
- one fourth of it should be mixed with sugar and honey
- And kept in a clean, strong and ghee smeared jar made of gold, silver or mud.

Following the prescribed procedure and taking into consideration the digestive power, this medicine should be administered in proper qualities, every morning and after digestion of Amalaka ghrita, the individual should be advised to take Shali or Shashtika types of rice with milk and ghee.

Benefits of Amalaki Ghrita:
- The person lives for 100 years free from old age.
- Shrutam Avatishtate – He remembers whatever he hears
- He is cured of all diseases.
- Acquires an unimpaired sexual potency and is blessed with progeny.

Thus it is said:
A Robust physique, strong like iron, stability and sharpness of sense organs, invincibility, exceeding charm, respect, honour, mental happiness, enormous strength, bright complexion, very sound voice resembling that of a thunderous cloud and healthy children in plenty- these are the outcomes of this therapy. [4-6]

Amalaki Avaleha:
आमलक सहस्रं पिप्पलीसहस्र सम्प्रयुक्तं पलाश तरुण क्षारोदकोत्तरं तिष्ठेत्, तदनुगत क्षारोदकमनातप शुष्कमनस्थि चूर्णीकृतं चतुर्गुणाभ्यां मधुसर्पिभ्यर्यां सन्नीय शर्कराचूर्ण चतुर्भाग सम्प्रयुक्तं घृतभाजनस्थं षण्मासान् स्थापयेदन्तर्भूमेः |
तस्योत्तर कालमग्नि बलसमां मात्रां खादेत्, पौर्वाह्णिकः प्रयोगो नापराह्णिकः, सात्म्यापेक्षश्चाहार विधिः |
अस्य प्रयोगाद्वर्षशतमजरं वयस्तिष्ठतीति समानं पूर्वेण ||७||
(इत्यामलकावलेहः) |

Ingredients and procedure: 1000 fruits each of Amalaki (Amla, Indian gooseberry) and Pippali (Long pepper fruit – Piper longum) are impregnated with Palasha Ksharodaka – the water of Palasha Kshara.
The seeds of the fruits are removed and dried in shade and powdered. To this powder, four times of honey and ghee are added and 1/4th of powdered sugar is mixed. The recipe, thus prepared is kept inside a ghee-smeared jar and should be stored underground for 6 months.
It should be administered based on
Kala – season
Agni – digestion strength of the patient
Bala – strength and immunity.
Wholesome diet should be given to the patient.
This also carries the benefits explained in relation to the previous recipe. (Amalaka ghrita) [7].

Amalaka Churna:
आमलक चूर्णाढकमेकविंशति रात्रमामलक स्वरस परिपीतं मधु घृताढकाभ्यां द्वाभ्यामेकीकृतमष्टभाग पिप्पलीकं शर्कराचूर्ण चतुर्भाग सम्प्रयुक्तं घृतभाजनस्थं प्रावृषि भस्मराशौ निदध्यात्; तद्वर्षान्ते सात्म्यपथ्याशी प्रयोजयेत्; अस्य प्रयोगाद्वर्ष शतमजरमायुस्तिष्ठतीति समानं पूर्वेण ||८|| (इत्यामलकचूर्णम्) |

Procedure and the ingredients:
Amalaki (Indian gooseberry) Powder – 1 Adhaka – 3.072 kg, is impregnated with and Gooseberry (Amalaki) for 21 nights
To this one Adhaka (3.072 Litre) of honey and ghee each should be added.
The whole thing should be mixed properly, and to this,

- 1/8th powder of Pippali – Long pepper fruit and
- 1/4th powder of sugar is added and mixed.

This powder mix is kept inside a ghee-smeared jar and stored inside a heap of ash during the rainy season (Pravrushi). After the rains, it is administered to the patient who has a wholesome diet. Administration of this recipe allows a person to live for 100 years, free from old age. [8]

Vidangavaleha:
विडङ्ग तण्डुल चूर्णानामाढकमाढकं पिप्पली तण्डुलानामध्यर्धाढकं सितोपलायाः सर्पिस्तैलमध्वाढकैः षड्भिरेकीकृतं घृत भाजनस्थं प्रावृषि भस्म राशाविति सर्वं समानं पूर्वेण यावदाशीः ||९|| (इति विडङ्गावलेहः) |

Ingredients and procedure:
One Adhaka (3.072 kg) of the powder of the:
- grains of Vidanga – Embelia ribes
- Pippali – Long pepper fruit – Piper longum
1.5 Adhaka (4.608 Gm) of sugar, 6 Adhakas (18.432kg) of ghee, Sesame oil and honey, taken together, should be mixed well and kept inside a ghee- smeared jar. This jar should be stored inside a heap of ashes during the rainy season and given to the patient on the lines suggested above. It produces all the therapeutic effects mentioned in the preceding paragraph and verses [9]

AmalakiAvaleh – different version:
यथोक्त गुणानामामलकानां सहस्रमार्द्रं पलाश द्रोण्यां सपिधानायां बाष्पमनुद्वमन्त्यामारण्य गोमयाग्निभिरुपस्वेदयेत्, तानि सुस्विन्न शीतान्युद्धृत कुलकान्यापोथ्याढकेन पिप्पली चूर्णानामाढकेन च विडङ्ग तण्डुल चूर्णानामध्यर्धेन चाढकेन शर्कराया द्वाभ्यां द्वाभ्यामाढकाभ्यां तैलस्य मधुनः सर्पिषश्च संयोज्य शुचौ दृढे घृतभाविते कुम्भे स्थापयेदेकविंशति रात्रम्, अत ऊर्ध्वं प्रयोगः; अस्य प्रयोगाद्वर्ष शतमजरमायुस्तिष्ठतीति समानं पूर्वेण ||१०|| (इत्यामलकावलेहोऽपरः) |

Procedure and ingredients:
1000 fruits of Amalaki having the attributes described earlier (in paragraph 4) are kept inside a drum prepared of a green Palasha – Butea monosperma tree. It is covered air-tight and is ensured that the steam from inside does not go out through any opening. This drum is set on fire by the forest cow dung cake.

When these fruits are fully baked, it is allowed to cool down, and then, their seeds are removed. Pulp is made into paste and taken in the quantity of one Adhaka (3.072 kg).

To this:
- 1 Adhaka (3.072kg) of Pippali Choorna (Long pepper fruit powder)
- 1.5 Adhaka (4.608 kg) of the powder of Vidanga (False black pepper – Embelia ribes fruit)
- 2 Adhakas (6.144 kg) each of sugar, sesame oil, honey and ghee should be added.

The recipe is kept inside a clean, strong ghee-smeared jar for 21 nights. Thereafter, it is administered. By the use of these recipes, one lives 100 years free from old age and gets such other benefits as are described in Para 4 and verses 5 and 6 above.

Nagabala Rasayana:

धन्वनि कुशास्तीर्णे स्निग्ध कृष्ण मधुर मृत्तिके सुवर्ण वर्णमृत्तिके वा व्यपगत विषश्वापद पवन सलिलाग्निदोषे कर्षण वल्मीक श्मशान चैत्योषरावसथवर्जिते देशे यथर्तु सुख पवन सलिलादित्य सेविते जातान्यनुपहतान्यनध्यारूढान्य बालान्यजीर्णान्यधिगत वीर्याणि शीर्ण पुराण पर्णान्यसञ्जातान्यपर्णानि तपसि तपस्ये वा मासे शुचिः प्रयतः कृतदेवार्चनः स्वस्ति वाचयित्वा द्विजातीन् चले सुमुहूर्ते नागबलामूलान्युद्धरेत्, तेषां सुप्रक्षालितानां त्वक्पिण्डमाम्र मात्रमक्षमात्रं वा श्लक्ष्ण पिष्टमालोड्य पयसा प्रातः प्रयोजयेत्, चूर्णीकृतानि वा पिबेत् पयसा, मधु सर्पिभ्यां वा संयोज्य भक्षयेत्, जीर्णे च क्षीर सर्पिभ्यां शालिषष्टिकमश्नीयात् |
संवत्सर प्रयोगादस्य वर्षशतमजरं वयस्तिष्ठतीति समानं पूर्वेण ||११|| (इति नागबलारसायनम्) |

The herbs – Grewia populifolia, Sida spinosa, Urena lobata, Grewia hirsuta – all these are identified with the name Nagabala.

Roots of Nagabala should be collected from a field having the following characteristics:
It should be located in Jangala Desa (arid region)
Kusha plants – Desmostachya bipinnata should have thickly grown in this field
The earth of the field should be unctuous, black and sweet or it should be golden in colour
The field should be free from poisons, wild animals and the faults of wind, water and fire
It
- should not be a cultivated land
- should not have anthill
- should not be a crematorium
- should not have a Chattya (sacred temple)
- should not be grown in Usara (saline) land
- should not have residential houses
- This land should have been exposed to wind, water and sun according to different seasons.

The plants of Nagabala should have the following characteristics:
It should not have been injured. There should not be any big tree by their side (Adhyarudha) to afflict them. It should neither be too young, nor too old. It should be full of Veerya (potency).

Collection of the herb – Nagabala:
- Nagabala is to be uprooted in the month of Tapas or Magha (January- February) and Tapasya or Phalaguna (February-March)
- By a person, who is clean, Prayata (devoted) who has offered prayer to the Gods
- Persons who are Dvijatis (Brahmanas, Kshatriyas and Vaishyas) have recited Swasti – auspicious chants namely, the Chala or Indra Muhurta.
- The roots are made to a thin paste or powder and taken with milk or honey in the morning.
Pathya: The person is advised food consisting of Sali or Sastika type of rice mixed with milk and ghee.

If this recipe is taken for one year, then the person lives for one hundred years, free from old age and he will get such other benefits as are described in para 4 and verses 5 and 6 above [11]

Other anti ageing recipes:

बलातिबला चन्दनागुरु धव तिनिश खदिर शिंशपासन स्वरसाः पुनर्नवान्ताश्चौषधयो दश नागबलया व्याख्याताः|
स्वरसानामलाभे त्वयं स्वरस विधिः:- चूर्णानामाढकमाढकमुदकस्याहोरात्र स्थितं मृदितपूतं स्वरसवत् प्रयोज्यम्||१२||

Procedure:

The juice of

Bala – Sida cordifolia Linn.

Atibala – Abutilon indicum (Linn.)

Chandana – Santalum album

Aguru – Aquilaria agallocha

Dhava – Anogeissus latifolia

Tinisha – Lagerstroemia speciosa, Ougeinia dalbergioides Benth./oojeinensis

Khadira – Acacia catechu

Simshapa – Dalbergia latifolia and

Asana – Pterocarpus marsupium

And the ten drugs ending with Punarnava viz.

Amra – Mango – Mangifera indica

Abhaya – Harad – Terminalia chebula

Dhatri – Amalaki (Indian gooseberry fruit – Emblica officinalis Gaertn)

Mukta-Rasna – Pluchea lanceolata

Shreyasi – Pluchea lanceolata

Shveta Punarnava (Spreading Hogweed – Boerhaavia diffusa)

Atirasa

Mandukaparni – Gotu Kola

Sthira – Desmodium gangeticum and

Punarnava (Spreading Hogweed – Boerhaavia diffusa) should be used according to the method described for Nagabala.

If the juice of the above mentioned plants is not available, then for the preparation of their juice the following special methods should be adopted:

- One Adhaka (3.072kg) of the plant powder is taken and to this one Adhaka (3.072 lit) of water is added
- And kept for 24 hours.
- Thereafter, it should be squeezed by hand.
- The liquid that comes out after filtration should be used like juice.[12]

Bhallataka Ksheera:

भल्लातकान्यनुपहतान्यनामयान्यापूर्णरस प्रमाणवीर्याणि पक्व जाम्बव प्रकाशानि शुचौ शुक्रे वा मासे सङ्गृह्य यवपल्ले माषपल्ले वा निधापयेत्, तानि चतुर्मासस्थितानि सहसि सहस्ये वा मासे प्रयोक्तुमारभेत शीत स्निग्ध मधुरोपस्कृत शरीरः |

पूर्वं दश भल्लातकान्यापोथ्याष्टगुणेनाम्भसा साधु साधयेत्, तेषां रसमष्ट भागावशेषं पूतं सपयस्कं पिबेत् सर्पिषाऽन्तर्मुखमभ्यज्य |

तान्येकैक भल्लातकोत्कर्षापकर्षेण दशभल्लातकान्यात्रिंशतः प्रयोज्यानि, नातः परमुत्कर्षः |

प्रयोग विधानेन सहस्रपर एव भल्लातक प्रयोगः | जीर्णे च ससर्पिषा पयसा शालिषष्टिकाशनमुपचारः, प्रयोगान्ते च द्विस्तावत् पयसैवोपचारः | तत्प्रयोगाद्वर्ष शतमजरं वयस्तिष्ठतीति समानं पूर्वेण ||१३|| (इति भल्लातकक्षीरम्) |

Bhallataka is Marking Nut – Semecarpus anacardium.

Collection of fruits of Bhallataka:

The fruits
- which are not damaged,
- free from physical defects,
- full of Rasa (taste),
- having full size,

- ripe in potency (veerya)
- which resemble ripe fruits of Jambu (Jamun fruit)

Time when it is to be collected:
In the months of Suchi or Jyestha (May-June) and Shukra or Ashadha (June-July)

Storage:
It is stored for 4 months inside a heap of Yava – Barley (Hordeum vulgare) or Masha (Black gram).

Method of Administration of Bhallatak Rasayan:

- Is done in the month of Sahas or Agrahayana (November-December) or Sahasya, i.e. Pushya (December-January),
- It is administered to a patient after his body has been smeared with the cooling, unctuous and sweet herbs. (This is because, Bhallataka is very hot in nature and may cause excessive burning sensation in the patient).
- In the beginning, 10 fruits of Bhallataka should be well boiled in 8 parts of water.
- After boiling, when $1/8^{th}$ of water remains, it is filtered, added with milk and given to the patient after his mouth has been smeared with ghee.
- Ten fruits should be added every day by one fruit till the number becomes thirty and thereafter, it should be decreased by one fruit per day till it reaches the original number – ten.
- It should not be further increased because thirty fruits of Bhallataka is the maximum dose.
- Following this procedure, one thousand Bhallatakas can be administered.

   Pathya:

- After digestion, the person should take the rice of Shali or Shashtika along with milk and ghee.
- After administration for a few days, the person should take milk only twice per day. (Milk acts as coolant and will take away that hot effects of Bhallatak).

By the use of this recipe, one lives for one hundred years and gains such other excellent results as are described in paragraph 4, 5 and 6 above.[13]

Bhallataka Kshaudra:
भल्लातकानां जर्जरीकृतानां पिष्टस्वेदनं पूरयित्वा भूमावाकण्ठं निखातस्य स्नेहभावितस्य दृढस्योपरि कुम्भस्यारोप्योडुपेनापिधाय कृष्णमृत्तिकावलिप्तं गोमयाग्निभिरुपस्वेदयेत्; तेषां यः स्वरसः कुम्भं प्रपद्येत, तमष्ट भाग मधुसम्प्रयुक्तं द्विगुण घृतमद्यात्; तत्प्रयोगादूर्वष शतमजरं वयस्तिष्ठतीति समानं पूर्वेण||१४||
(इति भल्लातकक्षौद्रम्)|

The procedure:

- Fruits of Bhallataka are slightly crushed and kept inside Pishta Svedana apparatus.
- It is kept inside a strong earthen jar which is smeared inside with Sneha (ghee or oil).
- This earthen jar is kept inside a hole dug in the earth.
- The mouth of the jar is sealed by smearing with black coloured mud.
- Over this jar, the fire of cow dung cake should be ignited for heating.
- By this heat, the Svarasa (liquid fraction) of these fruits will percolate and get accumulated at the bottom of the earthen jar.
- This liquid is collected and taken by adding $1/8^{th}$ honey and double the quantity of ghee.

Benefits:

- Person attains longevity.
- Free from old age and gets such other benefits as are mentioned in paragraph 4, 5 and 6 above. [14]

BhallatakaTaila:

भल्लातक तैलपात्रं सपयस्कं मधुकेन कल्केनाक्ष मात्रेण शतपाकं कुर्यादिति समानं पूर्वेण ||१५|| (इति भल्लातकतैलम्) |

One adhaka (3.072) of the oil of Bhallataka (Semecarpus anacardium Linn.) is boiled along with milk and one Aksha (12 g) of the paste of Madhuka– Licorice – Glycyrrhiza glabra. This process is repeated 100 times. By taking this, a person lives for one hundred years and gets such other benefits as are described in paragraph 4 and verses 5 and 6 above [15]

Different recipes of Bhallataka (Semecarpus anacardium Linn.):

भल्लातक सर्पिः, भल्लातक क्षीरं, भल्लातक क्षौद्रं, गुड भल्लातकं, भल्लातक यूषः, भल्लातक तैलं, भल्लातक पललं, भल्लातक सक्तवः, भल्लातक लवणं, भल्लातक तर्पणम्, इति भल्लातक विधानमुक्तं भवति||१६||

Following are the ten recipes prepared out of Bhallataka (Semecarpus anacardium Linn.):

1. Bhallataka sarpi – medicated ghee prepared by boiling with Bhallataka.
2. Bhallataka Ksheera – medicated milk of Bhallataka.
3. Bhallataka Kshaudra or the preparation of bhallataka mixed with honey.
4. Guda Bhallataka or the preparation of Bhallataka (Semecarpus anacardium Linn.) by adding or by boiling with Guda – Jaggery.
5. Bhallataka Yusha – soup prepared by boiling other drugs with Bhallataka.
6. Bhalataka Taila – medicated oil prepared by boiling with Bhallataka.
7. Bhalataka Palala – preparation of Bhalataka by adding meat.
8. Bhallataka Saktu – preparation of Bhallataka by adding it with roasted corn flour.
9. Bhallataka Lavana – Medicine of Bhallataka prepared by adding salt. This can be prepared by taking Bhallataka and salt in equal quantity and making Paka by Antardhuma method (heating in closed container)
10. Bhallataka Tarpana – the preparation of Bhallataka by adding tarpana (roasted corn flour mixed with large quantity of water)

Thus ends the description of different methods of preparation of Bhallataka (Semecarpus anacardium Linn.).[16]

Summary:

भवन्ति चात्र-

भल्लातकानि तीक्ष्णानि पाकीन्यग्नि समानि च|

भवन्त्यमृत कल्पानि प्रयुक्तानि यथाविधि||१७||

एते दश विधास्त्वेषां प्रयोगाः परिकीर्तिताः|

रोगप्रकृति सात्म्यज्ञस्तान् प्रयोगान् प्रकल्पयेत्||१८||

कफजो न स रोगोऽस्ति न विबन्धोऽस्ति कश्चन|

यं न भल्लातकं हन्याच्छीघ्रं मेधाग्नि वर्धनम्||१९||

(इति भल्लातकविधिः)|

प्राणकामाः पुरा जीर्णाश्च्यवनाद्या महर्षयः|

रसायनैः शिवैरेतैर्बभूवुरमितायुषः||२०||

ब्राह्मं तपो ब्रह्मचर्यमध्यात्मध्यानमेव च|

दीर्घायुषो यथाकामं सम्भृत्य त्रिदिवं गताः||२१||

तस्मादायुःप्रकर्षार्थं प्राणकामैः सुखार्थिभिः|
रसायनविधिः सेव्यो विधिवत्सुसमाहितैः||२२||

The constituents of Bhallataka:
Fruits of Bhallataka (Semecarpus anacardium Linn.) are
Teekshna (sharp),
Paaki (corrosive) and
Agni Sama (like agni)
But when prepared according to the prescribed methods, they work like Amrita (ambrosia).

The ten recipes said above should be administered by a physician who is expert in the knowledge of
Roga (diseases)
Prakrti (physical constitutions)
Satmya (wholesomeness).
It cures diseases of Kapha and Vibandha (constipation) instantaneously. Bhallataka promotes Medha (intellect) and Agni (power of digestion and metabolism). In the days of yore, the old Maharishis, viz, Chyavana etc. desirous of attaining vitality, used these auspicious recipes for rejuvenation and succeeded in attaining a long life.

Benefits of taking these recipes:
They were able to pursue their religious studies, Tapas (Penance), Brahmacharya (celibacy), spiritual knowledge and meditation and also attained heaven.

Therefore, persons desirous of obtaining long life vitality and happiness should practise rejuvenation therapy with complete devotion according to the prescribed procedure. [17-22]

To sum up:
तत्र श्लोकः-
रसायनानां संयोगाः सिद्धा भूतहितैषिणा|
निर्दिष्टाः प्राणकामीये सप्तत्रिंशन्महर्षिणा ||२३||
Thirty-seven different recipes for rejuvenation therapy which are extremely effective are described for the welfare of the living being by the great sage in this quarter on the desire for vitality. [23]

इत्यग्निवेशकृते तन्त्रे चरकप्रतिसंस्कृते चिकित्सास्थाने रसायनाध्याये प्राणकामीयो नाम रसायनपादो द्वि‍तीयः||२||
Here ends the second quarter called Pranakameeya Rasayana Pada of the chapter on Rasayana of the Chikistsa Section in Agnivesha's work as redacted by Charaka.

3

Chikitsasthana Chapter 1.3 Kara Prachiteeya Rasayanam

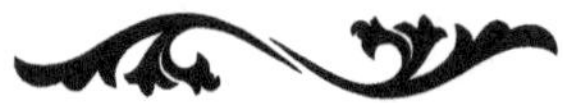

Charak Samhita Chikitsa sthana 1st chapter deals with anti-ageing treatments. It has 4 sections. The 3rd section is called Kara Prachiteeya Rasayana Pada. It deals with anti-aging recipes using Amla, Triphala, Long pepper and Shilajeet.

Third Quarter of the Chapter on Rejuvenation Therapy

अथातः करप्रचितीयं रसायनपादं व्याख्यास्यामः॥१॥

इति ह स्माह भगवानात्रेयः॥२॥

Now, we shall explore the quarter dealing with rejuvenation therapy by the administration of Amla fruit (Indian Gooseberry), being administered by hand – Kara Prachiteeya Rasayana Pada.

Thus said lord Atreya [1-2]

Amalakayasa Brahma Rasayana :

करप्रचितानां यथोक्तगुणानामामलकानामुद्धृतास्थ्नां शुष्क चूर्णितानां पुनर्माघे फाल्गुने वा मासे त्रिःसप्तकृत्वः स्वरस परिपीतानां पुनः शुष्क चूर्णीकृतानामाढकमेक ग्राहयेत्, अथ जीवनीयानां बृंहणीयानां स्तन्यजननानां शुक्रजननानां वयःस्थापनानां षड्विरेचनशताश्रितीयोक्तानामौषध गणानां चन्दनागुरु धव तिनिश खदिर शिंशपासनसाराणां चाणुशः कृतानामभया बिभीतक पिप्पली वचा चव्य चित्रक विडङ्गानां च समस्तानामाढकमेक दशगुणेनाम्भसा साधयेत्, तस्मिन्नाढकावशेषे रसे सुपूते तान्यामलक चूर्णानि दत्वा गोमयाग्निभिर्वेश विदल शर तेजनाग्निभिर्वा साधयेद्यावदपनयाद्रसस्य, तमनुपदग्धमुपहृत्यायसीषु पात्रीष्वास्तीर्य शोषयेत्, सुशुष्कं तत् कृष्णाजिनस्योपरि दृषदि श्लक्ष्णपिष्टमयःस्थाल्यां निधापयेत् सम्यक्, तच्चूर्णमयश्चूर्णाष्टभाग सम्प्रयुक्तं मधु सर्पिभ्र्यामग्निबलमभिसमीक्ष्य प्रयोजयेदिति ॥३॥

भवन्ति चात्र-

एतद्रसायनं पूर्वं वसिष्ठः कश्यपोऽङ्गिराः |

जमदग्निर्भरद्वाजो भृगुरन्ये च तद्विधाः ॥४॥

प्रयुज्य प्रयता मुक्ताः श्रम व्याधि जराभयात् |

यावदैच्छंस्तपस्तेपुस्तत्प्रभावान्महाबलाः ॥५॥

इदं रसायनं चक्रे ब्रह्मा वार्षसहस्रिकम् |

जरा व्याधि प्रशमनं बुद्धीन्द्रियबलप्रदम् ॥६॥

(इत्यामलकायसं ब्राह्मरसायनम्) |

Amalakayasa Brahma Rasayana :

Fruits of Amlaka are selected which are endowed with the attributes described earlier, separated from their seeds, dried and powdered. This is done during the month of Magha (January – February) or Phalguna (February- March) The powder is again impregnated with fruit juice of Amalaki fruits for 21 times. The dry powder is ground with its own juice extract till it dries. This is counted as one time. This process is repeated 21 times.

Thus prepared fortified Amla powder is taken in a quantity of one adhaka (3.072 Kg) kept separately.

One Adhaka (3.072 Kg) of all the following drugs taken together is boiled by adding ten times of water.

Jeevaneeya Gana – Enlivening, anti aging group of herbs

Jeevaka – Malaxis acuminata

Rishabhaka – Manilkara hexandra

Meda – Polygonatum cirrhifolium

Mahameda – Polygonatum verticillatum

Kakoli – Fritillaria roylei

Kshira Kakoli – Roscoea purpurea / Lilium polyphyllum

Mudgaparni – Phaseolus trilobus,

Mashaparni – Teramnus labialis,

Jivanti – Leptadenia reticulata and

Madhuka– Licorice – Glycyrrhiza glabra

Bruhmaneeya Gana – Nourishing, increasing weight

Ksheerini – Mimosops hexandra Roxb.

Rajakshavaka – Euphorbia microphylla,

Ashwagandha – Winter Cherry / Indian ginseng (root) – Withania somnifera,

Kakoli – Fritillaria roylei,

Ksheerakakoli – Roscoea purpurea / Lilium polyphyllum,

Vatyayani – Country mallow (root) – Sida cordifolia,

Bhadraudani - Sida cordifolia Linn.

Bharadvaji – Thespesia lampas,

Payasya – Ipomoea paniculata and

Rushyagandha

Stanyajanana – improving breast milk

Virana - Vetiveria zizanioides Nash.

Shali – Rice - Oryza sativa Linn.

Shastika – a variety of rice – Oryza sativa Linn.

Ikhsuvalika – Asteracantha longifolia Nees

Darbha – Desmostachya bipinnata Staff.

Kusha – Desmostachya bipinnata

Kasha – Saccharum spontaneum Linn.

Gundra – Saccharum sara

Itkata – Sesbania bispinosa

Katruna – Cymbopogon schoenanthus Spreng.

Shukrajanana – improving quality of semen and ovum

Jeevaka – Malaxis acuminata

Rishabhaka – Manilkara hexandra

Kakoli – Fritillaria roylei

Kshira Kakoli – Lilium polyphyllum

Mudgaparni – Phaseolus trilobus

Mashaparni – Teramnus labialis,

Meda – Polygonatum cirrhifolium,

Vriddharuha - Asparagus racemosus Willd.

Jatila – Nardostachys jatamamsi and

Kulinga – Rhus acuminata

Vayaha Sthapana -rejuvenating, anti-aging

Amruta – Tinspora cordifolia Miers.

Abhaya – Terminalia chebula,

Dhatri - Emblica - officinalis Gaertn.

Mukta (pearl),

Shveta – white variety of Clitoria ternatea

Jivanti – Leptadenia reticulata,

Atirasa – Asparagus root – Asparagus racemosus

Mandukaparni - Centella asiatica Urban

Sthira – Desmodium gangeticum and

Punarnava - Boerhaavia diffusa Linn.

The heartwood of

Chandana (Sandalwood – Santalum album)

Aguru – Aquilaria agallocha

Dhava – Anogeissus latifolia

Tinisha – Dalbergia latifolia

Khadira – Acacia catechu

Shimshapa – Dalbergia sissoo and

Asana cut into small pieces and

Abhaya – Terminalia chebula,

Bibhitaka – Terminalia bellerica

Pippali – Long pepper fruit – Piper longum,

Vacha – Acorus calamus Linn.

Chavya – Piper retrofractum and

Chitraka – Leadwort – Plumbago zeylanica.

• After boiling, when only one Adhaka (3.072 liter) of water remains (from 10 Adhaka, reduced to 1 Adhaka), it should be filtered.

• To this Kashaya, the powder of Amalaki prepared earlier is added.

• It is boiled by the fire of cow dung cake, or bamboo, or Shara or Tejana, till the liquid portion disappears.

• It is removed from the fire before it gets burnt and then spread over a plate made of iron till it gets dried up.

• After it is fully dried up, it is made to a fine paste in pestle and mortar and kept over a deer skin.

• This paste is kept in an iron container.

• This powder is mixed with eight times [some interpret as Ashta bhaga as 1/8th in quantity] of the powder of iron, honey and ghee and is administered to a person, keeping in view the limitations of his digestion strength.

Thus it is said:

By taking such recipes for rejuvenation, in the days of yore, sages viz, Vashishta, Kashyapa, Angeerasa, Jamadagni, Bharadvaja, Bhrugu and other sages like them became

• Free from the fear of fatigue, diseases and old age,

• Performed penance as long as they wished.

Because of its Prabhava (specific action) they were endowed with great strength.

This recipe is invented by Lord Brahma

Benefits of Amalakayasa Brahma Rasayan:

• A person lives for one thousand years

• Free from old age and diseases

• Promotes Buddhi (wisdom) and the strength of the sense organs (3-6)

Eligible beneficiaries:

तपसा ब्रह्मचर्येण ध्यानेन प्रशमेन च|
रसायन विधानेन कालयुक्तेन चायुषा||७||
स्थिता महर्षयः पूर्वं, नहि किञ्चिद्रसायनम्|
ग्राम्यानामन्यकार्याणां सिध्यत्यप्रयतात्मनाम्||८||

The great sages of the yester centuries were devoted to penance, celibacy (Brahmacharya), meditation and tranquility.

They did not have a limited span of life. The rejuvenation therapies administered to them according to the prescribed procedure enabled them to live for such a long time. Such excellent results of anti ageing Rasayana therapy will NOT be found when these recipes are administered to persons who resort to unethical habits (Gramya), who are engaged in worldly works, devoid of self control [7-8]

Kevala Amalaka Rasayana:

संवत्सरं पयोवृत्तिर्गवां मध्ये वसेत् सदा |
सावित्रीं मनसा ध्यायन् ब्रह्मचारी यतेन्द्रियः ||९||
संवत्सरान्ते पौषीं वा माघीं वा फाल्गुनीं तिथिम् |
त्र्यहोपवासी शुक्लस्य प्रविश्यामलकीवनम् ||१०||
बृहत्फलाढ्यमारुह्य द्रुमं शाखागतं फलम् |
गृहीत्वा पाणिना तिष्ठेज्जपन् ब्रह्मामृतागमात् ||११||
तदा ह्यवश्यममृतं वसत्यामलके क्षणम् |
शर्करामधुकल्पानि स्नेहवन्ति मृदूनि च ||१२||
भवन्त्यमृतसंयोगातानि यावन्ति भक्षयेत् |
जीवेद्वर्षसहस्राणि तावन्त्यागतयौवनः ||१३||
सौहित्यमेषां गत्वा तु भवत्यमरसन्निभः |
स्वयं चास्योपतिष्ठन्ते श्रीर्वेदा वाक् च रूपिणी ||१४||
(इति केवलामलकरसायनम्) |

Kevala Amalaka Rasayana:
• A person should live among the cows, living on cow milk for one year, mentally reciting Savitri Mantra following Celibacy (Brahmacharya) and having controlled senses should at the end of the year, on a suitable day of the bright fortnight (15 days, leading to full moon day) of Pushya (January- February), Magha (February- March) or Phalguna (March-April), observe fast for 3 days and enter into a garden of Amalaki – Indian gooseberry fruit – Emblica officinalis.
• He should then climb upon an Amalaki tree laden with big fruits.
• Holding one such fruit in hand, he should stay there reciting Brahma Mantra (Omkara chanting) till the fruit gets impregnated with Amruta (Ambrosia).
• Ambrosia will come to that fruit for a moment due to the Sacred effect of the Mantra, these fruits become sweet like sugar and honey in taste, unctuous and soft.
Benefits:
• Long life with youthfulness is regained, depending on number of Amla fruits he takes in this process.
• He becomes brilliant, like the Gods. He will be blessed with Shree (auspiciousness), the Vedas (knowledge) and Vak (Divine oration power) .[9-14]

Lauhadi Rasayana:

त्रिफलाया रसे मूत्रे गवां क्षारे च लवणे |
क्रमेण चेङ्गुदीक्षार किंशुकक्षार एव च ||१५||
तीक्ष्णायसस्य पत्राणि वह्निवर्णानि साधयेत् |
चतुरङ्गुलदीर्घाणि तिलोत्सेधतनूनि च ||१६||
ज्ञात्वा तान्यञ्जनाभानि सूक्ष्मचूर्णानि कारयेत् |
तानि चूर्णानि मधुना रसेनामलकस्य च ||१७||
युक्तानि लेहवत् कुम्भे स्थितानि घृतभाविते |
संवत्सरं निधेयानि यवपल्ले तथैव च ||१८||

दद्यादालोडनं मासे सर्वत्रालोडयन् बुधः |
संवत्सरात्यये तस्य प्रयोगो मधुसर्पिषा ||१९||
प्रातः प्रातर्बलापेक्षी सात्म्यं जीर्णे च भोजनम् |
एष एव च लौहानां प्रयोगः सम्प्रकीर्तितः ||२०||
नाभिघातैर्न चातङ्कैर्जरया न च मृत्युना |
स धृष्यः स्याद्गजप्राणः सदा चातिबलेन्द्रियः ||२१||
धीमान् यशस्वी वाक्सिद्धः श्रुतधारी महाधनः |
भवेत् समां प्रयुञ्जानो नरो लौहरसायनम् ||२२||
अनेनैव विधानेन हेम्नश्च रजतस्य च |
आयुःप्रकर्षकृत्सिद्धः प्रयोगः सर्वरोगनुत् ||२३||
(इति लौहादिरसायनम्)|

Teekshna Loha (a type of iron) is cut to thin leaves of 4 Angulas in length.

Their thickness should be of a sesame seed.

These thin iron sheets are heated. When red hot, they are immersed in following liquids separately –

Triphala Kashaya (decoction),

Gomutra – Cow urine,

Jyotishmati Kshara and Lavana (salt),

Ingudi Kshara – Balanites aegyptiaca and

Kimshuka Kshara – Butea monosperma

When the colour of these iron leaves becomes deep black like collyrium (Anjanaabha), it is ground to fine powder.

To this powder, honey and the fruit juice of Amalaki is added and stirred well to make it linctus (jam consistency).

This should be kept in an earthen jar, smeared with ghee, sealed, and kept inside a heap of Yava – Barley – Hordeum vulgare. This jar should be kept therein for one year.

Every month this linctus is thoroughly stirred.

After one year, this is given along with honey and ghee every morning.

Dosage:

• Is determined on the basis of the strength of the person.

• After its digestion, he is given wholesome food.

The same procedure should be followed for the administration of other types of Loha Bhasma.

Benefits:

By taking this recipe for one year, the person will

• Not succumb to any injury, fear, old age and death.

• Have the life span of an elephant.

• Be endowed with Dhi (intellect), Yashas (fame), Vak siddhi (what he speaks will come true), Srutadharatva (he will remember everything he hears) and Mahadhana (vast wealth).

Following the similar procedure, gold and silver can also be administered. These are the effective recipes that bring about longevity and freedom from all diseases. [15-23]

Aindra Rasayana

ऐन्द्री मत्स्याख्यको ब्राह्मी वचा ब्रह्मसुवर्चला |
पिप्पल्यो लवणं हेम शङ्खपुष्पी विषं घृतम् ||२४||
एषां त्रियवकान् भागान् हेम सर्पिर्विषैर्विना |
द्वौ यवौ तत्र हेम्नस्तु तिलं दद्यादिवषस्य च ||२५||
सर्पिषश्च पलं दद्यातदैकध्यं प्रयोजयेत् |
घृतप्रभूतं सक्षौद्रं जीर्णे चान्नं प्रशस्यते ||२६||

जराव्याधिप्रशमनं स्मृतिमेधाकरं परम् |
आयुष्यं पौष्टिकं धन्यं स्वरवर्णप्रसादनम् ||२७||
परमोजस्करं चैतत् सिद्धमैन्द्रं रसायनम् |
नैनत् प्रसहते कृत्या नालक्ष्मीर्न विषं न रुक् ||२८||
श्वित्रं सकुष्ठं जठराणि गुल्माः प्लीहा पुराणो विषमज्वरश्च|
मेधास्मृतिज्ञानहराश्च रोगाः शाम्यन्त्यनेनातिबलाश्च वाताः||२९||
(इत्यैन्द्रं रसायनम्)|

• Aindra – Abelia chinensis
• Matsyakhyaka
• Brahmi – Thyme leaved gratiola (whole plant) – Bacopa monnieri,
• Vacha – Acorus calamus
• Brahma Suvarchala,
• Pippali – Piper longum
• Saindhava Lavana – Rock salt
• Shankhapuspi – are to be taken in the quantity of three Yavas (one Yava = 1/6th g) each.
To this,
• two yava of gold,
• Visha of the quantity of one Tila – Sesame seed and
• 4 Palas (4 X 48 g) of ghee should be added and mixed together and administered based on digestion strength.
Pathya:
After this recipe is digested, intake of food mixed with ghee in large quantity and honey is indicated.
Benefits:
Promotes
• Memory as well as intellect par excellence.
• Longevity
• nourishment
• Dhana (wealth)
• Svara (voice)
Varna (complexion) and one cannot be victimized by Krutya (black magic), Alakshmi (inauspiciousness), Visha (poison) and Ruk (pain).
It prevents old age and diseases.
Cures these diseases:
• Shvitra – leucoderma
• Kustha – skin diseases
• Jathara – abdominal diseases, ascites
• Gulma – phantom tumor
• Purana Pleeha (chronic splenic disorder),
• Vishama Jvara (Intermittent fever),
• Psychic diseases afflicting Medha
• Excessive aggravation of Vayu
• It improves intelligence (intellect), Smrti(memory) and Jnana (knowledge) [24-29]

Medhya Rasayana:
मण्डूकपर्ण्याः स्वरसः प्रयोज्यः क्षीरेण यष्टीमधुकस्य चूर्णम् |
रसो गुडूच्यास्तु समूलपुष्प्याः कल्कः प्रयोज्यः खलु शङ्खपुष्प्याः ||३०||
आयुःप्रदान्यामयनाशनानि बलाग्निवर्णस्वरवर्धनानि |

मेध्यानि चैतानि रसायनानि मेध्या विशेषेण च शङ्खपुष्पी ||३१||
(इति मेध्यरसायनानि) |

Four rejuvenating recipes are given below:
1. Juice of Mandukaparni – Gotu Kola – Centella asiatica
2. Powder of Yastimadhu mixed with milk
3. Juice of Guduchi along with its root and flower
4. Paste of Shankhapushpi
Benefits:
• Increases longevity,
• Cures diseases, and
• Promote strength, Agni (power of Digestion and metabolism), Varna (complexion) and Svara (voice).
These rejuvenating recipes are Medhya (wholesome for intellect). Among them, Shankha Pushpi is the drug par excellence for the promotion of intellect.[30-31]

Pippali Rasayana:
पञ्चाष्टौ सप्त दश वा पिप्पलीर्मधुसर्पिषा |
रसायन गुणान्वेषी समामेकां प्रयोजयेत् ||३२||
तिस्रस्तिस्रस्तु पूर्वाह्णे भुक्त्वाऽग्रे भोजनस्य च |
पिप्पल्यः किंशुक क्षारभाविता घृतभर्जिताः ||३३||
प्रयोज्या मधु सम्मिश्रा रसायन गुणैषिणा |
जेतुं कासं क्षयं शोषं श्वासं हिक्कां गलामयान् ||३४||
अर्शांसि ग्रहणीदोषं पाण्डुतां विषमज्वरम् |
वैस्वर्यं पीनसं शोफं गुल्मं वातबलासकम् ||३५||
(इति पिप्पलीरसायनम्) |
Procedure and Ingredients used:
• A person desirous of rejuvenation should take five, eight, seven or ten Pippali – Long pepper fruits, along with honey and ghee for one year.
• Pippali should be impregnated with Kimshuka Kshara and fried with ghee.
• Three such Pippali are mixed with honey is taken in the morning twice- one before food and second time after food by a person who desires to be rejuvenated.
Cures the following diseases:
• Kasa – bronchitis
• Ksaya – pthisis
• Sosa – consumption
• Shvasa – asthma
• Hikka – Hiccup
• Galamaya – diseases on Neck
• Arshas – piles
• Grahani Dosha – Sprue syndrome
• Pandu – Anemia
• Vishama Jvara – intermittent fever
• Vaisvarya – hoarseness of voice
• Pinasa – chronic rhinitis
• Sopha – edema
• Gulma – Phantom tumor and
• Vata Balasaka – a type of fever [32-35]

Read more about Pippali Rasayan

Pippali Vardhamana Rasayan:
क्रमवृद्ध्या दशाहानि दशपैप्पलिकं दिनम्|
वर्धयेत् पयसा सार्धं तथैवापनयेत् पुनः||३६||
जीर्णे जीर्णे च भुञ्जीत षष्टिकं क्षीरसर्पिषा|
पिप्पलीनां सहस्रस्य प्रयोगोऽयं रसायनम्||३७||
पिष्टास्ता बलिभिः सेव्याः, शृता मध्यबलैर्नरैः|
चूर्णीकृता ह्रस्वबलैर्योज्या दोषामयान् प्रति||३८||
दशपैप्पलिकः श्रेष्ठो मध्यमः षट् प्रकीर्तितः|
प्रयोगो यस्त्रिपर्यन्तः स कनीयान् स चाबलैः||३९||
बृहणं स्वर्यमायुष्यं प्लीहोदरविनाशनम्|
वयसः स्थापनं मेध्यं पिप्पलीनां रसायनम्||४०||
(इति पिप्पलीवर्धमानं रसायनम्)|

• Pippali – Long pepper fruit – Piper longum is taken along with milk by gradually increasing the fruits of Pippalis to 10 per day.
• After 10 days, this is gradually decreased.
• Thus in total the person should take one thousand Pippali fruits for the purpose of rejuvenation.
After the digestion of the recipe, the person should take Sastika type of rice along with milk and ghee.
Depending upon the nature of Doshas and the diseases, these Pippalis should be taken in the form of –
paste by persons who are strong.
decoction (Kashaya) by persons having moderate strength and
Powder by persons having less strength.
Dosage:
• 10 Pippali fruits (as described above) – excellent,
• 6 Pippali fruits are of moderate dose and
• 3 Pippali fruits are smallest dose is given to persons who are very weak.
Benefits: The rejuvenation therapy through the recipe of Pippali – Long pepper fruit – Piper longum
• Is nourishing and promoter of voice and longevity
• It cures Pliha (Splenic disorders) and Udara (obstinate abdominal diseases including ascites).
• It restores youth and promotes intellect.[36-40]

Triphala Rasayana:
जरणान्तेऽभयामेकां प्राग्भुक्ताद् द्वे बिभीतके|
भुक्त्वा तु मधुसर्पिभ्यां चत्वार्यामलकानि च||४१||
प्रयोजयन् समामेकां त्रिफलाया रसायनम्|
जीवेद्वर्षशतं पूर्णमजरोऽव्याधिरेव च||४२||
(इति त्रिफलारसायनम्)|
The following are the four rejuvenating recipes of Triphala
1. Along with honey and ghee, a person should take the following after the previous meal is digested (i.e., early morning)
1 Abhaya – Haritaki – Terminalia chebula
2 Bibhitaki fruits before food (Terminalia bellirica) and
4 Amalaki fruits after food.
Duration: One year

Benefits: A person lives for one hundred years free from old age and diseases.

Triphal Rasayan – 2

त्रैफलेनायसीं पात्रीं कल्केनालेपयेन्नवाम्|
तमहोरात्रिकं लेपं पिबेत् क्षौद्रोदकाप्लुतम्||४३||
प्रभूतस्नेहमशनं जीर्णे तत्र प्रशस्यते|
अजरोऽरुक् समाभ्यासाज्जीवेच्चैव समाः शतम्||४४||
(इति त्रिफलारसायनमपरम्)|

A new iron vessel should be pasted with the Triphala paste (Kalka) for 24 hours.
This paste is administered with honey and water.
After its digestion, one should take a lot of fat (Prabhuta Sneha Ashanam)
By using this recipe continually for one year, one can live for one hundred years, free from aging and diseases.

Triphala Rasayanam – 3

मधुकेन तुगाक्षीर्या पिप्पल्या क्षौद्रसर्पिषा|
त्रिफला सितया चापि युक्ता सिद्धं रसायनम्||४५||
(इति त्रिफलारसायनमपरम्)|
Triphala mixed with
• Madhuka – Licorice – Glycyrrhiza glabra,
• Tugaksheeri
• Pippali – Long pepper fruit – Piper longum ,
• Honey, Ghee and Sugar, is an effective anti-ageing recipe.

Triphala Rasayanam – 3

सर्वलौहैः सुवर्णेन वचया मधुसर्पिषा|
विडङ्गपिप्पलीभ्यां च त्रिफला लवणेन च||४६||
संवत्सरप्रयोगेण मेधास्मृतिबलप्रदा|
भवत्यायुःप्रदा धन्या जरारोगनिबर्हणी||४७||
(इति त्रिफलारसायनमपरम्)|
Triphala along with
• Sarva Lauha,
• Suvarna (gold)
• Vacha – Acorus calamus
• honey, Ghee
• Vidanga – False black pepper – Embelia ribes,
• Pippali – Long pepper fruit – Piper longum and
• Lavana – Rock salt
The above mixture is administered continually for one year.
Benefits:
It is conducive to the advancement of
• Medha – intellect
• Smrti – memory
• Bala – Strength
• Ayus – longevity and
• Dhana – wealth.
It prevents ageing and diseases [41-47]

Shilajeet qualities and uses:

अनम्लं च कषायं च कटु पाके शिलाजतु|
नात्युष्णशीतं धातुभ्यश्चतुभ्र्यस्तस्य सम्भवः||४८||
हेम्नश्च रजताताम्राद्वरात् कृष्णायसादपि|
रसायनं तद्विधिभिस्तद्वृष्यं तच्च रोगनुत्||४९||
वातपित्तकफघ्नैश्च निर्यूहैस्तत् सुभावितम्|
वीर्योत्कर्षं परं याति सर्वैरेकैकशोऽपि वा||५०||

Shilajeet qualities:

Anamla – not very sour

Kashaya – astringent taste

Katu Paka – Undergoes pungent taste conversion after digestion

Na Ati ushna – neither too hot, nor too cold

It exudes from the stones / ores of four types of metals viz, gold, silver copper and black iron.

The Shilajeet from the black iron ore is the best.

If administered with proper procedure, it produces rejuvenating and aphrodisiac effects and cures diseases.

Its potency increases by impregnating it with the kashaya of herbs which alleviate Vayu, Pitta and Kapha.

Impregnation can be done by these drugs individually or by all of them taken together. [48-50]

Shilajit Rasayan:

प्रक्षिप्तोद्धृतमप्येनत् पुनस्तत् प्रक्षिपेद्रसे|
कोष्णे सप्ताहमेतेन विधिना तस्य भावना||५१||
पूर्वोक्तेन विधानेन लोहैश्चूर्णीकृतैः सह|
तत् पीतं पयसा दद्याद्दीर्घमायुः सुखान्वितम्||५२||
जराव्याधिप्रशमनं देहदाढर्यकरं परम्|
मेधास्मृतिकरं धन्यं क्षीराशी तत् प्रयोजयेत्||५३||
प्रयोगः सप्तसप्ताहास्त्रयश्चैकश्च सप्तकः|
निर्दिष्टस्त्रिविधस्तस्य परो मध्योऽवरस्तथा||५४||
पलमर्धपलं कर्षो मात्रा तस्य त्रिधा मता|५५|

Shilajeet Rasayanam:

• Shilajatu is immersed into the hot decoction of the drugs that are prescribed for alleviating the aggravation of Doshas and

• After it has absorbed the decoction, it should be immersed again.

• This process should be repeated for seven days.

• This processed Shilajatu mixed with the powder of iron should be administered with milk.

Benefits:

• This is an elixir for long life and happiness.

• It prevents ageing and diseases.

• It is an excellent drug for producing sturdiness of the body.

• It also promotes Medha (intellect), Smrti (memory) and Dhana (wealth).

Pathya: the person should live on milk.

Duration:

• 7 weeks – excellent effect

• 3 weeks – moderate effect and

• 1 week – very little effect

Classification: Depending upon the dose of the recipe

• 1 Pala (48 g) – highest potency

• 1/2 Pala (24g) – Moderate potency
• 1 Karsha (12 g) – lowest potency [51-55]

Varieties and their utility:

जातेर्विशेषं सविधिं तस्य वक्ष्याम्यतः परम्||५५||
हेमाद्याः सूर्यसन्तप्ताः स्रवन्ति गिरिधातवः|
जत्वाभं मृदु मृत्स्नाच्छं यन्मलं तच्छिलाजतु||५६||
मधुरश्च सतिक्तश्च जपापुष्पनिभश्च यः|
कटुविपाके शीतश्च स सुवर्णस्य निस्रवः||५७||
रूप्यस्य कटुकः श्वेतः शीतः स्वादु विपच्यते|
ताम्रस्य बर्हिकण्ठाभस्तिक्तोष्णः पच्यते कटु||५८||
यस्तु गुग्गुलुकाभासस्तिक्तको लवणान्वितः|
कटुविपाके शीतश्च सर्वश्रेष्ठः स चायसः||५९||
गोमूत्रगन्धयः सर्वे सर्वकर्मसु यौगिकाः|
रसायनप्रयोगेषु पश्चिमस्तु विशिष्यते||६०||
यथाक्रमं वातपित्ते श्लेष्मपित्ते कफे त्रिषु|
विशेषतः प्रशस्यन्ते मला हेमादिधातुजाः||६१||

Hereafter, varieties of Shilajit and the method of their use will be described.
• Stones of metals like gold etc, in the mountains get heated up by the sun and the exudate that comes out of them in the form of smooth and clean gum is called Silajatu.

Shilajeet from the stones containing gold,
• Shilajatu is sweet and has bitter aftertaste,
• like the flower of Japa in appearance,
• pungent in Vipaka

From the stone containing silver,
• pungent in taste
• white, cooling and
• Sweet in Vipaka.

From the stone containing copper,
• is like the peacock throat,
• bitter in taste
• Hot and pungent in Vipaka.

The exudates which looks like the gum of Guggulu (Commiphora mukul Engl.)
• Is bitter and Saline
• pungent in Vipaka, and cooling
• Is derived from the stone containing iron. This is the best among all.

All these types of Shilajeet having the smell of cow's urine are useful in all types of therapies. However, for rejuvenation therapy, the last variety (i.e. the one derived from the stone contain iron) in more useful.

In diseases caused by
• Vayu- Pitta – gold
• Kapha- Pitta – silver
• Kapha – copper and
• all the three Dosas – iron containing stones are useful

Prohibitions and Therapeutic effect:

शिलाजतुप्रयोगेषु विदाहीनि गुरूणि च|
वर्जयेत् सर्वकालं तु कुलत्थान् परिवर्जयेत्||६२||

ते ह्यत्यन्तविरुद्धत्वादश्मनो भेदनाः परम्।
लोके दृष्टास्ततस्तेषां प्रयोगः प्रतिषिध्यते॥६३॥
पयांसि तक्राणि रसाः सयूषास्तोयं समूत्रा विविधाः कषायाः।
आलोडनार्थं गिरिजस्य शस्तास्ते ते प्रयोज्याः प्रसमीक्ष्य कार्यम्॥६४॥
न सोऽस्ति रोगो भुवि साध्यरूपः शिलाह्वयं यं न जयेत् प्रसह्य।
तत् कालयोगैर्विधिभिः प्रयुक्तं स्वस्थस्य चोर्जां विपुलां ददाति॥६५॥
(इति शिलाजतुरसायनम्)।

Contraindicated foods while taking recipe of Silajatu,
• Vidahi foods (causing burning sensation) and Guru (heavy).
• Kulattha (horse gram) should be avoided forever (or till such time as the person has the effects of Silajatu in his body)
Reason for avoiding Kulattha:
• It is commonly seen that Kulattha is an excellent drug for breaking stones.
• By taking Shilajatu, the body of the person becomes like a stone to bring about sturdiness in it.
• Therefore, horse gram and Shilajatu have mutually contradicting effects, and is prohibited for a person who is using or who has used Shilajatu.
Ingredients which can be used with Shilajatu:
• Milk
• Butter milk
• Meat soup
• Vegetable soup
• Water
• Urine and
• decoction of different types of drugs
Benefits:
• There is no curable disease in the universe which is not effectively cured by Shilajatu when administered at the appropriate time, in combination with suitable drugs and by adopting the prescribed method.
• When administered to a healthy person, with similar conditions it produces immense energy. [62-65]

Summary:

तत्र श्लोकः:-
करप्रचितिके पादे दश षट् च महर्षिणा।
रसायनानां सिद्धानां संयोगः समुदाहृताः॥६६॥
In this quarter entitled 'Kara Pracitiya', the great sage has described 16 effective recipes for rejuvenation. [66]

इत्यग्निवेशकृते तन्त्रे चरकप्रतिसंस्कृते चिकित्सास्थाने रसायनाध्याये करप्रचितीयो नाम रसायनपादस्तृतीयः॥३॥
Thus ends the third quarter – Kara Prachiteeya Rasayana pada, of the first chapter on rejuvenation therapy in the Chikitsa section of the work of Agnivesha redacted by Master Charaka.

4

Chikitsasthana Chapter 1.4 Ayurveda Samutthaneeya Rasayanam

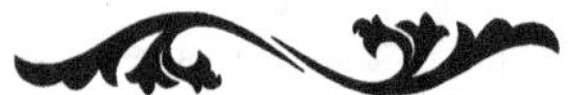

The fourth quarter of 1st chapter of Charaka Chikitsa Sthana deals with the origin of Ayurveda, anti-aging recipes with divine herbs, persons who can undergo rejuvenation (Rasayana) and who cannot, nobility of a doctor etc. This chapter is called Ayurveda Samutthaneeya Rasayana Paada.

Fourth Quarter of the Chapter on Rejuvenation Therapy

अथात आयुर्वेदसमुत्थानीयं रसायनपादं व्याख्यास्यामः॥१॥

इति ह स्माह भगवानात्रेयः॥२॥

Now we shall explore the quarter dealing with "Ayurveda Samutthaneeya – the original propagation of Ayurveda" of the chapter on Rejuvenation therapy. Thus said Lord Atreya [1-2]

Return of Sages to the Himalayas:

ऋषयः खलु कदाचिच्छालीना यायावराश्च ग्राम्यौषध्याहाराः सन्तः साम्पन्निका मन्दचेष्टा नातिकल्याश्च प्रायेण बभूवुः।

ते सर्वासामिति कर्तव्यतानामसमर्थाः सन्तो ग्राम्यवासकृतमात्मदोषं मत्वा पूर्व निवासमपगतग्राम्यदोषं शिवं पुण्यमुदारं मेध्यमगम्यमसुकृतिभिर्गङ्गाप्रभवममरगन्धर्व किन्नरानुचरितमनेक रत्ननिचयमचिन्त्याद्भुतप्रभावं ब्रह्मर्षिशिद्धचारणानुचरितं दिव्यतीर्थौषधि प्रभवमतिशरण्यं हिमवन्तममराधिपतिगुप्तं जग्मुर्भृग्वङ्गिरोऽत्रिवसिष्ठ कश्यपागस्त्य पुलस्त्य वामदेवासित गौतम प्रभृतयो महर्षयः॥३॥

Return of Sages to the Himalayas:

Sages who were formerly either Shalinas (residents of cottages in the woods) or Yayavaras (who moved from one place to the other) resorted to the herbs and diet of the ignorant villagers, as a result of which, they got interested in accumulation of wealth, became lazy, worldly and thus they could not maintain their health in good condition. They were therefore unable to attend to their regular meditation practices properly.

Then they realized the mistake of residing among such ignorant worldly people. Therefore, these great sages viz., Bhrigu, Angiras, Atri, Vasistha, Kashyapa, Agastya, Pulastya, Vamadeva, Asita, Gautama etc, returned to their old abodes in Himalayas which were free from Gramya dosha (unwholesome diet and habits).

Their abodes in the Himalayas were –

Auspicious, virtuous, altruistic

Conducive to the promotion of intellect

Not accessible to sinful persons

Original sources of the Holy Ganga

Inhabited by Amaras (the Gods), Gandharvas (Divine Persons) and Kinnaras

The receptacles of all types of gems

Have unimaginable and wonderful Prabhavas (specific features)
Surrounded by Brahma Rishis (great sages) and Siddhas
Had celestial holy places and herbs
Provided shelter par excellence and Protected by Lord Indra, the king of the Gods. [3]

Discussion with Indra:

तानिन्द्रः सहस्रदृगमरगुरुरब्रवीत्- स्वागतं ब्रह्मविदां ज्ञानतपोधनानां ब्रह्मर्षीणाम्।

अस्ति ननु वो ग्लानिरप्रभावत्वं वैस्वर्य वैवर्ण्य च ग्राम्यवासकृतमसुखमसुखानुबन्धं च; ग्राम्यो हि वासो मूलमशस्तानां, तत् कृतः पुण्यकृद्भिरनुग्रहः प्रजानां, स्वशरीरमवेक्षितुं कालः कालश्चायमायुर्वेदोपदेशस्य ब्रह्मर्षीणाम्; आत्मनः प्रजानां चानुग्रहार्थमायुर्वेदमश्विनौ मह्यं प्रायच्छतां, प्रजापतिरश्विभ्यां, प्रजापतये ब्रह्मा, प्रजानामल्पमायुर्जराव्याधिबहुलमसुखमसुखानुबन्धमल्पत्वादल्पतपोदमनियमदानाध्ययनसञ्चयं मत्वा पुण्यतममायुःप्रकर्षकरं जराव्याधिप्रशमनमूर्जस्करममृतं शिवं शरण्यमुदारं भवन्तो मत्तः श्रोतुमर्हताथोपधारयितुं प्रकाशयितुं च प्रजानुग्रहार्थमार्ष ब्रह्म च प्रति मैत्रीं कारुण्यमात्मनश्चानुत्तमं पुण्यमुदारं ब्राह्ममक्षयं कर्मेति॥४॥

तच्छ्रुत्वा विबुधपतिवचनमृषयः सर्व एवामरवरमृग्भिस्तुष्टुवुः, प्रहृष्टाश्च तद्वचनमभिननन्दुश्चेति॥५॥

Discussion with Indra:

Lord Indra, the one thousand eyed, the preceptor of the Gods, told them, "Welcome to the Divine sages, proficient of the Vedas endowed with the wealth of Knowledge and penance. Because of your association with people with the materialistic way of life, you have lost your strength, energy, voice and complexion as a result of which you are afflicted with ever growing unhappiness.

Association with materialistic people is the root cause of all sufferings. You pious souls have already accomplished the welfare of the people. Now is the time for you to look after your health. It is also the time for the Brahma Rishis (divine sages) to be imparted Ayurvedic instructions.

Origin of Ayurveda:

For the welfare of myself and people, the Ashwinis (twin divine doctors) imported sacred knowledge of Ayurveda from Daksha Prajapati and Prajapati received it from Lord Brahma. Now people have got a shorter span of life; and because of this, they are afflicted with old age, diseases, unhappiness and they have deviated from Tapas (Penance), Dama (control of senses), Niyama (observance of conduct rules), Dana (Charity), as well as Adhyayana (study).

Therefore, I am imparting to you this knowledge of Ayurveda which is

Punyatama (most scared),

Ayuh prakarsha kara (promoter of longevity),

Jara Vyadhi Prashamana (alleviator of old age and diseases),

Urjaskara (promoter of energy),

Amruta (ambrosia), Shiva (Auspicious), Sharanya (protector) and Udara (universal, sympathetic).

You may listen, absorb and propagate this scriptural knowledge for the welfare of the people – the knowledge in the process of successive transmission from Brahma out of friendly deposition and compassion, excellent piety and universal sympathy (Udara). Transmission of this knowledge constitutes a divine and immortal act.

After listening to the king of the Gods (Indra), all the sages offered prayers to him by reciting sacred hymns. The sages, extremely delighted, welcomed his statement. [4-5]

Indrokta Rasayana:

अथेन्द्रस्तदायुर्वेदामृतमृषिभ्यः सङ्क्रम्योवाच- एतत् सर्वमनुष्ठेयम्, अयं च शिवः कालो रसायनानां, दिव्याश्चौषधयो हिमवत्प्रभवः प्राप्तवीर्याः; तद्यथा- ऐन्द्री, ब्राह्मी, पयस्या, क्षीरपुष्पी, श्रावणी, महाश्रावणी, शतावरी, विदारी, जीवन्ती, पुनर्नवा, नागबला, स्थिरा, वचा, छत्रा, अतिच्छत्रा, मेदा, महामेदा, जीवनीयाश्चान्याः पयसा प्रयुक्ताः षण्मासात् परमायुर्वयश्च तरुणमनामयत्वं स्वर वर्ण सम्पदमुपचयं मेधां स्मृतिमुत्तम बलमिष्टांश्चापरान् भावानावहन्ति सिद्धाः॥६॥

(इतीन्द्रोक्तं रसायनम्)।

Thereafter, Indra imparted the knowledge of Ayurveda which is like ambrosia to the sages, "All these instruments should be followed. This is the auspicious time for rejuvenation. All the Divyausadhis (Celestial drugs) which grows in the Himalayas are matured with Veerya (Potency)."

For example,

Aindri – Colocynth – Citrullus colocynthis,

Brahmi – Bacopa monnieri

Payasya – Impomoea paniculata

Ksheerapushpi

Shravani, Maha Shravani(Alambusha) – Sphaeranthus indicus

Shatavari – Asparagus racemosus

Vidari (Ipomoea paniculata / Pueraria tuberosa)

Jivanti – Leptadenia reticulata

Punarnava – Boerhavia diffusa

Nagabala – Grewia populifolia, Sida spinosa, Urena lobata, Grewia hirsuta

Sthira – Shalaparni – Desmodium gangeticum,

Vacha – Acorus calamus

Chatra – Psalliota campestris

Atichatra (Madhurika)

Meda – Polygonatum cirrhifolium

Maha Meda – Polygonatum cirrhifolium and

Such other drugs which are Jeevaniya (promoter of Vitality) should be mixed with milk and taken for six months.

Benefits: The person is endowed with excellent longevity, youth, and freedom from diseases, voice, complexion, nourishment, intellect, memory, strength and such other desirable benefits. These are the drugs with infallible efficacy [6]

Recipe of other Divya Aushadhi – celestial herbs:

ब्रह्म सुवर्चला नामौषधिर्या हिरण्यक्षीरा पुष्कर सदृशपत्रा, आदित्यपर्णी नामौषधिर्या 'सूर्यकान्ता' इति विज्ञायते सुवर्णक्षीरा सूर्यमण्डलाकारपुष्पा च, नारीनामौषधिः 'अश्वबला' इति विज्ञायते या बल्वजसदृशपत्रा, काष्ठगोधा नामौषधिर्गोधाकारा, सर्पानामौषधिः सर्पाकारा, सोमो नामौषधिराजः पञ्चदशपर्वा स सोम इव हीयते वर्धते च, पद्मा नामौषधिः पद्माकारा पद्मरक्ता पद्मगन्धा च, अजा नामौषधिः 'अजशृङ्गी' इति विज्ञायते, नीला नामौषधिस्तु नीलक्षीरा नीलपुष्पा लताप्रतानबहुलेति; आसामोषधीनां यां यामेवोपलभेत तस्यास्तस्याः स्वरसस्य सौहित्यं गत्वा स्नेह भावितायामार्द्रे पलाशद्रोण्यां सपिधानायां दिग्वासाः शयीत, तत्र प्रलीयते, षण्मासेन पुनः सम्भवति, तस्याजं पयः प्रत्यवस्थापनं; षण्मासेन देवतानुकारी भवति वयोवर्ण स्वराकृति बलप्रभाभिः, स्वयं चास्य सर्ववाचोगतानि प्रादुर्भवन्ति, दिव्यं चास्य चक्षुः श्रोत्रं च भवति, गतिर्योजन सहस्रं दशवर्ष सहस्राण्यायुरनुपद्रवं चेति ॥७॥

Recipe of other Divya Aushadhi – celestial herbs:

In addition to the herbs described in the above passage, the following Divya Aushadhis (Celestial drugs) are also used for rejuvenation:

1. Brahma Suvarchala: it has golden coloured latex and its leaves are like those of Puskara.

2. Aditya Parni: it is also called Surya Kanta. It has golden coloured latex and its flowers are round like the sun.

3. Nari: it is known as Ashva Bala. Its leaves are like those of Balvaja.

4. Kasthagodha: It is like Goda (Iguana)

5. Sarpa: It is like a snake.

6. Soma: it is the king of drugs and has fifteen Parnas (leaves). Like the moon, these leaves decrease and increase.

7. Padma: It is like a lotus in shape. It is red like lotus and has the smell of Lotus.

8. Aja: It is known as Aja Shringi.

9. Neela: it has blue latex and their flowers are blue. It is a creeper with several branches.

Procedure:

• All or any of the above-mentioned herbs, depending on their availability, is collected.

• The person is given the juice of these herbs to fill his stomach.

• A Droni (a table specifically designed for the purpose) is prepared of the green wood of Palasha – Butea

monosperma and is smeared with Sneha (ghee or oil)
• The person should remove all his clothes and sleep in this Droni.
• He is then covered with the lid when he becomes unconscious.
• He regains consciousness after six months.
Pathya: The person is fed with goat's milk.
Benefits:
Within six months, He
• Gets youthfulness, complexion
• Good voice, shape, strength and luster like the Gods
• Gains mastery over his speech i.e., what he says comes true
• Is endowed with the divine vision and hearing
• Can walk for one thousand Yojanas
• Lives for ten thousand years free from all obstacles [7]

भवन्ति चात्र

दिव्यानामोषधीनां यः प्रभावः स भवदि्वधैः|
शक्यः सोढुमशक्यस्तु स्यात् सोढुमकृतात्मभिः||८||
ओषधीनां प्रभावेण तिष्ठतां स्वे च कर्मणि|
भवतां निखिलं श्रेयः सर्वमेवोपपत्स्यते||९||
वानप्रस्थैर्गृहस्थैश्च प्रयतैर्नियतात्मभिः|
शक्या ओषधयो ह्येताः सेवितुं विषयाभिजाः||१०||

Who can have the above-mentioned Rasayana:

Thus it is said:

Only the sages like you can withstand the specific action (Prabhava) of the divyausadhis (celestial herbs), described above, and not others who are devoid of self-control.

By the influence of these medicines, you will be able to perform your duties properly and be endowed with all their benefits.

Drugs which grown in sacred places can also be used by person in Vanaprastha Ashrama (the third stage of life in which the person leaves village and town and stays in forests for performance of meditation etc.) and Grahastha Ashrama (the second stage of life in which the person leads family life) provided he is sincere and is endowed with self- control [8-10]

यास्तु क्षेत्रगुणैस्तेषां मध्यमेन च कर्मणा |
मृदुवीर्यतरास्तासां विधिर्ज्ञेयः स एव तु ||११||
पर्येष्टुं ताः प्रयोक्तुं वा येऽसमर्थाः सुखार्थिनः |
रसायन विधिस्तेषामयमन्यः प्रशस्यते ||१२||

Depending upon the attribute of the land (other than the Himalayas) the effect of these drugs become moderate and their Virya (Potency) becomes mild. But they are to be administered, following the same method (as described above). The pleasure- seekers however, will not be able to search for them, for the method of rejuvenation is different which are described below. [11-12]

Indrokta Rasayana – another recipe described by Lord Indra:
बल्यानां जीवनीयानां बृंहणीयाश्च या दश |
वयसः स्थापनानां च खदिरस्यासनस्य च ||१३||
खर्जूराणां मधूकानां मुस्तानामुत्पलस्य च |
मृद्वीकानां विडङ्गानां वचायाश्चित्रकस्य च ||१४||
शतावर्याः पयस्यायाः पिप्पल्या जोङ्गकस्य च |

ऋध्द्या नागबलायाश्च द्वारदाया धवस्य च ||१५||

त्रिफलाकण्टकार्योश्च विदार्याश्चन्दनस्य च |

इक्षूणां शरमूलानां श्रीपर्ण्यास्तिनिशस्य च ||१६||

रसाः पृथक् पृथग्ग्राह्याः पलाशक्षार एव च |

एषां पलोन्मितान् भागान् पयो गव्यं चतुर्गुणम् ||१७||

द्वे पात्रे तिलतैलस्य द्वे च गव्यस्य सर्पिषः |

तत् साध्यं सर्वमेकत्र सुसिद्धं स्नेहमुद्धरेत् ||१८||

तत्रामलक चूर्णानामाढकं शतभावितम् |

स्वरसेनैव दातव्यं क्षौद्रस्याभिनवस्य च ||१९||

शर्कराचूर्णपात्रं च प्रस्थमेकं प्रदापयेत् |

तुगाक्षीर्याः सपिप्पल्याः स्थाप्यं सम्मूर्च्छितं च तत् ||२०||

सुचौक्षे मार्तिके कुम्भे मासार्धं घृतभाविते |

मात्रामग्निसमां तस्य तत ऊर्ध्वं प्रयोजयेत् ||२१||

हेमताम्र प्रवालानामयसः स्फटिकस्य च |

मुक्ता वैदूर्य शङ्खानां चूर्णानां रजतस्य च ||२२||

प्रक्षिप्य षोडशीं मात्रां विहायायासमैथुनम् |

जीर्णे जीर्णे च भुञ्जीत षष्टिकं क्षीरसर्पिषा ||२३||

सर्वरोग प्रशमनं वृष्यमायुष्यमुतमम् |

सत्त्वस्मृति शरीराग्नि बुद्धीन्द्रिय बलप्रदम् ||२४||

परमूर्जस्करं चैव वर्णस्वरकरं तथा |

विषालक्ष्मीप्रशमनं सर्ववाचोगतप्रदम् ||२५||

सिद्धार्थतां चाभिनवं वयश्च प्रजाप्रियत्वं च यशश्च लोके |

प्रयोज्यमिच्छद्भिरिदं यथावद्रसायनं ब्राह्ममुदारवीर्यम् ||२६||

(इतीन्द्रोक्तरसायनमपरम्) |

Indrokta Rasayana – another recipe described by Lord Indra:

48 ml of juice extract of each of the below mentioned herbs is collected.

Ten drugs belonging to each of Balya, Jeevaniya, Brumhaniya and Vayasthapana groups (vide Sutra 4:9, 10 & 18)

Balya Gana – improving strength

Aindri (Citrullus colocynthis),

Rishabhi – Rishabhaka – Manilkara hexandra

Atirasa – Asparagus root – Asparagaus racemosus,

Rishyaprokta – Teramnus labialis,

Payasya – Impomoea paniculata,

Ashwagandha – Winter Cherry / Indian ginseng (root) – Withania somnifera,

Sthira – Desmodium gangeticum,

Katukarohini – Picrorhiza kurroa,

Bala – Country mallow (root) – Sida cordifolia, and

Atibala – Abutilon indicum

Jeevaneeya Gana – – Enlivening, anti aging group of herbs

Jeevaka – Malaxis acuminata

Rishabhaka – Manilkara hexandra

Meda – Polygonatum cirrhifolium

Mahameda – Polygonatum verticillatum

Kakoli – Fritillaria roylei

Kshira Kakoli – Roscoea purpurea / Lilium polyphyllum

Mudgaparni – Phaseolus trilobus,

Mashaparni – Teramnus labialis,
Jivanti – Leptadenia reticulata and
Madhuka– Licorice – Glycyrrhiza glabra
Bruhmaneeya Gana – Nourishing, increasing weight
Ksheerini – Mimusops hexandra Roxb.
Rajakshavaka – Euphorbia microphylla,
Ashwagandha – Winter Cherry / Indian ginseng (root) – Withania somnifera,
Kakoli – Fritillaria roylei,
Ksheerakakoli – Roscoea purpurea / Lilium polyphyllum,
Vatyayani – Country mallow (root) – Sida cordifolia,
Bhadraudani (Sida cordifolia),
Bharadvaji – Thespesia lampas,
Payasya – Impomoea paniculata and
Rushyagandha - Withania coagulans
VayaSthapana -rejuvenating, anti aging.
Amruta (Tinospora cordifolia Miers.),
Abhaya – Terminalia chebula,
Dhatri (Emblica officinalis Gaertn.),
Mukta (pearl),
Shveta (white variety of Clitoria ternatea Linn.),
Jivanti – Leptadenia reticulata,
Atirasa – Asparagus root – Asparagus racemosus,
Mandukaparni (Centella asiatica),
Sthira – Desmodium gangeticum and
Punarnava (Boerhaavia diffusa)
Plus
Khadira – Acacia catechu
Asana – Indian Kino tree (heart wood) – Pterocarpus marsupium,
Kharjura – Dates – Phoenix dactylifera
Madhuka – Licorice – Glycyrrhiza glabra
Musta – Nut grass (root) – Cyperus rotundus,
Mrudveeka – Dry grapes
Vidanga – False black pepper – Embelia ribes,
Vacha – Acorus calamus
Chitraka – Plumbago zeylanica,
Shatavari –Asparagus racemosus
Payasya
Pippali – Long pepper fruit – Piper longum,
Jongaka – Aquilaria agallocha
Aguru – Aquilaria agallocha
Riddhi – Habenaria intermedia
Nagabala –,Grewia hirsuta
Dvarada (Shakataru or Kapi Kacchu),
Dhava – Anogeissus latifolia,
Triphala – Amla, Haritaki, Bibhitaki
Kantakari – Yellow berried nightshade (whole plant) – Solanum xanthcarpum
Vidari – Pueraria tuberosa
Chandana – Santalum album

Ikshu – Saccharum officinarum

Root of Shara – Saccharum munja

promotes natural movement of body fluids,

Shreeparni and

Tinisha – Lagerstroemia speciosa, Ougeinia dalbergioides Benth./ oojeinensis

48 ml of swarasa – juice extract is prepared individually from the above herbs.

48 ml of Palasha Kshar Jala (alkali water of Butea monosperma) is collected.

Cow milk is taken 4 times the cumulative amount of all of the above.

1 Adhaka (3.072 Lit) of sesame oil and cow's ghee each is added and the mixture is boiled together.

After the preparation is fully cooked and all the water content is evaporated, the obtained fat (medicated oil – ghee) is filtered.

Powder of Amalaki – Indian gooseberry fruit – Emblica officinalis – 1 Adhaka (3.072 kg), impregnated with amla juice for 100 times is added to it.

1 Adhaka – Old honey,

1 Adhaka (3.072 Kg) of the powder of Sugar and

1 Prastha (768 g) of Tugaksheeri – Bambusa bambos / Maranta arundinaceae and Pippali – Long pepper fruit – Piper longum are added.

This preparation is stored for 15 days in a clean earthen jar smeared with ghee.

To this, 1/16th in quantity of the powder of

Gold

Copper

Pravala Bhasma – Bhasma (Calx) of Coral,

Iron

Sphatika – Purified and processed Alum (crystal stone),

Pearl

Vaidurya (cat's eye),

Shankha (conch shell) and

Silver is added, mixed well and preserved.

Dosage: According to the power of digestion.

Pathya:

• During this period Aayaasa (exhaustion) and sexual intercourse should be avoided.

• After digestion of this medicine, he should take the Sastika type of rice with milk and ghee.

Benefits:

• Cures all diseases.

• An excellent medicine for virility, longevity and promoter of energy

• Promotes strength, Sattva (mental activities), memory, physique, Agni (power of digestion and metabolism) and Indriya (power of senses)

• It endows the person with good complexion and voice

• It alleviates poisoning or any other morbid condition

• It is conducive to an excellent power of expression

• It helps in the accomplishment of objects

• It restores youth

• It makes one endearing to the people

• It is conducive to the worldly name and fame (even otherwise)

Person desirous of availing themselves of the above mentioned and efficacy of this therapy should use this recipe for rejuvenation according to the prescribed procedure. It is Brahma (celestial) and Udara Virya with potency having no restrictions whatsoever (unlike those mentioned in connection with the prescription in the preceding paragraph) [13-26]

Suitability for rejuvenation therapy:
समर्थानामरोगाणां धीमतां नियतात्मनाम् |
कुटीप्रवेशः क्षणिनां परिच्छदवतां हितः ||२७||
अतोऽन्यथा तु ये तेषां सौर्यमारुतिको विधिः |
तयोः श्रेष्ठतरः पूर्वो विधिः स तु सुदुष्करः ||२८||
Kuti Praveshika type of rejuvenation therapy (vide Charaka Chikitsa 1:1 /17-24 – Wherein person is made to live in a house without being exposed to outside world) is useful for:
Samartha – persons who are able bodied
Aroga – whose bodies are free from diseases
Dheemataam – who are endowed with intellect
Niyata Atmavaan – whose bodies are self- controlled
Kshaninam pariccchadavatam hitah - who have sufficient time to spare and who have adequate wealth.
For others, the Saurya Marutika type (Vatatapika) of rejuvenation therapy, where a person is free to expose himself to the outside world, without being confined to a house, is useful. Between these two, the former is more useful, but it is far too difficult to accomplish.

Management of complications of Rasayana therapy:
रसायन विधिभ्रंशाज्जायेरन् व्याधयो यदि |
यथास्वमौषधं तेषां कार्यं मुक्त्वा रसायनम् ||२९||
If diseases appear due to wrong administration of rejuvenation therapy, then the medicine appropriate to those diseases should be administered leaving aside (at least temporarily) the rejuvenation therapy. [27-29]

Achara Rasayana – rejuvenates, anti-aging:
सत्यवादिनमक्रोधं निवृत्तं मद्यमैथुनात् |
अहिंसकमनायासं प्रशान्तं प्रियवादिनम् ||३०||
जपशौचपरं धीरं दाननित्यं तपस्विनम् |
देव गो ब्राह्मणाचार्य गुरुवृद्धार्चने रतम् ||३१||
आनृशंस्यपरं नित्यं नित्यं करुणवेदिनम् |
समजागरण स्वप्नं नित्यं क्षीरघृताशिनम् ||३२||
देशकाल प्रमाण ज्ञं युक्तिज्ञमनहङ्कृतम् |
शस्ताचारमसङ्कीर्णमध्यात्म प्रवणेन्द्रियम् ||३३||
उपासितारं वृद्धानामास्तिकानां जितात्मनाम् |
धर्मशास्त्रपरं विद्यान्नरं नित्यरसायनम् ||३४||
गुणैरेतैः समुदितैः प्रयुङ्क्ते यो रसायनम् |
रसायनगुणान् सर्वान् यथोक्तान् स समश्नुते ||३५||
(इत्याचाररसायनम्) |
Achara Rasayana – rejuvenation by means of good conduct / Who can get most out of Rasayana therapy:
Person who are
• Satyavadi – truthful
• Akrodha – free from anger
• Nivrutta Madya Maithunaat – devoid of alcohols and sex indulgence
• Ahimsaka - who do not indulge in violence (himsa) or exhaustion
• Anaayaasa – peaceful and pleasing in their speech
• Prashanta – calm
• Priyavaadi – who talk sweetly

• Japa Shaucha para – who do regular Mantra chanting and who are clean
• Dheera – courageous
• Daana nitya – who regularly donate
• Tapasvi – who meditate
• who regularly gives offerings to the Gods, cows , Brahmanas, teachers, preceptors,
• compassionate
• Sama Jaagarana Swapna – whose period of awakening and sleep are regular
• Nitya ksheera ghrutaashee – who habitually take milk and ghee
• Desha Kaala Pramanajna – who are acquainted with the measurement of (things appropriate to) the country and the time
• Yuktijna – who are experts in the knowledge of rationality
• Anahankruta – who are free from ego
• Shastaachaara – whose conduct is good
• Asankeerna – who are not narrow minded
• Adhyaatma – who have love for spiritual knowledge
• Pravanendriya – who have excellent sense organs
• Who have reverence for seniors Astikas (those who believe in the existence of God and validity of the knowledge of the Vedas), and
• Jitaatmana – having self- control and
• Who regularly study scriptures, get the best out of rejuvenation therapy.
Thus the rejuvenation effects of good conduct are described. [30-35]

Ineligible persons for Rasayana

यथास्थूलमनिर्वाह्य दोषाञ्छारीरमानसान् |
रसायन गुणैर्जन्तुर्युज्यते न कदाचन ||३६||
योगा ह्यायुःप्रकर्षार्था जरारोग निबर्हणाः |
मनःशरीरशुद्धानां सिध्यन्ति प्रयतात्मनाम् ||३७||
तदेतन्न भवेद्वाच्यं सर्वमेव हतात्मसु |
अरुजेभ्योऽद्विजातिभ्यः शुश्रूषा येषु नास्ति च ||३८||

In brief, a person, who is not free from the mental and physical defects, does never get the effects of rejuvenation therapy.
The recipes described here promote longevity and prevents old age (early ageing) as well as affliction by diseases.
These recipes produce effects in persons whose mind and body are clean and who are self- controlled.
The physician should never describe or speak anything about these recipes to a person with evil designs, who is not free from diseases, who is not a Dvijati (Brahmana, Ksatriya and Vaisya) and who has no faith in this therapy. [36-38]

Importance of a physician:

ये रसायनसंयोगा वृष्ययोगाश्च ये मताः |
यच्चौषधं विकाराणां सर्वं तद्वैद्यसंश्रयम् ||३९||
प्राणाचार्यं बुधस्तस्मादधीमन्तं वेदपारगम् |
अश्विनाविव देवेन्द्रः पूजयेदतिशक्तितः ||४०||
अश्विनौ देवभिषजौ यज्ञवाहाविति स्मृतौ |
यज्ञस्य हि शिरश्छिन्नं पुनस्ताभ्यां समाहितम् ||४१||
प्रशीर्णा दशनाः पूष्णो नेत्रे नष्टे भगस्य च |
वज्रिणश्च भुजस्तम्भस्ताभ्यामेव चिकित्सितः ||४२||
चिकित्सितश्च शीतांशुर्गृहीतो राजयक्ष्मणा |

सोमाभिपतितश्चन्द्रः कृतस्ताभ्यां पुनः सुखी ||४३||
भार्गवश्च्यवनः कामी वृद्धः सन् विकृतिं गतः |
वीतवर्णस्वरोपेतः कृतस्ताभ्यां पुनर्युवा ||४४||
एतैश्चान्यैश्च बहुभिः कर्मभिरभिषग्वुत्तमौ |
बभूवतुर्भृशं पूज्याविन्द्रादीनां महात्मनाम् ||४५||
ग्रहाः स्तोत्राणि मन्त्राणि तथा नानाहवींषि च |
धूम्राश्च पशवस्ताभ्यां प्रकल्प्यन्ते द्विजातिभिः ||४६||
प्रातश्च सवने सोमं शक्रोऽश्विभ्यां सहाश्नुते |
सौत्रामण्यां च भगवानश्विभ्यां सह मोदते ||४७||
इन्द्राग्नी चाश्विनौ चैव स्तूयन्ते प्रायशो द्विजैः |
स्तूयन्ते वेदवाक्येषु न तथाऽन्या हि देवताः ||४८||
अजरैरमरैस्तावद्दिवबुधैः साधिपैर्ध्रुवैः |
पूज्येते प्रयतैरेवमश्विनौ भिषजाविति ||४९||
मृत्युव्याधिजरावश्यैर्दुःखप्रायैः सुखार्थिभिः |
किं पुनर्भिषजो मर्त्यैः पूज्याः स्युर्नातिशक्तितः||५०||

Recipes for rejuvenation, aphrodisiacs and medicines for the treatment of diseases – all of them are dependent upon the physician. Therefore, a wise person should extend his utmost respectful regards to a Pranacharya (teacher of life science) who is endowed with intellect and the knowledge of the Vedas, as Indra offered prayers to the Ashwinis.

The Ashwinis are the twin physicians of the gods, who share the offerings in the Yajna (sacred oblation to the fire). When the head of Yajna (the name of mythical God) was decapitated, these two physicians connected the head to his body again.

They connected the loose teeth of Pusan (the sun),

They treated the eyes of Bhaga (one of the gods similar to Sun) and stiffness of the arm of Indra.

They treated and cured the moon when he was affected with Rajayakshma (tuberculosis) because of the depletion of his Soma (cooling essence); he was cured by them and was endowed with happiness again.

The sage Chyavana, the Son of Bhrigu, in his old age got afflicted by Kama (sex desire). As a result, he was deprived of his complexion and voice, the Ashwinis made him young again.

Because of these and many other activities, these two supreme divine physicians became objects of frequent prayers by the great souls like Indra etc. for this the Dvijats (Brahmanas, Ksatrias and Vaisyas) prescribe different types of Graha (vessels for taking Soma), Stotra (songs of prayers), Mantra (incantations), havis (oblations to fire) and Dhumra Pashu (brown coloured animals for sacrifice).

If the havana (oblation to fire) is offered in the morning, then the Soma (the juice of some plant), is shared by Shakra (Indra) along with the Asvins. In Sautramani (a type Yajna), the almighty God along with the Ashwinis, rejoice Indra, Agni and the Ashwinis- these are the three gods who are invariably offered prayers by Dvijas.

The Vedic chants are recited as prayers to them. No other God is respected so much.

So even the Gods, who are free from old age and death along with their king, sincerely offer prayers to these twin divine physicians, the Ashwinis, let alone the mortals in the world who are afflicted by miseries because of death, disease and old age, and who seek happiness. The mortals must specially extend their respectful regard to a physician.

Pranacharya – Physician who can save life:

शीलवान्मतिमान् युक्तो द्विजातिः शास्त्रपारगः |
प्राणिभिर्गुरुवत् पूज्यः प्राणाचार्यः स हि स्मृतः ||५१||

The physician who is endowed with good conduct and intellect and who is a Dvijathi (Brahmana, Kshatriya and Vaishya), and who is well versed in scriptures, may be considered as a preceptor and is offered respectful regards by the living beings. This physician is called Pranacharya (teacher of science of life). [39-51]

Definitions of Vaidya and Dvija:

विद्यासमाप्तौ भिषजो द्विवतीया जातिरुच्यते |
अश्नुते वैद्यशब्दं हि न वैद्यः पूर्वजन्मना ||५२||
विद्यासमाप्तौ ब्राह्मं वा सत्त्वमार्षमथापि वा |
ध्रुवमाविशति ज्ञानात्स्मादैद्यो द्विजः स्मृतः ||५३||
नाभिध्यायेन्न चाक्रोशेदहितं न समाचरेत् |
प्राणाचार्य बुधः कश्चिदिच्छन्नायुरनित्वरम् ||५४||

After the completion of the medical education, the physician takes a second birth (jati) and is called "Vaidya". This title is not given to him because of his expertise in the previous birth.

After the completion of the medical education, the physician is certainly endowed with either Brahma sattva (the mental faculty of Brahma) or Rushi Sattva (mental faculty of a Rishi). Therefore, he is called a "Vaidya" and "Dwija".

A person desirous of a happy life should never covet his possessions or show anger to the Pranacharya (a teacher of the science of life) or do any harm to him. [52-54]

चिकित्सितस्तु संश्रुत्य यो वाऽसंश्रुत्य मानवः |
नोपाकरोति वैद्याय नास्ति तस्येह निष्कृतिः ||५५||
भिषगप्यातुरान् सर्वान् स्वसुतानिव यत्नवान् |
आबाधेभ्यो हि संरक्षेदिच्छन् धर्ममनुत्तमम् ||५६||
धर्मार्थं चार्थकामार्थमायुर्वेदो महर्षिभिः |
प्रकाशितो धर्मपरैरिच्छद्भिः स्थानमक्षरम् ||५७||
नार्थार्थं नापि कामार्थमथ भूतदयां प्रति |
वर्तते यश्चिकित्सायां स सर्वमतिवर्तते ||५८||
कुर्वते ये तु वृत्त्यर्थं चिकित्सापण्यविक्रयम् |
ते हित्वा काञ्चनं राशिं पांशुराशिमुपासते ||५९||
दारुणैः कृष्यमाणानां गदैर्वैवस्वतक्षयम् |
छित्वा वैवस्वतान् पाशान् जीवितं यः प्रयच्छति ||६०||
धर्मार्थदाता सदृशस्तस्य नेहोपलभ्यते |
न हि जीवितदानादिध दानमन्यद्विशिष्यते ||६१||
परो भूतदया धर्म इति मत्वा चिकित्सया |
वर्तते यः स सिद्धार्थः सुखमत्यन्तमश्नुते ||६२||

Duties of patient and physician:

A person who has been treated by the physician should reciprocate by helping him (in some way or the other) whether such reciprocation was assumed in advance or not. If he does not do so, he has no redemption.

The physician should treat all his patients like his children. He should take care of their health and keep them away from miseries, if he is desirous of Dharma (Virtues) par excellence.

The great sages devoted to righteousness have propagated Ayurveda with their desire for attainment of Dharma (righteousness), Artha (wealth), Kama (satisfaction of the worldly desires) and Akshara Sthana (salvation).

A person who pursues medical profession just out of compassion for the living being and not for Artha (wealth) or Kama (satisfaction of the worldly desires) excels all others.

A physician, who practices his profession as a commercial commodity for earning wealth, is (as a matter of fact) running after a heap of ash instead of gold.

Patients suffering from serious diseases are dragged towards death by Yama (the God of death). Therefore, in this world, there is none equal to a physician, who can help an individual with both dharma (righteousness) and Artha (wealth). There is no other gift which excels the gift of life.

Compassion for the living creatures is the dharma (righteousness) par excellence. A physician, who enters into medical professions keeping this ideal in view, accomplishes his objects in the best possible way and gets happiness par excellence. [52-62]

Summary:
तत्र श्लोकौ-
आयुर्वेदसमुत्थानं दिव्यौषधिविधिं शुभम्।
अमृताल्पान्तरगुणं सिद्धं रत्नरसायनम्||६३||
सिद्धेभ्यो ब्रह्मचारिभ्यो यदुवाचामरेश्वरः|
आयुर्वेदसमुत्थाने तत् सर्वं सम्प्रकाशितम्||६४|||
In this quarter dealing with "the original propagation of Ayurveda", the following topics have been discussed in detail-
1. The original propagation of Ayurveda.
2. The method of use of celestial drugs which are auspicious
3. The effects of rejuvenation therapy contain gems and jewels which are like ambrosia but slightly less in quality.
4. The conversation of India with the Siddhas (the accomplished sage) and Brahmcharins (those observing celibacy) [63-64]
Colophon:

इत्यग्निवेशकृते तन्त्रे चरकप्रतिसंस्कृते चिकित्सितस्थाने रसायनाध्याये आयुर्वेदसमुत्थानीयो नाम रसायनपादश्चतुर्थः||४||
Thus, ends the fourth quarter of "Ayurveda samutthana" (original propagation of the science of life) of the chapter on Rasayana – rejuvenative; anti-aging (rejuvenation) of Chikitsa Section in Agnivesa's work, as redacted by Charaka.
समाप्तश्चायं रसायनाध्यायः||१||
Thus is the end of the chapter on rejuvenation therapy.

5

Chikitsasthana Chapter 2.1 Samyoga Sharamuliya Vajikaranam

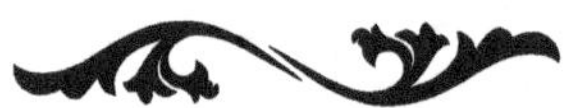

The 2nd chapter of Charak Samhita Chikitsa Sthana deals with Vajikarana – aphrodisiac therapy. It has 4 sub chapters. The first one, which deals with 15 aphrodisiac recipes, is called Samyoga Sharamuliya Vajikaran Pada.

अथातः संयोगशरमूलीयं वाजीकरणपादं व्याख्यास्यामः||१||

इति ह स्माह भगवानात्रेयः||२|||

Now we shall illustrate the quarter dealing with Samyoga sharamoola (recipe prepared by adding the root of Shara – Saccharum munja) of the chapter on aphrodisiacs. Thus said lord Atreya. [1-2]

Objects of Aphrodisiac therapy:

वाजीकरणमन्विच्छेत् पुरुषो नित्यमात्मवान्|

तदायत्तौ हि धर्मार्थौ प्रीतिश्च यश एव च||३||

पुत्रस्यायतनं ह्येतद्गुणाश्चैते सुताश्रयाः|४|

A person, should always seek the intake of aphrodisiacs, for he can earn

Dharma (righteousness),

Artha (wealth),

Preeti (love) and

Yashas (fame) through this therapy alone

A person gets these benefits through his progeny and the aphrodisiac therapy enables him to procreate children (literal meaning sons) [3-4]

The best Aphrodisiac:

वाजीकरणमग्र्यं च क्षेत्रं स्त्री या प्रहर्षिणी||४||

इष्टा ह्योकैकशोऽप्यर्था परं प्रीतिकरा स्मृताः|

किं पुनः स्त्रीशरीरे ये सङ्घातेन प्रतिष्ठिताः||७||

(सङ्घातो ह्येन्द्रियार्थानां स्त्रीषु नान्यत्र विद्यते)|

स्त्र्याश्रयो ह्येन्द्रियार्थ यः स प्रीतिजननोऽधिकम्|

स्त्रीषु प्रीतिर्विशेषेण स्त्रीष्वपत्यं प्रतिष्ठितम्||६||

धर्मार्थौ स्त्रीषु लक्ष्मीश्च स्त्रीषु लोकाः प्रतिष्ठिताः|

सुरूपा यौवनस्था या लक्षणैर्या विभूषिता||७||

या वश्या शिक्षिता या च सा स्त्री वृष्यतमा मता|८|

The best Aphrodisiac:

A sexually excited female partner is the best aphrodisiac. She is the receptacle of the sex act. Each individual item of beauty in a woman gives immense pleasure to an individual. This accounts for her excellence as an aphrodisiac.

All objects of beauty are assembled in a woman in a compact form, nowhere else.

All the objects of senses found in a woman evoke maximum delight in a man. The woman is, therefore, the most lovable for a man.

It is the woman who procreates children.

Dharma (righteousness), Artha (wealth), Lakshmi (auspiciousness) and the entire universe (loka) are established in a woman.

The woman who is

Suroopa – beautiful,

Youvanastha – young,

Lakshanairya Vibhooshita – endowed with auspicious signs

Vashya – who demands to get herself into control,

Shikshita – educated is the best aphrodisiac. [4-8]

Excellence of the Woman:

नानाभक्त्या तु लोकस्य दैवयोगाच्च योषिताम्||८||

तं तं प्राप्य विवर्धन्ते नरं रूपादयो गुणाः|

वयोरूपवचोहावैर्या यस्य परमाङ्गना||९||

प्रविशत्याशु हृदयं दैवाद्वा कर्मणोऽपि वा|

हृदयोत्सवरूपा या या समानमनःशया||१०||

समानसत्वा या वश्या या यस्य प्रीयते प्रियैः|

या पाशभूता सर्वेषामिन्द्रियाणां परैर्गुणैः||११||

यया वियुक्तो निस्त्रीकमरतिर्मन्यते जगत्|

यस्या ऋते शरीरं ना धत्ते शून्यमिवेन्द्रियैः||१२||

शोकोद्वेगारतिभयैर्या दृष्ट्वा नाभिभूयते|

याति यां प्राप्य विस्रम्भं दृष्ट्वा हृष्यत्यतीव याम्||१३||

अपूर्वामिव यां याति नित्यं हर्षातिवेगतः|

गत्वा गत्वाऽपि बहुशो यां तृप्तिं नैव गच्छति||१४||

सा स्त्री वृष्यतमा तस्य नानाभावा हि मानवाः|

Excellence of the Woman:

Women are as respectable as cows and Gods. People in this world have different types of liking as a result of the effects of their actions in the past life.

A person gets a woman of his liking, then his beauty and virtues grow.

By her youthfulness, body, speaking style, and erotic performances, the woman enters into the heart of the person as a result of either Daiva or Karma (effects of the actions in the past life).

She delights the heart; she is like Kama (God of sex); she bears similarity in her mental faculties with those of her husband; she is Vashya (amiable); she is loved by her lover and with her excellent qualities she works like a noose for sense organs.

A man who is deprived of her i.e., who does not have a wife, does not find any interest in this world. Without her, the person holds a body which is emptied of its senses.

In her presence, the person does not get seriously afflicted even when he faces grief, anxiety, detachment and frightful situations. Her very presence and looks are assuring and exciting to him.

He always rushes to her with excitement as if he has gained something unforeseen (pleasant). He is not satiated in spite of his repeated contacts with her. Such a woman is considered to be an aphrodisiac par excellence. Aphrodisiac qualities of a woman differ from one man to the other.

अतुल्यगोत्रां वृष्यां च प्रहृष्टां निरुपद्रवाम्||१५||
शुद्धस्नातां व्रजेन्नारीमपत्यार्थी निरामयः|१६|

How to get a progeny: A person who is healthy and who desires to have a child should enter into sexual intercourse with a woman who is

Atulya gotra (of a different clan)

Vrushya – Sexually strong

Prahrushta – Excited

Nirupadrava – Free from any ailments and

Shuddha snata – after she has taken bath completing her period of menses. [8-16]

In praise of many children:

अच्छायश्चैक शाखश्च निष्फलश्च यथा द्रुमः ||१६||
अनिष्ट गन्धश्चैकश्च निरपत्यस्तथा नरः |
चित्रदीपः सरः शुष्कमधातुर्धातुसन्निभः ||१७||
निष्प्रजस्तृणपूलीति मन्तव्यः पुरुषाकृतिः |
अप्रतिष्ठश्च नग्नश्च शून्यश्चैकेन्द्रियश्च ना ||१८||
मन्तव्यो निष्क्रियश्चैव यस्यापत्यं न विद्यते |
बहुमूर्तिर्बहुमुखो बहुव्यूहो बहुक्रियः ||१९||
बहुचक्षुर्बहु ज्ञानो बह्वात्मा च बहुप्रजः |
मङ्गल्येऽयं प्रशस्योऽयं धन्योऽयं वीर्यवानयम् ||२०||
बहुशाखोऽयमिति च स्तूयते ना बहुप्रजः |

In praise of many children:

A person without a child is like a tree just with one branch devoid of fruits and shadows and with an unwanted smell.

A person who does not have a child is just an idol made of grass wearing the grad of a man.

He is like a lamp in sketches

He is gold without any properties of gold.

A person who does not have a child is

Apratistha (not established)

Nagna (naked)

Shoonya (empty)

Ekendriya (having only one sense organ) and

Nishkriya (devoid of any useful activity)

A person who has many children, is

Bahu murti – having many images,

Bahu Mukha – having many faces,

Bahu Vyooha – having many dimensions;

Bahu Kriya – having multitude of activities,

Bahu chakshu – having many eyes,

Bahu Jnana – having multi-dimensional knowledge and

Bahu Atma – having a multitude of souls.

This type of person is

Auspicious

praise-worthy dhanya (blessed)

Veeryavan (having potency) and

Bahu shakha (having many branches).

Such people are hailed in this world.

Values of children:

प्रीतिर्बलं सुखं वृत्तिर्विस्तारो विपुलं कुलम् ||२१||

यशो लोका: सुखोदर्कास्तुष्टिश्चापत्यसंश्रिताः |

तस्मादपत्यमन्विच्छन् गुणांश्चापत्यसंश्रितान् ||२२||

वाजीकरणनित्यः स्यादिच्छन् कामसुखानि च |

उपभोगसुखान् सिद्धान् वीर्यापत्यविवर्धनान् ||२३||

वाजीकरणसंयोगान् प्रवक्ष्याम्यत उत्तरम् |२४|

Values of children:

Preeti – Love

Bala – Strength

Sukha – Happiness

Vrutti – Professional excellence

Vistara – Widespread influence

Vipula – Greatness

Yasha – success

Fame, utility and purpose in the world

Sukhodarka (which gives happiness at a later stage)

Pleasure – all these are dependent upon children.

Therefore, a person desirous of children and the qualities associated with them should use aphrodisiac therapy daily which bring about sexual delight known for their efficacy and promote semen and help in the procreation of many children. [16-24]

Brumhani Gutika:

शरमूलेक्षुमूलानि काण्डेक्षुः सेक्षुवालिका||२४||

शतावरी पयस्या च विदारी कण्टकारिका|

जीवन्ती जीवको मेदा वीरा चर्षभको बला||२५||

ऋद्धिर्गोक्षुरकं रास्ना सात्मगुप्ता पुनर्नवा|

एषां त्रिपलिकान् भागान् माषाणामाढकं नवम्||२६||

विपाचयेज्जलद्रोणे चतुर्भागं च शेषयेत्|

तत्र पेष्याणि मधुकं द्राक्षा फल्गूनि पिप्पली||२७||

आत्मगुप्ता मधुकानि खर्जूराणि शतावरी|

विदार्यामलकेक्षूणां रसस्य च पृथक् पृथक्||२८||

सर्पिषश्चाढकं दद्यात् क्षीरद्रोणं च तद्विभेषक्|

साधयेद्घृतशेषं च सुपूतं योजयेत् पुनः||२९||

शर्करायास्तुगाक्षीर्याश्चूर्णैः प्रस्थोन्मितैः पृथक्|

पलैश्चतुर्भिर्मागध्याः पलेन मरिचस्य च||३०||

त्वगेलाकेशराणां च चूर्णैरर्धपलोन्मितैः|

मधुनः कुडवाभ्यां च द्वाभ्यां तत्कारयेद्विभेषक्||३१||

पलिका गुलिकास्त्यानास्ता यथाग्नि प्रयोजयेत्|

एष वृष्यः परं योगो बृंहणो बलवर्धनः||३२||

अनेनाश्व इवोदीर्णो बली लिङ्गं समर्पयेत्|३३|

(इति बृंहणीगुटिका)|

3 palas (144 g) of each of the roots of:

shara and Ikshu

Kandekshu (bigger variety of Iksu)

Ikshuvalika

Shatavari – Asparagus racemosus

Payasya (ksheera vidari)

Shara – Saccharum munja

Ikshu – Sugarcane – Saccharum officinarum

Kandekshu – Bigger variety of sugarcane

Shatavari – Asparagus racemosus

Payasya (ksheera vidari) – Ipomoea mauritiana

Vidari – Pueraria tuberosa

Kantakari – Yellow berried nightshade (whole plant) – Solanum xanthcarpum

Jivanti – Leptadenia reticulata

Jivaka – Malaxis acuminata

Meda – Polygonatum cirrhifolium

Ksheerakakoli – Lilium polyphyllu

Rushabhaka – Manilkara hexandra

Bala – Country mallow (root) – Sida cordifolia

Riddhi – Habenaria intermedia

Goksuraka – Tribulus terrestris

Rasna – Alpinia galanga

Atmagupta – Velvet Bean (seed) – Mucuna pruriens and

Punarnava – Spreading Hogweed – Boerhaavia diffusa

1 Adhaka (3.072 Kg) of freshly harvested Masha (black gram) and boiled by adding one drona (12.288 Lit) of water till one- fourth (3.072 liters) remains.

To this, paste of

Madhuka – Licorice – Glycyrrhiza glabra,

Draksha – Raisins – Vitis vinifera

Phalgu – Ficus hispida

Pippali – Long pepper fruit – Piper longum

Atma Gupta – Kapikacchu – Mucuna pruriens

Kharjura – Dates – Phoenix dactylifera

Shatavari– Asparagus racemosus

Vidari – Pueraria tuberosa

Amalaki – Indian gooseberry fruit – Emblica officinalis Gaertn and

The juice of Ikshu (sugarcane) should be added to this.

Ghee should be boiled and filtered

To this ghee – 1 Adhaka – 3.072 Kg

1 Prastha (768 grams) of each of

sharkara – Sugar and

the powder of

Tugaksheeri – Bambusa bambos / Maranta arundinaceae

4 Palas (144 g) of Magadhi – Long pepper fruit – Piper longum

1 Pala (48 g) of Maricha – Black pepper

½ Pala (24 g) each of the powder of

Tvak – Cinnamon,

Ela – Cardamom and

Keshara – Mesua ferrea,

Eranda – Castor

2 Kudavas (192 g) of Honey, should be added

Dosage:

1 Pala (48 g) each semi solid gulikas (big tablet) is prepared.

It is administered in a suitable dose depending on the power of digestion of the person.

Benefits:

This recipe is exceedingly aphrodisiac, nourishing and promoter of strength.

The person gets exceedingly excited as a result of which he acquires stallion like vigor in sexual intercourse. [24-33]

Vajikarana Ghrita:

माषाणामात्मगुप्ताया बीजानामाढकं नवम्||३३||

जीवकर्षभकौ वीरां मेदामृद्धिं शतावरीम्|

मधुकं चाश्वगन्धां च साध्येत् कुडवोन्मिताम्||३४||

रसे तस्मिन् घृतप्रस्थं गव्यं दशगुणं पयः|

विदारीणां रसप्रस्थं प्रस्थमिक्षुरसस्य च||३५||

दत्त्वा मृद्वग्निना साध्यं सिद्धं सर्पिनिधापयेत्|

शर्करायास्तुगाक्षीर्याः क्षौद्रस्य च पृथक् पृथक्||३६||

भागांश्चतुष्पलांस्तत्र पिप्पल्याश्चावपेत् पलम्|

पलं पूर्वमतो लीढ्वा ततोऽन्नमुपयोजयेत्||३७||

य इच्छेदक्षयं शुक्रं शेफसश्चोत्तमं बलम्|३८|

(इति वाजीकरणं घृतम्)|

Vajikarana Ghrita:

Decoction of 1 Adhaka (3.072 kg) each of freshly collected

Masha – Black gram

seed of Atma gupta – Mucuna pruriens

Jivaka – Malaxis acuminata

Rishabhaka – Manilkara hexandra

Veera – Roscoea purpurea Royle / Ipomoea mauritiana Jacq.

Meda – Polygonatum cirrhifolium

Riddhi – Habenaria intermedia

Shatavari – Asparagus racemosus

Madhuka – Liquorice – Glycyrrhiza glabra and

Ashvagandha – Withania somnifera is prepared.

Into this decoction,

1 Prastha (768 ml) of cow's ghee

10 Prastha (768 ml) of milk

1 prastha (768 ml) of the juice of vidari – Ipomoea digitata and

1 prastha (768 ml)of the sugar- cane juice should be added.

Thereafter, this is boiled over mid fire and filtered.

To this prepared ghee,

4 Palas (144 g) of each of sugar, Tugaksheeri – Bambusa bambos / Maranta arundinaceae and honey and

1 Pala (48 g) of Pippali – Long pepper fruit – Piper longum are added.

Dosage: 1 Pala (48 g) of the medicated ghee is to be licked.

Benefits:

It prevents ejaculation of semen and

Provides excellent strength of his genital organ [33-37]

Vajeekaran Pinda Rasa :

शर्करा माष विदलास्तुगाक्षीरी पयो घृतम्||३८||

गोधूमचूर्णषष्ठानि सर्पिष्युत्कारिकां पचेत्|

तां नातिपक्वां मृदितां कौक्कुटे मधुरे रसे||३९||
सुगन्धे प्रक्षिपेदुष्णे यथा सान्द्रीभवेद्रसः|
एष पिण्डरसो वृष्यः पौष्टिको बलवर्धनः||४०||
अनेनाश्व इवोदीर्णो बली लिङ्गं समर्पयेत्|
शिखितित्तिरिहंसानामेवं पिण्डरसो मतः|
बलवर्णस्वरकरः पुमांस्तेन वृषायते||४१||
(इति वाजीकरणपिण्डरसा)|

An utkarika (a type of a preparation like linctus) is prepared by adding six drugs, namely
Sugar
Dehusked grains of Masha – Black gram
Tugaksheeri – Bambusa bambos / Maranta arundinaceae
Milk
Ghee
And the powder of wheat along with ghee.
When it is not fully boiled, it should be removed and squeezed.
To this, the meat soup of kukkuta (chicken soup), which is sweet, fragrant and hot, is added so that the whole thing becomes semi-solid.
This preparation is called "Pinda Rasa.
Benefits:
It promotes virility, nourishment and strength.
By the use of this recipe, a person gets extremely excited, as a result of which, he acquires the stallion like vigor.
In the same way, Pinda rasas can be prepared by
Adding the meat soup of Sikhi (peacock), Tittiri (female partridge) and Hamsa (swan).
Uses:
They promote strength, complexion and voice
Man becomes exceedingly excited [38-41]

Vrishya Mahisha Rasa:
घृतं माषान् सबस्ताण्डान् साधयेन्माहिषे रसे|
भर्जयेत्तं रसं पूतं फलाम्लं नवसर्पिषि||४२||
ईषत्सलवणं युक्तं धान्यजीरकनागरैः|
एष वृष्यश्च बल्यश्च बृंहणश्च रसोत्तमः||४३||
(इति वृष्यमाहिसरसः)|

Vrishya Mahisha Rasa:
Ingredients:
Ghee
Masha (black gram) and
Testicles of goat are boiled with soup of the meat of buffalo.
This is fried in freshly collected ghee, after adding sour fruits.
This recipe is then added with small quantity of
Salt
Dhanyaka – Coriander seed
Jiraka – Cumin – Cuminum cyminum and
Nagara – Ginger Rhizome
Benefits: This is an excellent recipe for the
Promotion of virility
Balya – promotes strength and immunity

Bruhmana – Nourishing [42-43]

Vrushya Rasa :

चटकांस्तितिरिरसे तितिरीन् कौक्कुटे रसे|
कुक्कुटान् बार्हिणरसे हांसे बार्हिणमेव च||४४||
नवसर्पिषि सन्तप्तान् फलाम्लान् कारयेद्रसान्|
मधुरान् वा यथासात्म्यं गन्धाढ्यान् बलवर्धनान्||४५||
(इत्यन्ये वृष्यरसाः)|

Vrushya Rasa :
In the freshly collected ghee, the following ingredients should be added:-
Chataka (sparrow) along with the soup of the meat of Tittiri (Female partridge)
Tittiri (female partridge) along with the soup of meat of Kukkuta (sparrow)
Kukkuta along with the soup of meat of Barhina (peacock)
Barhi (peacock) along with the soup of meat of Hamsa (swan)
After these are boiled, the juice of sweet or sour fruits is added and depending upon the liking of the person, fragrant ingredients are also added.
Benefits: Promotes strength. [44-45]

Vrusya Mamsa:

तृप्तिं चटकमांसानां गत्वा योऽनुपिबेत् पयः|
न तस्य लिङ्गशैथिल्यं स्यान्न शुक्रक्षयो निशि ||४६||
(इति वृष्यमांसम्) |

Vrusya Mamsa:
If a person takes the meat of Chataka (sparrow) to his satisfaction, and thereafter takes milk,
Benefits:
His genital organ will become sturdy, and
There will be no ejaculation of semen even if he indulges in sexual intercourse for the whole night. [46]

Vrushya Masha yoga:

माषयूषेण यो भुक्त्वा घृताढ्यं षष्टिकौदनम्|
पयः पिबति रात्रिं स कृत्स्नां जागर्ति वेगवान्||४७||
(इति वृष्यमाषयोगः)|

Ingredients : Rice of Shastika along with the soup of Masha (black gram), added with liberal quantity of ghee, and takes milk.
Benefit: Remains awake for the whole night with urge for sexual intercourse [47]

Vrushya Kukkuta Mamsa Prayoga:

न ना स्वपिति रात्रिषु नित्यस्तब्धेन शेफसा|
तृप्तः कुक्कुटमांसाना भृष्टानां नक्ररेतसि||४८||
(इति वृष्यः कुक्कुटमांसप्रयोगः)|

Ingredient: If a man eats the meat of Kukkuta (cock), fried with the semen of nakra (Crocodile) to his satisfaction
Uses: He does not sleep at night because of the strong erection of his genital organ. [48]

Vrushya Anda Rasa:

निःस्राव्य मत्स्याण्डरसं भृष्टं सर्पिषि भक्षयेत्|
हंसबर्हिण दक्षाणामेवमण्डानि भक्षयेत्||४९||

(इति वृष्योऽण्डरसः)|

Recipe: A person takes the extract of the eggs of fish, fried with ghee.

Similarly, the eggs of Hamsa (swan), Barhina (Peacock) and Daksha are described to be taken separately. But this is treated as only one recipe.

This makes 15 aphrodisiac recipes in total, which will be described in verse no 53. [49]

Importance of Panchakarma ahead of Aphrodisiac therapy:

भवतश्चात्र-

स्रोतःसु शुद्धेष्वमले शरीरे वृष्यं यदा ना मितमत्ति काले|

वृषायते तेन परं मनुष्यस्तद्बृंहणं चैव बलप्रदं च||५०||

तस्मात् पुरा शोधनमेव कार्यं बलानुरूपं न हि वृष्ययोगाः|

सिध्यन्ति देहे मलिने प्रयुक्ताः क्लिष्टे यथा वाससि रागयोगाः||५१||

Importance of Panchakarma ahead of Aphrodisiac therapy:

Thus it is said

If a person takes aphrodisiac recipes in appropriate quantity and in proper time, when the channels of circulation of his body are clean (by means of Panchakarma treatment), then they help in the promotion of virility, nourishment and strength.

Therefore, depending on the strength of the person, cleansing Panchakarma therapies should be administered to him, before he resorts to these aphrodisiac recipes.

As a dirty cloth does not get properly coloured similarly in an unlearned body, the aphrodisiac recipes do not produce the desired effects. [50-51]

तत्र श्लोकौ-

वाजीकरण सामर्थ्यं क्षेत्रं स्त्री यस्य चैव या|

ये दोषा निरपत्यानां गुणाः पुत्रवतां च ये||५२||

दश पञ्च च संयोगा वीर्यापत्यविवर्धनाः|

उक्तास्ते शरमूलीये पादे पुष्टिबलप्रदाः||५३||

Summary:

In this quarter on SaraMuliya, the following topics have been discussed:-

1. The utility of aphrodisiac therapies

2. The woman as the receptacle

3. The suitability of a woman for a particular man

4. Doshas (faults) of persons who are childless

5. The utility of persons having many children and

6. 15 recipes for increasing semen and children and promotion of nourishment as well as strength. [52-53]

इत्यग्निवेशकृते तन्त्रे चरकप्रतिसंस्कृते चिकित्सास्थाने वाजीकरणाध्याये संयोगशरमूलीयो नाम वाजीकरणपादः प्रथमः||१||

Thus, ends the first quarter on Samyoga Sharamula (recipe prepared by adding the root of Sara) of the chapter on aphrodisiacs of the Chikitsa section of Agnivesha's work, as redacted by Charak.

6

Chikitsasthana Chapter 2.2 Asikta Kshiriya Vajikaranam

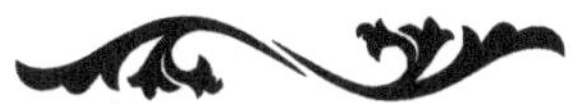

The second section of Charaka's chapter on aphrodisiac therapy deals with eight recipes for infertility and sexual disorders. Rice is used as the main content in many of them. This is the second section of the second chapter of Charaka Samhita Sutrasthana – Called Asikta Ksheerika Vajikarana Paada.

Chapter 2.2

Second Quarter of the Chapter on Aphrodisiacs

वाजीकरणाध्यये द्विवतीय पादः ।

अथात आसिक्तक्षीरिकं वाजीकरणपादं व्याख्यास्यामः||१||

इति ह स्माह भगवानात्रेयः||२||

We shall now illustrate the quarter on "Asikta Ksheerika" (herbs impregnated with milk) of the chapter on aphrodisiacs.

Thus said lord Atreya [1-2]

Apatyakari Shashtikadi Gutika:

आसिक्त क्षीरमापूर्णमशुष्कं शुद्ध षष्टिकम्|

उदूखले समापोथ्य पीडयेत् क्षीरमर्दितम्||३||

गृहीत्वा तं रसं पूतं गव्येन पयसा सह|

बीजानामात्मगुप्ताया धान्य माष रसेन च||४||

बलायाः शूर्पपर्ण्योश्च जीवन्त्या जीवकस्य च |

ऋद्ध्यर्षभक काकोली श्वदंष्ट्रा मधुकस्य च||५||

शतावर्या विदार्याश्च द्राक्षा खर्जूरयोरपि|

संयुक्तं मात्रया वैद्यः साधयेत्तत्र चावपेत्||६||

तुगाक्षीर्याः समाषाणां शालीनां षष्टिकस्य च|

गोधूमानां च चूर्णानि यैः स सान्द्रीभवेद्रसः||७||

सान्द्रीभूतं च कुर्यात् प्रभूत मधु शर्करम्|

गुलि(टि)का बदरैस्तुल्यास्ताश्च सर्पिषि भर्जयेत्||८||

ता यथाग्नि प्रयुञ्जानः क्षीरमांसरसाशनः|

पश्यत्यपत्यं विपुलं वृद्धोऽप्यात्मजमक्षयम्||९||

(इत्यपत्यकरी षष्टिकादिगुटिका)|

Apatyakari (male fertility promoting) Shashtikadi Gutika:

The Shashtika rice (white coloured) is first cleaned.

The rice grains are impregnated with milk by filling the rice vessel with milk.

When these grains are still wet, they are crushed in pestle and mortar.

Then it is ground with milk, and sought in a piece of cloth, the paste is squeezed to collect its juice.

To this juice, cow milk and the juice of the seeds of

Atmagupta – Velvet Bean (seed) – Mucuna pruriens

Dhanya – Coriander and

Masha – Black gram is added and boiled.

While boiling, the decoctions of

Bala – Country mallow (root) – Sida cordifolia,

Surpaparni

Jivanti – Leptadenia reticulata

Jivaka – Malaxis acuminata

Riddhi

Rishabhaka – Manilkara hexandra

Kakoli – Fritillaria roylei

Shvadamstra – Tribulus terrestris

Madhuka – Licorice – Glycyrrhiza glabra,

Shatavari – Asparagus racemosus

Vidari – Pueraria tuberosa

Draksha – Raisins – Vitis vinifera and

Kharjura – Dates – Phoenix dactylifera is added.

At the end of the boiling, the powders of

Tugaksheeri – Bambusa bambos / Maranta arundinaceae

Masha – Black gram

Shali Shashtika – rice

Godhuma – Wheat are added so that the whole recipe becomes semi- solid.

When it becomes semi-solid, honey and sugar is added in adequate quantity, and pills are prepared with ghee.

Dosage: Depending upon the power of digestion of the individual, these and the soup of the meat are to be taken.

Benefits: By taking this potion, even an old man becomes capable of procreating many children and he does not get exhausted during sexual intercourse. [3-9]

Vrushya Pupalikadi Yoga:
चटकानां सहंसानां दक्षाणां शिखिनां तथा|
शिशुमारस्य नक्रस्य भिषक् शुक्राणि संहरेत्||१०||
गव्यं सर्पिर्वराहस्य कुलिङ्गस्य वसामपि|
षष्टिकानां च चूर्णानि चूर्णं गोधूमकस्य च||११||
एभिः पूपलिकाः कार्याः शष्कुल्यो वर्तिकास्तथा|
पूपा धानाश्च विविधा भक्ष्याश्चान्ये पृथग्विधाः||१२||
एषां प्रयोगाद्भक्ष्याणां स्तब्धेनापूर्णरेतसा|
शेफसा वाजिवद्याति यावदिच्छं स्त्रियो नरः||१३||
(इति वृष्यपूपलिकादियोगाः) |
Vrushya Pupalikadi Yoga: Aphrodisiac sweet cake:
The physician should collect the semen of

Chataka – Sparrow

Daksha

Shikhi – peacock

Shishumaara – Alligator, Gangetic porpoise, dolphin

Nakra – Crocodile.

He should also take the

Vasa (Fat) of Kulinga – A variety of mouse / Fork-tailed Shrike and

The powders of Shashtika rice, as well as Godhuma (wheat).

Out of these ingredients,

Pupalika (sweet cake)

Shashkula (Chakkuli – spiral shaped dish)

Vartika – (Kodu bale – round shaped dish)

Pupa – Cake

Dhana and such other varieties of dishes are prepared.

Benefits:

A man becomes fully potent, and

With strongly erected genital organ enjoys optimum sexual delight in women with good vigour. [10-13]

Apatyakara svarasa:

आत्मगुप्ताफलं माषान् खर्जूराणि शतावरीम्।

शृङ्गाटकानि मृद्वीकां साधयेत् प्रसृतोन्मितम्॥१४॥

क्षीरप्रस्थं जलप्रस्थमेतत् प्रस्थावशेषितम्।

शुद्धेन वाससा पूतं योजयेत् प्रसृतैस्त्रिभिः॥१५॥

शर्करायास्तुगाक्षीर्याः सर्पिषोऽभिनवस्य च।

तत् पाययेत सक्षौद्रं षष्टिकान्नं च भोजयेत्॥१६॥

जरापरीतोऽप्यबलो योगेनानेन विन्दति।

नरोऽपत्यं सुविपुलं युवेव च स हृष्यति॥१७॥

(इत्यपत्यकरः स्वरसः)।

Apatyakara svarasa – Fertility promoting juice extract:

The fruit of

Atmagupta – Velvet Bean (seed) – Mucuna pruriens,

Masha – Black gram

Kharjura – Dates – Phoenix dactylifera ,

Shatavari – Asparagus racemosus

Shringataka – Trapa bispinosa

and

Mrudvika – raisins are taken in the quantity of 1 Prasruta – 8 Tola = 96 ml.

1 Prastha (768 ml) of milk and water is added and to this,

3 Prasthas (2.304 kg) of Sharkara (sugar) and Tugaksheeri (Bambusa bambos) and freshly collected ghee are added.

Dosage: This is given to the person along with honey.

Pathya: He is given Shashtika type of rice to eat.

Benefits: Even an old and a weak person becomes capable of procreating many children and gets excited like a young man. [14-17]

Vrusya Ksheera: Aphrodisiac milk

खर्जूरीमस्तकं माषान् पयस्यां च शतावरीम्।

खर्जूराणि मधूकानि मृद्वीकामजडाफलम्॥१८॥

पलोन्मितानि मतिमान् साधयेत् सलिलाढके।

तेन पादावशेषेण क्षीरप्रस्थं विपाचयेत्॥१९॥

क्षीरशेषेण तेनाद्याद् घृताढ्यं षष्टिकौदनम्।

सशर्करेण संयोग एष वृष्यः परं स्मृतः॥२०॥

(इति वृष्यक्षीरम्) |
Vrusya Ksheera: Aphrodisiac milk
1 pala (48 g) each of these fruits:
Kharjuri Mastaka (top portion of dates tree),
Masha – Black gram
Payasya – Ipomoea paniculata,
Shatavari – Asparagus racemosus
Kharjura – Phoenix sylvestris – Dates
Madhuka– Licorice – Glycyrrhiza glabra,
Mrudvika – Raisins and
Boiled with 1 Adhaka (3.072 liters) of water till 1/4th remains.
To this decoction, 1 Prastha (768 ml) of milk is added and boiled till only milk remains.
To this, sugar should be added.
Pathya: Shashtika type of rice along with liberal quantity of ghee.
Uses: This is an excellent aphrodisiac. [18-20]

Vrushya Ghrita: Aphrodisiac ghee:
जीवकर्षभकौ मेदां जीवन्तीं श्रावणीद्वयम्|
खर्जूरं मधुकं द्राक्षां पिप्पलीं विश्वभेषजम्||२१||
शृङ्गाटकं विदारीं च नवं सर्पिः पयो जलम्|
सिद्धं घृतावशेषं तच्छर्कराक्षौद्र पादिकम्||२२||
षष्टिकान्नेन संयुक्तमुपयोज्यं यथाबलम्|
वृष्यं बल्यं च वर्ण्यं च कण्ठ्यं बृंहणमुत्तमम्||२३||
(इति वृष्यघृतम्) |
Vrushya Ghrita: Aphrodisiac ghee:
Jivaka
Rishabhaka
Meda
Jivanti – Leptadenia reticulata
both the type of Sravani
Kharjura – Phoenix sylvestris
Madhuka – Liquorice
Draksha – Raisin – Vitis vinifera,
Pippali – Long pepper fruit – Piper longum,
Vishvabhesaja – Ginger
Shringataka – Trapa bispinosa
Vidari Pueraria tuberosa),
Freshly collected ghee, milk and water should be boiled together till ghee remains.
To this, 1/4th quantity of sugar and honey should be added.
Dosage: Depending upon the strength of the man
Pathya: Shashtika type of rice.
Benefit: This is an excellent recipe to promote virility, strength, complexion, Kanta (voice) and nourishment [21-23]

Vrusya Dadhisara: Aphrodisiac curd recipe
दध्नः सरं शरच्चन्द्रसन्निभं दोषवर्जितम्|
शर्करा क्षौद्र मरिचैस्तुगाक्षीर्या च बुद्धिमान्||२४||
युक्त्या युक्तं ससूक्ष्मैलं नवे कुम्भे शुचौ पटे|

मार्जितं प्रक्षिपेच्छीते घृताढ्ये षष्टिकौदने॥२५॥
पिबेन्मात्रां रसालायास्तं भुक्त्वा षष्टिकौदनम् ।
वर्णस्वरबलोपेतः पुमांस्तेन वृषायते॥२६॥
(वृष्यो दधिसरप्रयोगः)।

Vrusya Dadhisara: Aphrodisiac curd recipe
The cream of curd which is like the moon of autumn and is free from impurities is added with
Sugar
honey
Maricha – Black pepper fruit – Piper nigrum and
Tugaksiri – Bambusa bambos / Maranta arundinaceae
by a wise physician.
To this Sukshma Ela (lesser cardamom) is added in appropriate quantities.
This is properly mixed in a fresh earthen jar or clean rice mixed with liberal quantity of ghee.
Dosage and Pathya: This Rasala is taken in appropriate quantity, and thereafter, the person should eat Sastika type of rice.
Benefits: it promotes the complexion, voice, strength and Virility of the man. [24-26]

Vrushya shashtikaudana: Aphrodisiac rice dish:
चन्द्रांशुकल्पं पयसा घृताढ्यं षष्टिकौदनम् ।
शर्करामधुसंयुक्तं प्रयुञ्जानो वृषायते॥२७॥
(इति वृष्यः षष्टिकौदनप्रयोगः)।
Vrushya shashtikaudana: Aprhodisiac rice dish:
By taking the rise of Shashtika which is white like the rays of moon, along with ghee in liberal quantity, sugar and honey, a man become sexually excited. [27]

Vurshya Pupalika:
तप्ते सर्पिषि नक्राण्डं ताम्रचूडाण्डमिश्रितम् ।
युक्तं षष्टिकचूर्णेन सर्पिषाऽभिनवेन च॥२८॥
पक्त्वा पूपलिकाः खादेद्वारुणीमण्डपो नरः।
य इच्छेदश्ववद्गन्तुं प्रसेक्तुं गजवच्च यः॥२९॥
(इति वृष्यपूपलिकाः)।
Vurshya Pupalika: Aphrodisiac cake:
The eggs of Nakra – Crocodile and Tamrachuda – Cock, are fried in ghee.
The powder of Shashtika is added and is boiled in ghee.
Out of this, Pupalikas (cake) should be prepared.
After eating these Pupalikas, the man should drink the Manda (scum or the upper portion) of Varuni (wine), if he wants to indulge in it with the vigour of an elephant. [28-29]

भवतश्चात्र-
एतैः प्रयोगैर्विधिवद्वपुष्मान् वीर्योपपन्नो बलवर्णयुक्तः।
हर्षान्वितो वाजिवदष्टवर्षो भवेत् समर्थश्च वराङ्गनासु॥३०॥
यद्यच्च किञ्चिन्मनसः प्रियं स्याद्रम्या वनान्ताः पुलिनानि शैलाः।
इष्टाः स्त्रियो भूषणगन्धमाल्यं प्रिया वयस्याश्च तदत्र योग्यम् ॥३१॥
Thus it is said:-
By the use of these recipes, according to the prescribed procedure,
The man is endowed with an adequate quantity of semen, strength and complexion.

With excitement and stallion vigour, he becomes capable of sexual intercourse with beautiful women for eight years. The parks in the fringe of the forest, ponds, mountains, pleasing women, ornaments, scents, garlands, friendly companions and such other things which are liked by the man, should be provided for getting the prescribed effects of these rejuvenating recipes. [30-31]

Summary:
A person who is desirous of manliness (adequate quantity of semen) and children should use these eight recipes described in the quarter called "Asikta Ksirika" [32]

तत्र श्लोकः-
आसिक्तक्षीरिके पादे ये योगाः परिकीर्तिताः|
अष्टावपत्यकामैस्ते प्रयोज्याः पौरुषार्थिभिः||३२||
The Yogas explained in this chapter are useful for people seeking conception and maleness.

इत्यग्निवेशकृते तन्त्रे चरकप्रतिसंस्कृते चिकित्सास्थाने वाजीकरणाध्याये आसिक्तक्षीरिको नाम वाजीकरणपादो द्वितीयः||२||
Thus, ends the second quarter on "Asika Ksheerika" (drugs impregnated with milk) of the chapter on aphrodisiacs of Chikitsa section of Agnivesa's work, as redacted by Charaka.

7

Chikitsasthana Chapter 2.3
Mashaparna Bhrutiyam

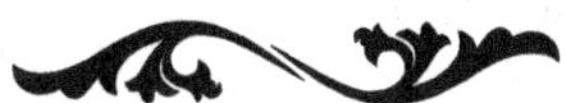

The third quarter of Charaka's chapter on sexual health deals with factors that lead to excitation, many aphrodisiac recipes with milk, liquorice, ghee, and honey and sex vigour promoting articles based on season etc. This quarter is called Mashaparna Bhrutiya Adhyaya.

Charaka Chikitsa Sthana – Chapter 2.3

Third Quarter of the Chapter on Aphrodisiacs

अथातो माषपर्णभृतीयं वाजीकरणपादं व्यख्यास्यामः||१||

इति ह स्माह भगवानात्रेयः||२||

Now, we shall explore the quarter on "Mashaparna Bhrtiya" (dealing with recipes prepared of the milk of a cow fed with the leaves of Masha – Black gram, etc) of the chapter on aphrodisiacs.

Thus said lord Atreya. [1-2]

Cow milk Aphrodisiac recipe:

माषपर्णभृतां धेनुं गृष्टिं पुष्टां चतुःस्तनीम् |

समानवर्णवत्सां च जीवद्वत्सां च बुद्धिमान् ||३||

रोहिणीमथवा कृष्णामूर्ध्वशृङ्गीमदारुणाम् |

इक्ष्वादामर्जुनादां वा सान्द्रक्षीरां च धारयेत् ||४||

केवलं तु पयस्तस्याः शृतं वाऽशृतमेव वा |

शर्कराक्षौद्रसर्पिभिर्युक्तं तद्वृष्यमुत्तमम् ||५||

Cow milk recipe for sexual strength:

Milk should be collected from a cow who is fed with the

Leaves of Masha – Black gram

Stalks of sugarcane or Leaves of Arjuna (terminalia arjuna)

The cow should be delivered only once,

Is well-nourished

Has 4 nipples in her udder

Has a calf having identical colour

Whose calf is alive

Who is red or black in colour

Whose horns are projected upwards

Who is not ferocious and

Whose milk is thick.

Dosage: Such a cow's milk can be taken after boiling or even without it by adding sugar, honey and ghee.

This is an excellent diet to promote virility – Vrushyam – Uttamam. [3-5]
Milk recipe to improve semen and sperm – Shukrala

शुक्रलैर्जीवनीयैश्च बृंहणैर्बलवर्धनैः।
क्षीरसञ्जननैश्चैव पयः सिद्धं पृथक् पृथक्||६||
युक्तं गोधूमचूर्णेन सघृतक्षौद्र शर्करम्।
पर्यायेण प्रयोक्तव्यमिच्छता शुक्रमक्षयम्||७||

Milk recipe to improve semen and sperm – Shukrala
Milk boiled with herbs belonging to Shukrajanana (sperm production promoting), Jeevaniya (enlivening), Brumhana (nourishing) and Stanya Janana (lactation promoting) – these groups should be administered separately.
Shukrala Shukrajanana -improving quality of semen and ovum
Jeevaka
Rishabhaka
Kakoli – Fritillaria roylei
Kshira Kakoli – Lilium polyphyllum
Mudgaparni - Phaseolus trilobus
Mashaparni – Teramnus labialis,
Meda
Vriddharuha
Jatila (Nardostachys jatamansi DC.)
Kulinga
Jeevaneeya Gana – Enlivening, anti-aging group of herbs
Jeevaka
Rishabhaka
Meda
Mahameda
Kakoli – Fritillaria roylei
Kshira Kakoli – Lilium polyphyllum
Mudgaparni – Phaseolus trilobus,
Mashaparni – Teramnus labialis,
Jivanti – Leptadenia reticulata and
Madhuka– Licorice – Glycyrrhiza glabra
Bruhmaneeya Gana – Nourishing, increasing weight
Ksheerini
Rajakshavaka – Euphorbia microphylla,
Ashwagandha – Winter Cherry / Indian ginseng (root) – Withania somnifera,
Kakoli – Fritillaria roylei,
Ksheerakakoli Lilium polyphyllum,
Vatyayani – Country mallow (root) – Sida cordifolia,
Bhadraudani
Bharadvaji
Payasya – Impomoea paniculata and
Rushyagandha
Bala Vardhana – Balya Gana – improving strength
Aindri
Rishabhi – Rishabhaka
Atirasa – Asparagus root – Asparagaus racemosus,
Rishyaprokta

Payasya – Impomoea paniculata,
Ashwagandha – Winter Cherry / Indian ginseng (root) – Withania somnifera,
Sthira – Desmodium gangeticum,
Katukarohini – Picrorhiza kurroa,
Bala – Country mallow (root) – Sida cordifolia, and
Atibala – Abutilon indicum
Ksheera Samjanana – Stanyajanana – improving breast milk
Virana - Vetiveria zizanioides
Shali – Rice (Oryza sativa Linn.),
Shastika (a variety of rice – Oryza sativa Linn.),
Ikhsuvalika
Darbha
Kusha
Kasha (Saccharum spontaneum Linn.),
Gundra
Itkata – and
Katruna
Before administration of such processed milk with any of above-group of herbs, heat flour, ghee, honey and sugar are added.
These 5 recipes are administered separately to a person who is desirous of inexhaustible semen. [6-7]

Sex power improving Ayurvedic recipe:
मेदां पयस्यां जीवन्तीं विदारीं कण्टकारिकाम्|
श्वदंष्ट्रां क्षीरिकां माषान् गोधूमाञ्छालिषष्टिकान्||८||
पयस्यर्धोदके पक्त्वा कार्षिकानाढकोन्मिते|
विवर्जयेत् पयःशेषं तत् पूतं क्षौद्रसर्पिषा||९||
युक्तं सशर्करं पीत्वा वृद्धः सप्ततिकोऽपि वा|
विपुलं लभतेऽपत्यं युवेव च स हृष्यति||१०||
Sex power improving Ayurvedic recipe:
1 Karsha – 12 g of
Meda
Payasya – Impomoea paniculata
Jivanti - Leptadenia reticulata
Vidari (Pueraria tuberosa)
Kantakarika – Solanum xanthocarpum
Svadamshtra – Gokshura – Tribulus terrestris
Ksheerika
Masha – Black gram
Godhuma – wheat – Triticum sativum,
Shali Shastika – Rice – are boiled in
1 Adhaka – 3.072 litre of milk and
1/2 Adhaka – 1.536 litres of water.
After boiling, 1 Adhaka – 3.072 litre of liquid should remain.
This is filtered and the liquid is added with honey, ghee and sugar.
Uses: By taking this medicated milk, even an old man and a person who is 70 years old, gets large number of children and in sex acts he gets sex vigour like that of a young person. [8-10]

Sex recipe with milk ghee and honey:
मण्डलैर्जातरूपस्य तस्या एव पयः शृतम्|
अपत्यजननं सिद्धं सघृतक्षौद्रशर्करम्||११||
Milk of a cow, whose skin has been marked by a heated ring of gold, is boiled and added with ghee, honey and sugar.
Benefits: It is an effective recipe for procreation of children. [11]

Vrushya Pippali: – Aphrodisiac remedy using long pepper fruit:
त्रिंशत् सुपिष्टाः पिप्पल्यः प्रकुञ्चे तैलसर्पिषोः|
भृष्टाः सशर्कराक्षौद्राः क्षीरधारावदोहिताः||१२||
पीत्वा यथाबलं चोर्ध्वं षष्टिकं क्षीरसर्पिषा|
भुक्त्वा न रात्रिमस्तब्धं लिङ्गं पश्यति ना क्षरत्||१३||
(इति वृष्यः पिप्पलीयोगः)|
Vrushya Pippali: – Aphrodisiac remedy using long pepper fruit:
30 Pippali fruits are made into a fine paste and fried with 1 Prakuncha (Pala = 48 ml) of oil and ghee.
This is added with sugar and honey and to this; milk is poured directly from the nipple of the cow.
Dosage: according to the strength of the individual
Pathya: By taking Sastika rice along with the milk and ghee
Benefits:
The genital organ of the man remains strongly erected all through the night and it does not become laxed even after ejaculation of semen. [12-13]

Vrushya Payasa – Aphrodisiac kheer – sweet soup:
श्वदंष्ट्राया विदार्याश्च रसे क्षीरचतुर्गुणे|
घृताढ्यः साधितो वृष्यो माष षष्टिक पायसः||१४||
(इति वृष्यपायसयोगः)|
To the juice (decoction) of
Svadamshtra – Tribulus terrestris and
Vidari (Ipomoea paniculata / Pueraria tuberosa) 4 times of milk is added.
To this, ghee is added in liberal quantity and boiled by adding
Masha – Black gram and Shashtika – Rice.
Benefits: This payasa (a type of milk preparation) promotes virility. [14]

Vrushya Pupalika:
फलानां जीवनीयानां स्निग्धानां रुचिकारिणाम्|
कुडवश्चूर्णितानां स्यात् स्वयंगुप्ताफलस्य च||१५||
कुडवश्चैव माषाणां द्वौ द्वौ च तिलमुद्गयोः|
गोधूमशालिचूर्णानां कुडवः कुडवो भवेत्||१६||
सर्पिषः कुडवश्चैकस्तत् सर्वं क्षीरमर्दितम्|
पक्त्वा पूपलिकाः खादेद्बह्व्यः स्युर्यस्य योषितः||१७||
(इति वृष्यपूपलिकाः)|
The powder of fruits which are
Jivaniya (Promoters of longevity), Snigdha (Snehopaga) and Ruchikara (Ruchya) are taken
1 Kudava – 192 g of each of the powders of the fruits
Svayamgupta – Mucuna pruriens and
Masha – Black gram and
2 Kudavas each of

Tila – Sesame (Sesamum indicum) and
Mudga – Green gram
1 Kudava – 192 g of each of the powder of
Godhuma – wheat and
Shali – Rice, and
1 Kudava – 192 g of ghee is added.
All these powders are kneaded by adding milk.
By boiling this dough, Pupalikas are prepared.
These Pupalikas are taken by a person who has many wives. [15-17]

Vrushya Shatavari Ghrita:
घृतं शतावरी गर्भं क्षीरे दशगुणे पचेत्|
शर्करा पिप्पली क्षौद्र युक्तं तद्वृष्यमुत्तमम्||१८||
(इति वृष्यं शतावरीघृतम्)|
Ingredients and Procedure:
Ghee boiled with Shatavari
10 times of milk along with
Sugar,
Pippali – Long pepper fruit – Piper longum and
Honey
Benefit: makes an excellent aphrodisiac recipe. [18]

Vrushya Madhuka Yoga – Licorice recipe:
कर्ष मधुक चूर्णस्य घृत क्षौद्र समांशिकम् |
प्रयुङ्क्ते यः पयश्चानु नित्यवेगः स ना भवेत्||१९||
(इति वृष्य मधुक योगः)|
One Karsha – 12 g of the powder of Madhuka– Licorice – Glycyrrhiza glabra is added with equal quantities of ghee and honey. The man, who takes this recipe followed by the intake of milk, gets sexual urge every day. [19]

Factors contributing to improved sex vigour:
घृत क्षीराशनो निर्भीर्निर्व्याधिर्नित्यगो युवा|
सङ्कल्प प्रवणो नित्यं नरः स्त्रीषु वृषायते||२०||
कृतैक कृत्याः सिद्धार्था ये चान्योऽन्यानुवर्तिनः|
कलासु कुशलास्तुल्याः सत्त्वेन वयसा च ये||२१||
कुलमाहात्म्यदाक्षिण्य शील शौच समन्विताः|
ये काम नित्या ये हृष्टा ये विशोका गत व्यथाः||२२||
ये तुल्य शीला ये भक्ता ये प्रिया ये प्रियंवदाः|
तैर्नरः सह विस्रब्धः सुवयस्यैर्वृषायते||२३||
अभ्यङ्गोत्सादन स्नान गन्धमाल्यविभूषणैः|
गृहशय्यासनसुखैर्वासोभिरहतैः प्रियैः||२४||
विहङ्गानां रुतैरिष्टैः स्त्रीणां चाभरणस्वनैः|
संवाहनैर्वरस्त्रीणामिष्टानां च वृषायते||२५||
Factors contributing to improved sex vigour:
A person gets sex vigour with women by the doing the following:
Ghrita Ksheerashana – who takes ghee and milk
Is free from fear, complexion and diseases

who indulges in sex every day
who is youthful and
Sankalpa – who has determination
Ideal partner:
who has friends with similar profession,
who are accomplished in their objectives
Anuvarti – who are attached to each other
Kalasu Kushala – who are skilful in arts
Satvena Vayasa – who are similar in mind and age
who have noble lineage, expertise, good conduct and purity
who regularly indulge in sex acts
who are excited
who are free from grief and pain
who have similar conduct
Who have lovable and pleasant disposition as well as speech - friendship with such good companions

Factors that sexually excite a man:

अभ्यङ्गोत्सादन स्नान गन्धमाल्यविभूषणैः|
गृहशय्यासनसुखैर्वासोभिरहतैः प्रियैः||२४||
विहङ्गानां रुतैरिष्टैः स्त्रीणां चाभरणस्वनैः|
संवाहनैर्वरस्त्रीणामिष्टानां च वृषायते||२५||

Factors that sexually excite a man:
A man gets sexually excited by
Abhyanga – massage,
Utsadana – unction, dry massage, without any oil
Snana – bath
Gandha Mala Vibhushana – use of scents, garlands and ornaments,
Gruha Shayya Asana Sukha – comfortable home, bed and seat,
happiness, wearing of clothes which are not worn out and to the liking of the person, pleasing sound of the birds,
sounds of the ornaments of women an Samvahana (Kneading) by beautiful woman.[20-25]

The following erotic articles work as sex stimulants in different seasons:-

मत्तद्विरेफाचरिताः सपद्माः सलिलाशयाः|
जात्युत्पलसुगन्धीनि शीत गर्भगृहणि च||२६||
नद्यः फेनोत्तरीयाश्च गिरयो नीलसानवः|
उन्नतिर्नीलमेघानां, रम्यचन्द्रोदया निशाः||२७||
वायवः सुखसंस्पर्शाः कुमुदाकरगन्धिनः|
रतिभोगक्षमा रात्र्यः सङ्कोचागुरुवल्लभाः||२८||
सुखाः सहायाः परपुष्टघुष्टाः फुल्ला वनान्ता विशदान्नपानाः|
गान्धर्व शब्दाश्च सुगन्ध योगाः सत्त्वं विशालं निरुपद्रवं च||२९||
सिद्धार्थता चाभिनवश्च कामः स्त्री चायुधं सर्वमिहात्मजस्य|
वयो नवं जातमदश्च कालो हर्षस्य योनिः परमा नराणाम्||३०||

The following erotic articles work as sex stimulants in different seasons:-
Summer season
Big ponds having lotus flowers,
Surrounded by intoxicated Dvirepha (black bee), Fragrance of Jati (Jasmine) and Utpala (Nymphaea alba) and
underground rooms which are cold.

Rainy season:
River with waves of foam, mountains with blue peaks and the onset of black clouds
Autumn season:
Rise of a beautiful moon at night, wind which is pleasant to touch and which has the small pond full of Kumuda (Water Lily).
Early and late winter:
Nights which are long enough for sexual indulgence and women smeared with saffron and Aguru.
Spring:
Pleasing companions,
Cooling sound of the cuckoo bird,
Flowers in the ridge of the forests,
Pleasing diet and drinks,
Sound of the music,
Mind which is broad and free from afflictions,
Accomplishment of the objective,
Freshly initiated love affair and women- these are weapons of cupid (the god of sex).
All seasons in general

तत्र श्लोकः:-
प्रहर्षयोनयो योगा व्याख्याता दश पञ्च च|
माषपर्णभृतीयेऽस्मिन् पादे शुक्र बल प्रदाः ||३१||
Beginning of youth, sexual excitement, and pleasing time - these are excellent erotic factors for men. [26-30]
Summary:
In this quarter on Masha Parna Bhritiya, 15 recipes which help in sexual excitement and which promote semen as well as strength are described [31]

इत्यग्निवेशकृते तन्त्रे चरकप्रति संस्कृते चिकित्सास्थाने वाजीकरणाध्याये माषपर्णभृतीयो नाम वाजीकरणपादस्तृतीयः||३||
Thus, ends the third quarter on Masha Parna Bhrtiya (recipes prepared by the milk of cow fed with the leaves of Masha etc) of the chapter on aphrodisiacs of the Chikitsa section of Agnivesa's work, as redacted by Caraka.

8

Chikitsasthana Chapter 2.4 Puman Jata Baladhika Vajikaranam

Charaka Chikitsa 2.4 Puman Jata Baladhika Vajikarana Pada

The last quarter of Charaka's chapter on sexual health details the right age for intercourse, qualities of semen, causes for lack of sexual vigour and low-quality semen, definition of Vajikarana, factors contributing to ejaculation etc.

Fourth Quarter of the Chapter on Aphrodisiacs

अथातः पुमाञ्जातबलादिकं वाजीकरणपादं व्याख्यास्यामः॥१॥ इति ह स्माह भगवानात्रेयः॥२॥

We shall now explore the quarter dealing with aphrodisiacs, called "Puman jata baladika" Thus said lord Atreya [1-2]

Different types of men based on sexual strength:

पुमान् यथा जातबलो यावदिच्छं स्त्रियो व्रजेत् |

यथा चापत्यवान् सद्यो भवेतदुपदेक्ष्यते ||३||

न हि जातबलाः सर्वे नराश्चापत्यभागिनः |

बृहच्छरीरा बलिनः सन्ति नारीषु दुर्बलाः ||४||

सन्ति चाल्पाश्रयाः स्त्रीषु बलवन्तो बहुप्रजाः|

प्रकृत्या चाबलाः सन्ति सन्ति चामयदुर्बलाः||५||

नराश्चटकवत् केचिद् व्रजन्ति बहुशः स्त्रियम्|

गजवच्च प्रसिञ्चन्ति केचिन्न बहुगामिनः||६||

काल योगबलाः केचित् केचिदभ्यसनध्रुवाः|

केचित् प्रयत्नैर्व्यज्यन्ते वृषाः केचित् स्वभावतः||७||

तस्मात् प्रयोगान् वक्ष्यामो दुर्बलानां बल प्रदान्|

Different types of men based on sexual strength:

Now, we shall explore the procedure which instantaneously produces strength in the person and enables him to have sexual intercourse with women in order to procreate children.

It is not that all men possessing strong physical strength are capable of procreating children.

There are persons having stout and strong physique who are sexually very weak, there are physically lean and thin persons but they are very strong with women and procreate many children.

There are some people who are weak by nature and there are others who have become weak due to diseases.

There are people who indulge in women very frequently, like a sparrow.

There are others who, like an elephant, ejaculate lots of semen during sexual intercourse, but they do not indulge in sex too frequently.

There are persons who gain sexual vitality (only) at appropriate time (Kala Yoga).

There are others, who are capable of indulging in sex because of their regular habit and by taking aphrodisiacs

There are persons, who are divine by nature

Therefore, we shall now describe recipes which give strength to the weak, which help the strong enjoy the sex act and which add to their virility.

Basti Panchakarma treatment to improve sex power and fertility:

सुखोपभोगान् बलिनां भूयश्च बल वर्धनान्||८||

पूर्वं शुद्ध शरीराणां निरूहैः सानुवासनैः|

बलापेक्षी प्रयुञ्जीत शुक्रापत्य विवर्धनान्||९||

घृत तैल रस क्षीर शर्करा मधु संयुताः |

बस्तयः संविधातव्याः क्षीर मांस रसाशिनाम्||१०||

First of all, the physical system of the person is corrected by the administration of

Niruha type of Basti – decoction enema along with honey, rock salt etc.

and

Anuvasana Basti – Oil / fat enema.

Depending upon the strength, recipes of medicated enema consisting of ghee, oil, Rasa (juice and soup), milk, sugar and honey is administered.

These recipes promote semen and help a person in procreation of offspring.

Diet: The person is given milk and meat soup to take. [3-10]

Vrushya Mamsa Gutika:

पिष्ट्वा वराह मांसानि दत्वा मरिच सैन्धवे|

कोलवद्गुलिकाः कृत्वा तप्ते सर्पिषि वर्तयेत्||११||

वर्तनस्तम्भितास्ताश्च प्रक्षेप्याः कौक्कुटे रसे|

घृताढ्ये गन्ध पिशुने दधि दाडिम सारिके||१२||

यथा न भिन्द्याद्गुलि(टि)कास्तथा तं साधयेद्रसम्|

तं पिबन् भक्षयंस्ताश्च लभते शुक्रमक्षयम्||१३||

मांसानामेवमन्येषां मेद्यानां कारयेद्भिषक्|

गुटिकाः सरसास्तासं प्रयोगः शुक्रवर्धनः||१४||

(इति वृष्या मांसगुटिकाः)|

Pork paste is added with Maricha – Black pepper fruit – Piper nigrum and rock salt.

Out of this, Gulikas (round pills) the size of a Kola (bear fruit) are prepared.

These pills are fried in boiled ghee.

When they become hard after boiling, they are poured into the chicken soup, which is added with liberal quantity of ghee, powdered spices, curd and the juice of pomegranate.

This is cooked with care, so that the pills do not break. By drinking this soup and eating these pills, a person acquires exhaustive semen.

Similarly, following the same procedure, the meat soup and pills of the meat of other animals that are fatty, is prepared and administered.

Uses: These recipes are promoters of semen.

Vrushya Mahisha Rasa:

माषानङ्कुरितांछुद्धान् वितुषान् साजडाफलान्|

घृताढ्ये माहिष रसे दधि दाडिम सारिके||१५||

प्रक्षिपेन्मात्रया युक्तो धान्य जीरक नागरैः|

भुक्तः पीतश्च स रसः कुरुते शुक्रम क्षयम्||१६||

(इति वृष्यो माहिषरसः) |

Grains of Masha are cleaned and made to germinate. Thereafter, their husk is removed. To this, the fruits of Ajad (Shuka Shimbi) are added. These are added to the soup of buffalo meat, mixed with liberal quantities of ghee, curd and the juice of Dadima – Pomegranate – Punica granatum.

This preparation is further added with coriander, cumin and ginger. This portion is given to a person to eat and drink in appropriate quantity which endows him with inexhaustible semen. [15-16]

Aphrodisiac meat and fish, fried in ghee:

आर्द्राणि मत्स्य मांसानि शफरीर्वा सुभार्जिताः|

तप्ते सर्पिषि यः खादेत् स गच्छेत् स्त्रीषु न क्षयम्||१७||

घृत भृष्टान् रसे च्छागे रोहितान् फलसारिके|

अनुपीतरसान् स्निग्धानपत्यार्थी प्रयोजयेत्||१८||

(इति वृष्यघृतभृष्टमत्स्यमांसानि)|

Fish (Rohita) and meat when they are wet (not dry), or Saphari (name of the type of a fish) is well fried in boiling ghee.

After taking them, if a person indulges in women, he does not get exhausted.

Rohita fish fried in ghee and mixed with the soup of the meat of the goat and the juice of fruits, is used by a person who desires to procreate offspring.

After taking the recipe, he should take the unctuous soup. [17-18]

Two recipes of Vrushya Pupalika – aphrodisiac sweet cakes:

कुट्टकं मत्स्य मांसानां हिङ्गु सैन्धव धान्यकैः|

युक्तं गोधूम चूर्णेन घृते पूपलिकाः पचेत्||१९||

माहिषे च रसे मत्स्यान् स्निग्धाम्ल लवणान् पचेत्|

रसे चानुगते मांसं पोथयेत्तत्र चावपेत्||२०||

मरिचं जीरकं धान्यमल्पं हिङ्गु नवं घृतम्|

माष पूपलिकानां तद्गर्भार्थमुपकल्पयेत्||२१||

एतौ पूपलिका योगौ बृंहणौ बलवर्धनौ|

हर्ष सौभाग्यदौ पुत्र्यौ परं शुक्राभिवर्धनौ||२२||

(इति वृष्यौ पूपलिकायोगौ)|

1st pupalika yoga:

The fish and meat is made to a paste by crushing.

To this Hingu – Asa foetida, Saindhava – rock salt and Dhanyaka – coriander are added.

This is mixed with the wheat flour and boiled in ghee for the preparation of Pupalikas.

2nd Pupalika yoga:

Different types of fish are added with unctuous, sour and saline spices, and are boiled in the soup of the meat of buffalo. When the liquid portion of it is evaporated, the meat (of fish) is made into a paste.

To this, Black pepper fruit powder, cumin and coriander, small quantities of Asafoetida and freshly collected ghee are added. This is used for stuffing the Pupalikas made of black gram

Benefits:

They are – nourishing, promote strength, aphrodisiac and auspicious. They help in the procreation of male offspring by increasing the quantity of semen.

Vrushya Mashadi Pupalika – Black gram sweet cake:

माषात्मगुप्ता गोधूम शालि षष्टिक पैष्टिकम्|

शर्कराया विदार्याश्च चूर्णमिक्षुरकस्य च||२३||
संयोज्य मसृणे क्षीरे घृते पूपलिकाः पचेत्|
पयोऽनुपानास्ताः शीघ्रं कुर्वन्ति वृषतां पराम्||२४||
(इति वृष्या माषादिपूपलिकाः)|

The powders of these drugs are taken:

Masha – Black gram

Atmagupta – Mucuna pruriens

Godhuma – wheat – Triticum sativum,

Shali Shashtika – Rice

Sharkara – Sugar

Vidari (Ipomoea paniculata / Pueraria tuberosa),

Ikshuraka (Kokilaksha) – Asteracantha longifolia

And to this, milk having fat is added for preparation of the dough.

This is boiled in ghee for the preparation of Pupalikas.

Benefits and dosage: By taking these Pupalikas and taking milk thereafter, the man instantaneously gets excellent sexual vigour.

Sex recipe:

शर्करायास्तुलैका स्यादेका गव्यस्य सर्पिषः|
प्रस्थो विदार्याश्चूर्णस्य पिप्पल्याः प्रस्थ एव च||२५||
अर्धाढकं तुगाक्षीर्याः क्षौद्रस्याभिनवस्य च|
तत्सर्वं मूर्च्छितं तिष्ठेन्मार्तिके घृतभाजने||२६||
मात्रामग्निसमां तस्य प्रातः प्रातः प्रयोजयेत्|
एष वृष्यः परं योगो बल्यो बृंहण एव च||२७||

1 Tula of each of the sugar and cow's ghee,

1 Prastha each of the powder of

Vidari (Ipomoea paniculata / Pueraria tuberosa) and

Pippali – Long pepper fruit – Piper longum and

1/2 Adhaka each of Tugaksheeri – Bambusa bambos and freshly collected honey- all these drugs should be mixed and preserved in an earthen jar smeared with ghee.

Dosage: Depending upon the power of digestion, this potion is taken in appropriate quantities every morning.

Benefits: This is an excellent aphrodisiac recipe. This promotes strength and nourishment also. [25-27]

Apatyakara Ghrita:- Fertility promoting herbal ghee:

शतावर्या विदार्याश्च तथा माषात्मगुप्तयोः|
श्वदंष्ट्रायाश्च निष्क्वाथाञ्जलेषु च पृथक् पृथक्||२८||
साधयित्वा घृत प्रस्थं पयस्यष्टगुणे पुनः|
शर्करा मधु युक्तं तदपत्यार्थी प्रयोजयेत्||२९||
(इत्यपत्यकरं घृतम्)|

Decoction is prepared of

Shatavari – Asparagus racemosus

Vidari (Pueraria tuberosa),

Masha – Black gram

Atmagupta – Mucuna pruriens and

Svadamshtra – Tribulus terrestris by boiling them separately in water

Along with this decoction, 1 Prastha of ghee is cooked by adding 8 times of milk.

To this, sugar and honey is added.

This is taken by men desirous of procreating offspring. [28-29]

Vrushya Gutika:

घृत पात्रं शतगुणे विदारी स्वरसे पचेत्‌|
सिद्धं पुनः शतगुणे गव्ये पयसि साधयेत्‌||३०||
शर्करायास्तुगाक्षीर्या क्षौद्रस्येक्षुरकस्य च|
पिप्पल्याः साजडायाश्च भागैः पादांशिकैर्युतम्‌||३१||
गुलि(टि)काः कारयेद्वैद्यो यथा स्थुलमुदुम्बरम्‌|
तासां प्रयोगात् पुरुषः कुलिङ्ग इव हृष्यति||३२||
(इति वृष्यगुटिकाः)|

One Patra (vessel) of ghee is boiled with 100 times the juice of Vidari (Ipomoea paniculata / Pueraria tuberosa).
When it is cooked, it is again boiled with 100 times the milk of a cow.
This is added with 1/4th in quantity of
sugar,
Tugaksheeri – Bambusa bambos,
Honey,
Ikshuraka – Asteracantha longifolia,
Pippali – Long pepper fruit – Piper longum, and Ajada.
From these, pills are prepared by the physician.
The size of the pills should be like the fruit of Udaumbara.
By taking this recipe, the man gets excited like a Kulinga (sparrow).[30-32]

Vrushya Utkarika:

सितोपला पल शतं तदर्धं नव सर्पिषः|
क्षौद्रं पादेन संयुक्तं साधयेज्जलपादिकम्‌||३३||
सान्द्रं गोधूम चूर्णानां पादं स्तीर्णे शिलातले|
शुचौ श्लक्ष्णे समुत्कीर्य मर्दनेनोपपादयेत्‌||३४||
शुद्धा उत्कारिकाः कार्यश्चन्द्र मण्डल सन्निभाः|
तासां प्रयोगाद्गजवन्नारीः सन्तर्पयेन्नरः||३५||
(इति वृष्योत्कारिका) |

Vrushya Utkarika:
100 Palas of crystal sugar (Sitopala)
50 Palas of freshly collected ghee and
25 Palas of Honey are mixed together and boiled in 25 Palas of water.
When it becomes semi-solid, 25 Palas of wheat flour should be added.
The paste, thus prepared, should be spread over a stone, which is clean and smooth.
It is kneaded by repeatedly spreading it.
From this dough, Utkarikas are prepared by boiling.
These Utkarikas will appear like the moon.
Benefits: By the use of these Utkarikas, the man becomes capable of indulging in sex acts with women, in an elephant's vigour [33-35]

Definition of Vrushya – aphrodisiac, vigour enhancement:

यत् किञ्चिन्मधुरं स्निग्धं जीवनं बृंहणं गुरु|
हर्षणं मनसश्चैव सर्वं तद्वृष्यमुच्यते||३६||
द्रव्यैरेवंविधैस्तस्मादभावितः प्रमदां व्रजेत्‌|

आत्मवेगेन चोदीर्णः स्त्रीगुणैश्च प्रहर्षितः||३७||

Articles which are sweet, unctuous, Jivana (promoters of life), nourishing and heavy and which cause excitement of the mind- all these are called aphrodisiacs. Therefore, a person is first of all impregnated with these articles before sexual intercourse. He thus, gets excited by his own urge and also by the erotic attributes of woman.

'After-sex' regimen:

गत्वा स्नात्वा पयः पीत्वा रसं वाऽनु शयीत ना|

तथाऽस्याप्यायते भूयः शुक्रं च बलमेव च||३८||

After sexual indulgence, one should take bath and drink milk or Rasa (juice or meat soup) before going to sleep. By doing so, his semen and strength both increase.

Right age for sex:

यथा मुकुल पुष्पस्य सुगन्धो नोपलभ्यते|

लभ्यते तद्विकाशात्तु तथा शुक्रं हि देहिनाम्||३९||

नर्ते वै षोडशाद्वर्षात् सप्ततयाः परतो न च|

आयुष्कामो नरः स्त्रीभिः संयोगं कर्तुमर्हति||४०||

अतिबालो ह्यसम्पूर्णसर्वधातुः स्त्रियं व्रजन्|

उपशुष्येत सहसा तडागमिव काजलम्||४१||

शुष्कं रूक्षं यथा काष्ठं जन्तुदग्धं विजर्जरम्|

स्पृष्टमाशु विशीर्येत तथा वृद्धः स्त्रियो व्रजन्||४२||

Right age for sex:

There is no fragrance in a bud. Fragrance appears only when the flower blossoms. Similarly, a person desirous of longevity should not enter into sexual intercourse with women before the age of sixteen years and after the age of seventy years.

A young boy of very tender age does not possess all the tissue elements in their matured form. If he enters into sex act with a woman, his body gets dried up like a pond having very little water.

A piece of wood which is dried and unctuous, eaten away by insects and has become porous, gets broken immediately by a little pressure (of touch). Similarly, the body of the old man gets decayed by sexual intercourse with a woman.

Cause for diminishing sexual strength:

जरया चिन्तया शुक्रं व्याधिभिः कर्म कर्षणात्|

क्षयं गच्छत्यनशनात् स्त्रीणां चातिनिषेवणात्||४३||

क्षयाद्भयादविश्रम्भाच्छोकात् स्त्रीदोष दर्शनात्|

नारीणामरसज्ञत्वाद विचारादसेवनात्||४४||

तृप्तस्यापि स्त्रियो गन्तुं न शक्तिरुपजायते|

देह सत्व बलापेक्षी हर्षः शक्तिश्च हर्षजा||४५||

The sex power gets reduced by

Jaraya – old age,

Chintya – worry, stress

Vyadhibhihi – due to diseases,

Karma Karshanaat – excessive hard work, exertion, exhaustion

Anashana – continuous fasting,

Streenam cha ati nishevanaat – excessive sexual indulgence,

Kshayat – due to depleted body tissues,

Bhayaat – fear,

Avishrambha – suspicion

Shoka – grief,

Stri Dosha Darshanaat – finding faults in women,

non-excitation and complete avoidance of sex acts

A person, who is satisfied after sex act, does not possess power of entering into sex act with the woman again. Because, this power is dependent upon excitement and excitement, in turn is dependent upon the strength of the body and the mind.

Omnipresent Shukra Dhatu:

रस इक्षौ यथा दध्नि सर्पिस्तैलं तिले यथा|

सर्वत्रानुगतं देहे शुक्रं संस्पर्शने तथा||४६||

तत् स्त्रीपुरुषसंयोगे चेष्टासङ्कल्पपीडनात्|

शुक्रं प्रच्यवते स्थानाज्जलमार्द्रात् पटादिव||४७||

Omnipresent Shukra Dhatu:

The entire sugarcane plant is filled with its sweet juice. Ghee is available in the whole curd and oil is available in all parts of the sesame seed. Similarly, semen pervades the entire body which has the sensation of touch.

As water comes out of a wet cloth when squeezed, similarly, the semen trickles out from its site during copulation, because of sexual act (Chesta), determination (Sankalpa) and physical pressure (Peedana).

Factors contributing to ejaculation:

हर्षात्तर्षात् सरत्वाच्च पैच्छिल्याद्गौरवादपि|

अणुप्रवणभावाच्च द्रुतत्वान्मारुतस्य च||४८||

अष्टाभ्य एभ्यो हेतुभ्यः शुक्रं देहात् प्रसिच्यते|

चरतो विश्वरूपस्य रूपद्रव्यं यदुच्यते||४९|

The semen is ejaculated because of 8 factors, namely,

Harshaat – excitement

Tarshaat – passionate desire

Saratvaat – fluidity

Paicchillya – sliminess

Gaurava – heaviness

Anu Bhava (Atomicity)

Pravana Bhava (the tendency to flow out) and

The force of Vata Dosha.

The un-manifested soul which takes different forms in this world, manifest itself in the form of semen. [46-49]

Qualities of Semen:

बहलं मधुरं स्निग्धमविस्रं गुरु पिच्छिलम्|

शुक्लं बहु च यच्छुक्रं फलवत्तदसंशयम्||५०||

Semen which is

Bahala – thick, voluminous,

Madhura – sweet,

Snigdha – Oily, unctuous,

Avisra – without any putrid smell,

Guru – heavy,

Picchila – slimy,

Shukla – white and in

Bahu – large quantity, invariably helps in procreation of offspring. There is no doubt about it. [50]

Definition of Vajikarana:
येन नारीषु सामर्थ्यं वाजीवल्लभते नरः|
व्रजेच्चाभ्यधिकं येन वाजीकरणमेव तत्||५१||
The factors which make a man capable of entering into sexual intercourse with women with stallion vigour and which makes him capable of performing excessive sexual intercourse are called "Vajikarana". [51]

तत्र श्लोकौ-
हेतुर्योगोपदेशस्य योगा द्वादश चोत्तमाः|
यत् पूर्व मैथुनात् सेव्यं सेव्यं यन्मैथुनादनु||५२||
यदा न सेव्याः प्रमदाः कृत्स्नः शुक्रविनिश्चयः|
निरुक्तं चेह निर्दिष्टं पुमाञ्जातबलादिके||५३||
To sum up:
In this quarter called "Puman-Jata Baladika" the following topics are discussed:
The purpose for which the aphrodisiac recipes have been prescribed.
Twelve excellent recipes for virility
regimens to be adopted before after sexual intercourse
Regimens to be adopted after sexual intercourse.
the time (age) when the sexual intercourse with the woman is prohibited 'determination of all semen and
Definition of the term "Vajikarana" [52-53]

इत्यग्निवेशकृते तन्त्रे चरक प्रतिसंस्कृते चिकित्सा स्थाने वाजीकरणाध्याये पुमाञ्जातबलादिको नाम वाजीकरणपादश्चतुर्थः||४||
Thus, ends the fourth quarter called "Puman Jata Baladika" of the chapter on aphrodisiacs of Cikitsa section of Agnivesa's work, as redacted by Charaka.
समाप्तश्चायं द्वितीयो वाजीकरणाध्यायः||२||
Thus ends the last quarter of the second chapter on Aphrodisiacs.

9

Chikitsasthana Chapter 3 Jwara Chikitsitam

The third chapter of Charaka Chikitsasthana is called Jwara Chikitsa. It deals with management of different types of fever. Jvara in general terms can be translated as fever.

अथातो ज्वरचिकित्सितं व्याख्यास्यामः||१||

इति ह स्माह भगवानात्रेयः||२||

We shall now explore the chapter on the treatment of Jwara (different types of fever). Thus said Lord Atreya [1–2]

Agnivesha's approach to Punarvasu:

विज्वरं ज्वर सन्देहं पर्यपृच्छत् पुनर्वसुम्|

विविक्ते शान्तमासीनमग्निवेशः कृताञ्जलिः||३||

Punarvasu, who is free from 3 types of Jwaras (miseries) was sitting in a lonely place and had absolute tranquillity of mind. Agnivesha, with folded hands approached him with his queries about Jwara [3]

Agnivesha's Query:

देहेन्द्रिय मनस्तापी सर्व रोगाग्रजो बली|

ज्वरः प्रधानो रोगाणामुक्तो भगवता पुरा||४||

तस्य प्राणिसपत्नस्य ध्रुवस्य प्रलयोदये|

प्रकृतिं च प्रवृतिं च प्रभावं कारणानि च||५||

पूर्वरूपमधिष्ठानं बलकालात्मलक्षणम्|

व्यासतो विधिभेदाच्च पृथग्भिन्नस्य चाकृतिम्||६||

लिङ्गमामस्य जीर्णस्य सौषधं च क्रिया क्रमम्|

विमुञ्चतः प्रशान्तस्य चिह्नं यच्च पृथक् पृथक्||७||

ज्वरावसृष्टो रक्ष्यश्च यावत्कालं यतो यतः|

प्रशान्तः कारणैर्यैश्च पुनरावर्तते ज्वरः||८||

याश्चापि पुनरावृतं क्रियाः प्रशमयन्ति तम्|

जगदिहितार्थं तत् सर्व भगवन्! वक्तुमर्हसि||९||

तदग्निवेशस्य वचो निशम्य गुरुरब्रवीत्|

ज्वराधिकारे यद्वाच्यं तत् सौम्य! निखिलं शृणु||१०||

Oh! Lord! You have already stated earlier (in Nidana Sthana 1:6) that "Jwara is the most painful among the diseases. It afflicts the body, the senses and the mind. It is exceedingly powerful. This enemy of human beings is invariably associated with dissolutions, birth and death. (It is said that one gets fever during birth and death). Therefore kindly explain the following points for the benefit of the living being:–

Prakruti or nature of the disease

Pravrtti or origin of the disease

Prabhava or the manifestations of the disease

Karana or causative factors

Purva Rupa or premonitory signs and symptoms

Adhisthana or place of manifestation

Bala Kala or its power and the time of its manifestation

Atma Laksana or signs and symptoms which are invariably associated with this disease

Details of classification

Signs and symptoms of each variety of this disease

Signs and symptoms of Ama Jwara i.e primary stage of the disease

Signs and symptoms of Jeerna Jwara or chronic disease

medicines for the treatment of the disease

Line of treatment

Signs and symptoms that are manifested when the fever is getting cured, or when it is being alleviated – both separately

The duration for which the patient who has become free from Jvara should avoid certain regimens, and the reasons for that

The reason for the re-attack / recurrence of the fever after it has subsided

The therapies administered in order to alleviate this re-attack of fever

After bearing the treatment of Agnivesha, the preceptor said: "All these will be explained in this chapter on the description of fever, Oh affectionate one! Hear them in detail". [4:2:10]

Synonyms of Jwara:

ज्वरो विकारो रोगश्च व्याधिरातङ्क एव च|

एकोऽर्थो नाम पर्यायैर्विविधैरभिधीयते||११||

The synonyms of Jwara are – Jwara (fever), Vikara (ailment), Roga (disease), Vyadhi (disease) and Atanka (fear inducing factor) [11]

Nature of Jwara:

तस्य प्रकृतिरुद्दिष्टा दोषाः शारीर मानसाः|

देहिनं न हि निर्दोषं ज्वरः समुपसेवते||१२||

Factors which are responsible for the manifestation of Jwara, in brief are –

the 3 physical Doshas – Vata, Pitta and Kapha

and 2 Doshas of the mind namely – Rajas and Tamas

Living beings do not get afflicted with Jwara without the involvement of these Doshas. [12]

Specific features of Jwara – Jwara Prakruti

क्षयस्तमो ज्वरः पाप्मा मृत्युश्चोक्ता यमात्मकाः|

पञ्चत्व प्रत्ययान्नृणां क्लिश्यतां स्वेन कर्मणा||१३||

इत्यस्य प्रकृतिः प्रोक्ता, ...|१४|

Specific features of Jwara:

Kshaya – depletion of body tissues, weight loss,

Tamas – entering into internal darkness

Papma – manifestation of the sinful acts and

Mrutyu – death

The specific feature of disease is:
Jwara is like Yama (God of death). Being afflicted by his own actions, the individual succumbs to death after suffering from fever. [13–14]

Origin of the disease – Jwara Pravrutti

... प्रवृत्तिस्तु परिग्रहात्‌।
निदाने पूर्वमुद्दिष्टा रुद्रकोपाच्च दारुणात्‌॥१४॥

The origin of Jwara is because of the attachment (Parigraha).
In the Nidana section, it has been described that Jwara is originated because of the ferocious wrath of Rudra. [14]

Mythology about the origin of Jwara:

द्वितीये हि युगे शर्वमक्रोधव्रतमास्थितम्‌।
दिव्यं सहस्रं वर्षाणामसुरा अभिदुद्रुवुः॥१५॥
तपोविघ्नाशनाः कर्तुं तपोविघ्नं महात्मनः।
पश्यन् समर्थश्चोपेक्षां चक्रे दक्षः प्रजापतिः॥१६॥
पुनर्माहेश्वरं भागं ध्रुवं दक्षः प्रजापतिः।
यज्ञे न कल्पयामास प्रोच्यमानः सुरैरपि॥१७॥
ऋचः पशुपतेर्याश्च शैव्या आहतयश्च याः।
यज्ञसिद्धिप्रदास्ताभिर्हीनं चैव स इष्टवान्‌॥१८॥
अथोत्तीर्णव्रतो देवो बुद्ध्वा दक्ष व्यतिक्रमम्‌।
रुद्रो रौद्रं पुरस्कृत्य भावमात्मविदात्मनः॥१९॥
सृष्ट्वा ललाटे चक्षुर्वै दग्ध्वा तानसुरान् प्रभुः।
बालं क्रोधाग्नि सन्तप्तमसृजत् सत्रनाशनम्‌॥२०॥
ततो यज्ञः स विध्वस्तो व्यथिताश्च दिवौकसः।
दाहव्यथापरीताश्च भ्रान्ता भूतगणा दिशः॥२१॥
अथेश्वरं देवगणः सह सप्तर्षिभिर्विभुम्‌।
तमृग्भिरस्तुवन् यावच्छैवे भावे शिवः स्थितः॥२२॥
शिवं शिवाय भूतानां स्थितं ज्ञात्वा कृताञ्जलिः।
भिया भस्मप्रहरणस्त्रिशिरा नवलोचनः॥२३॥
ज्वालामालाकुलो रौद्रो ह्रस्वजङ्घोदरः क्रमात्‌।
क्रोधाग्निरुक्तवान् देवमहं किं करवाणि ते॥२४॥
तमुवाचेश्वरः क्रो धं ज्वरो लोके भविष्यसि।
जन्मादौ निधने च त्वमपचारान्तरेषु च॥२५॥

During the second age (Treta Yuga), Lord Shiva took a vow not to manifest wrath for 1,000 celestial years. During this time, the Asuras (demons), who indulged in creating obstruction to the penance of sages, made mischief. Daksha Prajapati was capable of combating their obstructions to the penance of this great soul (Shiva). But he did not make any effort in this direction. Again, in the Yajna (Homa), Daksha Prajapati did not offer a share to Maheshvara even though he was requested to do by the Gods. These are also the descriptions of giving Ahuti (pouring of ghee in the sacrificial fire) for Shiva. These 2 rituals are necessary for proper accomplishment of the Yajna and for achieving the desired objectives. Daksha Prajapati, however, did not perform these 2 rituals during his Yajna.
Lord Shiva is endowed with the power to know everything by himself. When he completed the penance and got up, he realized the evasion of the duty by Daksha and became angry. He touched his third eye in his forehead, and from this third eye emanated the wrathful fire which burnt all those Asuras (demons). From this fire a child called Veerabhadra took birth. He was dazzling with the fire produced because of Shiva's anger. He pursues the mission of destroying the enemies and destroying the Homa of Daksha prajapati. As a result of this, the Gods got afflicted with burning sensation and pain. The living beings all around became unconscious.

Thereafter, the Gods along with sages offered prayers to the Omnipotent and Omnipresent Lord Shiva by the help of Ahutis described in the Rig Veda. This alleviated the wrath of Lord Shiva and endowed Him with the compassionate as well as auspicious disposition.

When it was known that Lord Shiva has developed an auspicious disposition, Veerabhadra who was produced from the wrathful fire, who had 3 heads and 9 eyes, who had ash as his weapon, who had the flame of fire as his garland, who was wrathful and who had slender legs and stomach, approached Lord Shiva and inquired him about his future work.

Lord Shiva replied to that incarnation of his anger, "You will become Jwara in this world and afflict people at the time of birth and death and also afflict those who will resort to erratic regimens". [15–25]

Manifestations of Jwara – JwaraPrabhava

सन्तापः सारुचिस्तृष्णा साङ्गमर्दो हृदि व्यथा|

ज्वरप्रभावो, जन्मादौ निधने च महत्तमः||२६||

प्रकृतिश्च प्रवृतिश्च प्रभावश्च प्रदर्शितः|२७|

The special manifestations of Jwara:

Santapa – temperature

Aruchi – Anorexia

Trushna – excessive thirst

Angamarda – malaise, body ache with heaviness

Hrudi Vyatha – pain in cardiac region

In the beginning of the birth and during death, it is manifested in the form of Tamas (entering into darkness).

Thus, the Prakruti (nature), Pravrutti (origin) and Prabhava (special manifestation) of Jwara are described. [26–27]

Etiological factors of Jwara:

निदाने कारणान्यष्टौ पूर्वोक्तानि विभागशः||२७||

In the Nidana section, the etiological factors of each of the 8 types of Jwara are described separately. [27]

Premonitory Signs and Symptoms:

आलस्यं नयने सास्रे जृम्भणं गौरवं क्लमः|

ज्वलनातपवाय्वम्बुभक्तिद्वेषावनिश्चितौ||२८||

अविपाकास्य वैरस्ये हानिश्च बलवर्णयोः|

शील वैकृतमल्पं च ज्वर लक्षणमग्रजम्||२९||

Alasyam – Lethargy

Nayana aasre – excessive lacrimation

Jrambhana – yawning

Gauravam – heaviness

Klama – Mental fatigue

Jwalana, Aatapa, Vayu and Ambu Bhakti Dwesha – Uncertainty about liking and disliking for fire, sun, wind and water

Avipaka – Indigestion

Vairasya – Anorexia

Bala Hani – Depletion in strength and complexion, and

Alpa Sheela Vikruti – Slight change in conduct [28–29]

Site of Manifestation of fever:

केवलं समनस्कं च ज्वराधिष्ठानमुच्यते|

शरीरं, बलकालस्तु निदाने सम्प्रदर्शितः||३०||

JwaraAdhishtana:

The entire body along with the mind

The strength and the time of manifestation of Jwara are already described in Nidana 1:21, 24 and 27. [30]

Classical feature of fever:

ज्वर प्रत्यात्मिकं लिङ्गं सन्तापो देह मानसः|

ज्वरेणाविशता भूतं न हि किञ्चिन्न तप्यते||३१||

Jwara Pratyatmaka Linga:

The signs and symptoms invariably associated with Jwara are

Santapa Deha Manasa – The increase in the temperature of the body and mental unhappiness.

There is no living being which is not afflicted by Jwara [31]

Jwara Bheda – Classification:

द्विव विधो विधि भेदेन ज्वरः शारीर मानसः|

पुनश्च द्विविधो दृष्टः सौम्यश्चाग्नेय एव वा||३२||

अन्तर्वेगो बहिर्वेगो द्विविधः पुनरुच्यते|

प्राकृतो वैकृतश्चैव साध्यश्चासाध्य एव च||३३||

पुनः पञ्च विधो दृष्टो दोष काल बलाबलात्|

सन्ततः सततोऽन्येद्युस्तृतीयक चतुर्थकौ||३४||

पुनराश्रय भेदेन धातूनां सप्तधा मतः|

भिन्नः कारण भेदेन पुनरष्ट विधो ज्वरः||३५||

Jwara is classified into 2 categories, each on the basis of the following criteria:–

1. Sharira (Physical) and Manasa (mental)

2. Saumya (caused by cold) and Agneya (caused by heat).

3. Antarvega (internal) and Bahirvega (external)

4. Prakruta (natural, seasonal) and Vaikruta (Unseasonal) and

5. Sadhya (curable) and Asadhya (incurable).

Jwara is again classified into 5 categories depending upon the strength and weakness of Doshas and the time. These are

Satata, Santata, Anyedyuska, Trtiyaka and Chaturthaka.

Depending upon the Ashraya (site of manifestation) in the 7 Dhatus (basic tissue elements), Jwara is also classified into 7 categories. [32–35]

Signs and symptoms of each variety of Jwara:

शारीरो जायते पूर्व देहे, मनसि मानसः|

वैचित्यमरतिर्ग्लानिर्मनसस्ताप लक्षणम्||३६||

इन्द्रियाणां च वैकृत्यं ज्ञेयं सन्ताप लक्षणम्|३७|

The Sharira (Physical) type of Jwara first appears in the body and the Manasa (mental) type first appears in the mind.

The Manas Taapa – mental discomfort manifests as –

Vaichitya – mental instability

Arati – disliking for everything and

Glani – feeling of weakness in the body

The Santapa of the Indriyas (sense organs) in indicated by their morbidity. [36–37]

वात पित्तात्मकः शीतमुष्णं वात कफात्मकः||३७||

इच्छत्युभयमेतत्तु ज्वरो व्यामिश्रलक्षणः|३८|

The patient suffering from Jwara caused by:

Pitta desires cold things.

Vayu and Kapha desire hot things.

When, however, these Doshas get mixed up, both the types of symptoms are manifested. [37–38]

Vata Dosha is a Yogavahi

योगवाहः परं वायुः संयोगादुभयार्थकृत्||३८||

दाह कृतेजसा युक्तः, शीतकृत् सोम संश्रयात्|३९|

Vata is exceedingly Yogavahi (which accentuates the properties of others) in nature.

In combination, it produces both the types of effects.

For example, when combined with Tejas (fire), it produces burning sensation and when combined with Soma (water) it produces cooling effects. [38–39]

Antarvega and Bahirvega symptoms of Jwara:

अन्तर्दाहोऽधिकस्तृष्णा प्रलापः श्वसनं भ्रमः||३९||

सन्ध्यस्थिशूलमस्वेदो दोष वर्चो विनिग्रहः|

अन्तर्वेगस्य लिङ्गानि ज्वरस्यैतानि लक्षयेत्||४०||

सन्तापोऽभ्यधिको बाह्यस्तृष्णादीनां च मार्दवम्|

बहिर्वेगस्य लिङ्गानि सुखसाध्यत्वमेव च||४१||

The signs and symptoms of Antarvega (internal) type of Jwara:

Antardaha – Burning sensation inside the body

Trishna – Excessive thirst

Pralapa – delirium, irrelevant talk

Shwasana – dysponea, difficulty in breathing

Bhrama – giddiness,

Sandhi asthishoola – pain in bones and joints

Asveda – Absence of sweating

A-varchas – non excretion n of Doshas and feaces

The signs and symptoms of Bahirvega (external) type of Jwara:

Excessive temperature in the ext the patient suffering from Jwara caused by: erior of the body, and less thirst etc symptoms. This type of Jwara is easily curable. [39–41]

Prakruti Jwara – seasonal fever:

प्राकृतः सुख साध्यस्तु वसन्त शरदुद्भवः|

उष्णमुष्णेन संवृद्धं पित्तं शरदि कुप्यति||४२||

चितः शीते कफश्चैवं वसन्ते समुदीर्यते|

वर्षास्वम्ल विपाकाभिरद्भिरोषधिभिस्तथा||४३||

सञ्चितं पित्तमुद्रिक्तं शरद्यादित्य तेजसा|

ज्वरं सञ्जनयत्याशु तस्य चानुबलः कफः||४४||

प्रकृत्यैव विसर्गस्य तत्र नानशनाद्भयम्|

अद्भिरोषधिभिश्चैव मधुराभिश्चितः कफः||४५||

हेमन्ते, सूर्यसन्तप्तः स वसन्ते प्रकुप्यति|

वसन्ते श्लेष्मणा तस्माज्ज्वरः समुपजायते||४६||

आदान मध्ये तस्यापि वात पित्तं भवेदनु|४७|

Prakruta Jwara – seasonal fever:

The Jwara that manifests in Vasanta (spring season) and Sharat (autumn season), is called Prakruta (seasonal). It is easily curable.

Kapha which gets aggravated in winter gets excited during Vasanta (spring) season.

Pitta is hot in nature and it gets aggravated during Sharat (autumn) season.

Jwara during Varsha Rutu (Rainy season):

During the rainy season the water, herbs and dishes become sour in Vipaka (taste that emerges after digestion). This results in the accumulation of Pitta. This accumulated Pitta gets excited or aggravated in autumn because of the exposure to hot Sun rays. This may immediately produce Jwara.

Kapha is the secondary associate in the manifestation of Jwara. Autumn is the Visarga Kala (time of elimination). Therefore, fasting (which is the first step for the treatment of Jwara) does not create any problem.

During Hemanta (first part of the winter season), the water, herbs and dishes become sweet in taste. This helps in the accumulation of Kapha. The Kapha gets aggravated in the subsequent spring season because of strong rays of the sun. Therefore, during the Vasanta (spring) season Kaphaja Jwara is manifested.

Spring season is a part of Adana Kala (time of absorption) and in any type of Jwara that is caused during this period, Vata and Pitta constitute its secondary associates. [42–47]

आदावन्ते च मध्ये च बुद्ध्वा दोष बलाबलम्||४७||

शरद्वसन्तयोर्विद्वाञ्ज्वरस्य प्रतिकारयेत्|४८|

The wise should treat a patient suffering from Jwara keeping in view the strength or weakness of Doshas in the beginning, at the end and in the middle of Sharat (autumn) and Vasanta (spring) seasons. [47–48]

VaikrutaJwara:

काल प्रकृतिमुद्दिश्य निर्दिष्टः प्राकृतो ज्वरः||४८||

प्रायेणानिलजो दुःखः कालेष्वन्येषु वैकृतः|

हेतवो विविधास्तस्य निदाने सम्प्रदर्शिताः||४९||

Depending upon the nature of the season, seasonal (Prakruta) type of Jvara is described.

Generally the Jwara caused by Vata Dosha is difficult to cure. The following types of Jwara are to be treated as Vaikruta:

• Vatika Jwara irrespective of its season of occurrence.

• Paittika Jwara if it occurs during seasons other than autumn.

• Kapha Jwara if it occurs during seasons other than spring.

The causative factors of different types of Jwara are described in the Nidana section. [48–49]

SadhyaJwara – Easily curable fever:

बलवत्स्वल्प दोषेषु ज्वरः साध्योऽनुपद्रवः|५०|

In a person with strong physique, if Jwara occurs by the vitiation of fewer amounts (number) of Doshas and if there is no complication; then it is easily curable. [50]

Incurable type of Jwara – Asadhya

हेतुभिर्बहुभिर्जातो बलिभिर्बहु लक्षणः||५०||

ज्वरः प्राणान्तकृद्यश्च शीघ्रमिन्द्रिय नाशनः|५१|

The Jwara having the following characteristics leads to death, which:

Caused by strong etiological factors

Associated with many signs and symptoms and

Destroys the sense organs immediately

Bad prognosis:

सप्ताहाद्वा दशाहाद्वा द्वादशाहात्तथैव च||५१||

स प्रलाप भ्रम श्वासस्तीक्ष्णो हन्याज्ज्वरो नरम्|५२|

Acute fever (Teekshna Jwara) associated with

Pralapa – delirium,

Bhrama – Giddiness and

Shwasa – difficulty in breathing, asthma causes death of the patient on the seventh, tenth or twelfth days. [51–52]

ज्वरः क्षीणस्य शूनस्य गम्भीरो दैर्घरात्रिकः||५२||

असाध्यो बलवान् यश्च केशसीमन्तकृज्ज्वरः|५३|

If deep seated (Gambhira) and strong fever occurs in a weak and in an emaciated patient, and continues for several nights (Dairgha Ratrika), then it is incurable. In such diseases; the hairs of the head fall apart to produce a straight line (Kesha SemantaKrut) [52–53]

Vishama Jwara:

This type of fever is recurrent in nature with certain time gap in between.

Visham Jwara is of 5 types.

SantatakaJwara – Affects Rasavaha Srotas, either gets cured or kills the patient on 12th, 10th or 7th day.

SatataJwara – Affects Rakta Dhatu, Satataka Jwara occurs twice in a day and night

AnyedyushkaJwara – Affects Rakta dhatu and Medovaha Srotas. Jwara occurs once per day.

Truteeyaka – Occurs on every third day (on alternate days). Asthi Dhatu and Mamsavaha srotas are involved.

Chaturtaka – occurs with a gap of two days. Afflicts Majja Dhatu and Medovaha Srotas

SantatakaJwara:

स्रोतोभिर्विसृता दोषा गुरवो रसवाहिभिः||५३||

सर्व देहानुगाः स्तब्धा ज्वरं कुर्वन्ति सन्ततम्|

दशाहं द्वादशाहं वा सप्ताहं वा सुदुःसहः||५४||

स शीघ्रं शीघ्रकारित्वात् प्रशमं याति हन्ति वा|

कालदूष्यप्रकृतिभिर्दोषस्तुल्यो हि सन्ततम्||५५||

निष्प्रत्यनीकः कुरुते तस्माज्ज्ञेयः सुदुःसहः|

यथा धातूंस्तथा मूत्रं पुरीषं चानिलादयः||५६||

युगपच्चानुपद्यन्ते नियमात् सन्तते ज्वरे|

स शुद्ध्या वाऽप्यशुद्ध्या वा रसादीनामशेषतः||५७||

सप्ताहादिषु कालेषु प्रशमं याति हन्ति वा|

यदा तु नातिशुध्यन्ति न वा शुध्यन्ति सर्वशः||५८||

द्वादशैते समुद्दिष्टाः सन्ततस्याश्रयास्तदा|

विसर्ग द्वादशे कृत्वा दिवसेऽव्यक्त लक्षणम्||५९||

दुर्लभोपशमः कालं दीर्घमप्यनुवर्तते|

इति बुद्ध्वा ज्वरं वैद्य उपक्रामेत्तु सन्ततम्||६०||

क्रिया क्रम विधौ युक्तः प्रायः प्रागपतर्पणैः|६१|

The imbalanced Doshas spread all across the body through Rasavaha Srotas causing stiffness. Such a fever is called Santata Jwara. It manifests its symptoms very quickly and either gets cured or kills the patient on 12th, 10th or 7th day. It is extremely difficult to tolerate this type of fever.

If the Doshas involved in the Santata type of Jwara are similar in property to the season (Kala), Dhatus (Dushya) and physical constitution (Prakruti), then it is Asadhya (incurable).

If the Dhatus and waste products (urine, stool and flatus) are purified, then on 7th, 10th, or 12th days the fever gets subsided. However, if Dhatus and Malas are not purified then fever kills the patient on those days. The death of the patient occurs even if these Dhatus are partially purified.

The Santata Jwara is thus located on 12 factors namely, 7 Dhatus, 3 Doshas, Urine and stool. Even if the fever subsides on 12th day etc. the symptoms of Jwara may become latent. It may continue for a longer period and cure of this disease is extremely difficult. Therefore, the physician should first administer Apatarpana (fasting) treatment, followed by other treatments for fever. [53–61]

Satataka Jwara – Fever that occurs twice in a day

रक्तधात्वाश्रयः प्रायो दोषः सततकं ज्वरम्||६१||

सप्रत्यनीकः कुरुते कालवृद्धि क्षयात्मकम्|

अहोरात्रे सततको द्वौ कालावनुवर्तते||६२||

In Satataka Jwara, Dosha is mostly located in the Rakta Dhatu. It can be treated with success.

It gets aggravated and subsided depending upon the nature of the time.

In a day and night, Satataka Jwara occurs twice. [61–62]

Anyeduska, Truteeyaka and Chaturthaka Jwara:

काल प्रकृति दूष्याणां प्राप्यैवान्यतमाद्बलम्|

अन्येद्युष्कं ज्वरं दोषो रुद्ध्वा मेदोवहाः सिराः||६३||

सप्रत्यनीको जनयत्येककालमहर्निशि|

दोषोऽस्थिमज्जगः कुर्यात्तृतीयक चतुर्थकौ||६४||

गतिद्र्व्येकान्तराऽन्येद्युर्दोषस्योक्ताऽन्यथा परैः|

अन्येद्युष्कं ज्वरं कुर्यादपि संश्रित्य शोणितम्||६५||

मांस स्रोतांस्यनुगतो जनयेत्तु तृतीयकम्|

संश्रितो मेदसो मार्ग दोषश्चापि चतुर्थकम्||६६||

अन्येद्युष्कः प्रतिदिनं दिनं हित्वा तृतीयकः|

दिनद्वयं यो विश्रम्य प्रत्येति स चतुर्थकः||६७||

AnyedyuskaJwara: Fever that occurs every day

Occurrence: Due to the support of the strength of any one from among the Kala (time), Prakruti (physical constitution) and Dushya (Dhatus). It occurs every day. It affects Medovaha Sira (fat channels). Here Rakta is vitiated.

TrtiyakaJwara – Fever that occurs on alternate days

It occurs when Doshas afflict Asthi Dhatu (bone tissue). In this type of fever, Mamsavaha Srotas are also involved.

Chaturthaka Jwara: Fever that repeatedly occurs after every 2 days. Here Doshas afflict Majja Dhatu (marrow) and Medovaha Srotas (Fat channels).

According to some scholars different types of Jwara viz, Anyedyuska, Trtiyaka and Chaturthaka are manifested because of the affliction of alternate Dhatu by the Dosha. [63–67]

Why does the fever spike in Trutiyaka and ChaturtakaJwara?

अधिशेते यथा भूमिं बीजं काले च रोहति|

अधिशेते तथा धातुं दोषः काले च कुप्यति||६८||

स वृद्धिं बल कालं च प्राप्य दोषस्तृतीयकम्|

चतुर्थकं च कुरुते प्रत्यनीक बल क्षयात्||६९||

As a seed in the soil waits for the right time to germinate, similarly, imbalanced Dosha remain inactive in the Dhatus till suitable time. When the Dosha gains strength in time and when the power of the inhibiting factors (immunity) is subsided, then Trutiyaka and Chaturthaka types of Jwara occur. [68–69]

Explanation for day gaps in Trutiyaka and ChaturthakaJwara:

कृत्वा वेगं गतबलाः स्वे स्वे स्थाने व्यवस्थिताः|

पुनर्विवृद्धाः स्वे काले ज्वरयन्ति नरं मलाः||७०||

The Doshas, after manifesting their aggravated signs and symptoms, lose their strength and get located in their respective places. At the appropriate time, they again get aggravated to afflict the person with fever. [70]

Trutiyaka type of Jwara is of three types as follows:

कफ पित्तात्रिकग्राही पृष्ठाद्वात कफात्मकः|

वात पित्ताच्छिरोग्राही त्रिविधः स्यात्तृतीयकः||७१||

चतुर्थको दर्शयति प्रभावं द्विविधं ज्वरः|

जङ्घाभ्यां श्लैष्मिकः पूर्वं शिरस्तोऽनिलसम्भवः||७२||

When manifested by the aggravation of

Trikagrahi – Kapha and Pitta, it afflicts the Trika (lumbo–sacral joint)

Prushtagrahi – Vata and Kapha, it afflicts the Prushta (back)

Shirograhi – Vata and Pitta, it afflicts the Shiras (head)

Similarly, Chaturthaka Jwara is of 2 types as follows, when manifested by the vitiation of

Kapha – afflicts the calf– region in the beginning.

Vata – afflicts the head in the beginning. [71–72]

विषम ज्वर एवान्यश्चतुर्थक विपर्ययः|

त्रिविधो धातुरेकैको द्विधातुस्थः करोति यम्||७३||

Another variety of Vishama Jwara (irregular or intermittent fever) is called Chaturthaka Viparayaya.

Each of the 3 Doshas viz. Vata, Pitta and Kapha cause this disease by afflicting 2 Dhatus viz., Asthi (bone) and Majja (bone marrow) [73]

Causative factor for Vishama Jwara:

प्रायशः सन्निपातेन दृष्टः पञ्च विधो ज्वरः|

सन्निपाते तु यो भूयान् स दोषः परिकीर्तितः||७४||

ऋत्वहोरात्रदोषाण मनसश्च बलाबलात्|

कालमर्थवशाच्चैव ज्वरस्तं तं प्रपद्यते||७५||

The 5 types of Jwara are caused by Sannipata (Simultaneous vitiation of all the 3 Doshas). However, the Dosha which is predominant among 3 is considered the causative factor. [74]

Manifestation of Jwara in a particular time happens because of the following factors:

Rutu – season

Ahoratra Dosha – variation of Doshas in day and night

Manasabalaabalat – mind's strength or weakness

Dhatugata Jwara: Features of Jwara when it afflicts individual Dhatus:

Rasa Dhatu Gata Jwara:

गुरुत्वं दैन्यमुद्वेगः सदनं छर्द्यरोचकौ|

रस स्थिते बहिस्तापः साङ्गमर्दो विजृम्भणम्||७६|||

Gurutva – heaviness,

Dainya – miserable feeling, being humbled by the effect of disease

Udvega – restlessness

Sadana – malaise, lack of strength
Chardi – Vomiting
Arochaka – anorexia
Bahistapa – warm body and extremities, increase in external body temperature
Angamarda – bodyache
Vijrumbhana – yawning

Rakta Dhatugata Jwara:
रक्तोष्णाः पिडकास्तृष्णा सरक्तं ष्ठीवनं मुहुः|
दाह राग भ्रम मद प्रलापा रक्त संस्थिते||७७||
Signs and symptoms manifested when the vitiated Doshas causing Jwara are located in the Rakta Dhatu (hemoglobin fraction of blood):
RaktaUshna – excess hotness of blood
Pidaka – Pimples
Trushna – Thirst
Sa RaktaSthivana – Frequent spitting of blood – hemoptysis
Daha –Burning sensation
Raga – redness
Bhrama – Giddiness
Mada – Intoxication and
Pralapa – Irrelevant talk

MamsagataJwara:
अन्तर्दाहः सतृण्मोहः सग्लानिः सृष्ट विट्कता|
दौर्गन्ध्यं गात्र विक्षेपो ज्वरे मांस स्थिते भवेत्||७८||
Signs and symptoms manifested when the vitiated Doshas causing Jwara are located in the Mamsa Dhatu (muscle tissue):
Antardaha – Burning sensation inside the body (in internal organs)
Trushna – Thirst
Sammoha – Unconsciousness
Glani – tiredness
SrushtaVitkata – Diarrhea
Daurgandhyam – Foul smell and strong movement of the limbs and the body
Gatra Vikshepa – body shivering

Medodhatugata Jwara:
स्वेदस्तीव्रा पिपासा च प्रलापो वम्यभीक्षणशः|
स्वगन्धस्यासहत्वं च मेदःस्थे ग्लान्यरोचकौ||७९||
Signs and symptoms manifested when the vitiated Doshas causing Jwara are located in the Medo Dhatu (fat tissue):
Teevra sweda – Excessive sweating
Pipasa – Thirst
Pralapa – Delirium
Vamana – Frequent vomiting
Swagandhasyāsahatvaṃ – Inability to tolerate the smell of one's own body
Glani – lassitude, debility
Arochaka – Anorexia

Asthidhatugata Jwara:

विरेक वमने चोभे सास्थिभेदं प्रकूजनम्|
विक्षेपणं च गात्राणां श्वासश्चास्थिगते ज्वरे||८०||

Signs and symptoms manifested when the vitiated Doshas causing Jwara are located in the Asthi Dhatu (bone tissue):

Vireka and Vamana – Both diarrhea and vomiting

Asthibheda – Pain in the bones

Prakujanam – Production of Kujana (cooing) sound

Gatra Vikshepa – Strong movement of the body and its limbs

Shwasa – difficulty in breathing

Majja Dhatugata Jwara:

हिक्का श्वासस्तथा कासस्तमसश्चातिदर्शनम्|
मर्मच्छेदो बहिः शैत्यं दाहोऽन्तश्चैव मज्जगे||८१||

Signs and symptoms manifested when the vitiated Doshas causing Jwara are located in the Majja Dhatu (bone marrow):

Hikka – Hiccup

Shwasa – Asthma, difficulty in breathing

Kasa – cough

Tama darshana – Frequently entering into the darkness, blindness,

Marmacheda – Pain in vital organs

Bahir shaityam – Cold extremities

Antardaha – Internal burning sensation

Shukra Dhatugata Jwara:

शुक्र स्थानगतः शुक्र मोक्षं कृत्वा विनाश्य च|
प्राणं वाय्वग्निसोमैश्च सार्धं गच्छत्यसौ विभुः||८२||

Signs and symptoms manifested when the vitiated Doshas causing Jwara are located in the Shukra Dhatu (semen including sperm & ovum):

Shukra Moksham – Ejaculation and

Shukra Vinasham – Destruction of Shukra (semen) resulting in the extinction of life along with Vayu, Agni and Soma of the subtle body (Sookshma Sharira)

Curability of Dhatu Jwara (fever afflicting body tissues):

रस रक्ताश्रितः साध्यो मेदो मांसगतश्च यः|
अस्थि मज्जगतः कृच्छः शुक्रस्थो नैव सिद्ध्यति||८३||

Fevers located in –

Rasa Rakta, Mamsa and Medas are Sadhya (curable)

Asthi and Majja are Kastasadhya (difficult to cure)

Shukra is Asadhya (incurable)

Eight types of Jwara based on Dosha:

Based on Dosha involvement, there are eight types of fever. Viz:

Vataja, Pittaja, Kaphaja,

Vata-Pittaja, Vata – Kaphaja, Pitta-Kaphaja

Sannipataja – Vata, Pitta and Kapha – all the three are involved.

Agantuja – fever due to external factors such as injury

Among these eight types of fever, Vataja, Pittaja, and Kaphaja fevers (caused by individual Doshas) are explained in detail in Jwara Nidana Chapter). The fever caused due to combination of Doshas is explained here –

Vata-Pittaja Jwara:

हेतुभिर्लक्षणैश्चोक्तः पूर्वमष्टविधो ज्वरः|

समासेनोपदिष्टस्य व्यासतः शृणु लक्षणम्||८४||

शिरो रुक् पर्वणां भेदो दाहो रोम्णां प्रहर्षणम्|

कण्ठास्य शोषो वमथुस्तृष्णा मूर्च्छा भ्रमोऽरुचिः||८५||

स्वप्न नाशोऽतिवाग्जृम्भा वातपित्त ज्वराकृतिः|

Fever that occurs due to vitiation of Vata and Kapha Dosha exhibits following symptoms:

Shiro ruk – Headache

Parvanambheda – breaking pain in fingers and toes

Daha – burning sensation

Romanam Praharshanam – horripilation

Kanthasyashosho – dryness of throat and mouth

Aruchi – anorexia

Swapna nasha – sleeplessness

AtiVak – excessive talk and

Vijrumbha – Yawning

Vata Kaphatmaka Jwara:

शीतको गौरवं तन्द्रा स्तैमित्यं पर्वणां च रुक्||८६||

शिरोग्रहः प्रतिश्यायः कासः स्वेदाप्रवर्तनम्|

सन्तापो मध्यवेगश्च वातश्लेष्मज्वराकृतिः||८७||

The signs and symptoms of Jwara caused by the vitiation of vata and kapha:

Sheeta – Feeling of cold

Gauravam – heaviness

Tandra – drowsiness

Staimityam – timidity, stiffness, as if covered by a wet cloth

Parvaṇām ruk – Pain in the joints of fingers and toes

Shiro graha – rigidity of head, stiffness

Pratishyāyaḥ – coryza, running nose

Kasa – cough

Asweda – absence of sweating and

Madhyavega Santapa – moderate rise in temperature

Kapha Pittaja Jwara:

मुहुर्दाहो मुहुः शीतं स्वेदस्तम्भो मुहुर्मुहुः|

मोहः कासोऽरुचिस्तृष्णा श्लेष्म पित्त प्रवर्तनम्||८८||

लिप्त तिक्तास्यता तन्द्रा श्लेष्म पित्त ज्वराकृतिः|

इत्येते द्वन्द्वजाः प्रोक्ताः ...|८९|

The signs and symptoms of the Jwara caused by the vitiation of Kapha and Pitta:

Muhurdāho muhuḥshitam – Frequent feeling of burning sensation and cold

Svedastambha Muhurmuhuḥ – repeated episodes of sweating and no-sweating

moha– unconsciousness

Kasa – cough

Aruchi – anorexia

Trushna – thirst

Shleṣma pitta pravartanam – elimination of phlegm and bile,

Liptatiktāsya – coated tongue and bitterness in the mouth

Tandra – drowsiness

Thus different type of fever (Jwara) caused by the simultaneous vitiation of 2 Doshas (Dvandvaja) are described {84–89}

Sannipata Jwara – due to imbalance of all the three Doshas:

... सन्निपातज उच्यते||८९||

सन्निपात ज्वरस्योर्ध्वं त्रयोदश विधस्य हि|

प्राक्सूत्रितस्य वक्ष्यामि लक्षणं वै पृथक् पृथक्||९०||

Based on individual Dosha strength, Sannipataja Jwara is of 13 types.

Manda Kapha Jwara:

भ्रमः पिपासा दाहश्च गौरवं शिरसोऽतिरुक्|

वातपित्तोल्बणे विद्याल्लिङ्गं मन्द कफे ज्वरे||९१||

Sannipata Jwara – all 3 Doshas are involved, but Kapha Dosha is mild in imbalance. Symptoms are –

Bhrama – Giddiness

Pipasa – thirst,

Dāha – burning sensation,

Gaurava – heaviness,

Shiras ati ruk – excessive headache

Manda Pitta Sannipata Jwara:

शैत्यं कासोऽरुचिस्तन्द्रा पिपासा दाहरुग्व्यथाः|

वात श्लेष्मोल्बणे व्याधौ लिङ्गं पित्तावरे विदुः||९२||

SannipataJwara in which vitiation of both Vayu and Kapha predominates over the vitiation of Pitta:

Shaityaṃ – Coldness

Kasa – cough

Aruchi – anorexia

Tandra – drowsiness

Pipasa – thirst

Daha – burning sensation

Vyatha – pain

Manda Vata Sannipata Jwara:

छर्दिः शैत्यं मुहु दाहस्तृष्णा मोहोऽस्थिवेदना|

मन्दवाते व्यवस्यन्ति लिङ्गं पित्त कफोल्बणे||९३||

The signs and symptoms of sannipata Jwara in which the vitiation of Pitta and Kapha predominates over the vitiation of Vata:

Chardi – Emesis

Shaityam – coldness

Muhurdaha – frequent burning sensation

Trishna – thirst

Moha – unconsciousness and

Asthi vedana– pain in the bones

Vatolbana Sannipata Jwara – When Vata is dominant than Pitta and Kapha:

सन्ध्यस्थिशिरसः शूलं प्रलापो गौरवं भ्रमः|

वातोल्बणे स्याद् द्रव्यनुगे तृष्णा कण्ठास्य शुष्कता||९४||

Sandhishoola – joint pain

Asthishoola – bone pain

Shiroshoola – headache

Pralapa – irrelevant talk

Gaurava – heaviness

Bhrama – dizziness, psychosis

Trushna – Excessive thirst

Kanthashosha – dry throat

Asyashosha – dry mouth

Pittolbana Sannipata Jwara: When Pitta dominates other Doshas in Sannipata Jwara:

रक्त विण्मूत्रता दाहः स्वेदस्तृड् बलसङ्क्षयः|

मूर्च्छा चेति त्रिदोषे स्याल्लिङ्गं पित्ते गरीयसि||९५||

Raktavit – blood in stools

Raktamootrata – blood in urine

Daha – Burning sensation

Sveda – excess sweating

Trut – excess thirst

Balakshaya – depleted strength and immunity

Murcha – unconsciousness, fainting

Kapholbana Sannipata Jwara - When Kapha dominates other Doshas in Sannipata Jwara:

आलस्यारुचि हुल्लास दाहवम्यरतिभ्रमैः|

कफोल्बणं सन्निपातं तन्द्रा कासेन चादिशेत्||९६||

Alasya – laziness, lethargy

Aruchi – Anorexia, lack of interest in food

Hrullasa – nausea

Daha – Burning sensation

Vami – vomiting

Arati – lack of interest

Bhrama – dizziness, psychosis

Tandra – drowsiness

Kasa – cold, cough

Heena Vata Madhya Pitta ShleshmaAdhika:

प्रतिश्या छर्दिरालस्यं तन्द्राऽरुच्यग्निमार्दवम्|

हीन वाते पित्त मध्ये लिङ्गं श्लेष्माधिके मतम्||९७||

In Sannipata Jwara, where Vata is mild, Pitta is moderately dominant and Kapha is very dominant, it produces below symptoms:

Pratishyaya – Running nose, coryza

Chardi – vomiting

Alasya – laziness, lethargy

Tandra – drowsiness, weakness in sense organs

Aruchi – Anorexia, lack of interest in food

Agnimardava – weak digestion strength

Heena Vata, Madhya Kapha Pitta Adhika Sannipata Jwara:

हारिद्र मूत्र नेत्रत्वं दाहस्तृष्णा भ्रमोऽरुचिः|
हीनवाते मध्यकफे लिङ्गं पित्ताधिके मतम्||९८||

In Sannipata Jwara, where Vata is mildly dominant, Kapha is moderate and Pitta is highly dominant, it produces below symptoms.

Haridramutra – Excessive yellow colored urine

Haridranetra – Yellow sclera (eyes)

Daha – Burning sensation

Trushna – Excessive thirst

Bhrama – dizziness, psychosis

Aruchi – Anorexia, lack of interest in food

Heenapitta Madhyakapha Maruta Adhika:

शिरोरुग्वेपथुः श्वासः प्रलापश्छर्द्यरोचकौ|
हीनपित्ते मध्यकफे लिङ्गं स्यान्मारुताधिके||९९||

In Sannipat Jvara, where Pitta is mildly dominant, Kapha is moderate and Vata is high, it produces below symptoms –

Shiroruk – headache

Vepathu – trembling, quivering

Shwasa – asthma, respiratory disorders involving difficulty in breathing

Pralapa – irrelevant talk, delirium

Chardi – vomiting

Arochaka – anorexia, lack of interest in food

Heena Pitta Vata Madhya ShleshmaAdhika:

शीतको गौरवं तन्द्रा प्रलापोऽस्थिशिरोऽतिरुक्|
हीनपित्ते वातमध्ये लिङ्गं श्लेष्माधिके विदुः||१००||

In SannipataJwara, where Pitta is mild, Vata is moderate and Kapha is high –

Sheetaka – feeling cold

Gaurava – heaviness

Tandra – drowsiness, weakness in sense organs

Pralapa – irrelevant talk, delirium

Asthiruk – bone pain

Shiroruk – headache

Heena Kapha, Pitta Madhya, Vata Adhika –

श्वासः कासः प्रतिश्यायो मुखशोषोऽतिपार्श्वरुक्|
कफहीने पित्तमध्ये लिङ्गं वाताधिके मतम्||१०१||

In SannipataK Jwara, where Kapha is mild, Pitta is moderate and Vata is aggressive –

Shwasa – asthma, respiratory disorders involving difficulty in breathing

Kasa – cold, cough

Pratishyaya – Running nose, coryza

Mukhashosha – dry mouth

Ati Parshwa ruk – severe pain in flanks

Heenakapha Madhya Vata Pitta Adhika –

वर्चोभेदोऽग्निनदौर्बल्यं तृष्णा दाहोऽरुचिर्भ्रमः|

कफ हीने वातमध्ये लिङ्गं पित्ताधिके विदुः||१०२||

In SannipataJwara where Kapha is mild, Vata is moderate and Pitta is high –

Varchabheda –Diarrhea

Agnidaurbalyaṃ – loss in the power of digestion

Tṛṣṇā – thirst

Daha – burning sensation,

Aruchi – anorexia and

Bhrama – giddiness

Sannipata Jwara with all the Three Doshas are equally dominant:

सन्निपातज्वरस्योर्ध्वमतो वक्ष्यामि लक्षणम्|

क्षणे दाहः क्षणे शीतमस्थिसन्धिशिरोरुजा||१०३||

सास्रावे कलुषे रक्ते निर्भुग्ने चापि दर्शने |

सस्वनौ सरुजौ कर्णौ कण्ठः शूकैरिवावृतः||१०४||

तन्द्रा मोहः प्रलापश्च कासः श्वासोऽरुचिर्भ्रमः|

परिदग्धा खर स्पर्शा जिह्वा सस्ताङ्गता परम्||१०५||

ष्ठीवनं रक्तपितस्य कफेनोन्मिश्रितस्य च|

शिरसो लोठनं तृष्णा निद्रानाशो हृदि व्यथा||१०६||

स्वेद मूत्र पुरीषाणां चिराद्दर्शनमल्पशः|

कृशत्वं नातिगात्राणां प्रततं कण्ठकूजनम्||१०७||

कोठानां श्याव रक्तानां मण्डलानां च दर्शनम्|

मूकत्वं स्रोतसां पाको गुरुत्वमुदरस्य च||१०८||

चिरात् पाकश्च दोषाणां सन्निपात ज्वराकृतिः||१०९|

In the Sannipata Jwara in which all the three Doshas are simultaneously vitiated in a similar manner, the signs and symptoms are as follows:

1. Kshaṇedāhaḥ kṣaṇeśītam – The patient at times has burning sensation and at times feels cold.

2. Asthi sandhi śirorujā– Pain in bones, joints and head.

3. Sāsrāve kaluṣhe rakte nirbhugne cha api darśane – excessive lacrimation and eyes will be cloudy and red. The eye balls are wrinkled.

4. Sasvanau sarujau karṇau – There will be sound (tinnitus) and pain in the ears.

5. Kaṇṭhaḥ shukaiivaavruta – The throat will feel as if covered with sharp edged bristles.

6. Tandrā mohaḥ pralāpascha kāsaḥ śvāso'rucir bhramaḥ – There will be drowsiness, unconsciousness, delirium, cough, asthma, anorexia and giddiness.

7. Paridagdhā kharasparśājihvā – The tongue will appear as if burnt (black) and the tongue will be rough to touch.

8. Sṭhīvanaṃ – There will be expectoration

9. Raktapittasya kaphenonmiśrita – Spitting of blood and bile mixed with phlegm

10. Shirasoloṭhanaṃ tṛṣṇā nidrānāśo hṛdivyathā – The patient will move here and there, there will be thirst, sleeplessness and pain in the cardiac region

11. Sveda mūtrapurīṣāṇām chiratdarśhanam alpaśaḥ – Sweet, urine and stool will appear very late and they will be in small quantity.

12. Kṛśatvaṃ nātigātrāṇām – The body will not be emaciated in excess.

13. Kaṇṭha kūjanam–rumbling sound from the throat.

14. Koṭhānāṃ śyāvaraktānām maṇḍalānām ca darśanam – In the skin, urticaria and patches heaving bluish–black and red color will appear.

15. Mūkatvaṃ srotasāmp āko –The patient will be dumb (absence of speech or difficulty in speech) and there will be inflammation of the channels of circulation.

16. Udara gurutvam – There will be heaviness in the abdomen.

17. The Doshas will undergo Paka (metabolic transformation) after a long time. [89–109]

Incurability of Sannipata Jwara:

दोषे विबद्धे नष्टेऽग्नौ सर्व सम्पूर्ण लक्षणः||१०९||

सन्निपात ज्वरोऽसाध्यः कृच्छ्रसाध्यस्त्वतोऽन्यथा|११०|

If there is obstruction or non–elimination of imbalanced Doshas, if the Agni (enzymes which are responsible for digestion and metabolism) are completely destroyed and if all the signs and symptoms are fully manifested, then Sannipata Jwara is incurable; otherwise it is difficult of cure. [109– 110]

निदाने त्रिविधा प्रोक्ता या पृथग्जज्वराकृतिः||११०||

संसर्ग सन्निपातानां तया चोक्तं स्व लक्षणम्|१११|

In the Nidana section, the signs and symptoms of Jwaras caused individually by Vata Pitta and Kapha are described separately. From these signs and symptoms, those of the Dvandvaja types (where 2 Doshas are simultaneously vitiated) and of the Sannipata type (where all the 3 Doshas are simultaneously vitiated) are determined. [110–111]

Agantuja Jwara – Fever by Exogenic factors:

आगन्तुरष्टमो यस्तु स निर्दिष्टश्चतुर्विधः||१११||

अभिघाताभिषङ्गाभ्यामभिचाराभिशापतः|

Agantuj (which is caused by external factors) is the 8th type of Jwara. AgantuJwara is of 4 varieties Viz,

Abhighataja – due to external injury

Abhishangaja – due to excess lust, anger, grief, poison, etc

Abhicharaja – Due to evil tantric rituals

Abhishapaja – due to Shapa (curse) of elderly

Abhighataja Jwara – Due to injury:

शस्त्र लोष्टक शाकाष्ठमुष्ट्यरत्निलदिवजैः||११२||

तद्विधैश्च हते गात्रे ज्वरःस्यादभिघातजः|

तत्राभिघातजे वायुः प्रायो रक्तं प्रदूषयन्||११३||

सव्यथा शोफ वैवर्ण्य करोति सरुजं ज्वरम्|११४|

(1) Abhighataja – The Jwara caused by the injury of

Shastra – weapons,

Loshtaka – stone, hunter,

Shaka – wood,

Mushti – fist, sole of the palm, teeth and such other factors.

By this injury, Vata vitiates blood resulting in pain, swelling, discoloration and painful fever.

(2) Abhisangaja – The Jwara caused by the affliction of passion, grief, fear, anger and evil spirits including germs.

काम शोक भय क्रोधैरभिषक्तस्य यो ज्वरः||११४||

सोऽभिषङ्गाज्वरो ज्ञेयो यश्च भूताभिषङ्गजः|

काम शोकभयाद्वायुः, क्रोधात् पित्तं, त्रयो मलाः||११५||

भूताभिषङ्गात् कुप्यन्ति भूत सामान्य लक्षणाः|

भूताधिकारे व्याख्यातं तदष्टविध लक्षणम्||११६||

विष वृक्षानिल स्पर्शात्तथाऽन्यैर्विष सम्भवैः|

अभिषक्तस्य चाप्याहुर्ज्वरमेकेऽभिषङ्गजम्||११७||

चिकित्सया विषघ्न्यैव स शमं लभते नरः|

Abhishangajajwara occurs due to –
Kama – lust
Shoka – grief
Bhaya – fear
Krodha – anger,
Bhuta – evil spirits, microorganisms
Visha – toxins
Due to lust, grief and fear, Vata increases. Due to anger, Pitta aggravates, due to Bhuta (evil spirits / microbes), all the Three Doshas aggravate.
Vishaja Abhishangaja Jwara can occur due to touch or consumption of toxic plants, toxic air, and toxic animals.
(3) Abhicharja – The Jwara caused by the contact of the poisonous air of the toxic plants and such other toxins. This type of Jwara gets cured by the administration of antidotes of these poisons.

Abhicharaja and Abhishapaja Jwara:
अभिचाराभिशापाभ्यां सिद्धानां यः प्रवर्तते||११८||
सन्निपात ज्वरो घोरः स विज्ञेयः सुदुःसहः|
सन्निपात ज्वरस्योक्तं लिङ्गं यत्तस्य तत् स्मृतम्||११९||
चित्तोन्द्रिय शरीराणामर्तयोऽन्याश्च नैकशः|
प्रयोगं त्वभिचारस्य दृष्ट्वा शापस्य चैव हि||१२०||
स्वयं श्रुत्वाऽनुमानेन लक्ष्यते प्रशमेन वा|
वैविध्यादभिचारस्य शापस्य च तदात्मके||१२१||
Abhicharaja fever occurs due to evil deeds and evil tantric rituals. It has Sannipata (aggravation of all the three Doshas).
Abhishapaja is cursed. It has Sannipata (aggravation of all the three Doshas).
In both the above types, all the features of Sannipata Jwara can be appreciated. Mind, senses, organs and body are affected.
Several signs and symptoms caused by the affliction of mind, sense organs and body are also manifested. Abhicaraja and Abhisapaja types of Jwara can be determined from the following:
1. By the direct observation of the performance of evil tantric ritual (Abhicara) and curse (Abhishapa)
2. By hearing from others about it
3. By inference (Anumana) and
4. By the alleviation of Jwara after counteracting their effects.

Different types of Abhishangaja Jwara:
यथा कर्म प्रयोगेण लक्षणं स्यात् पृथग्विधम्|
ध्यान निःश्वास बहुलं लिङ्गं काम ज्वरे स्मृतम्||१२२||
शोकजे बाष्प बहुलं त्रास प्रायं भय ज्वरे|
क्रोधजे बहु संरम्भं भूतावेशे त्वमानुषम्||१२३||
मूर्च्छा मोह मद ग्लानि भूयिष्ठं विष सम्भवे|
केषाञ्चिदेषां लिङ्गानां सन्तापो जायते पुरः||१२४||
पश्चात्तुल्यं तु केषाञ्चिदेषु काम ज्वरादिषु|
कामादिजानामुद्दिष्टं ज्वराणां यद्विशेषणम्||१२५||
कामादिजानां रोगाणामन्येषामपि तत् स्मृतम्|
मनस्यभिहते पूर्वं कामाद्यैर्न तथा बलम्||१२६||
ज्वरः प्राप्नोति वाताद्यैर्देहो यावन्न दूष्यति|
देहे चाभिह(द्रु)ते पूर्वं वाताद्यैर्न तथा बलम्||१२७||

ज्वरः प्राप्नोति कामाद्यैर्मनो यावन्न दूष्यति|१२८|

In Kama AbhishangajaJwara, due to excess lust, patient will have

Dhyana – excessive thoughts, restless

Nishwasa – excess breathing

In Shoka Abhishangaja Jwara, due to grief, crying spells are seen.

In Bhaya Jwara, due to fever, excess tiredness is seen

In Krodhaja Jwara, Pitta symptoms such as redness of face is seen.

In Bhuta Jwara – due to evil spirits /microbes, varied symptoms are observed.

In VishaJwara –

Murcha – unconsciousness, Moha – confusion

Mada – intoxication

Glani – excess tiredness of sense organs are seen.

In some of these Jwaras, they appear first and then the signs and symptoms of Kama (passion) etc. are manifested, and in others, it happens the other way.

The specific features of Kama (passion) etc. described in the present context of Jwara are also manifested in other diseases (like Unmada or insanity) caused by these factors.

In Kama Jwara etc. the mind is first afflicted by passion etc. but Jwara does not gain strength till such time as the Doshas viz, Vayu etc of the body are not vitiated. Similarly, vitiation of Vayu etc. in the body does not gain power for the production of Jwara till such time as the mind is not afflicted by Kama (passion) etc. [114–128]

ते पूर्वं केवलाः पश्चान्निजैर्व्यामिश्रलक्षणाः||१२८||

हेत्वौषध विशिष्टाश्च भवन्त्यागन्तवो ज्वराः|१२९|

The AgantujaJwaras caused by external factors are in the beginning independent; manifest individual independent signs and symptoms based on cause (fear, anger etc).

Subsequently, they get mixed up with the signs and symptoms of Nija (endogenous) types of Jwara. However, these Agantu Jwaras have their own specific etiological factors and medicines. [128–129]

Jwara Samprapti – Pathogenesis in general:

संसृष्टाः सन्निपतिताः पृथग्वा कुपिता मलाः||१२९||

रसाख्यं धातुमन्वेत्य पक्तिं स्थानान्निरस्य च|

स्वेन तेनोष्मण चैव कृत्वा देहोष्मणो बलम्||१३०||

स्रोतांसि रुद्ध्वा सम्प्राप्ताः केवलं देहमुल्बणाः|

सन्तापमधिकं देहे जनयन्ति नरस्तदा||१३१||

भवत्यत्युष्णसर्वाङ्गो ज्वरितस्तेन चोच्यते|१३२|

The aggravated Doshas – Vata, Pitta and Kapha– either individually or in the combinations of two (samsrushta) or all the 3 Doshas (Sannipata) spread through the Rasa Dhatu and dislodge the Jatharagni (digestive fire present in stomach) from its own place. Being supplemented with their own heat and the heat of the Jatharagni, the heat of the body gets increased. Due to this, the body channels (Srotas) get obstructed by the imbalanced Doshas. This leads to further increase in the internal temperature. Thus Jwara manifests with increase in body temperature as its unique sign. [129–132]

Why is there no sweating in the initial stages of fever?

स्रोतसां सन्निरुद्धत्वात् स्वेदं ना नाधिगच्छति||१३२||

स्वस्थानात् प्रच्युते चाग्नौ प्रायशस्तरुणेज्वरे|१३३|

Generally a person suffering from Taruna Jwara (first stage of Jwara), does not sweat because of the obstruction to the channels of circulation and the displacement of the Agni (fire). [132–133]

Ama Jwara and Pachyamana Jwara – Stages of fever:

Ama and Pachyamana are the two stages of fever. In the Ama stage, the digestion strength is very low and it produces Ama – (altered digestion and metabolism).

During the Pachyamana stage of Jwara, the Ama slowly starts weaking leading to improved digestion strength.

Ama Jwara – Ama stage of fever:

अरुचिश्चाविपाकश्च गुरुत्वमुदरस्य च||१३३||

हृदयस्याविशुद्धिश्च तन्द्रा चालस्यमेव च|

ज्वरोऽविसर्गी बलवान् दोषाणामप्रवर्तनम्||१३४||

लालाप्रसेको हुल्लासः क्षुन्नाशो विरसं मुखम्|

स्तब्ध सुप्त गुरुवं च गात्राणां बहुमूत्रता||१३५||

न विड् जीर्णा न च ग्लानिर्ज्वरस्यामस्य लक्षणम्|

Aruchi – Anorexia, lack of interest in food

Avipaka – Altered metabolism

Udara gurutva – heaviness of stomach

Hrudaya Avishuddhi – lack of clarity and purity at heart

Tandra – drowsiness, weakness in sense organs

Alasya – laziness, lethargy

Avisargi, Balavaan – fever has good strength, there is no decrease of temperature

Doshanam Apravartanam – The doshas do not get eliminated out of body

Lala Praseka – excess salivation

Hrullasa – nausea

KshutNasha – absence of hunger

VirsaMukha – tastelessness in the mouth

Stabda – body stiffness

Supta – numbness

Gurugatrata – heaviness

Bahu mutrata – Excessive urination

Na vit – ill formed feces or no feces

Jeernana cha – abscess of digestion process

Glani – debility, fatigue

Pachyamana Jwara Lakshana:

ज्वर वेगोऽधिकस्तृष्णा प्रलापः श्वसनं भ्रमः||१३६||

मलप्रवृत्तिरुत्क्लेशः पच्यमानस्य लक्षणम्|१३७|

The signs and symptoms of Pacyamana stage of Jwara:

Once the Jwara gets past the Ama stage,

Adhika Jwara Vega – Excessive fever

Trushna – thirst

Pralapa – delirium, irrelevant talk

Shwasa – dyspnoea

Bhrama – giddiness

Mala and Shleshma pravrutthi –elimination of feces as well as Phlegm [133–137]

Nirama Jwara Lakshana – Stage of fever when Ama subsides:

क्षुत् क्षामता लघुत्वं च गात्राणां ज्वर मार्दवम्||१३७||

दोषप्रवृत्तिरष्टाहो निरामज्वरलक्षणम्|१३८|

Ksut kshamata – Appearance of the appetite,

Gatra laghutvam – lightness of the body,

Jwara mardavam – reduction in temperature,

Dosha Pravritti – elimination of Doshas along with waste products from the body [137–138]

Avoid these things during fever of recent origin – Navajware Apathya:

नवज्वरे दिवास्वप्न स्नानाभ्यङ्गान्न मैथुनम्||१३८||

क्रोध प्रवात व्यायामान् कषायांश्च विवर्जयेत्|१३९|

During Nava Jwara (first stage of Jwara), one should avoid

Divaswapna – Sleep during day time

Snana – bath,

Abhyanga – massage

Guru Anna – heavy food

Maithuna – sexual intercourse

Krodha – anger

Pravata – exposure to wind,

Vyayama – exercise and

Kashaya – medicines having astringent taste. [138–139]

Langhana or fasting:

ज्वरे लङ्घनमेवादावुपदिष्टमृते ज्वरात्||१३९||

क्षयानिल भय क्रोध काम शोकश्रमोद्भवात्|१४०|

In the first stage of Jwara, Langhana or fasting is prescribed.

It is however, not indicated in the Jwaras caused by Kshaya (depletion of body tissue), aggravation of Vayu, due to fear, anger, lust, grief and physical exertion. [139–140]

Effects of Langhana:

लङ्घनेन क्षयं नीते दोषे सन्धुक्षितेऽनले||१४०||

विज्वरत्वं लघुत्वं च क्षुच्चैवास्योपजायते |

प्राणाविरोधिना चैनं लङ्घनेनोपपादयेत्||१४१||

बलाधिष्ठानमारोग्यं यदर्थोऽयं क्रियाक्रमः|१४२|

Langhana (fasting) alleviates the aggravated Doshas and stimulates the Agni (power of digestion). As a result of this, Jwara subsides, the body becomes light and there is appetite.

Langhana is prescribed to the extent that it does not go against physical strength (Prana Avirodhi). The aim of all therapeutic measures is to maintain the strength of the body by which the patient becomes free from the disease. [140–141]

Nava Jwara Chikitsa:

लङ्घनं स्वेदनं कालो यवाग्वस्तिक्तको रसः||१४२||

पाचनान्य विपक्वानां दोषाणां तरुणे ज्वरे|१४३|

Langhana (fasting),

Svedana (fomentation), Kala (time or passage of eight day),

Yavagu (medicated gruels) with Tikta rasa (medicines having bitter taste) – these help in the Pachana (metabolic transformation) of Avipakva Doshas in Taruna Jwara (first stage of fever). [142–143]

Administering hot water to the patient:

तृष्यते सलिलं चोष्णं दद्याद्वातकफज्वरे ||१४३||

मद्योत्थे पैतिके चाथ शीतलं तिक्तकैः शृतम्|

दीपनं पाचनं चैव ज्वरघ्नमुभयं हि तत्||१४४||
स्रोतसां शोधनं बल्यं रुचिस्वेदकरं शिवम्|१४५|

If a Jwara patient feels thirsty, then hot water is given if the Jwara is due to Vata or Kapha, or Vata and Kapha simultaneously aggravated.

If the thirst occurs because of Paittik Jwara or as a result of the intake of alcohol, then cold water is given to drink. This cold water should, however, be boiled with bitter medicines.

Both the hot water and cold water (boiled with bitter medicines) are Dipana (digestive stimulant), Pachana (carminative) and alleviator of Jwara.

Srotasam Shodhana – They help in the cleansing of the channels of circulation. Balya – They promote strength,

Ruchikara – increase appetite,

Swedakara – promote sweating and

Shivam – auspiciousness. [143–145]

Shadang Paniya:

मुस्त पर्पटकोशीर चन्दनोदीच्य नागरैः||१४५||
शृत शीतं जलं दद्यात् पिपासा ज्वर शान्तये|१४६|

For the alleviation of thirst and Jwara, the patient is given water boiled with –

Musta (Cyperus rotundus)

Parpataka – Fumaria parviflora

Ushira – Vetiver – Vetiveria zizanioides,

Chandana (Sandalwood – Santalum album),

Udichya – Pavonia odorata;

Nagara- ginger

After boiling, the water is cooled before administration [145– 146]

Vamana treatment for Jwara:

कफ प्रधानानुत्क्लिष्टान् दोषानामाशय स्थितान्||१४६||
बुद्ध्वा ज्वरकरान् काले वम्यानां वमनैर्हरेत्|१४७|

If the Jwara is dominated by Kapha and if it is located in the Amasaya (stomach and small intestine), is in a stage of Utklesa (detached or about to come out), then it is removed by administration of emetics – Vamana.

The state of Kapha is carefully ascertained before the administration of Vamana. [146–147]

Adverse effects of Emetic therapy – Akale Vamana PrayogaPhala:

अनुपस्थित दोषाणां वमनं तरुणे ज्वरे||१४७||
हृद्रोगं श्वासमानाहं मोहं च जनयेद्भृशम्|
सर्व देहानुगाः सामा धातुस्था असुनिर्हराः ||१४८||
दोषाः फलानामामानां स्वरसा इव सात्यया:|१४९|

If in Taruna (first stage) Jwara, Emetic therapy is administered to a patient in whom the Doshas have not reached the above–mentioned state, then it causes

Hrdrogam – acute heart disease,

Shwasa – Asthma,

Anaha – obstruction in the movement of flatus, and feces in the intestine and colon and

Moha – unconsciousness

Simily: As it is difficult, rather impossible, to take out juice from an unripe fruit, similarly, it is extremely difficult to take out the Ama Dosha pervading all over the body from out of the Dhatus in which they are located. It is likely to cause serious complications. [147–149]

Yavagu and Manda Pana in Jwara:

वमितं लङ्घितं काले यवागूभिरुपाचरेत्||१४९||

यथास्वौषधसिद्धाभिर्मण्डपूर्वाभिरादितः|

यावज्ज्वरमृदूभावात् षडहं वा विचक्षणः||१५०||

तस्याग्निर्दीप्यते ताभिः समिद्भिरिव पावकः|

ताश्च भेषजसंयोगाल्लघुत्वाच्चाग्निदीपनाः||१५१||

वात मूत्र पुरीषाणां दोषाणां चानुलोमनाः|

स्वेदनाय द्रवोष्णत्वाद्द्रवत्वात्तृट्प्रशान्तये||१५२||

आहारभावात् प्राणाय सरत्वाल्लाघवाय च|

ज्वरघ्नो ज्वरसात्म्यत्वात्तस्मात् पेयाभिरादितः||१५३||

ज्वरानुपचरेद्धीमानृते मद्य समुत्थितात्|

मदात्यये मद्यनित्ये ग्रीष्मे पित्त कफाधिके||१५४||

ऊर्ध्वगे रक्तपित्ते च यवागूर्न हिता ज्वरे|१५५|

Administration of Yavagu (gruel) and Manda (thin gruel) –

After the patient has been administered with Vamana treatment, the patient is made to fast. Then Yavagu prepared with Shadanga Paneeya herbs (Musta, Parpata, Usheera, Chandana, Udeechya and Nagara) is administered at an appropriate time.

Before administering Yavagu, the patient is given Manda (extremely thin rice gruel). Yavagu and Manda are administered for 6 days or till fever subsides.

As the fire becomes more inflamed by the addition of fuel (Samit), similarly by the administration of gruels, the digestive fire becomes stimulated. These gruels are light for digestion.They help in Anulomana (elimination through downward track) of flatus, urine, feces and Doshas.

Because they are liquid and hot they cause sweating.

Because they are watery in nature, they alleviate thirst.

They sustain Prana (vital force of life) because of their nourishing properties. Because of their laxative property they bring about lightness to the body.

They are wholesome for Jwara.

In view of the above, to a patient suffering from Jwara the wise should administer, in the beginning, with different types of Peya (thin gruel).

Gruel, however, is contra-indicated in fever caused by the intake of alcohol, in summer season, when there is predominance of Pitta and Kapha and in Urdhvaga Rakta Pitta (a disease characterized by bleeding from different upper body channels). [149–155]

Tarpana Chikitsa for Jwara:

तत्र तर्पणमेवाग्रे प्रयोज्यं लाज सक्तुभिः||१५५||

ज्वरापहैः फल रसैर्युक्तं समधु शर्करम्|१५६|

In such cases where administration of Yavagu is prohibited (In high Pitta, in alcoholics etc), the physician should administer in the beginning tarpana prepared of the Laja Saktu (power of field paddy) mixed with honey, sugar and juices which have properties alleviate the Jwara. [155–156]

Procedure to be followed after Tarpana treatment:

ततः सात्म्यबलापेक्षी भोजयेज्जीर्णतर्पणम्||१५६||

तनुना मुद्गयूषेण जाङ्गलानां रसेन वा|

अन्नकालेषु चाप्यस्मै विधेयं दन्तधावनम्||१५७||

योऽस्य वक्त्ररसस्तस्मादिवपरीतं प्रियं च यत्|

तदस्य मुखवैशद्यं प्रकाङ्क्षां चान्नपानयोः||१५८||

धत्ते रसविशेषाणामभिज्ञत्वं करोति यत्|
विशोध्य द्रुमशाखाग्रैरास्यं प्रक्षाल्य चासकृत्||१५९||
मस्तिवक्षुरसमद्याद्यैर्यथाहारमवाप्नुयात्|१६०|

Post Tarpana procedure:

After the Tarpana is digested, depending upon the wholesomeness and strength of the patient, he is given Mudgayusha – green gram thin soup or meat soup of wild animals (Jangala mamsarasa). Before giving food, the patient's teeth are cleared with the twigs of plants. Such plants whose taste can counteract the taste of the mouth of the patient, and which would be relishing, are selected for this purpose.

Importance of cleaning teeth – Danta Dhawana

By the cleaning of teeth with the help of twigs, the patient feels freshness in the mouth and appetite for diet and drinks. He becomes capable of appreciating the taste of the food to be taken. After cleaning the teeth with the twigs of the plants, the mouth is cleaned with water several times. Therefore, he is given Mastu (thin buttermilk) juice of sugarcane, alcoholic drinks etc, along with an appropriate diet. [156– 160]

Administration for Kashaya:

पाचनं शमनीयं वा कषायं पाययेद्विभषक्||१६०||
ज्वरितं षड्दहेऽतीते लघ्वन्नप्रतिभोजितम्|१६१|

After the 6th day, having light diet to eat, the patient is administered decoctions which are either Pachana (stimulant of digestion) or Shamana (alleviator of Doshas) [160– 161]

Adverse effects of astringent Kashaya in TarunaJwara:

स्तभ्यन्ते न विपच्यन्ते कुर्वन्ति विषम ज्वरम्||१६१||
दोषा बद्धाः कषायेण स्तम्भित्वातरुणे ज्वरे|
न तु कल्पनमुद्दिश्य कषायः प्रतिषिध्यते||१६२||
यः कषायकषायः स्यात् स वर्ज्यस्तरुणज्वरे|१६३|

If astringent decoctions are administered in Taruna (first stage of) Jwara, before the 6th day, then, the Doshas get adhered because of stickiness, and do not undergo Paka. This leads to the onset of Vishama Jwara – fever (irregular fever).

The former is not prohibited, but the decoction having astringent taste, is prohibited in Taruna (first stage of Jwara – fever [161– 163]

Administration of light Diet:

यूषैरम्लैरनम्लैर्वा जाङ्गलैर्वा रसैर्हितैः||१६३||
दशाहं यावदशनीयाल्लघ्वन्नं ज्वरशान्तये|१६४|

For the alleviation of Jwara – fever, up to the 10th day the patient is given light foods along with Yusha (soup) prepared of vegetables and Pulses and mamsarasa (meat soup) of animals dwelling in the forests (Jangala Mamsarasa). These Yushas and Rasas may or may not be added with sour things. [163– 164]

Administration of Ghee:

अत ऊर्ध्वं कफे मन्दे वात पित्तोतरे ज्वरे||१६४||
परिपक्वेषु दोषेषु सर्पिष्पानं यथाऽमृतम्|१६५|

Thereafter, Ghee is administered when there is less Kapha aggravation with dominant Vata and Pitta Doshas. Ghee should only be adminstered after fever has crossed pachyamana stage (as explained above).

Contribution of ghee and administration of Meat soup:

निर्देशाहमपि ज्ञात्वा कफोतरमलङ्घितम्||१६५||
न सर्पिः पाययेद्वैद्यः कषायैस्तमुपाचरेत्|

यावल्लघुत्वादशनं दद्यान्मांसरसेन च||१६६||
बलं ह्यलं निग्रहाय दोषाणां, बलकृच्च तत्|१६७|

Ghee should not be administered

if the patient has Kapha dominance and

if the Langhana (lightning) treatment is not appreciated even after the 10th day of fever. To such a patient, Kashaya (decoction) is given till the body becomes light.

The food in such cases is Mamsa Rasa (meat soup) because it promotes strength, which is capable of inhibiting the Doshas. [165–167]

Administration of Milk:

दाह तृष्णा परीतस्य वात पित्तोत्तरं ज्वरम्||१६७||
बद्धप्रच्युतदोषं वा निरामं पयसा जयेत्|१६८|

When there is an excess of burning sensation and thirst.

When the Jwara is dominated by Vata and Pitta Dosha and

When the Doshas are either Badhha (Adhered), or Pracyuta (slightly dislodged), or

when there is Nirama stage (Pachyamana or Vipakwa stage of Jwara) – in these conditions, milk can be administered. [167–168]

Administration of Virechana – Purgation treatment:

क्रियाभिरभिः प्रशमं न प्रयाति यदा ज्वरः||१६८||
अक्षीण बल मांसाग्नेः शमयेत्तं विरेचनैः|१६९|

When the fever does not subside by the therapies described earlier, then,

If the patient has good Bala (immunity), Mamsa (muscle strength) and Agni (digestion strength), then Virechana can be administered. [168–169]

Administration of Milk and Niruha Basti:

ज्वर क्षीणस्य न हितं वमनं न विरेचनम्||१६९||
कामं तु पयसा तस्य निरूहैर्वा हरेन्मलान्|
निरूहो बलमग्निं च विज्वरत्वं मुदं रुचिम्||१७०||
परिपक्वेषु दोषेषु प्रयुक्तः शीघ्रमावहेत्|१७१|

For patients who are severely emaciated by fever, neither Vamana (emesis) nor Virechana is useful. Therefore, it is desirable to remove Malas (waste products) of this patient by the oral administration of milk or Niruha Basti (herbal decoction enema).

If Niruha is administered to a patient when Doshas are in the stage of Paripakva (well cooked), it immediately promotes strength & the power of digestion, alleviates fever and causes happiness as well as relish for food. [169–171]

Importance of Sramsana& Basti:

पित्तं वा कफपित्तं वा पित्ताशयगतं हरेत्||१७१||
संसनं त्रीन्मलान् बस्तिर्हरेत् पक्वाशय स्थितान्|१७२|

Sramsana (Purgation) eliminates either Pitta or Kapha or both of them from the pittashaya (lower stomach and small intestine). Basti eliminates all the 3 Doshas lodged in the Pakvsaya (Colon). [171–172]

Administration of Anuvasana:

ज्वरे पुराणे सङ्क्षीणे कफपित्ते दृढाग्नये||१७२||
रूक्षबद्धपुरीषाय प्रदद्यादनुवासनम्|१७३|

In chronic fever, Anuvasana (oil / fat of enema) is given in the following conditions:

When Kapha & Pitta are alleviated

When there is strong digestion strength

When there is constipation or dry feces.

In the present context, the treatment of chronic fever only is being described. Thus Anuvasana is useful in very chronic cases. [172– 173]

Administration of Nasya – Shiro Virechana treatment:

गौरवे शिरसः शूले विबद्धेष्विन्द्रियेषु च||१७३||

जीर्णज्वरे रुचिकरं कुर्यान्मूर्ध विरेचनम्|१७४||

In Jeerna Jwara (when ama is not there), Shiro Virechana (Nasya treatment to eliminate Doshas from mouth and nose) is administered in the following conditions:

When there is heaviness and pain in the head and

When there is inactivity (vibaddha) of the sense organs, as a result of which these are not able to perceive their objects.[173–174]

Massage etc therapies for fever:

अभ्यङ्गांश्च प्रदेहांश्च परिषेकावगाहने||१७४||

विभज्य शीतोष्णकृतं कुर्याज्जीर्णे ज्वरे भिषक्|

तैराशु प्रशमं याति बहिर्मार्गगतो ज्वरः||१७५||

लभन्ते सुखमङ्गानि बलं वर्णश्च वर्धते|१७६|

In JeernaJwara, (after passing Ama stage), the following are administered keeping in view, their heating and cooling natures.

Abhyanga (massage)

Pradeha (ointment / unction)

Parisheka (sprinkling of medicated water) and

Avagahana (tub Bath / immersion with medicated water).

By these therapies, the Bahirmarga Gata Jwara (the fever lodged in the external channels of the body) gets alleviated instantaneously.

There is a feeling of ease in the limbs and promotion of strength as well as complexion. [174–176]

Administration of Dhupana, Anjana:

धूपनाञ्जनयोगैश्च यान्ति जीर्ण ज्वराः शमम्||१७६||

त्वङ्मात्रशेषा येषां च भवत्यागन्तुरन्वयः|१७७|

Jeerna jwara gets alleviated by the administration of Dhupana (fumigation) and Anjana (collyrium) therapies.

It is especially useful for the residual fever remaining confined only to the skin and is associated with Agantu (extraneous) factors. [176–177]

Ingredients for therapies:

इति क्रियाक्रमः सिद्धो ज्वरघ्नः सम्प्रकाशितः||१७७||

येषां त्वेष क्रमस्तानि द्रव्याण्यूर्ध्वमतः शृणु|

रक्तशाल्यादयः शस्ताः पुराणाः षष्टिकैः सह||१७८||

यवाग्वोदनलाजार्थ ज्वरितानां ज्वरापहाः|१७९|

For the accomplishment of the alleviation of Jwara, proper treatment has been described above. The ingredients used for the therapies described in accordance with this line of treatment are being elaborated henceforth.

Yavagu (rice gruel), Odana (boiled rice) and Laja (fried paddy) are used to mitigate the fever. For these preparations, Rakta Shali (red variety of rice), along with Shashtika type of rice are given after they have become Purana (preserved over one year). [177–179]

Yavagu – Medicated gruels for Jwara:

लाजपेयां सुख जरां पिप्पली नागरैः शृताम्||१७९||

पिबेज्ज्वरी ज्वरहरां क्षुद्वानल्पाग्निरादितः|

अम्लाभिलाषी तामेव दाडिमाम्लां सनागराम्||१८०||

सृष्टविट् पैत्तिको वाऽथ शीतां मधुयुतां पिबेत्|

पेयां वा रक्तशालीनां पार्श्व बस्ति शिरो रुजि||१८१||

श्वदंष्ट्रा कण्टकारिभ्यां सिद्धां ज्वरहरां पिबेत्|

ज्वरातिसारी पेयां वा पिबेत् साम्लां शृतां नरः||१८२||

पृश्निपर्णी बला बिल्व नागरोत्पल धान्यकैः|

शृतां विदारीगन्धाद्यैर्दीपनीं स्वेदनीं नरः||१८३||

कासी श्वासी च हिक्की च यवागूं ज्वरितः पिबेत्|

विबद्धवर्चाः सयवां पिप्पल्यामलकैः शृताम्||१८४||

सर्पिष्मतीं पिबेत् पेयां ज्वरी दोषानुलोमनीम्|

कोष्ठे विबद्धे सरुजि पिबेत् पेयां शृतां ज्वरी||१८५||

मृद्वीका पिप्पलीमूल चव्यामलक नागरैः|

पिबेत् सबिल्वां पेयां वा ज्वरे सपरिकर्तिके||१८६||

बला वृक्षाम्ल कोलाम्लकलशीधावनीशृताम्|

अस्वेदनिद्रस्तृष्णार्तः पिबेत् पेयां सशर्करराम्||१८७||

नागरामलकैः सिद्धां घृतभृष्टां ज्वरापहाम्|१८८|

Ten types of Yavagus (gruels) used in Jwara are described below:

1. Lajapeya – The drink prepared of fried paddy and boiled with Pippali – Long pepper fruit – Piper longum and ginger is light for digestion. It alleviates Jwara and is given to the patient in the beginning stage of fever when there is less digestion strength.

2. Amla Peya – If the patient is desirous of sour things and if there is movement of bowel, then the Peya described above is made sour by adding Dadima – Pomegranate. It is given along with ginger.

3. In a Paittika type of patient, the above mentioned Peya is cooled and added with honey before administration.

4. The Peya prepared of red variety of rice (Raktashali) and boiled with Gokshura (Tribulus) and Kantakari (Solanum surattense Burm – Solanum xanthocarpum) alleviates fever and it is taken by the patient suffering from pain in Parsva (sides of the chest), Basti (urinary bladder) and Shiras (head).

5. The Peya which is sour and which is boiled with Prishnaparni – Uraria picta, Bala – Country mallow (root) – Sida cordifolia, Bilva – Bael, ginger, Utpala (Nymphaea alba) and coriander, is taken by a person suffering from Jwara-atisara (fever associated with diarrhea).

6. The Yavagu prepared by boiling with the group of medicines belonging to Vidarigandhadi Gana is a stimulant of digestion and it promotes sweating. This Yavagu is taken by a patient suffering from Jwara associated with Kasa (cough), Shvasa (Asthma) and Hikka (hiccup).

7. The Peya prepared of Yava – Barley (Hordeum vulgare) boiled with Pippali – Long pepper fruit – Piper longum and Amalaki causes the Anulomana (which helps in the downward movement of doshas), this Peya, mixed with ghee is taken by a patient suffering from Jwara associated with constipation.

8. The Peya prepared by boiling with raisins, long pepper root, Chavya (Piper chaba), Amalki and ginger is taken by a patient suffering from Jwara associated with constipation and pain.

9. If there is pain in a patient suffering from Jwara then he should take Peya boiled with Bala – Country mallow (root) – Sida cordifolia,Vruksamla (Citron fruit), Kolamla, Kakasi (Simha Pucchi), and Dhavani (Kantakari – Solanum surattense Burm – Solanum xanthocarpum) along with Bilva – Bael.

10. The Peya prepared by boiling with Nagara and Amalaka, fried with ghee and mixed with sugar alleviates Jwara. It is given to the patient suffering from Asveda (absence of sweating), Anidra (sleeplessness) and Trsna (Morbid

thirst). [179–188]

Use of Yusa:

मुद्गान्मसूरांश्चणकान् कुलत्थान् समकुष्टकान्||१८८||
यूषार्थं यूषसात्म्यानां ज्वरितानां प्रदापयेत्|१८९|

For some patients suffering from Jwara, Yusha gruel prepared with green gram, Masoor dal, Chanaka, horse gram and Makushtaka is useful. [188–189]

Vegetables:

पटोलपत्रं सफलं कुलकं पापचेलिकम्||१८९||
कर्कोटकं कठिल्लं च विद्याच्छाकं ज्वरे हितम्|१९०|

The leaves and fruits of Patola (pointed gourd), Kulaka (Karavallaka – Bitter gourd), Papachelika (Patha – Cissampelos pareira), Karkotaka, Kathilla (red variety of Punarnava – Boerhaavia diffusa Linn, these vegetables are useful in Jwara. {189–190}

Meat Soup:

लावान् कपिञ्जलानेणांश्चकोरानुपचक्रकान्||१९०||
कुरङ्गान् कालपुच्छांश्च हरिणान् पृषताञ्छशान्|
प्रदद्यान्मांससात्म्याय ज्वरिताय ज्वरापहान्||१९१||
ईषदम्लाननम्लान् वा रसान् काले विचक्षणः|
कुक्कुटांश्च मयूरांश्च तित्तिरिक्रौञ्चवर्तकान्||१९२||
गुरूष्णत्वान्न शंसन्ति ज्वरे केचिच्चिकित्सकाः|
लङ्घनेनानिलबलं ज्वरे यद्यधिकं भवेत्||१९३||
भिषङ्मात्राविकल्पज्ञो दद्यात्तानपि कालवित्|१९४|

The soup prepared of Lava, Kapinjala (white variety of sparrow), Ena (Krishna Shara), Chakora, Upacakraka (a variety of Chakora), Kuranga, Kala– Puccha (coppery colored dear), Prasata (spotted deer) and Shasha (Rabbit) are best in alleviating jwara. These meat soups may be slightly sour or many are free from any sourness. The wise physician should administer these soups at appropriate times.

Some physicians do not advise the use of the soup prepared of the meat of Kukkuta (cock), Mayura (peacock), Tittiri, Kraunca and Vartaka, because they are heavy and hot. In Jwara if Vata gets aggravated because of Langhana (Fasting), then the physician acquainted with the signs of Doshas gives the meat soup of these animals at appropriate times. [190–194]

Anupana (co-Drink):

घर्माम्बु चानुपानार्थं तृषिताय प्रदापयेत्||१९४||
मद्यं वा मद्य सात्म्याय यथादोषं यथाबलम्|१९५|

To a thirsty patient, hot water is given to drink. Depending upon the Doshas involved and the strength of the patient for whom it is wholesome. [194–195]

Diet contraindications:

गुरूष्ण स्निग्ध मधुरान् कषायांश्च नव ज्वरे||१९५||
आहारान् दोषपक्त्यर्थं प्रायशः परिवर्जयेत्|
अन्नपान क्रमः सिद्धो ज्वरघ्नः सम्प्रकाशितः||१९६||

In Nava Jwara (first stage of fever) food ingredients which are heavy, hot, unctuous, sweet and astringent are mostly avoided with a view to facilitate the Paka (metabolic transformation) of Doshas.

Thus, the diet and drinks which are appropriate for the alleviation of Jwara are described. [195–196]

Kashayas for Jwara – water decoctions

अत ऊर्ध्वं प्रक्ष्यन्ते कषाया ज्वर नाशनाः।

पाक्यं शीत कषायं वा मुस्त पर्पटकं पिबेत्||१९७||

सनागरं पर्पटकं पिबेद्वा सदुरालभम्।

किरालतिक्तकं मुस्तं गुडूची विश्वभेषजम्||१९८||

पाठामुशीरं सोदीच्यं पिबेद्वा ज्वर शान्तये।

ज्वरघ्ना दीपनाश्चैते कषाया दोष पाचनाः||१९९||

तृष्णारुचि प्रशमना मुखवैरस्य नाशनाः।|२००|

Hereafter, will be described the decoctions to alleviate Jwara. These are as follows:

1, 2 - Musta and Parpataka are taken either in the form of decoction (Pakya) or Sheeta Kashaya (keeping the medicines overnight in water and taking this water in the morning after filtering).

3 The decoction of Parapataka may be given to the patient along with ginger or Duralabha.

4 .The decoction of KirataTikta (Swertia chirata), Musta (Cyperus rotundus), Guduchi (Tinospora cordifolia) and ginger.

5 The decoction of Patha and Ushira – Vetiver – Vetiveria zizanioides along with Udichya.

These kashayas stimulate the power of digestion and help in the Pachana (metabolic transformation) of Doshas. They alleviate thirst, anorexia and cure MukhaVairasya (bad taste in the mouth) [197– 200]

Kashaya for Vishama Jwara:

कलिङ्गकाः पटोलस्य पत्रं कटुक रोहिणी||२००||

पटोलः सारिवा मुस्तं पाठा कटुक रोहिणी।

निम्बः पटोलस्त्रिफला मृद्वीका मुस्त वत्सकौ||१०१||

किरालतिक्तममृता चन्दनं विश्वभेषजम्।

गुडूच्यामलकं मुस्तमर्धश्लोकसमापनाः||२०२||

कषायाः शमयन्त्याशु पञ्च पञ्चविधाञ्ज्वरान्।

सन्ततं सततान्येद्युस्तृतीयक चतुर्थकान्||२०३||

The five types of Vishama Jwara (recurrent fever) namely, the Santata, Satata, Anyedyuska, Trtiyaka and Chaturthaka, are immediately cured by the five types of decoctions of medicines enumerated below:–

1. Kalingaka, leaf of Patola (pointed gourd) and Katukarohini – Picrorhiza kurroa

2. Patola, Sariva – Indian Sarsaparilla – Hemidesmus indicus, Musta (Cyperus rotundus), Patha, and Katukarohini – Picrorhiza kurroa

3. Nimba – Neem (Azadirachta indica), Patola (pointed gourd), Triphala, raisins, Musta (Cyperus rotundus) and Vatsaka (Holarrhena antidysenterica Wall.)

4. Kiratatikta, Amruta, Chandana (Sandalwood – Santalum album) and ginger and

5. Guduchi (Giloy), Amalaka and Musta (Cyperus rotundus) [200–203]

Jwarahara Kashaya:

वत्सकारग्वधौ पाठां षड्ग्रन्थां कटुरोहिणीम्।

मूर्वां सातिविषां निम्बं पटोलं धन्वयासकम्||२०४||

वचां मुस्तमुशीरं च मधुकं त्रिफलां बलाम्।

पाक्यं शीतकषायं वा पिबेज्ज्वरहरं नरः||२०५||

मधूकमुस्तमृद्वीकाकाश्मर्याणि परूषकम्।

त्रायमाणामुशीरं च त्रिफलां कटुरोहिणीम्||२०६||

पीत्वा निशिस्थितं जन्तुर्ज्वराच्छीघ्रं विमुच्यते।२०७।

The decoctions or Sheeta Kashaya of the following medicines is taken by a person for the cure of Jvara:

1. Vatsaka (Holarrhena antidysenterica Wall.), Aragvadha, Patha, SasGrantha and Katukarohini – Picrorhiza kurroa

2. Murva along with Ativisa, Nimba – Neem (Azadirachta indica), Patola and Dhanvayasaka and

3. Vacha (Acorus calamus Linn), Musta (Cyperus rotundus), Ushira – Vetiver – Vetiveria zizanioides, Madhuka– Licorice – Glycyrrhiza glabra, Musta (Cyperus rotundus), raisins, Kashmarya, Parushaka, Trayamana, Ushira – Vetiver – Vetiveria zizanioides, Triphala and Katukarohini – Picrorhiza kurroa, prepared by keeping overnight, immediately cures the Jwara of living beings. [204–207]

जात्यामलकमुस्तानि तद्वद्धन्वयवासकम्||२०७||

विबद्धदोषो ज्वरितः कषायं सगुडं पिबेत्।

त्रिफलां त्रायमाणां च मृद्वीकां कटुरोहिणीम्||२०८||

पित्तश्लेष्महरस्त्वेष कषायो ह्यानुलोमिकः।

त्रिवृताशर्करायुक्तः पित्तश्लेष्मज्वरापहः||२०९||

When Doshas are in a state of Vibaddha (adhered to Dhatus) the patient suffering from Jwara should take the decoction of either Jati, Amalaki and Musta (Cyperus rotundus), or that of Dhanvayasaka along with Guda (Jaggery). The decoction prepared of Triphala, Trayamana, raisins and Katukarohini – Picrorhiza kurroa alleviates Pitta and Sleshma. It causes Anulomana (elimination through downward tract) of Doshas. This decoction when taken along with Trivrut and sugar cures Jwara caused by the aggravation of Pitta and Sleshma. [207– 209]

Kashayam for Sannipata Jwara:

बृहत्यौ वत्सकं मुस्तं देवदारु महौषधम्।

कोलवल्ली च योगोऽयं सन्निपातज्वरापहः||२१०||

शटी पुष्करमूलं च व्याघ्री शृङ्गी दुरालभा।

गुडूची नागरं पाठा किरातं कटुरोहिणी||२११||

एष शट्यादिको वर्गः सन्निपातज्वरापहः।

कासहृद्ग्रहपार्श्वार्तिश्वासतन्द्रासु शस्यते||२१२||

बृहत्यौ पौष्करं भार्गी शटी शृङ्गी दुरालभा।

वत्सकस्य च बीजानि पटोलं कटुरोहिणी||२१३||

बृहत्यादिर्गणः प्रोक्तः सन्निपातज्वरापहः।

कासादिषु च सर्वेषु दद्यात् सोपद्रवेषु च||२१४||

kashaya prepared of both Brihati – Solanum indicum, Kantakari, Vatsaka (Holarrhena antidysenterica Wall.), Musta (Cyperus rotundus), Devadaru, Mahaushadha and Kolavalli cures Sannipata type of Jwara.

The kashaya of ShatyadiVarga:

Shati, Puskaramula, Srungi, Duralabha, Guduchi, ginger, Patha, Kirata, Katukarohini – Picrorhiza kurroa.

Cures: Sannipata Jwara along with Kasa (cough), Hrut graha (stiffness in cardiac region), Parshva arti (pain in the sides of the chest), Shvasa (asthma) and Tandra (drowsiness).

Bruhatyadigana:

Both the varieties of Brihati – Solanum indicum, Pauskara, Shati, Srungi, Duralabha, Seeds of Vatsaka (Holarrhena antidysenterica Wall), Patola and Katukarohini – Picrorhiza kurroa

Cures: Sannipata Jwara, Kasa (cough) etc. and all types of complications. [210–214]

कषायाश्च यवाग्वश्च पिपासा ज्वर नाशनाः।

निर्दिष्टा भेषजाध्याये भिषक्तानपि योजयेत्||२१५||

Different types of decoctions and gruels for the cure of thirst and fever described in first four chapters of Sutra Sthana. Those decoctions can also be used by the physicians for the treatment of Jwara. [215]

Use of Herbal Ghee:

ज्वराः कषायैर्वमनैर्लङ्घनैर्लघुभोजनैः|
रूक्षस्य ये न शाम्यन्ति सर्पिस्तेषां भिषग्जितम्||२१६||
रूक्षं तेजो ज्वरकरं तेजसा रूक्षितस्य च|
यः स्यादनुबलो धातुः स्नेहवध्यः स चानिलः||२१७||

If, in a person having excess dryness, the fever does not get alleviated by the use of Kashayas, Vamana, fasting and by light diet, then it is treated by medicated ghee.

Rooksha – dryness and Tejas – fire elements – both these can cause or worsen fever. So, in a patient with dryness and excess hotness, unctuous foods like ghee are very useful. [216–217]

कषायाः सर्व एवैते सर्पिषा सह योजिताः|
प्रयोज्या ज्वरशान्त्यर्थमग्निसन्धुक्षणाः शिवाः||२१८||

All the above Kashayas can be administered with ghee as Anupana (co drink) for the allevation of Jwara – fever. They stimulate the power of digestion and endow auspiciousness. [218]

Jwarahara Pippalyadi Ghrita:
पिप्पल्यश्चन्दनं मुस्तमुशीरं कटुरोहिणी|
कलिङ्गकास्तामलकी सारिवाऽतिविषा स्थिरा||२१९||
द्राक्षामलकबिल्वानि त्रायमाणा निदिग्धिका|
सिद्धमितैर्घृतं सद्यो जीर्णज्वरमपोहति||२२०||
क्षयं कासं शिरःशूलं पार्श्वशूलं हलीमकम्|
अंसाभितापमग्निं च विषमं सन्नियच्छति||२२१||

The medicated Ghee prepared by boiling with
Pippali – Piper longum
Chandana – Santalum album
Musta – Cyperus rotundus
Usheera – Vetiver
Katurohini
Kalingaka
Tamalaki (Bhumyamalaki)
Sariva
Ativisha
Sthira – Desmodium gangeticum
Draksha – grapes
Amalaki (Indian gooseberry fruit – Emblica officinalis Gaertn)
Bilva – Aegle marmelos,
Trayamana and
Nidigdhika
Cures:
Chronic fever instantaneously
Kshaya (Consumption)
Kasa – cough, Cold
Shirashula – Headache,
Parshvashula – pain in the sides of the chest
Halimaka – a type of Jaundice
Amsabhitapa – burning sensation in the scapular region and
Vishama Agni – irregularity in the power of digestion [219–221]

Vasakadi Ghrita:

वासां गुडूचीं त्रिफलां त्रायमाणां यवासकम्|
पक्त्वा तेन कषायेण पयसा द्विगुणेन च||२२२||
पिप्पली मुस्त मृद्वीका चन्दनोत्पल नागरैः|
कल्कीकृतैश्च विपचेद्धृतं जीर्णज्वरापहम्||२२३||

Decoction is prepared by boiling

Vasa – Adhatoda vasica,

Guduchi – Tinospora cordifolia

Triphala,

Trayamana and

Yavasaka

Milk is added to it in double the quantity.

To this the paste of

Pippali – Piper longum

Musta – Cyperus rotundus

Raisin

Chandana – Santalum album

Utpala and ginger are added.

Along with these medicines, ghee is prepared by boiling. This medicated ghee cures Jeerna Jwara (chronic fever). [222–223]

Baladi Ghrita:

बलां श्वदंष्ट्रां बृहतीं कलसीं धावनीं स्थिराम्|
निम्बं पर्पटकं मुस्तं त्रायमाणां दुरालभाम्||२२४||
कृत्वा कषायं पेष्यार्थे दद्यातामलकीं शटीम्|
द्राक्षां पुष्करमूलं च मेदामामलकानि च||२२५||
घृतं पयश्च तत् सिद्धं सर्पि ज्वरहरं परम्|
क्षय कास शिरःशूल पार्श्वशूलांसतापनुत्||२२६||

A decoction of

Bala – Sida cordifolia

Svadamstra – Gokshura

Bhavani,

Sthira,

Nimba – neem,

Parpataka,

Mustaka,

Trayamana and

Duralabha is prepared.

Paste of the medicines:

Tramalaki – Bhui Amla

Shati – Hedychium spicatum

Draksa – raisins

Pushkaramula – Inula racemosa

Meda and

Amalaka

To the above mentioned decoction and paste ghee and milk is added and boiled.

The medicated ghee, thus prepared, is an excellent medicated for the cure of Jwara – fever.

It also cures

Kshaya (chronic bronchitis, tuberculosis)

Kasa – cough,

Cold (Bronchitis),

Sirah Sula (Headache),

Parsvasula (pain in the sides of the chest) and

Amsa Tapa (burning sensation in the scapular region) [224– 226]

Panchakarma for fever – Elimination of Therapy:

ज्वरिभ्यो बहुदोषेभ्य ऊर्ध्वं चाधश्च बुद्धिमान्।

दद्यात् संशोधनं काले कल्पे यदुपदेक्ष्यते॥२२७॥

मदनं पिप्पलीभिर्वा कलिङ्गैर्मधुकेन वा।

युक्तमुष्णाम्बुना पेयं वमनं ज्वरशान्तये॥२२८॥

क्षौद्राम्बुना रसेनेक्षोरथवा लवणाम्बुना।

ज्वरे प्रच्छर्दनं शस्तं मद्यैर्वा तर्पणेन वा॥२२९॥

मृद्वीकामलकानां वा रसं प्रस्कन्दनं पिबेत्।

रसमामलकानां वा घृतभृष्टं ज्वरापहम्॥२३०॥

लिह्याद्वा त्रैवृतं चूर्णं संयुक्तं मधुसर्पिषा।

पिबेद्वा क्षौद्रमावाप्य सघृतं त्रिफलारसम्॥२३१॥

आरग्वधं वा पयसा मृद्वीकानां रसेन वा।

त्रिवृतां त्रायमाणां वा पयसा ज्वरितः पिबेत्॥२३२॥

ज्वरादिवमुच्यते पीत्वा मृद्वीकाभिः सहाभयाम्।

पयोऽनुपानमुष्णं वा पीत्वा द्राक्षारसं नरः॥२३३॥

To a patient suffering from Jwara and having highly aggravated doshas; the wise physician should administer elimination therapies in appropriate time for the elimination of Doshas both through the upward and downward tracts.

Administration of Vamana therapy (emesis) by hot water and Madanaphala (Randia dumentorum) mixed with Pippali (long pepper), Kalinga or Madhuka alleviates Jwara – fever.

The Vamana therapy administered by giving water mixed with honey, sugarcane juice, water mixed with rock salt, alcoholic drinks and Tarpana (roasted flour of corn diluted with water) is useful in Jwara – fever.

A patient suffering from Jwara can be given the juice of raisins and amalaka for Purgation.

Administration of the juice of Amalaka fried with ghee cures Jwara – fever.

The following recipes are also useful for a patient suffering from Jwara – fever:

1. Avaleha prepared of the powder of Trivrt mixed ghee and honey

2. The Juice of Triphala mixed with honey and Ghee

3. Aragvadha along with milk or the juice of Mrdvika

4. Trivrit and Trayamana along with milk

5. Raisins and Abhaya (Haritaki) along with Warm milk or the juice of Draksha as Anupana (Post prandial milk) [227– 233]

Medicated milk:

कासाच्छ्वासाच्छिरःशूलात्पार्श्वशूलाच्चिरज्वरात्।

मुच्यते ज्वरितः पीत्वा पञ्चमूलीशृतं पयः॥२३४॥

एरण्डमूलोत्क्वथितं ज्वरात् सपरिकर्तिकात्।

पयो विमुच्यते पीत्वा तद्वदिबल्वशलाटुभिः॥२३५॥

त्रिकण्टक बला व्याघ्री गुड नागर साधितम्।

वर्चो मूत्र विबन्धध्नं शोफ ज्वरहरं पयः||२३६||

सनागरं समृद्वीकं सघृत क्षौद्र शर्करम्|

शृतं पयः सखर्जूरं पिपासा ज्वर नाशनम्||२३७||

चतुर्गुणेनाम्भसा वा शृतं ज्वरहरं पयः|

धारोष्णं वा पयः सद्यो वातपित्तज्वरं जयेत्||२३८||

जीर्ण ज्वराणां सर्वेषां पयः प्रशमनं परम्|

पेयं तदुष्णं शीतं वा यथास्वं भेषजैः शृतम्||२३९||

By taking milk boiled with Pancamula (Bilva – Aegle marmelos, Synonaka, Gambhari, Patala – Stereospermum suaveolens and Ganikarika), the patient suffering from Jwara gets cured of

Kasa – cough

Shvasa – Asthma

Sirah Sula – headache

Parsva Sula – pain in the sides of the chest and

ChiraJwara – chronic pyrexia

The milk is boiled either with the castor root or the Shalatu (Unripe fruit cut into pieces) of Bilva – Aegel marmelos, when taken, cures fever along with Parikartika (itchy pain) in the abdomen.

The milk boiled with Trikantaka (Gokshura), Bala – Country mallow (root) – Sida cordifolia, Vyaghri, jaggery and ginger cures Jwara along with Sopha (oedema). It also cures the Vibandha (obstruction) of feces and urine.

The liquid prepared by boiling milk with Nagara, Mrdvika and Khajura and added with ghee, honey and sugar cures Jwara associated with thirst.

Milk boiled by adding 4 times of water cures Jwara.

The milk which is Dharoshna (freshly milked from the cow when it is warm) immediately cures Jwara caused by the aggravation of Vayu and Pitta.

Milk alleviates all types of chronic fever. It may be taken either hot or cold, and it can be taken after boiling with medicines appropriate to the type of fever. [234–239]

Niruhabasti for Jwara – Decoction enema:

प्रयोजयेज्ज्वरहरान्निरूहान् सानुवासनान्|

पक्वाशय गते दोषे वक्ष्यन्ते ये च सिद्धिषु||२४०||

पटोलारिष्टपत्राणि सोशीरश्चतुरङ्गुलः|

ह्रीबेरं रोहिणी तिक्ता श्वदंष्ट्रा मदनानि च||२४१||

स्थिरा बला च तत् सर्वं पयस्यर्धोदके शृतम्|

क्षीरावशेषं निर्यूहं संयुक्तं मधुसर्पिषा||२४२||

कल्कैर्मदनमुस्तानां पिप्पल्या मधुकस्य च|

वत्सकस्य च संयुक्तं बस्तिं दद्याज्ज्वरापहम्||२४३||

शुद्धे मार्गे हृते दोषे विप्रसन्नेषु धातुषु|

गताङ्गशूलो लघ्वङ्गः सद्यो भवति विज्वरः||२४४||

आरग्वधमुशीरं च मदनस्य फलं तथा|

पिप्पलीफलमुस्तानां कल्केन मधुकस्य च||२४८||

ईषत्सलवणं युक्त्या निरूहं मधुसर्पिषा|

ज्वरप्रशमनं दद्याद्बलस्वेदरुचिप्रदम्||२४९||

Niruhabasti for Jwara – Decoction enema:

For the cure of Jwara, when the Doshas are lodged in Pakvasaya (colon), Niruha and Anuvasana, types of medicated enema which will be described in Siddhi Sthana, is administered.

All these medicines are boiled in milk by adding water which latter is taken in half the quantity of milk:

Patola

Leaves of Arista
Ushira – Vetiver – Vetiveria zizanioides
Chaturangula (Cassia fistula)
Hrivera
Katukarohini – Picrorhiza kurroa
Tikta
Svadamstra – Gokshura
Madanaphala
Sthira – Desmodium gangeticum and
Bala – Country mallow (root) – Sida cordifolia
After boiling the residue is equal to the quantity of milk.
To this liquid, honey and ghee are added along with the Kalka (paste) of
Madanaphala – Randia dumentorum
Musta (Cyperus rotundus)
Pippali – Long pepper fruit – Piper longum
Madhuka– Licorice – Glycyrrhiza glabra and
Vatsaka (Holarrhena antidysenterica Wall.).
This potion is administered in the form of enema for the cure of Jwara.
When the channels are cleaned, Doshas are eliminated and Dhatus (tissue elements) are refreshed, the pain in the body disappears and the body becomes light and instantaneously free from fever.
A decoction of
Aragvadha (Cassia fistula), Ushira – Vetiver, Madanaphala, Shalaparni, Prishnaparni, Mashaparni Mudgaparni is prepared.
To this, the paste of
Priyangu
Madana
Musta
Shatahva and
Madhuyasti are added, and it is used.
This is an excellent recipe of enema to cure Jwara.
Herbs used for the preparation of the decoction:
Guduchi
Trayamana
Madhuka– Licorice – Glycyrrhiza glabra
Vrusha – Vasa,
Sthira – Desmodium gangeticum,
Bala – Country mallow (root) – Sida cordifolia
Prishnaparni – Uraria picta and
Madana
To this the Meat soup of Jangala type of animals (those inhabiting arid land) is to be added.
And the paste of
Pippali – Long pepper fruit – Piper longum,
Musta - Cyperus rotundus and Madhuka – Licorice – Glycyrrhiza glabra are added.
To this potion, a small quantity of rock salt should also be added along with honey and ghee.
This potion is administered as a Niruha type of medicated enema for the alleviation of Jwara.
It promotes Strength, Sweating and appetite [240–249]

Snehabasti – Oil or fat enema:

जीवन्तीं मधुकं मेदां पिप्पलीं मदनं वचाम्।
ऋद्धिं रास्नां बलां विश्वं शतपुष्पां शतावरीम्।।२५०।।
पिष्ट्वा क्षीरं जलं सर्पिस्तैलं च विपचेद्भिषक्।
आनुवासनिकं स्नेहमेतं विद्याज्ज्वरापहम्।।२५१।।
पटोलपिचुमर्दाभ्यां गुडूच्या मधुकेन च।
मदनैश्च शृतः स्नेहो ज्वरघ्नमनुवासनम्।।२५२।।
चन्दनागुरुकाश्मर्यपटोलमधुकोत्पलैः।
सिद्धः स्नेहो ज्वरहरः स्नेहबस्तिः प्रशस्यते।।२५३।।

A paste of
Jivanti, Madhuka, Meda,, Pippali, Madana, Vacha, Ruddhi, Rasna, Bala, Bilva, Shatapuspa and Shatavari is prepared.
To this, milk, water, ghee and oil is added and boiled.
This medicated ghee is used for Anuvasana type of enema to cure Jwara.
The Sneha (ghee and oil) is boiled with Patola, Pichumarda, Guduchi , Madhuka and, Madana
This portion is used as an Anuvasana type of enema for the cure of Jwara.
The Sneha (oil and ghee) is boiled with
Chandana – Santalum album
Aguru – Aquilaria agallocha,
Kashmarya
Patola
Madhuka and
Utpala
This potion is exceedingly useful for being administratered as Sneha basti to cure Jwara [250– 253]

Shiro Virechana treatment for Jwara:
यदुक्तं भेषजाध्याये विमाने रोगभेषजे।
शिरोविरेचनं कुर्याद्युक्तिज्ञस्तज्ज्वरापहम्।।२५४।।
यच्च नावनिकं तैलं याश्च तैलं याश्च प्राग्धूमवर्तयः।
मात्राशितीये निर्दिष्टाः प्रयोज्यास्ता ज्वरेष्वपि।।२५५।।

Recipes for inhalation therapy are already described in the 2nd chapter of Sutra Sthana (Bhesajadhyaya) and 8th chapter of Vimana Sthana (Roga– Bhesagitiya). A Physician who is well versed with Rationality of the administration of these therapies should give them to the patient for the cure of Jwara.
In the 5th chapter of Sutra Sthana (Matrashiteeya), the medicated oil (Anu Taila) for use as Nasal drop and DhumaVarti (Cigars for smoking) are described. These should also be administered for the cure of Jwara. [254–255]

Massage etc:

अभ्यङ्गांश्च प्रदेहांश्च परिषेकांश्च कारयेत्।
यथाभिलाषं शीतोष्णं विभज्य द्विविधं ज्वरम्।।२५६।।
Abhyanga (Massage), Pradeha (Unction) and Pariseka medicated bath) is done, either hot or cold, as per the requirement of thr two types of Jwara.[256]
सहस्रधौतं सर्पिर्वा तैलं वा चन्दनादिकम्।
दाह ज्वर प्रशमनं दद्यादभ्यञ्जनं भिषक्।।२५७।।
Medicated ghee called Sahasra Dhauta ghruta and medicated oil called Chandanadya Taila which alleviate fever associated with burning sensation may be given for massage by the Physician [257]

Chandanadya Taila

अथ चन्दनाद्यं तैलमुपदेक्ष्यामः– चन्दन भद्र श्रीकालानुसार्य कालीयक पद्मापद्मकोशीर सारिवा मधुक प्रपौण्डरीक नागपुष्पोदीच्यवन्यपद्मोत्पलनलिनकुमुद– सौगन्धिक पुण्डरीक शतपत्र बिस मृणाल शालूक शैवालक शेरुकानन्ताकुशकाशेक्षुदर्भशरनल शालिमूल जम्बु वेतस वानीरगुन्द्रा– ककुभासनाश्वकर्णस्यन्दनवातपोथशालतालधवतिनिशखदिरकदरकदम्बकाश्मर्यफलसर्जप्लक्षवटकपीतनोदुम्बराश्वत्थ– न्यग्रोध धातकीदूर्वेत्कट शृङ्गाटक मञ्जिष्ठा ज्योतिष्मती पुष्करबीज क्रौञ्चादन बदरी कोविदार कदली– संवर्तकारिष्ट शतपर्वा शीतकुम्भिका शतावरी श्रीपर्णी श्रावणी महाश्रावणी रोहिणी शीतपाक्योदनपाकीकालबलापयस्या विदारी– जीवकर्षभक मेदा महामेदा मधुरसर्ष्यप्रोक्ता तृणशून्य मोचरसाटरूषक बकुल कुटज पटोल निम्ब शाल्मली नारिकेल– खर्जूर मृद्वीका प्रियाल प्रियङ्गु धन्वनात्मागुप्ता मधूकानामन्येषां च शीतवीर्याणां यथालाभमौषधानां कषायं कारयेत्।

तेन कषायेण द्विगुणित पयसा तेषामेव च कल्केन कषायार्धमात्रं मृद्वग्निना साधयेतैलम्।

एतत्तैलमभ्यङ्गात् सद्यो दाह ज्वरमपनयति।

एतैरेव चौषधैरश्लक्ष्णपिष्टैः सुशीतैः प्रदेहं कारयेत्।

एतैरेव च शृतशीतं सलिलमवगाह परिषेकार्थ प्रयुञ्जीत॥२५८॥

इति चन्दनाद्यं तैलम्।

मध्वारनाल क्षीर दधि घृत सलिल सेकावगाहाश्च सद्यो दाह ज्वरमपनयन्ति शीतस्पर्शत्वात्॥२५९॥

Here after the preparation of Chandanadya Taila will be explained. A decoction is prepared of

Chandana (red variety)

Bhadrasri (white variety of Chandana)

Kalanusarya, Kaliyaka, Padma (Prapaundarika), Padmaka, Usheera, Sariva, Madhuka, Magapushpa, Udeechya, Vanya, padma, Utapala, Nalima (a variety of Padma), Kumuda, Saugandhika, Pundarika, Sala Patra Bisa (thread of lotus stalk), Mruvala, Shaivala, Kasheruka, Ananta, Kusha, Kasha, Ikshu, Darbha, Shara, Nala– root of Shali, Jambu, Vetasa, Vanira (a variety of Vetasa having roots which are not fragrant), Gundra, Kakubha, Asana, Ashvakarna (A variety of Sala), Syandana (NemiVruksa), Vatapotha (Palasa), Shala, Tala, Dhava, Tinisha, Khadira, Kashara, Vitkhala– dira, Kadamba, Fruit of Kasmarya, Sarja, Vata (the variety without any adventitious root), Kapitana (which popularly known as Gandhamunda), Udambara, Asvattha, Nyagrodha, Dhataki, Durva, Itkata, Shrungataka, Manjistha, Jyotismati (Kanganika), Seeds of Puskara, Krauncadana, Badari (Ber fruit), Kovidara, Kasali, Samvartaka, Arista (a variety of Nimba growing in hills), Shataparva (Bibitaka), Sita Kumbhika (KasthaPatala), Shatavari, Sriparni, Sravani, MahaSravani (alambusa having big fruits), Rohini, Sita Paki (Gandhadurva), Odanapaki (NilaBhendi), Kala (Kakoli), Bala, Payasya, Vidari, Jivaka, Rishabhaka, Meda, Mahameda, Madhurasa, Rushyaprokta, Truna Shunya, Ketaki, Macarsa, Tarusaka, Bakula, Kutaja, Patola, Shalmali, Narikela, Kharjura, Mrudveeka – raisins, Priyala, Priyangu, Dhanvana, Atmagupta, Madhuka and such other medicines which are cold in potency.

All these medicines which are readily available are taken for the preparation of this decoction.

This decoction is prepared by adding double the quantity of water.

All the above-mentioned medicines can also be used as Kalka (paste).

Oil mixed with the above mentioned decoction and paste is boiled over mild fire till it is reduced to half the quantity of decoction. Massage of this medicated oil instantaneously cures Daha Jwara (fever associated with burning sensation).

The above-mentioned medicines are made into a coarse paste and used for unction when it is very cold. The water boiled with these medicines and cooled is used for Avagaha (bath) and Pariseka (Sprinkling over the body).

The Seka (sprinkling over body) and Avagaha (bath) with Madhu (honey), Aranala (sour Gruel), milk, curd, ghee and water instantaneously cure Daha Jwara (fever associated with burning sensation) because of their cold touch. [258–259]

Regimens of fever associated with burning sensation:

भवन्ति चात्र–

पौष्करेषु सुशीतेषु पद्मोत्पलदलेषु च।
कदलीनां च पत्रेषु क्षौमेषु विमलेषु च॥२६०॥

चन्दनोदक शीतेषु शीते धारागृहेऽपि वा|
हिमाम्बु सिक्ते सदने दाहार्तः संविशेत् सुखम्||२६१||
हेमशङ्ख प्रवालानां मणीनां मौक्तिकस्य च|
चन्दनोदक शीतानां संस्पर्शानुरसान् स्पृशेत्||२६२||
स्रग्भिर्नीलोत्पलैः पद्मैर्व्यजनैर्विविधैरपि|
शीतवातावहैर्व्यज्ज्येच्चन्दनोदकवर्षिभिः ||२६३||
नद्यस्तडागाः पद्मिन्यो ह्रदाश्च विमलोदकाः|
अवगाहे हिता दाह तृष्णा ग्लानि ज्वरापहाः||२६४||
प्रियाः प्रदक्षिणाचाराः प्रमदाश्चन्दनोक्षिताः|
सान्त्वययुः परैः कामैर्मणिमौक्तिकभूषणाः||२६५||
शीतानि चान्नपानानि शीतान्युपवनानि च|
वायवश्चन्द्रपादाश्च शीता दाहज्वरापहाः||२६६||

Regimens of fever associated with burning sensation:

A patient suffering from Jwara with burning sensation, should reside in a house cooled by the leaves of Pushkara (Inula racemosa, lotus, Utpala, banana or Kshauma.

The house can also be cooled by the cold water of Sandalwood.

The patient can also stay in a Dhara Gruha (a house which is cooled by a stream of water flowing over or from its roof).

The house can also be cooled by sprinkling snow water around it. This gives pleasure to the patient. His body is touched with the pleasant touch of gold, conch shell, coral, jewels and pearls which are cooled by the water of sandalwood.

He is consoled by ladies smeared with sandalwood paste and wearing the desirable jewels and pearls. These ladies are affectionate and expert in polite manners.

Diet and drinks which are cold, cooling gardens, cold wind and cold rays of the moon– these alleviate Jwara with burning sensation. [260–266]

Aguruvadya Taila:

अथोष्णाभि प्रायिणां ज्वरितानामभ्यङ्गादीनुपक्रमानुपदेक्ष्यामः– अगुरु कुष्ठ तगर पत्र नलद शैलेयध्यामक हरेणुकास्थौणेयकक्षेमकैलावराङ्गदलपुरतमालपत्रभूतीक रोहिष सरल शल्लकी– देवदार्वग्निमन्थ बिल्व स्योनाक काश्मर्य पाटला पुनर्नवावृश्चीर कण्टकारी बृहती शालपर्णी पृश्निपर्णी माषपर्णी मुद्गपर्णी गोक्षुरकैरण्ड– शोभाञ्जनक वरुणार्क चिर बिल्व तिल्वक शटी पुष्करमूल गण्डीरोरुबूकपतूराक्षीवाश्मान्तक शिगु मातुलुङ्ग पीलुक मूलकपर्णी– तिलपर्णी पीलुपर्णी मेषशृङ्गीहिंसादन्तशठैरावतक भल्लातकास्फोतकाण्डीरात्मजैकेषीका करञ्ज धान्यकाजमोद– पृथ्वीका सुमुख सुरस कुठेरक कालमालक पर्णासक्षवक फणिज्झक भूस्तृण शृङ्गवेर पिप्पली सर्षपाश्वगन्धा रास्नारुहारोहा वचा बलातिबला– गुडूची शतपुष्पा शीतवल्ली नाकुली गन्धनाकुली श्वेताज्योतिष्मती चित्रकाध्यण्डाम्ल चाङ्गेरी– तिल बदर कुलत्थ माषाणामेवंविधानामन्येषां चोष्णवीर्याणां यथालाभमौषधानां कषायं कारयेत्, तेन कषायेण तेषामेव च कल्केन सुरासौवीरक तुषोदकमैरेयमेदकदधिमण्डारनालकट्वरप्रतिविनीतेन तैलपात्रं विपाचयेत्|

तेन सुखोष्णेन तैलेनोष्णाभिप्रायिणं ज्वरितमभ्यञ्ज्यात्, तथा शीतज्वरः प्रशाम्यति; एतैरेव चौषधैः श्लक्ष्णपिष्टैः सुखोष्णैः प्रदेहं कारयेत्, एतैरेव च शृतं सुखोष्णं सलिलमवगाहनार्थं परिषेकार्थं च प्रयुञ्जीत शीतज्वरप्रशमार्थम्||२६७||

इत्यगुर्वाद्यं तैलम्|

Now we shall explain the therapies like massage etc. for patients suffering from Jwara and for whom hot treatment is diserable.

A decoction is prepared of:

Aguru – Aquilaria agallocha

Kushta – Saussurea lappa

Tagara – Valeriana wallichii

Patra – Cinnamomum tamala

Nalada

Shaileya, Dhyamaka, Harenuka, Sthaauneyaka, Ksemaka (Choraka), Ela – Elettaria cardamomum, Varanga, Bala, Pura – Guggulu, Tamala Patra, Bhutaika, Rohisha (popularly known as Rama Karpura), Sarala – Pinus roxburghii, Shallaki – Boswellia serrata, Devadaru – Cedrus deodara, Agnimantha – Clerodendrum phlomidis Linn.f., Bilva – Aegel marmelos, Shyonaka – Oroxylum indicum (Linn) Vent, Kashmarya (Gambhari), Patala – Stereospermum suaveolens, Punarnava – Boerhaavia diffusa Linn, Vrushcheera, Kantakari – Solanum surattense Burm, Brihati – Solanum indicum Linn, Shalaparni, Prushnaparni, Mashaparni, MudgaParni, Gokshuraka – Tribulus, Eranda – Castor, Sobhanjana, Varuna – Crataeva nurvala, Arka – Calotropis gigantea, Cira Bilva Tilvaka, Shati, PuskaraMula – Inula racemosa, Gandira (a Variety of Ramatha), Urubuka, Pattura, Aksiva, Ashmantaka , Shigru , Matulunga – Citrus medica, Piluka, MulakaParni (a variety of Sobhanjana), TilaParni, PiluParni (Morata or Murva), MesaSrngi – Gymnema sylvestre, Himsra, DantaShata, Aravata, Bhallataka – Semecarpus anacardium, Asphotaka, Andrira, Atmaja (Putranjana), Ekaisika (Ambastha), Karanja – Pongamia pinnata (Linn), Dhanyaka – Coriandrum sativum, Ajamoda – Apium graveolens, Prthvika, Sumakha, Surasa, Kutheraka, Asphotaka, Andira, Atmaja (Putranjama), Ekaisika (Ambastha), Phanijjhaka, Bhustruna, Srungavera, Pippali – Piper longum, mustard, Ashvagandha – Withania somnifera, Rasna, Ruha (VrukshaRuha), Roha (Anjalikarika), Yava, Bala, Atibala, Guduchi, Shatapushpa, Sitavalli (VrksaKalambuka), Nakuli (Chavika), GandhaNakuli (a variety of Rasna), Sveta jyotismati, Citraka – Plumbago zeylanica, Adhyanda (Sukasimbi), Amla Cangeri, Tila – Sesamum indicum, Badara, Kulattha – Dolichos biflorus, Masha and such other medicines which are hot in potency

All these medicines or those amongst them which are available are taken for the preparation of this decoction.

Paste of these medicines is also prepared.

This decoction and paste is added with

Sura – alcoholic drinks

Sauviraka – Vinegar

Tushodaka – a type of vinegar

Maireya – a type of alcoholic drink

Medaka – a type of alcoholic drink also called Jagala

Dadhi Manda – scum of the curd

Aranala – sour gruel and

Katvara – curd made watery along with fat is boiled in one Patra (3.072 Ltr) of oil.

Indications: When this oil is Lukewarm, it is used for giving massage to a patient suffering from Jwara and for whom hot therapy is indicated.

For the cure of Sita Jwara, the lukewarm water boiled with medicines can also be used for Avagaha (bath) and Pariseka (sprinkling). [267]

Remedy for sheetajwara – fever associated with chill, cold:

भवन्ति चात्र–
त्रयोदशविधः स्वेदः स्वेदाध्याये निदर्शितः।
मात्राकालविदा युक्तः स च शीतज्वरापहः॥२६८॥
सा कुटी तच्च शयनं तच्चावच्छादनं ज्वरम्।
शीतं प्रशमयन्त्याशु धूपाश्चागुरुजा घनाः॥२६९॥
चारूपचितगात्र्यश्च तरुण्यो यौवनोष्मणा।
आश्लेषाच्छमयन्त्याशु प्रमदाः शिशिरज्वरम्॥२७०॥
स्वेदनान्यन्नपानानि वातश्लेष्महराणि च।
शीतज्वरं जयन्त्याशु संसर्गबलयोजनात्॥२७१॥

Remedy for sheetajwara – fever associated with chill, cold:

In the fourteenth chapter of sutra Sthana, 13 varieties of Sveda (fomentation therapy) have been described. A physician who is well–versed with their dose and time should administer them for the bed as well as the apparel described. They immediately alleviate Sita (cold). Similarly, the thick fumigation of Aguru – Aqualaria agallocha alleviates Sheeta – cold.

Passionate ladies, who are beautiful, having a plump body and young, should embrace the patient. Because of the heat of their youth, the Sheeta Jwara is cured.

Different types of diet and drinks which cause fomentation and alleviate Vata and Kapha, instantaneously alleviates Sita Jwara. These should, however, be administered keeping in view the Samsarga (combination of 2 Doshas) and the Bala (strength) of each of these Doshas. (268–271)

Line of treatment:

वातजे श्रमजे चैव पुराणे क्षतजे ज्वरे|
लङ्घनं न हितं विद्याच्छमनैस्तानुपाचरेत्||२७२||
विक्षिप्यामाशयोष्माणं यस्मादगत्वा रसं नृणाम्|
ज्वरं कुर्वन्ति दोषास्तु हीयतेऽग्निबलं ततः||२७३||
यथा प्रज्वलितो वह्निः स्थाल्यामिन्धनवानपि|
न पचत्योदनं सम्यगनिलप्रेरितो बहिः||२७४||
पक्तिस्थानात्तथा दोषैरूष्मा क्षिप्तो बहिर्नृणाम्|
न पचत्यभ्यवहृतं कृच्छ्रात् पचति वा लघु||२७५||
अतोऽग्निबलरक्षार्थं लङ्घनादिक्रमो हितः|
सप्ताहेन हि पच्यन्ते सप्तधातुगता मलाः||२७६||
निरामश्चाप्यतः प्रोक्तो ज्वरः प्रायोऽष्टमेऽहनि|
उदीर्णदोषस्त्वल्पाग्निरश्नन् गुरु विशेषतः||२७७||
मुच्यते सहसा प्राणैश्चिरं क्लिश्यति वा नरः|
एतस्मात्कारणादिवद्वान् वातिकेऽप्यादितो ज्वरे||२७८||
नाति गुर्वति वा स्निग्धं भोजयेत् सहसा नरम्|
ज्वरे मारुतजे त्वादावनपेक्ष्यापि हि क्रमम्||२७९||
कुर्यान्निरनुबन्धानामभ्यङ्गादीनुपक्रमान्|
पाययित्वा कषायं च भोजयेद्रसभोजनम्||२८०||
जीर्णज्वरहरं कुर्यात् सर्वशश्चाप्युपक्रमम्|
श्लेष्मलानामवातानां ज्वरोऽनुष्णः कफाधिकः||२८१||
परिपाकं न सप्ताहेनापि याति मृदूष्मणाम्|
तं क्रमेण यथोक्तेन लङ्घनाल्पाशनादिना||२८२||

Contra indication for Langhana treatment:

Langhana (fasting) is not useful for patients suffering from Jwara caused by aggravated Vata, and by exhaustion, in chronic fever and also in fever caused by Kshata (external cut injury). Such patients are treated by Shamana (alleviation therapy).

For causing the fever, the aggravated Doshas afflict the Rasa Dhatu and decrease Agni (fire) from the Amashaya (Stomach and Small intestine). Therefore, such patients have less of Agni Bala (power of digestion). Even if a rice pot is kept over the burning fire with sufficient fuel, the rice will not get cooked if the flame of the fire is blown away by a strong wind. Similarly, in a person suffering from fever, the aggravated Doshas throw the Usma (digestive fire) out of the Pakti sthana (place of digestion).

In this condition the eaten food is not digested. If however, the food is light, it gets digested with difficulty. Therefore, for the preservation of the power of digestion, the line of treatment in the order of Langhana (fasting) etc. is useful.

The Malas (waste Products) of 7 Dhatus (tissue elements) get cooked or metabolised in 7 days. Therefore, generally on the 8th day the Jwara becomes Nirama (free from Ama or Accumulated metabolic waste products).

In the stage, when the Doshas are aggravated and the power of digestion is suppressed, if a person takes food which is especially heavy, he then succumbs to death immediately, or becomes miserable for a long time.

If the Jwara is caused by Vata Dosha, and other Doshas are not associated, then in suppression of the prescribed general rule, the patient is given massage and such other therapies. He is given decoctions and meat or vegetable soup to drink. All the therapies prescribed for the treatment of chronic fever are useful in this condition.

Extended Langhana till 10th day:

|In persons, having Sleshmala type of physical constitution, if fever is caused by excessive Kapha, if Vayu is not aggravated and if there is mild temperature, then because of the excessively mild digestive fire, the stage of Ama Paripaka (metabolic transformation of Ama) is not reached even within a week time. Such patients are kept on fast or are given light food or such other measures till the 10th day. Hereafter, they are treated by the administration of decoction etc. [272–283]

Langhana Therapy:

सामा ये ये च कफजाः कफपित्तज्वराश्च ये||२८३||

लङ्घनं लङ्घनीयोक्तं तेषु कार्यं प्रति प्रति|२८४|

Langana therapy (fasting) and similar other therapies described in the 22nd chapter of Sutra Sthana should invariably be administered in the following conditions:

1. When the Jwara is in its Sama stage
2. When Kapha is aggravated to produce the Jwara and
3. When both the Kapha and Pitta are aggravated together. [283–284]

Elimination therapies:

वमनैश्च विरेकैश्च बस्तिभिश्च यथाक्रमम्||२८४||

ज्वरानुपचरेद्धीमान् कफपित्तानिलोद्भवान्|२८५|

For the cure of Jwara caused by the aggravation of Vayu, Pitta and Kapha, Vamana (emesis), Virecana (purgation) and Basti (enema) therapies is administered respectively. [284–285]

Line of treatment of Samsrsta and SannipatikaJwara – fever:

संसृष्टान् सन्निपतितान् बुद्ध्वा तरतमैः समैः||२८५||

ज्वरान् दोषक्रमापेक्षी यथोक्तैरौषधैर्जयेत्|

वर्धनेनैकदोषस्य क्षपणेनोच्छ्रितस्य वा||२८६||

कफस्थानानुपूर्व्या वा सन्निपातज्वरं जयेत्|२८७|

Having ascertained the Samsrsta (Simultaneous vitiation of two Doshas) and Sannipatika (Simultaneous vitiation of all the three Doshas) nature of the disease, the Tara and Tama of the vitiation of dosha or either dual vitiation, the disease fever is treated with appropriate medicines keeping in view the line of treatment prescribed for each Dosha. Sannipata Jwara is treated by increasing 1 Dosha, by reducing the excessively aggravated one or by correcting the sites of Doshas in order, beginning with the site of Kapha. [285– 287]

Parotitis

सन्निपातज्वरस्यान्ते कर्णमूले सुदारूणः||२८७||

शोथः सञ्जायते तेन कश्चिदेव प्रमुच्यते|

रक्तावसेचनैः शीघ्रं सर्पिष्पानैश्च तं जयेत्|२८८||

प्रदेहैः कफपित्तघ्नैर्नावनैः कवलग्रहैः|२८९|

Inflamations near the root of the ear as a sequel of Sannipata Jwara is a serious condition and very few such patients survive. Therefore, efforts are made immediately to cure it by therapeutic measures which alleviate Kapha and Pitta like bloodletting, intake of Ghee, Pradeha (application of unction), Navana (inhalation therapy) and Kavala Graha (therapy in which medicines are kept in the mouth, gargles, rinse). [287–289]

Sakhanusari Jwara – fever:

शीतोष्ण स्निग्ध रूक्षाद्यैर्ज्वरो यस्य न शाम्यति|२८९||

शाखानुसारी रक्तस्य सोऽवसेकात् प्रशाम्यति|२९०|

When the Jwara does not get subsided by therapies which are cold, hot unctuous, unctuous etc, then it is diagnosed as Sakhanusari (which is located in the peripheral region of the body) such type of fever gets cured by the administration of bloodletting therapy. [289–290]

Jwara – fever as a Complication of Visarpa – herpes etc:

विसर्पणाभिघातेन यश्च विस्फोटकैर्ज्वरः||२९०||
तत्रादौ सर्पिषः पानं कफपित्तोत्तरो न चेत्|२९१|

The fever which has been caused due to visarpa – herpes, abhighata – trauma and visphota – eruptions, boils – and if there is no predominance of kapha and pitta in these fevers, ghee should be given to drink (oral administration) at the beginning.

Diet for Chronic fever:

दौर्बल्याद्देहधातूनां ज्वरो जीर्णोऽनुवर्तते||२९१||
बल्यैः सम्बृंहणैस्तस्मादाहारैस्तमुपाचरेत्|२९२|

The chronic fever persists if there is weakness of the Dhatus (Tissue elements) inside the body. Therefore, such patient is given such food which is strength promoting and nourishing [291–292]

Treatment of Trtiyaka and ChaturthakaJwara:

कर्म साधारणं जह्यात्तृतीयकचतुर्थकौ ||२९२||
आगन्तुरनुबन्धो हि प्रायशो विषमज्वरे|
वातप्रधानं सर्पिर्भिर्बस्तिभिः सानुवासनैः||२९३||
स्निग्धोष्णैरन्नपानैश्च शमयेद्विषमज्वरम्|
विरेचनेन पयसा सर्पिषा संस्कृतेन च||२९४||
विषमं तिक्तशीतैश्च ज्वरं पित्तोत्तरं जयेत्|
वमनं पाचनं रूक्षमन्नपानं विलङ्घनम्||२९५||
कषायोष्णं च विषमे ज्वरे शस्तं कफोत्तरे|२९६|

Treatment of Trtiyaka and ChaturthakaJwara:

In the Tritiyaka and Chaturthaka type of Visama Jwara, the line of treatment suggested for the Jwaras in general should not be followed because these 2 types of fever are mostly associated with Agantu or exogenic factors viz, dhatus or evil spritis including germs.

When in these two types of Jwara, Vayu is predominantly aggravated, then it is cured by the administration of ghee, Niruha and Anuvasana types of enema and unctuous as well as hot diet and drinks.

When Pitta is predominant, then the patient is given purgation therapy, medicated milk and ghee and articles which are bitter and cold.

When however, Kapha is predominant, then for the patient, emetic therapy, Pachana (the therapy which promotes metabolism), un-unctuous diet and drinks, fasting and hot decoctions are useful [292–296]

Recipes for different types of visamaJwara:

योगाः पराः प्रवक्ष्यन्ते विषम ज्वर नाशनाः||२९६||
प्रयोक्तव्या मतिमता दोषादीन् प्रविभज्य ते|
सुरा समण्डा पानार्थे भक्ष्यार्थे चरणायुधः||२९७||
तित्तिरिश्च मयूरश्च प्रयोज्या विषमज्वरे|
पिबेद्वा षट्पलं सर्पिरभयां वा प्रयोजयेत्|२९८||
त्रिफलायाः कषायं वा गुडूच्या रसमेव वा|
नीलिनीमजगन्धां च त्रिवृतां कटुरोहिणीम्||२९९||

पिबेज्ज्वरागमे युक्त्या स्नेहस्वेदोपपादितः।
सर्पिषो महतीं मात्रां पीत्वा वा छर्दयेत् पुनः॥३००॥
उपयुज्यान्नपानं वा प्रभूतं पुनरुल्लिखेत्।
सान्नं मद्यं प्रभूतं वा पीत्वा स्वप्याज्ज्वरागमे॥३०१॥
आस्थापनं यापनं वा कारयेद्विषमज्वरे।
पयसा वृषदंशस्य शकृद्वा तदहः पिबेत्॥३०२॥
वृषस्य दधिमण्डेन सुरया वा ससैन्धवम्।
पिप्पल्यास्त्रिफलायाश्च दध्नस्तक्रस्य सर्पिषः॥३०३॥
पञ्चगव्यस्य पयसः प्रयोगो विषमज्वरे।
रसोनस्य सतैलस्य प्राग्भक्तमुपसेवनम्॥३०४॥
मेद्यानामुष्णवीर्याणामामिषाणां च भक्षणम्।
हिङ्गुतुल्या तु वैयाघ्री वसा नस्यं ससैन्धवा॥३०५॥
पुराणसर्पिः सिंहस्य वसा तद्वत् ससैन्धवा।
सैन्धवं पिप्पलीनां च तण्डुलाः समनःशिलाः॥३०६॥
नेत्राञ्जनं तैलपिष्टं शस्यते विषमज्वरे।
पलङ्कषा निम्बपत्रं वचा कुष्ठं हरीतकी॥३०७॥
सर्षपाः सयवाः सर्पिर्धूपनं ज्वरनाशनम्।
ये धूमा धूपनं यच्च नावनं चाञ्जनं च यत्॥३०८॥
मनोविकारे निर्दिष्टं कार्यं तद्विषमज्वरे।
मणीनामोषधीनां च मङ्गल्यानां विषस्य च॥३०९॥
धारणादगदानां च सेवनान्न भवेज्ज्वरः।३१०।

Recipes which are very effective in curing Visama Jwara are being described. A wise physician should administer them keeping in view their suitability for the type of Doshas involved. These recipes are as follows:

1. Sura (alcoholic preparation) along with its Manda (upper layer) for use as a drink

2. The meat of cock, Tittiri and peacock for use as food.

3. Intake of (1) the medicated ghee called Satpala, (2) Abhaya (3) decoction of Triphala, (4) Juice of Guduchi, and preparation of nilini (Nilika or Nilabuhna), Ajagandha, Trivrta and Katurohini during the onset of fever. These preparations are administered appropriately after the patient is given Snehana (oleation) and Svedana (fomentation) therapies

4. Emesis after the administration of ghee in large quantity

5. Emesis after taking large quantity of food and drinks

6. Sleeping after taking large quantity of alcohol along with food when the attack of fever

7. Administration of Asthapana and Yapana types of medicated enema

8. Intake of the stool of the cat mixed with milk on the same day.

9. Intake of the stool of the cat mixed with either Dadhi Manda (Scum of the curd), alcohol, rock salt, Pippali, Triphala, curd, butter, milk ghee, Pancagavya (mixture of five products of cow or milk).

10. Intake of Rasona along with oil immediately before food

11. Intake of the meat of animals which are fatty and which are hot in potency

12. Inhalation of Hingu and Vasa (muscle fat) of Vyaghra (tiger) taken in equal quantity and mixed with rock salt

13. Inhalation of old ghee and the Vasa of Simha (lion) along with rock salt

14. Application of Anjana (collyrium) prepared of rock salt, seeds of Pippali and Manahsila mixed with oil

15. Fumigation by Palankasa, Leaves of Nimba, Vacha, Kushta – Saussurea lappa, Haritaki, Sarsapa, Yava and ghee

16. Administration of recipes of Dhuma (smoking), Dhupana (fumigation), Navana (Nasal inhalation) and ANjana (Collyrium), which are prescribed in the treatment of Manovikara or psychic ailments like Unmada (insanity) and apasmara (epilepsy)

17. Wearing of Mani (jewels),Ausadha (medicines), Mangalya (auspicious talisman) and Visa (poisonous

substances)
18. Intake of Agada (medicines)

Religious Rites:
सोमं सानुचरं देवं समातृगणमीश्वरम्||३१०||
पूजयन् प्रयतः शीघ्रं मुच्यते विषमज्वरात्|
विष्णुं सहस्रमूर्धानं चराचरपतिं विभुम्||३११||
स्तुवन्नामसहस्रेण ज्वरान् सर्वानपोहति|
ब्रह्माणमश्विनाविन्द्रं हुतभक्षं हिमाचलम्||३१२||
गङ्गां मरुद्गणांश्चेष्ट्य पूजयञ्जयति ज्वरान्|
भक्त्या मातुः पितुश्चैव गुरूणां पूजनेन च||३१३||
ब्रह्मचर्येण तपसा सत्येन नियमेन च|
जपहोमप्रदानेन वेदानां श्रवणेन च||३१४||
ज्वरादिवमुच्यते शीघ्रं साधूनां दर्शनेन च|
ज्वरे रसस्थे वमनमुपवासं च कारयेत्||३१५||

Prayer is offered to Lord Isvara along with Uma, their retinues and Matrs which immediately cures VisamaJwara.

Recitation of the Sahasra namas (One thousand names) of Lord Vishnu who has 1000 heads, who is the chief of the caracara (moving and non– moving things of the universe) and who is omnipresent, cures all types of Jwara.

Offering prayer (puja) through Isti or Yajna (fire ritual) to Brahma, the Asvins, Indra, Agni, the Himalayas, the Gangas and the retinue of Maruta cures Jwara.

Devotion of father and mother, prayer to gurus, observance of celibacy, practice of penace (tapa) truthfulness, and Niyama (religious rites), Japa (recitation of matras or increations), Homa (offering oblation to fire), hearing the recitation of the Vedas and Darsana (seeing or visiting) of saints immediately cures Jwara. [310–315]

Treatment of Dhatugata Jwara – fever:
सेकप्रदेहौ रक्तस्थे तथा संशमनानि च|
विरेचनं सोपवासं मांसमेदःस्थिते हितम्||३१६||
अस्थिमज्जगते देया निरूहाः सानुवासनाः|३१७|

When the Doshas causing are located in the Rasadhatu, then Vamana (emesis) and Upavasa (fasting) is done.

If they are located in the Rakta Dhatu then Seka (fomentation) and Pradeha (application of ointments) is done.

Virecana (purgation) and Upavasa (fasting) are done when the Doshas causing Jwara are located in Mamsa and Medas.

If Asthi and Majja Dhatus are pervaded by these Doshas, then Niruha and Anuvasana types of medicated enema is administered. (315– 317)

Agantuja Jwara Chikitsa – Line of treatment of Jwara caused by exogenic factors:
शापाभिचारादभूतानामभिषङ्गाच्च यो ज्वरः||३१७||
दैवव्यपाश्रयं तत्र सर्वमौषधमिष्यते|
अभिघातज्वरो नश्येत् पानाभ्यङ्गेन सर्पिषः||३१८||
रक्तावसेकैर्मद्यैश्च सात्म्यैर्मांसरसौदनैः|
सानाहो मद्यसात्म्यानां मदिरा रस भोजनैः||३१९||
क्षतानां व्रणितानां च क्षत व्रण चिकित्सया|
आश्वासेनेष्ट लाभेन वायोः प्रशमनेन च||३२०||
हर्षणैश्च शमं यान्ति काम शोक भय ज्वराः|
काम्यैरर्थैर्मनोज्ञैश्च पित्तघ्नैश्चाप्युपक्रमैः||३२१||
सद्वाक्यैश्च शमं याति ज्वरः क्रोध समुत्थितः|

कामात् क्रोधज्वरो नाशं क्रोधात् काम समुद्भवः||३२२||
याति ताभ्यामुभाभ्यां च भय शोक समुत्थितः|३२३|

For the Jwara caused by Shapa, Abhichara (black magic), Bhuta (microbes) and Abhishanga (affliction by lust, anger, fear), DaivaVyapashraya chikitsa (performance of religious rites) is the most preferred therapy.

Jwara caused by Abhighata (external injury) gets cured by the intake and massage of ghee and bloodletting. For patients who are suffering from anaha – constipation associated with fever caused by external injury, foods given along with pleasing alcohol and meat soup for those accustomed to alcohol would relieve these conditions.

For the treatment of Jwara caused by Ksata (injury like cuts) and Vrana (Ulcers), the line of treatment suggested for the treatment of Kshata (injury) and Vrana (ulcer) is adopted.

The Jwara caused by Kama (passion), Shoka (grief) and Bhaya (fear) gets treated by Ashvasa (consolation), Ishtalabha (providing KamyaArtha (described object), Manojna Artha (Pleasant object), therapies for the alleviation of Pitta and Sadvakya (correct advice, counselling).

The Jwara caused by Krodha (anger) subsides by Kama (passion) and Jwara caused by Kama (passion) gets subsided by Krodha (anger). Jwaras caused by Bhaya (fear) and Shoka (Grief) get subsided by Kama and krodha. . (317– 323)

Psychological fever:

ज्वरस्य वेगं कालं च चिन्तयञ्ज्वर्यते तु यः||३२३||
तस्येष्टैस्तु विचित्रैश्च विषयैर्नाशयेत् स्मृतिम्|३२४|

If the patient gets Jwara just by the thought of the time of onset of the disease, then his mind shall be diverted. [323–324]

Jwara Pramoksha Lakshana – signs that indicate fever is gradually relieving:

ज्वर प्रमोक्षे पुरुषः कूजन् वमति चेष्टते|
श्वसन्निवर्णः स्विन्नाङ्गो वेपते लीयते मुहुः||३२४||
प्रलपत्युष्णसर्वाङ्गः शीताङ्गश्च भवत्यपि|
विसञ्ज्ञो ज्वरवेगार्तः सक्रोध इव वीक्ष्यते ||३२५||
सदोषशब्दं च शकृद्द्रवं स्रवति वेगवत्|
लिङ्गान्येतानि जानीयाज्ज्वरमोक्षे विचक्षणः||३२६||
बहुदोषस्य बलवान् प्रायेणाभिनवो ज्वरः|
सत्क्रियादोषपक्त्या चेद्विमुञ्चति सुदारुणम्||३२७||
कृत्वा दोषवशाद्वेगं क्रमादुपरमन्ति ये|
तेषामदारुणो मोक्षो ज्वराणां चिरकारिणाम्||३२८||

Jwara Pramoksha Lakshana – signs that indicate fever is gradually relieving:

Production of Kujana (rumbling) sound, vomiting, Chesta (purposeless movements of limbs), heavy breathing, discolouration, Svinnanga (prostration), trembling, frequent fainting, delirium, at times the whole body becoming hot and at times cold, unconsciousness, more rise of temperature, angry appearance and passage of liquid motion with Doshas and sound along with force– these signs and symptoms are manifested at the time of remission of (Sannipata) Jwara. The wise physician should know them.

If a serious type of fever in which Doshas are aggravated in excess is treated with appropriate therapy, then because of Dosha Paka (metabolic changes) there will be sudden (Daruna) remission. This mostly happens in Abhinava (freshly attacked) fever.

In chronic types of fever, because of the Doshas, the temperature rise and then there is gradual remission (Adaruna Moksha) [324–328]

Jwaramuktalakshana:

Signs and symptoms when the patient becomes free from Jwara – fever:

विगत क्लम सन्तापमव्यथं विमलेन्द्रियम्|

युक्तं प्रकृतिसत्त्वेन विद्यात् पुरुषमज्वरम्||३२९||

Disappearance of Klama (mental fatigue) and Santapa (temperature), Absence of Pain, clarity of Senses, and Gaining of natural mental faculty, these are the signs and symptoms of a person who has become free from Jwara. [329]

Prohibitions during fever relief period:

सज्वरो ज्वरमुक्तश्च विदाहीनि गुरूणि च|
असात्म्यान्यन्नपानानि विरुद्धानि च वर्जयेत्||३३०||
व्यवायमतिचेष्टाश्च स्नानमत्यशनानि च|
तथा ज्वरः शमं याति प्रशान्तो जायते न च||३३१||
व्यायामं च व्यवायं च स्नानं चङ्क्रमणानि च|
ज्वरमुक्तो न सेवेत यावन्न बलवान् भवेत्||३३२||

Prohibitions during fever relief period:

Food and drinks which are Vidahi (causing burning sensation) Guru (heavy) Asatmya (Unwholesome) and Viruddha (mutually contradictory), sexual intercourse excessively shall be avoided by a patient suffering from fever and also when he has become free from fever. By observing thes rules, fever gets alleviated and it does not attack again. Exercise, sexual intercourse, bath, Chankraman (brisk walk) –these are avoided by the person who has become free from fever till he regains strength. [330–332]

PunaravartitaJwara – Reccurence of fever and its Management:

असञ्जात बलो यस्तु ज्वर मुक्तो निषेवते|
वर्ज्यमेतन्नरस्तस्य पुनरावर्तते ज्वरः||३३३||
दुर्हतेषु च दोषेषु यस्य वा विनिवर्तते|
स्वल्पेनप्यपचारेण तस्य व्यावर्तते पुनः||३३४||
चिरकाल परिक्लिष्टं दुर्बलं हीनतेजसम् |
अचिरेणैव कालेन स हन्ति पुनरागतः||३३५||
अथवाऽपि परीपाकं धातुष्वेव क्रमान्मलाः|
यान्ति ज्वरमकुर्वन्तस्ते तथाऽप्यपकुर्वते||३३६||
दीनतां श्वयथुं ग्लानिं पाण्डुतां नान्नकामताम्|
कण्डूरुक्तोठपिडकाः कुर्वन्त्यग्निं च ते मृदुम्||३३७||
एवमन्येऽपि च गदा व्यावर्तन्ते पुनर्गताः|
अनिर्घातेन दोषाणामल्पैरप्यहितैर्नृणाम्||३३८||
निर्वृत्तेऽपि ज्वरे तस्माद्यथावस्थं यथाबलम्|
यथाप्राणं हरेद्दोष प्रयोगैर्वा शमं नयेत्||३३९||
मृदुभिः शोधनैः शुद्धिर्यापना बस्तयो हिताः|
हिताश्च लघवो यूषा जाङ्गलामिषजा रसाः||३४०||
अभ्यङ्गोद्वर्तनस्नानधूपनान्यञ्जनानि च|
हितानि पुनरावृते ज्वरे तिक्तघृतानि च||३४१||
गुर्व्यभिष्यन्द्यसात्म्यानां भोजनात् पुनरागते|
लङ्घनोष्णोपचारादिः क्रमः कार्यश्च पूर्ववत्||३४२||
किराततिक्तकं तिक्ता मुस्तं पर्पटकोऽमृता|
घ्नन्ति पीतानि चाभ्यासात् पुनरावर्तकं ज्वरम्||३४३||

PunaravartitaJwara – Reccurence of fever and its Management:

If a person, who has become free from fever, resorts prohibited factors described above, before gaining strength, the Jwara reappears. If a person becomes free from fever when the Doshas have not been eliminated properly, then, even with mild irregularity in regimens (Apachara), it reappears. There is weakness and loss of vitality in them. If the fever reappears in them then this certainly leads to their death.

Sometimes, Doshas (Malas) undergo Paripaka (metabolic transformation) in the Dhatus (tissue elements) gradually and the fever subsides. The doshas which have been left over in the body might not prove to be dangerous by causing recurrence of fever. These doshas will gradually undergo suppuration in the cells. These doshas on gaining entry into the deeper tissues will not cause fever but will still harm the body. The harmful effects include symptoms like Dinata (uneasiness), Shvayathu (odema), Glani (a feeling as if covered with a wet cloth), Panduta (anemia), loss of appetite, itching, urticaria, pimples and supression of the power of digestion.

Similarly, other diseases which are already cured reappear in the individual by not eliminating the Doshas properly and by not following proper regimen after the cure of the disease. Therefore, even after the fever subsides, the Doshas are removed either by elimination or Alleviation therapies depending upon the stage and strength of Doshas. For this purpose, mild elimination therapies and Yapana type of Basti is administered. Yusa (vegetable soups) and Rasa (meat soups) of the meat of Jangala type of animals, which are light, are useful in this condition. Abhyanga (massage), Udvartana (Unction), Snana (bath), dhupana (fumigation), Anjana (Collyrium) and ghee prepared by boiling with bitter medicines are useful in the treatment of Jwara which has reappeared.

If the fever reappears because of the intake of food which is Guru (heavy), Abhisyandi (which obstructs the channels of circulation) and

Unwholesome, the below mentioned treatment should be done.

Treatment:
Langhana (fasting) and
Hot therapies are administered as described before.
Intake of the decoction of KirataTiktaka, Tikta, Musta (Cyperus rotundus), Parpataka and Amrta cures reappeared fever. [333–343]

तस्यां तस्यामवस्थायां ज्वरितानां विचक्षण:|
ज्वराक्रियाक्रमापेक्षी कुर्यात्तत्तच्चिकित्सितम्||३४४||
In different stages of Jwara, the wise physician should treat the patient by the therapies suggested in the line of treatment. [344]

रोगराट् सर्वभूतानामन्तकृद्दारुणो ज्वर:|
तस्मादिवशेषतस्तस्य यतेत प्रशमे भिषक्||३४५||
Jwara is the king of diseases.
It causes the death of all creatures and is of serious nature. Therefore, the physician should make special efforts for its cure. [345]

To sum up:–
तत्र श्लोक:–
यथाक्रमं यथाप्रश्नमुक्तं ज्वरचिकित्सितम्|
आत्रेयेणाग्निवेशाय भूतानां हितकाम्यया||३४६||
With a desire for the welfare of the living creatures, Atreya has furnished the replies to the queries of Agnivesha regarding the treatment of Jwara. [346]

इत्यग्निवेशकृते तन्त्रे चरक प्रतिसंस्कृते चिकित्सित स्थाने ज्वर चिकित्सितं नाम तृतीयोऽध्याय:||३|
Thus, ends the 3rd chapter on the treatment of Jwara (fever) of the Chikitsa section of Agnivesha's work as redacted by Charaka.

10

Chikitsasthana Chapter 4
Raktapitta Chikitsitam

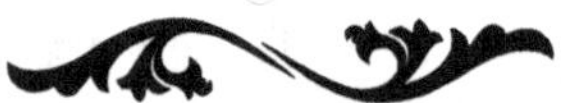

The fourth chapter of Charaka Chikitsa sthana is called Raktapitta Chikitsa. Raktapitta disease is a collection of bleeding disorders such as nasal bleeding, bleeding through ear, nose, heavy periods, rectal bleeding, urethral bleeding etc.

For easy understanding, read about bleeding disorders and Ayurvedic treatment

अथातो रक्तपित्तचिकित्सितं व्याख्यास्यामः||१||

इति ह स्माह भगवानात्रेयः||२||

Now we shall expound the chapter on the treatment on RaktaPitta (a condition characterized by bleeding from different parts of the body)

Thus said lord Atreya [1-2]

विहरन्तं जितात्मानं पञ्चगङ्गे पुनर्वसुम्|

प्रणम्योवाच निर्मोहमग्निवेशोऽग्निवर्चसम्||३||

भगवन् रक्तपित्तस्य हेतुरुक्तः सलक्षणः|

वक्तव्यं यत् परं तस्य वक्तुमर्हसि तद्गुरो||४||

Lord Punarvasu, who is Jitatma – having self control, was on a stroll in a place called Pancha Ganga. Agnivesha, who was free from attachment, and whose speech was like fire, paid obeisance to him and enquired, "Oh Lord; you have already described the aetiology, signs and symptoms of RaktaPitta. Oh Preceptor! Please tell us further details on this subject" [3-4]

Lord Punarvasu replied:

गुरुरुवाच-

महागदं महावेगमग्निवच्छीघ्रकारि च|

हेतु लक्षणविच्छीघ्रं रक्तपित्तमुपाचरेत्||५||

तस्योष्णं तीक्ष्णमम्लं च कटूनि लवणानि च|

घर्मश्चान्नविदाहश्च हेतुः पूर्व निदर्शितः||६||

RaktaPitta is a serious disease and it afflicts the patient with great speed. Like fire, it manifests itself and affects swiftly. Therefore, the physician who is well versed in the aetiology, signs and symptoms of this disease, should immediately take steps for its treatment.

Causes for RaktaPitta:

Diet and activities that are

Ushna – hot

Tikshna – sharp

Amlam – sour

Katu – pungent

Lavana – saline

Heat of the sun and

Vidaha – Improper digestion leading to burning sensation of food [5-6]

Raktapitta Samprapti – Pathogenesis:
तैर्हेतुभिः समुत्क्लिष्टं पित्तं रक्तं प्रपद्यते।
तद्योनित्वात् प्रपन्नं च वर्धते तत् प्रदूषयत्॥७॥
तस्योष्मणा द्रवो धातुर्धातोर्धातोः प्रसिच्यते।
स्विद्यतस्तेन संवृद्धिं भूयस्तदधिगच्छति॥८॥

Because of the above causative factors, Pitta gets vitiated and reaches Raktha (blood). Pitta and Rakta are directly related. Therefore, when it reaches Rakta and vitiates it, Rakta gets further aggravated because of the heating property of Pitta, these tissue elements get heated, as a result of which , there is exudation of more liquids from these elements. These liquids get heated, as a result of which, their liquids get mixed up with Rakta (blood). This leads to increase in volume of blood and its expulsion. [7-8]

Definition of Rakta Pitta:-
संयोगाद्दूषणात्तु सामान्याद्गन्धवर्णयोः।
रक्तस्य पित्तमाख्यातं रक्तपित्तं मनीषिभिः॥९॥

The disease is called RaktaPitta by the Wise because

Pitta combines with Rakta

Both Pitta and Rakta have hotness as a common feature.

Pitta imparts its odour and colour to Rakta.

Hence, this disease is called as Raktapitta.[9]

Adhishtana for Raktapitta – Location of Raktapitta:
प्लीहानं च यकृच्चैव तदधिष्ठाय वर्तते।
स्रोतांसि रक्तवाहीनि तन्मूलानि हि देहिनाम्॥१०॥

Adhishtana – root place for the disease Raktapitta is Pleeha – spleen and Yakrut – liver.

This disease affects Raktavaha Srotas – blood channels.

RakptaPitta types and Lakshana – Specific signs and symptoms:
सान्द्रं सपाण्डु सस्नेहं पिच्छिलं च कफान्वितम्।
श्यावारुणं सफेनं च तनु रूक्षं च वातिकम्॥११॥
रक्तपित्तं कषायाभं कृष्णं गोमूत्रसन्निभम्।
मेचकागार धूमाभमञ्जनाभं च पैत्तिकम्॥१२॥
संसृष्टलिङ्गं संसर्गात्त्रिलिङ्गं सान्निपातिकम्॥१३॥

Kaphaja Raktapitta:

When the disease has Kapha dominance, the blood will be

Sandra – dense, viscous

Sa pandu – whitish discoloration

Sasneha – oiliness, unctuousness

Picchila – Sticky, Slimy

Vataja Raktapitta:

When it is associated with Vata dominance, the blood will be

Shyava – Aruna – brownish red

Saphena – frothy

Tanu – thin

Rooksha – dry

Pittaja Raktapitt:

When associated with Pitta, blood becomes

Kashaya (or pink red, like the colour of the Patala flower),

Black like the cow's urine, Mechaka (greasy- black), Agara Dhuma (house soot) and Anjana (Black collyrium).

Samsarga – When vitiated by 2 Doshas, the signs and symptoms of the aggressive 2 Doshas are manifested in the blood

Sannipata – When vitiated by all the 3 Doshas, the signs and symptoms of all the 3 Doshas are manifested. [11-13]

Prognosis – Sadhya Asadhyatva:

एकदोषानुगं साध्यं द्विदोषं याप्यमुच्यते||१३||

यत्त्रिदोषमसाध्यं तन्मन्दाग्नेरतिवेगवत्|

व्याधिभिः क्षीणदेहस्य वृद्धस्यानशनतश्च यत्||१४||

The Rakta Pitta, associated with:

1 Dosha is curable.

2 Doshas it is palliable, or Yapya.

All the 3 Doshas, is incurable;

It also becomes incurable in the following conditions:

1. If the patient is having Mandagni (less power of digestion and metabolism)

2. Ativegavat – If the disease has an acute attack

3. If the patient is emaciated by diseases

4. Ksheena Deha – if the patient is debilitated

5. Vruddha – if the patient is aged

6. Anashna – If the patient is not able to eat. [13-14]

Determination of prognosis on the basis of movement through different tracks:

गतिरूर्ध्वमधश्चैव रक्तपित्तस्य दर्शिता|

ऊर्ध्वा सप्त विधद्वारा द्विद्वारा त्वधरा गतिः||१५||

सप्त छिद्राणि शिरसि द्वे चाधः, साध्यमूर्ध्वगम्|

याप्यं त्वधोगं, मार्गौ तु द्वावसाध्यं प्रपद्यते||१६||

यदा तु सर्वच्छिद्रेभ्यो रोमकूपेभ्य एव च|

वर्तते तामसङ्ख्येयां गतिं तस्याहुरान्तिकीम्||१७||

यच्चोभयाभ्यां मार्गाभ्यामतिमात्रं प्रवर्तते|

तुल्यं कुणपगन्धेन रक्तं कृष्णमतीव च||१८||

संसृष्टं कफवाताभ्यां कण्ठे सज्जति चापि यत्|

यच्चाप्युपद्रवैः सर्वैर्यथोक्तैः समभिद्रुतम्||१९||

हारिद्रनीलहरितताम्रैर्वर्णैरुपद्रुतम्|

क्षीणस्य कासमानस्य यच्च तच्च न सिध्यति||२०||

यद्द्विदोषानुगं यद्वा शान्तं शान्तं प्रकुप्यति|

मार्गान्मार्गं चरेद्यद्वा याप्यं पित्तमसृक् च तत्||२१||

The movement of RaktaPitta through upward (Urdhwaga Raktapita) and downward tracks (Adhoga Raktapita) has been described. There are 7 openings (Dvara) in upward track. There are 2 openings in the downward track. In the head (3), 7 holes namely, two eyes, two ears, two nostrils and oral cavity. Similarly, there are 2 openings downwards namely the anus and the genito- urinary tract.

Sadhyam Urdhwagam – RakthaPitta having upward movement is curable.

Yapyam tu Adhogam – If it moves downward then it is palliable.

If it moves through both the upward and downward tracks, then it becomes incurable.

Sometimes, Rakta Pitta also becomes incurable in the following conditions: -

1. When bleeding takes place in excess through either of the upward and downward tracks;

2. When the blood has a smell like that of the dead body (Kunapa gandhi)

3. When it is exceedingly black

4. When it gets associated with both Kapha and Vata

5. When it gets obstructed in the throat

6. When it is associated with all the complications described in Nidanasthana

7. When an emaciated patient has continuous coughing and the phlegm that comes out is yellow, blue, green or coppery in color.

Rakta Pitta becomes palliable in the following conditions:-

1. When it is associated with 2 Doshas while moving through the tracks;

2. When it gets repeatedly alleviated and aggravated and

3. When it leaves one channel and gets manifested in another.[15-21]

Curability:

एकमार्गं बलवतो नातिवेगं नवोत्थितम्।

रक्तपित्तं सुखे काले साध्यं स्यान्निरुपद्रवम्॥२२॥

RaktaPitta is curable in the following conditions:-

1. When it is manifested only through 1 track (here it is to be interpreted as only upward track)

2. When the patient is physically strong

3. When the attack of the disease is not very acute

4. When the treatment is immediately after the attack

5. When the treatment is initiated immediately after the attack

6. When the disease is free from complications. [22]

Specific etiological factors:

स्निग्धोष्णमुष्णरूक्षं च रक्तपित्तस्य कारणम्।

अधोगस्योत्तरं प्रायः, पूर्वं स्यादूर्ध्वगस्य तु॥२३॥

ऊर्ध्वगं कफ संसृष्टमधोगं मारुतानुगम्।

द्विमार्गं कफ वाताभ्यामुभाभ्यामनुबध्यते॥२४॥

Factors which are Snigdha (unctuous, oily) and Ushna (hot) and those which are Ushna (hot) and Rooksha (dry) cause Rakta Pitta. The hot and dryness cause the disease and oiliness and hotness are generally responsible for its upward movement.

Upward movement of the disease mostly leads to the association of Kapha and downward movement of the disease mostly leads to the association Vata.

Urdhwaga is associated with Kapha and Adhoga is associated with Vata.

When the disease moves through both the tracks then both Kapha and Vayu become associated [23-24]

Raktapitta Chikitsa: Avoid Stambhana Chikitsa in the beginning stage:

अक्षीण बल मांसस्य रक्तपित्तं यदश्नतः।

तद्दोषदुष्टमुत्क्लिष्टं नादौ स्तम्भनमर्हति॥२५॥

गलग्रहं पूतिनस्यं मूर्च्छायमरुचिं ज्वरम्।

गुल्मं प्लीहानमानाहं किलासं कृच्छ्रमूत्रताम्॥२६॥

कुष्ठान्यर्शांसि वीसर्पं वर्णनाशं भगन्दरम्।

बुद्धीन्द्रियोपरोधं च कुर्यात् स्तम्भितमादितः||२७||
तस्मादुपेक्ष्यं बलिनो बलदोषविचारिणा |
रक्तपित्तं प्रथमतः प्रवृद्धं सिद्धिमिच्छता||२८||

Raktapitta Chikitsa: Avoid Stambhana Chikitsa in the beginning stage:

If Rakta Pitta occurs as a result of over nourishment (santarpana) and if the strength and the muscle and tissues of the patient are not depleted, then Stambhana treatment (blockage) treated may not be administered at first.

If the bleeding is stopped by Sthambha treatment at the beginning then it may cause:

Galagraha – obstruction in throat

Putinasya – putrid smell in the nose

Murcha – Fainting

Aruchi – Anorexia

Jvara – fever

Gulma – Phantom tumour

Plihan – enlargement of spleen

Anaha – constipation

Kilasa – a type of skin disease

Mutra Krcchra – dysuria

Kustha – skin diseases

Arshas – piles

Visarpa – erysipelas,

Varna Nasha – loss of complexion

Bhagandara – fistula in ano and

Inhibition of the functions of the senses

Therefore, a physician who is acquainted with body strength and Doshas, should at the beginning, refrain from stopping the bleeding in the patient suffering from Rakta Pitta.

A Physician who desires success in treatment should do so even if the attack of the disease is acute [25-28]

Langhana treatment:

प्रायेण हि समुत्क्लिष्टमामदोषाच्छरीरिणाम्|
वृद्धिं प्रयाति पितासृक्तस्मात्तल्लङ्घ्यमादितः||२९||
मार्गौ दोषानुबन्धं च निदानं प्रसमीक्ष्य च|
लङ्घनं रक्तपित्तादौ तर्पणं वा प्रयोजयेत्||३०||

Urdhwaga Raktapitta (bleeding from upper orifices) is associated with Pitta and Kapha. It occurs due to Snigdha – unctuous, oily and Ushna – hot qualities.

To counter Kapha, in the initial stages, Langhana – lightening therapy (to bring about lightness to the body, via fasting etc) is advocated.

Adhoga Raktapitta (bleeding through lower orifices), is due to Vata and Pitta. Here, Tarpana treatment (nourishing) is advocated. Tarpana is achieved by giving nourishing Yavagu (gruels). [29-30]

Diet and Drinks:

ह्रीबेर चन्दनोशीर मुस्त पर्पटकैः शृतम्|
केवलं शृतशीतं वा दद्यात्तोयं पिपासवे||३१||
ऊर्ध्वगे तर्पणं पूर्व पेयां पूर्वमधोगते|
काल सात्म्यानुबन्ध ज्ञो दद्यात् प्रकृति कल्पवित्||३२||
जल खर्जूर मृद्वीका मधूकैः सपरूषकैः|
शृत शीतं प्रयोक्तव्यं तर्पणार्थे सशर्करम्||३३||
तर्पणं सघृतक्षौद्रं लाजचूर्णैः प्रदापयेत्|

ऊर्ध्वगं रक्तपितं तत् पीतं काले व्यपोहति||३४||
मन्दाग्नेरम्लसात्म्याय तत् साम्लमपि कल्पयेत्|
दाडिमामलकैर्विद्वानम्लार्थं चानुदापयेत्||३५||

If the patient is thirsty, he is given water boiled with

Hrivera – Pavonia odorata

Chandana – Santalum album

Usira – Vetiveria zizanioides

Musta – Cyperus rotundus

And Parpataka – Fumaria parviflora.

Or simple boiled and cooled water (sruta Sheeta) can also be given in this condition.

In Urdhwaga Raktapitta, Tarpana (nourishing drink) is given in the beginning.

In Adhoga Raktapitta, Peya (thin liquid drink) is given in the beginning.

The drug that is used for the preparation of Tarpana or Peya is determined by a physician who is acquainted with time, Satmya, associated Doshas, nature of the drugs and Kalpa (method of preparation).

For the purpose of Tarpana, water is boiled with

Kharjura – dates - Phoenix dactylifera

Mrdvika – Grapes – Vitis vinifera

Madhuka – Madhuca longifolia and

Parushaka – Grewia asiatica

This water is cooled and added with sugar before administration.

The above recipe is prepared based on Shadanga Paneeya procedure – 1 part of herbs plus 64 parts of water, boiled and reduced to 32 parts, and filtered.

Tarpana prepared with the powder of Laja (fried paddy) along with ghee and honey, is given to the patient to drink, in appropriate time. This potion cures Urdhvaga RaktaPitta.

This Tarpana is made sour in taste for a person whose digestion is suppressed and who has a liking for the sour taste. For making its sour,

Dadima – Pomegranate - Punica granatum and

Amalaka – Emblica officinalis is used by a wise physician [31-35]

Raktapiita Pathyam:

शालि षष्टिक नीवार कोरदूष प्रशान्तिकाः|
श्यामाकश्च प्रियङ्गुश्च भोजनं रक्तपितिनाम्||३६||
मुद्गा मसूराश्चणकाः समकुष्ठाढकीफलाः|
प्रशस्ताः सूपयूषार्थं कल्पिता रक्तपितिनाम्||३७||
पटोल निम्ब वेत्राग्र प्लक्ष वेतस पल्लवाः|
किराततिक्तकं शाकं गण्डीरः सकठिल्लकः||३८||
कोविदारस्य पुष्पाणि काश्मर्यस्याथ शाल्मले:|
अन्नपानविधौ शाकं यच्चान्यद्रक्तपितनुत्||३९||
शाकार्थं शाक सात्म्यानां तच्छस्तं रक्तपितिनाम्|
स्विन्नं वा सर्पिषा भृष्टं यूषवद्वा विपाचितम्||४०||
पारावतान् कपोतांश्च लावान् रक्ताक्षवर्तकान्|
शशान् कपिञ्जलानेणान् हरिणान्कालपुच्छकान्||४१||
रक्तपित्ते हितान् विद्याद्रसांस्तेषां प्रयोजयेत्|
ईषदम्लाननम्लान् वा घृतभृष्टान् सशर्करान्||४२||
कफानुगे यूषशाकं दद्याद्वातानुगे रसम्|
रक्तपित्ते यवागूनामतः कल्पः प्रवक्ष्यते||४३||

पद्मोत्पलानां किञ्जल्कः पृश्निपर्णी प्रियङ्गुकाः।
जले साध्या रसे तस्मिन् पेया स्याद्रक्तपित्तिनाम्॥४४॥
चन्दनोशीर लोध्राणां रसे तद्वत् सनागरे।
किरात तिक्तकोशीर मुस्तानां तद्वदेव च॥४५॥
धातकी धन्वयासाम्बुबिल्वानां वा रसे शृता।
मसूर पृश्निपर्ण्योर्वा स्थिरामुद्गरसेऽथ वा॥४६॥
रसे हरेणुकानां वा सघृते सबलारसे।
सिद्धाः पारावतादीनां रसे वा स्युः पृथक्पृथक्॥४७॥
इत्युक्ता रक्तपित्तघ्न्यः शीताः समधुशर्कराः।
यवाग्वः कल्पना चैषा कार्या मांसरसेष्वपि॥४८॥

Foods used by a patient suffering from RaktaPitta:

Shali – rice

Shastika – a type of rice

Neevara –

Koradusha

Prasantika

Shyamaka and

Priyangu – Callicarpa macrophylla

Drugs useful for the preparation of Supa (soup) and Yusha (drink) for a patient suffering from Rakta Pitta:

Mudga – Green gram

Masura – Masoor dal

Chanaka – Bengal gram

Makustha – Phaseolus aconitifolius and

Fruits of Adhaki – Cajanus cajan

Vegetables to be given to patients suffering from Rakta pitta:

Patola – Trichosanthes dioica

Nimba – Neem – Azadirachta indica

Vetragra

Plaksha – Ficus lacor

Leaves of Vetasa – Salix caprea

Kirata Tikta – Swertia chirata

Gandira – Canthium parviflorum

Kathillaka

Flowers of Kovidara – Bauhinia variegata and

Shalmali – Salmalia malabarica

These vegetables can be prepared by steam boiling, or by frying with ghee.

These can also be given in the form of vegetable soup.

The meat or meat soup of Paravata, Kapota (pigeon), Lava, Raktaksha, Vartaka, Shasha (rabbit), Kapinjala, Ena, Harina (deer), Kalapucchaka shall be administered. The meat should be fried with ghee and added with sugar.

If the disease is associated with Kapha, then vegetable soup (Yusha shaka) is preferred and if it is associated with Vata, then meat soup is preferred.

Different Yavagu – medicated gruels:

1. Padmakinjalka (lotus androecium) and Utpala, Parni and Priyangu should be boiled in water. With this water, gruel is prepared.

2. Similar gruel can also be prepared with Chandana (sandalwood), Usheera (Vetiver), Lodhra (Symplocos racemosa) and ginger.

3. Gruel can also be prepared with water of Kiratatikta (Swertia chirata), Usheera and Musta (Cyperus rotundus).

4. Yavagu prepared with Masura and Prishniparni is useful
5. Yavagu prepared with extract of Dhataki, Dhanvayasa, Ambu and Bilva
6. Yavagu of Sthira and Mudga – Green gram
7. Yavagu of Harenuka
8. Yavagu prepared with ghee and Bala (Sida cordifolia)
These gruels should be administered after self cooling and added with honey and sugar. Yavagu can also be prepared using meat soups.

Diet based on RaktaPitta stages:
शशः सवास्तुकः शस्तो विबन्धे रक्तपितिनाम्|
वातोल्बणे तितिरिः स्यादुदुम्बररसे शृतः||४९||
मयूरः प्लक्ष निर्यूहे न्यग्रोधस्य च कुक्कुटः|
रसे बिल्वोत्पलादीनां वर्तकक्रकरौ हितौ||५०||
तृष्यते तिक्तकैः सिद्धं तृष्णाघ्नं वा फलोदकम्|
सिद्धं विदारिगन्धाद्यैरथवा शृतशीतलम्||५१||
If the patient suffering from RaktaPitta develops constipation, then the meat of Shasha (rabbit) along with Vastuka is useful.
If there is predominance of Vayu, then Tittiri – Partridge boiled with the extract of udumbara (Ficus racemosa) is useful.
Following medicines are also useful.
1. Mayura (peacock) boiled with the decoction of Plaksha – Ficus lacor
2. Kukkuta (cock) boiled with the decoction of Nyagrodha – Ficus bengalensis
3. Vartaka and Krakra, boiled with the decoction of Bilva – Aegle marmelos ; Utpala etc:
If the patient is suffering from thirst, then, the following recipes are useful
1. Water boiled with bitter herbs
2. Fruit juice
3. Water boiled Vidarigandha etc. (Laghu Panca Mula) (49-51)

Drinks
ज्ञात्वा दोषावनुबलौ बलमाहारमेव च|
जलं पिपासवे दद्यादिवसर्गादल्पशोऽपि वा||५२||
After ascertaining that nature of the subsidiary Doshas, the strength and diet of the patient, water is given to him when he is thirsty till the limit of satisfaction is reached or in small quantities.[52]

Advice to avoid causative factors:
निदानं रक्तपित्तस्य यत्किञ्चित् सम्प्रकाशितम्|
जीवितारोग्यकामैस्तन्न सेव्यं रक्तपित्तिभिः||५३||
इत्यन्नपानं निर्दिष्टं क्रमशो रक्तपित्तनुत्|५४|
In Nidana 2:4, the causative factors of RaktaPitta are described. A patient of RaktaPitta who desires life and health should not resort to these factors.
Thus the diet and drinks for a person suffering from RaktaPitta are described. [53-54]

Shodhana for Raktapitta – Panchakarma procedures:
वक्ष्यते बहुदोषाणां कार्यं बलवतां च यत्||५४||
अक्षीण बल मांसस्य यस्य सन्तर्पणोत्थितम्|
बहुदोषं बलवतो रक्तपित्तं शरीरिणः||५५||
काले संशोधनार्हस्य तद्धरेन्निरुपद्रवम्|

विरेचनेनोर्ध्वभागमधोगं वमनेन च॥५६॥
त्रिवृतामभयां प्राज्ञः फलान्यारग्वधस्य वा।
त्रायमाणां गवाक्ष्या वा मूलमामलकानि वा॥५७॥
विरेचनं प्रयुञ्जीत प्रभूतमधुशर्करम्।
रसः प्रशस्यते तेषां रक्तपित्ते विशेषतः॥५८॥
वमनं मदनोन्मिश्रो मन्थः सक्षौद्रशर्करः।
सशर्करं वा सलिलमिक्षूणां रस एव वा॥५९॥
वत्सकस्य फलं मुस्तं मदनं मधुकं मधु।
अधोवहे रक्तपित्ते वमनं परमुच्यते॥६०॥
ऊर्ध्वगे शुद्धकोष्ठस्य तर्पणादिः क्रमो हितः।
अधोगते यवाग्वादिर्न चेत्स्यान्मारुतो बली॥६१॥

Let us know about the therapies that are administered to persons having exceedingly aggravated Doshas and physical strength.

Virechana (purgation) is given to a patient suffering from Urdhvaga Rakta Pitta and

Vamana (Emesis) is given to a patient suffering from Adhoga Rakta PItta, in the following circumstances:

1. If the strength and muscle tissue of the patient are not reduced,

2. If disease is caused because of Santarpana (over-nourishment)

3. If there is excess of aggravated Doshas

4. If the patient is physically strong because of seasonal effects.

5. If the time is conducive to the administration of elimination therapy i.e. if the reason is neither very hot nor very cold.

6. If the patient is suitable for the administration of these therapies

7. If the patient is free from complications, or if the recipe, to be administered, is not associated with any complications

For the purpose of Virechana (Purgation) a wise physician should administer along with liberal quantity of honey and sugar, the following recipes:

1. Trivrit – Ipomoea turpethum and Abhaya – Terminalia chebula

2. Fruits of Aragvadha – Cassia fistula

3. Trayamana – Gentiana kurroo

4. Gavakshi

5. Mulaka – Radish and Amalaki – Emblica officinalis

For Adhoga Raktapita, Vamana is an excellent therapy and it is administered by the following recipes:

1. Mantha prepared of Madana (Randia dumetorum) and added with honey and Sugar along with additional sugar and water

2. Mantha prepared of Madana (Randia dumetorum) and added with honey and sugar and added with sugarcane juice

3. The fruits of Vatsaka – Kutaja – Holarrhena antidysenterica

Musta – Cyperus rotundus

Madana – Randia dumetorum

Madhuka—Madhuca longifolia and

Madhu – honey

In Urdhvaga Rakta Pitta, when the bowels are cleaned by the administration of purgation, Tarpana etc. is gradually given to the patient.

In adhoga type of Rakta pitta, when the alimentary tract is cleaned by emesis, Yavagu etc, is given to the patient, if Vayu is not aggravated in excess [54-46]

Shamana Chikitsa – Alleviation therapy:

बल मांस परिक्षीणं शोकभाराध्व कर्शितम्।

ज्वलनादित्य सन्तप्तमन्यैर्वा क्षीणमामयैः||६२||
गर्भिणीं स्थविरं बालं रूक्षाल्प प्रमिताशिनम्|
अवम्यम विरेच्यं वा यं पश्येद्रक्तपितिनम्||६३||
शोषेण सानुबन्धं वा तस्य संशमनी क्रिया|
शस्यते रक्तपित्तस्य परं साऽथ प्रवक्ष्यते||६४||
अटरूषक मृद्वीकापथ्याक्वाथः सशर्करः|
मधुमिश्रः श्वास कास रक्तपित्त निबर्हणः||६५||
अटरूषक निर्यूहे प्रियङ्गुं मृतिकाञ्जने|
विनीय लोध्रं क्षौद्रं च रक्तपित्तहरं पिबेत्||६६||
पद्मकं पद्मकिञ्जल्कं दूर्वा वास्तूकमुत्पलम्|
नागपुष्पं च लोध्रं च तेनैव विधिना पिबेत्||६७||
प्रपौण्डरीकं मधुकं मधु चाश्वशकृद्रसे|
यवासभृङ्गरजसोर्मूलं वा गोशकृद्रसे||६८||
विनीय रक्तपित्तघ्नं पेयं स्यात्तण्डुलाम्बुना|
युक्तं वा मधुसर्पिभ्यां लिह्याद्गोश्वशकृद्रसम्||६९||
खदिरस्य प्रियङ्गूणां कोविदारस्य शाल्मलेः|
पुष्पचूर्णानि मधुना लिह्यान्ना रक्तपित्तिकः||७०||
शृङ्गाटकानां लाजानां मुस्तखर्जूरयोरपि|
लिह्याच्चूर्णानि मधुना पद्मानां केशरस्य च||७१||
धन्वजानामसृग्लिह्यान्मधुना मृगपक्षिणाम्|
सक्षौद्रं ग्रथिते रक्ते लिह्यात् पारावतं शकृत्||७२||

Shamana Chikitsa – Alleviation therapy:

Alleviation therapy is useful for a patient suffering from RaktaPitta in the following conditions:

1. If there is loss of strength and muscle tissue in the patient

2. If the patient is emaciated because of grief, carrying heavy load and walking long distance

3. If the patient is afflicted with the heat of the fire or sunrays;

4. If the patient is emaciated because of other diseases

5. If the patient is a pregnant lady, person of old age or very young

6. If the patient is habituated with taking unctuous food or if he takes small quantity of food for less number of times

7. If the patient is not suitable for emesis or Purgation therapies and

8. If the patient is suffering from consumption,

Recipes for alleviation therapy are being described below:

1. The Kashaya of

Atarusaka – Vasa – Adhatoda vasica

Mrdvika – raisins and

Pathya – Terminalia chebula along with sugar and honey

Cures

Shvasa – Asthma

Kasa – bronchitis and

Rakta Pitta.

2. In the decoction of Atarusaka, the paste of

Priyangu – Callicarpa macrophylla

Mrttika – mud

Anjana – Collyrium

Lodhra – Symplocos racemosa and

Honey are added. This Kashaya cures Rakta Pitta.

3. A Kashaya prepared of

Padmaka Kinjalka (androecium) or Padma – Nelumbo nucifera

Durva – Cynodon dactylon

Vastuka

Utpala

Nagapuspa – Mesua ferrea and

Lodhra – Symplocos racemosa is taken along with the decoction of Vasa and honey.

4. A medicated liquid prepared of

Prapaundarika

Madhuka – Madhuca longifolia and

Madhu – honey

In root of

Yavasa – Alhagi pseudalhagi and

Bhrngaraja – Eclipta alba

In the juice of the stool of horse or the one prepared of the root of

Yavasa – Alhagi pseudalhagi and

Bhrngaraja – Eclipta alba

In the juice of the stool of the cow is taken along with Tandulambu (rice-wash).

5. Avaleha prepared of the powder of

Khadira – Acacia catechu

Priyangu – Callicarpa macrophylla

Kovidara – and

The flower of Shalmali – Salmalia malabarica

By adding honey it is given to the patient suffering from raktapitta.

6. Avaleha prepared of the powders of

Shringataka – Trapa bispinosa

Laja – Fried paddy

Musta – Cyperus rotundus

Kharjura – Phoenix dactylifera and

Kesara (androecium) of Padma (Nelumbo nucifera) by adding honey is given to the patient.

7. The blood of animals and birds habiting in arid land (Jangala) is taken as linctus by adding honey.

8. A linctus is prepared of the juice of the stool of horse and taken along with honey and ghee

9. If the blood is clotted, then the stool of Paravata mixed with honey is given to the patient in the form of a linctus. [62-72]

उशीर कालीयक लोध्र पद्मक प्रियङ्गुका कट्फलशङ्ख गैरिकाः।
पृथक् पृथक् चन्दन तुल्यभागिकाः सशर्करास्तण्डुलधावनाप्लुताः॥७३॥
रक्तं सपित्तं तमकं पिपासां दाहं च पीताः शमयन्ति सद्यः।
किराततिक्तं क्रमुकं समुस्तं प्रपौण्डरीकं कमलोत्पले च॥७४॥
ह्रीबेर मूलानि पटोलपत्रं दुरालभा पर्पटको मृणालम्।
धनञ्जयोदुम्बरवेतसत्वङ्न्यग्रोधशालेयय वासकत्वक्॥७५॥
तुगालतावेतस तण्डुलीयं ससारिवं मोचरसः समङ्गा।
पृथक् पृथक् चन्दनयोजितानि तेनैव कल्पेन हितानि तत्र॥७६॥
निशि स्थिता वा स्वरसीकृता वा कल्कीकृता वा मृदिताः शृता वा।
एते समस्ता गणशः पृथग्वा रक्तं सपित्तं शमयन्ति योगाः॥७७॥

Usira – Vetiveria zizanioides

Kaliyaka –

Lodhra – Symplocos racemosa

Padma – Nelumbo nucifera

Priyanguka – Callicarpa macrophylla

Katphala – Myrica nagi

Shankha and

Gairika- these drugs taken separately, is added with equal quantity of Chandana (Santalum album) and given to the patient along with sugar (in equal quantity) and Tandula Dhavana (rice wash).

These preparations instantaneously cure Rakta Pitta, Tamaka (Asthma), Pipasa (Morbid thirst) and Daha (burning sensation)

Kiratatikta – Swertia chirata

Kramuka (Pattika Lodhra)

Musta – Cyperus rotundus

Prapaundarika

Kamala – Nelumbo nucifera

Utpala

The roots of Hribera – Pavonia odorata

Leaves of Patola – Trichosanthes dioica

Duralabha –

Parpataka –

Mrnala –

Dhananjaya (Arjuna) — Terminalia arjuna

Udumbara – Ficus racemosa

Bark of Vetasa – Salix caprea

Nyagrodha – Ficus bengalensis

Shaleya

Bark of Yavasaka – Alhagi pseudalhagi

Tunga

Lata (Priyangu)

Vetasa – Salix caprea

Tanduliya

Sariva – Cordia latifolia

Mocharasa—Salmalia malabarica and

Samangi (Varadha Kranta or Lajjalu) – Mimosa pudica

These drugs taken separately, along with equal quantities of Chandana (Santalum album), are given to the patient with sugar (in equal quantity) and Tandula Dhavana (rice wash).

These drugs can be administered in the form of Sita Kasaya (Keeping the powder in water overnight in the water and then filtering), Svarasa (Juice), Kalka (paste or powder) Mrudita (infusion) or Sheeta (decoction).

Recipes prepared by taking all these drugs together or drugs of each of these groups separately, cure Rakthapitta [73-77]

मुद्गाः सलाजाः सयवाः सकृष्णाः सोशीरमुस्ताः सह चन्दनेन।
बलाजले पर्युषिताः कषाया रक्तं सपित्तं शमयन्त्युदीर्णम्।।७८।।

These drugs are soaked in the decoction of Bala and kept overnight:

Mudga – Vigna radiata

Laja – Fried paddy

Yava –

Krushna –

Usira -Vetiveria zizanioides

Musta – Cyperus rotundus and

Chandana – Santalum album

This recipe, if administered, cures acute form of Rakta Pitta[78]

वैदूर्य मुक्ता मणि गैरिकाणां मृच्छइखहेमामलकोदकानाम्|
मधूदकस्येक्षुरसस्य चैव पानाच्छमं गच्छति रक्तपितम्||७९||
उशीर पद्मोत्पल चन्दनानां पक्वस्य लोष्टस्य च यः प्रसादः|
सशर्करः क्षौद्रयुतः सुशीतो रक्तातियोग प्रशमाय देयः||८०||
प्रियङ्गुका चन्दन लोध्र सारिवा मधूक मुस्ताभय धातकी जलम्|
समृत्प्रसादं सह यष्टिकाम्बुना सशर्करं रक्तनिबर्हणं परम्||८१||

By taking the water soaked with

Vaidurya,

Mukta – Pearl

Manigairika,

Mrut – mud

Shankha – conch

Hema – gold and

Amalaka, the water mixed with honey and sugarcane juice- rakta pitta is cured.

In the decoction of

Usira – Vetiveria zizanoides

Padma – Nelumbo nucifera

Utpala and

Chandana – Santalum album

Red hot coal of earth is immersed.

Then the decoction is filtered and cooled.

To this decoction, sugar and honey is added and administered to the patient for the cure of bleeding in excess, in Rakta Pitta.

The water soaked with

Priyanguka – Callicarpa marophylla

Chandana – Santalum album

Lodhra – Symplocos racemosa

Sariva – Sarsaparilla

Madhuka – Madhuca longifolia

Musta – Cyperus rotundus

Abhaya, Usheera and

Dhataki – Woodfordia fruticosa

Is taken along with Mrt Pradada (water soaked with red hot clot of earth and cooled), decoction of Yastika and sugar.

These are the excellent recipes for the stoppage of bleeding [79-81]

कषाययोगैर्विविधैर्यथोक्तैर्दीप्तेऽनले श्लेष्मणि निर्जिते च|
यद्रक्तपितं प्रशमं न याति तत्रानिलः स्यादनु तत्र कार्यम्||८२||
छागं पयः स्यात् परमं प्रयोगे गव्यं शृतं पञ्चगुणे जले वा|
सशर्करं माक्षिक सम्प्रयुक्तं विदारिगन्धादिगणैः शृतं वा||८३||
द्राक्षाशृतं नागरकैः शृतं वा बलाशृतं गोक्षुरकैः शृतं वा|
सजीवकं सर्षभकं ससर्पिः पयः प्रयोज्यं सितया शृतं वा||८४||

If Rakta Pitta does not get alleviated even after the administration of the various types of Kashaya described before and by stimulation of the power of digestion as well as alleviation of Kapha, then, the physician should understand

that Vayu is aggravated. For cure of this condition, the following are the excellent recipes:
1. Goat milk
2. Cow's milk boiled with five times of water to be taken along with sugar and honey.
3. Cow's milk is boiled with herbs belonging to Vidari Gandhadi gana group of herbs
4. Cow's milk boiled with raisins and ginger
5. Cow's milk boiled with Bala (Sida cordifolia) and Goksuraka (Tribulus terrestris)
6. Cow's milk is boiled with Jivaka and Rishabhaka added with ghee and sugar. [82-84]

शतावरी गोक्षुरकैः शृतं वा शृतं पयो वाऽप्यथ पर्णिनीभिः|
रक्तं निहन्त्याशु विशेषतस्तु यन्मूत्रमार्गात् सरुजं प्रयाति||८५||
Milk boiled with
Shatavari – Asparagus racemosus and
Goksuraka – Tribulus terrestris or with
Shalaparni – Desmodium gangeticum
Prishniparni – Uraria picta and
Mudgaparni – Phaseolus trilobus immediately stops bleeding especially when blood comes out through the urinary tract along with pain [85]

विशेषतो विट्पथसम्प्रवृत्ते पयो मतं मोचरसेन सिद्धम्|
वटावरोहैर्वटशुङ्गकैर्वा ह्रीबेर नीलोत्पल नागरैर्वा||८६||
कषाययोगान् पयसा पुरा वा पीत्वाऽनु चाद्यात् पयसैव शालीन्|
कषाययोगैरथवा विपक्वमेतैः पिबेत् सर्पिरतिस्रवे च||८७||
When there is bleeding, especially through the Anus, then the following recipes are useful:
1. Milk boiled with Mocharasa
2. Milk boiled with either Vatavaroha (adventitious root of Vata) or Vata- Sunga (leafy buds of Vata)
3. Milk boiled with Hribera, Nilotapala and Nagara
4. Recipes of drugs described before (vide verse no 65-71) shall be administered along with milk.
After taking these recipes the patient should take Sali rice along with milk.
If there is excessive bleeding, then ghee boiled with the decoctions described above is administered [86-87]

Vasa Ghruta:
वासां सशाखां सपलाशमूलां कृत्वा कषायं कुसुमानि चास्याः|
प्रदाय कल्कं विपचेद्घृतं तत् सक्षौद्रमाश्वेव निहन्ति रक्तम्||८८||
इति वासाघृतम्|
Decoctions are prepared of Vasa (Adhathoda vasica) along with its twigs, leaves, roots and flowers. Along with this decoction and the paste of Vasa, ghee is boiled and honey is added to it. Administration of this recipe immediately stops bleeding [88]

पलाश वृन्त स्वरसेन सिद्धं तस्यैव कल्केन मधु द्रवेण|
लिह्याद्घृतं वत्सक कल्क सिद्धं तद्वत् समङ्गोत्पल लोध्र सिद्धम्||८९||
स्यात्रायमाणाविधिरेष एव सोदुम्बरे चैव पटोलपत्रे|
सर्पींषि पित्तज्वरनाशनानि सर्वाणि शस्तानि च रक्तपित्ते||९०||
For the alleviation of Rakta pitta, all the following recipes are useful:
1. The ghee is prepared by boiling with the juice and paste of the stalk of Palasha. This is used as linctus by liquefying with honey.
2. Similarly, ghee prepared with the paste of Vatsaka
3. Ghee is prepared with the paste of Samanga, Utpala and Lodhra in a similar manner.

4. Ghee prepared in a similar manner, with Trayamana

5. Ghee prepared in a similar manner by Udumbara and leaves of Patola

6. Medicated ghee described earlier (in Cikistsa 3) for the alleviation of Pitta Jvara.[89-90]

अभ्यङ्ग योगाः परिषेचनानि सेकावगाहाः शयनानि वेश्म|
शीतो विधिर्बस्तिविधानमग्र्यं पित्त ज्वरे यत् प्रशमाय दिष्टम्||९१||
तद्रक्तपित्ते निखिलेन कार्यं कालं च मात्रां च पुरा समीक्ष्य|
सर्पिर्गुडा ये च हिताः क्षतेभ्यस्ते रक्तपित्तं शमयन्ति सद्यः||९२||

Excellent recipes of Abhyanga (massage), Parisecana (sprinkling), Seka (spray), Avagaha (bath), Sayana (bed), Veshma (residence), Sita Vidhi (method of cooling), Basti (medicated enema) described for the alleviation of Pitta is used in their entirety for the treatment of RaktaPitta. Before administration, the physician should keep in view the time and the dose of these recipes.

Sarpis (medicated ghee) and Guda (recipes prepared out of Jaggery), which are useful for patients suffering from Kshata (phithsis) are also useful in alleviating Rakta Pitta instantaneously.[91-92]

कफानुबन्धे रुधिरे सपित्ते कण्ठागते स्याद्ग्रथिते प्रयोगः|
युक्तस्य युक्त्या मधुसर्पिषोश्च क्षारस्य चैवोत्पलनालजस्य||९३||
मृणाल पद्मोत्पल केशराणां तथा पलाशस्य तथा प्रियङ्गोः|
तथा मधूकस्य तथाऽसनस्य क्षाराः प्रयोज्या विधिनैव तेन||९४||

If in Rakta Pitta there is Kaphanubandha (vitiation of Kapha as a secondary pathology), and if it gets clotted while passing through the throat, then appropriately (in appropriate quantity) honey and ghee is used.

In the same manner, the Ksaras (alkali preparations) is prepared of the stalk of Utpala, Mrnala, Kesara (androecium) of Padma and Utpala, Priyangu, Madhuka and Asana is administered in the above mentioned conditions [93-94]

Shatavaryadi Ghrita:
शतावरी दाडिम तिन्तिडीकं काकोलि मेदे मधुकं विदारीम्|
पिष्ट्वा च मूलं फलपूरकस्य घृतं पचेत् क्षीर चतुर्गुणं ज्ञः||९५||
कास ज्वरानाह विबन्ध शूलं तद्रक्तपित्तं च घृतं निहन्यात्|
यत् पञ्चमूलैरथ पञ्चभिर्वा सिद्धं घृतं तच्च तदर्थकारि||९६||
इति शतावर्यादिघृतम्|

The recipe prepared by boiling ghee with the paste of

Shatavari – Asparagus racemosus

Dadima – Punica granatum

Tintidika – Rhus parviflora

Kakoli – Roscoea purpurea

Both the varieties of Meda – Polygonatum verticillatum

Madhuka – Madhuca longifolia

Vidari – Pueraria tuberosa

Root of Phala Puraka (Bija Puraka) — Citrus medica and

4 times of milk, is used by a physician

For curing:

Kasa – cough

Jvara – fever

Anaha – flatulence

Vibandha – constipation

Sula – colic pain and

Rakta Pitta.

Medicated ghee prepared by the five varieties of Pancha Mula (described in Chikista 1:1;41:45) has also got the above mentioned properties.[95-96]

कषाययोगा य इहोपदिष्टास्ते चावपीडे भिषजा प्रयोज्याः|
घ्राणात् प्रवृत्तं रुधिरं सपित्तं यदा भवेन्निःसृतदुष्टदोषम्||९७||
रक्ते प्रदुष्टे ह्यवपीडबन्धे दुष्टप्रतिश्याय शिरोविकाराः|
रक्तं सपूयं कुणपश्च गन्धः स्याद् घ्राणनाशः कृमयश्च दुष्टाः||९८||
नीलोत्पलं गैरिक शङ्खयुक्तं सचन्दनं स्यातु सिताजलेन|
नस्यं तथाऽऽमास्थिरसः समङ्गा सधातकीमोचरसः सलोध्रः||९९||
द्राक्षारसस्येक्षुरसस्य नस्यं क्षीरस्य दूर्वास्वरसस्य चैव|
यवासमूलानि पलाण्डुमूलं नस्यं तथा दाडिमपुष्पतोयम्||१००||
प्रियालतैलं मधुकं पयश्च सिद्धं घृतं माहिषमाजिकं वा|
आम्रास्थिपूर्वैः पयसा च नस्यं ससारिवैः स्यात् कमलोत्पलैश्च||१०१||

In Rakta Pitta, when there is bleeding from the nose, the physician should administer the recipes of decoctions described here (verse nos. 73-74 of this chapter) in the form of Avapida (vide commentary for the meaning of this term) types of inhalation therapy.

This therapy is administered only when all the vitiated Doshas are excreted. If the Doshas are present then this leads to Dusta Pratisyaya (serious type of rhinitis) and Siro Vikara (diseases of the head). From the nose of the patient, bad smell of blood, pus and Kunapa gandha (smell of dead body) appears. He loses the sense of smell and dangerous types of Krmi (maggots) appear in his nose.

The following recipes for inhalation are also recommended in this condition:

1. The paste of Nilotpala, Gairika, Sankha and Chandana, mixed with sugar solution
2. The juice of Amrasthi (the pulp inside the mango seed) and Samanga along with Dhataki, Moca Rasa, Lodhra, juice of Draksa and sugar cane Juice.
3. The juice of Durva along with milk
4. The paste of root of Yavasaka, and Palandu along with the juice of the flower of Dadima
5. Ghee of either buffalo or goat, or the oil of Priyala prepared by boiling with the paste of madhuka and milk
6. Drugs like amrasthi described before along with milk.
7. Sariva, Kamala and Utpala along with Milk. [97-101]

भद्रश्रियं लोहित चन्दनं च प्रपौण्डरीकं कमलोत्पले च|
उशीरवानीरजलं मृणालं सहस्रवीर्या मधुकं पयस्या||१०२||
शालीक्षुमूलानि यवास गुन्द्रामूलं नलानां कुशकाशयोश्च|
कुचन्दनं शैवलमप्यनन्ता कालानुसार्या तृणमूलमृद्धिः||१०३||
मूलानि पुष्पाणि च वारिजानां प्रलेपनं पुष्करिणीमृदश्च|
उदुम्बराश्वत्थ मधूक लोध्राः कषायवृक्षाः शिशिराश्च सर्वे||१०४||
प्रदेह कल्पे परिषेचने च तथाऽवगाहे घृततैलसिद्धौ|
रक्तस्य पित्तस्य च शान्तिमिच्छन् भद्रश्रियादीनि भिषक् प्रयुञ्ज्यात्||१०५||
धारागृहं भूमिगृहं सुशीतं वनं च रम्यं जलवातशीतम्|
वैदूर्य मुक्तामणिभाजनानां स्पर्शाश्च दाहे शिशिराम्बुशीताः||१०६||
पत्राणि पुष्पाणि च वारिजानां क्षौमं च शीतं कदलीदलानि|
प्रच्छादनार्थं शयनासनानां पद्मोत्पलानां च दलाः प्रशस्ताः||१०७||
प्रियङ्गुका चन्दनरूषितानां स्पर्शाः प्रियाणां च वराङ्गनानाम्|
दाहे प्रशस्ताः सजलाः सुशीताः पद्मोत्पलानां च कलापवाताः||१०८||
सरिद्ध्रदानां हिमवद्दरीणां चन्द्रोदयानां कमलाकराणाम्|

मनोऽनुकूलाः शिशिराश्च सर्वाः कथाः सरक्तं शमयन्ति पित्तम्||१०९||

Bhadra sirya, Lohita Chandana, praundaka, Kamala, Utpala, Usira, Vanira (a variety of Usira), Jala, Mrnala, Sahasra virya, Madhuka, Payasya, root of Trna , Radhi, Roots and flowers of aquatic plants and of the pond, astringent trees like Udumbara, Asvattha, Madhuka and Lodhra and all the cooling drugs are used as Pralepana (ointment) for the treatment of Rakta PItta.

The above mentioned drugs are used by the physician in recipes of Pradeha (thick ointment) for Shecana (sprinkling), Avagaha (bath) Ghrta (medicated ghee) and Taila (medicated oil) if he desires to cures Rakta Pitta.

If there is Daha (burning sensation), the patient should resort to Dhara Grhia (the house which is cooled by the flow of water), Bhumi Grha (underground cellar) which is exceedingly cold, forests which are beautiful and cooled by water as well as wind and the touch of utensils prepared of Vaidurya, Mukta and Mani, which are cooled by cold water. For covering the beds, and seats, the leaves and flowers of aquatic plants, cooling silken clothes and leaves of Kadali, Padma as well as Utpal are very useful.

If there is burning sensation, then the following are useful:-

1. The touch of the paste of Priyanguka and Chandana
2. The touch of the beautiful and pleasing women
3. The wind caused by fan prepared of Padma and Utpala which is cooled by water

Raktapitta is also alleviated by the following:

1. Sea shore and the bank of Lakes
2. Caves of Himalayas covered by snow:
3. Rising of the moon
4. Lotus pond
5. All things which are pleasing to the mind; and
6. Pleasant stories [102-109]

Summary:

तत्र श्लोकौ-

हेतुं वृदि्धं सञ्ज्ञां स्थानं लिङ्गं पृथक् प्रदुष्टस्य|
मार्गौ साध्यमसाध्यं याप्यं कार्यक्रमं चैव||११०||
पानान्नमिष्टमेव च वर्ज्यं संशोधनं च शमनं च|
गुरुरुक्तवान्यथावच्चिकित्सिते रक्तपित्तस्य||१११||

1. Hetu or causative factors
2. Vrddhi or mode or aggravation
3. Sanja or definition
4. Sthana or location
5. Linga or signs and symptoms of each variety
6. Marga or the channels of manifestation
7. Curability, incurability and palliability
8. Karya karma or the line of treatment
9. Useful diet and drinks
10. Harmful diet and drinks
11. Samshodhana or elimination therapy and
12. Shamana or alleviation therapy.[110-111]

इत्यग्निवेशकृते तन्त्रे चरकप्रतिसंस्कृते चिकित्सितस्थाने रक्तपित्तचिकित्सितं नाम चतुर्थोऽध्यायः||४||

Thus ends the 4th chapter dealing with the treatment of Raktapitta in Chikitsa Sthana of the text by Agnivesha, as redacted by Charaka.

11

Chikitsasthana Chapter 5 Gulma Chikitsitam

The 5th Chapter of Chikitsa Sthana of Charak Samhita deals with Gulma Chikitsa – treatment of different types of abdominal tumors. This chapter has very useful Ayurvedic medicines like Ksheera shatpal Ghruta, Lashuna ksheerapaka, Shatyadi Churna, Trayamana Ghrita etc.

For a simple version of this chapter, read here

अथातो गुल्मचिकित्सितं व्याख्यास्यामः||१||
इति ह स्माह भगवानात्रेयः||२||
We shall now expound the chapter on the treatment of Gulma (Tumor)
Thus, said Lord Atreya [1-2]

सर्वप्रजानां पितृवच्छरण्यः पुनर्वसुर्भूतभविष्यदीशः|
चिकित्सितं गुल्मनिबर्हणार्थं प्रोवाच सिद्धं वदतां वरिष्ठः||३||
Punarvasu, the foremost among teachers, who is courteous like the father of all living beings, the paramount seer of the past and the future, expounded the effective treatment for the cure of Gulma (tumor) [3]

Gulma Nidana – Causative Factors:
विट्श्लेष्मपित्तातिपरिस्रवाद्वा तैरेव वृद्धैः परिपीडनाद्वा|
वेगैरुदीर्णैर्विहतैरधो वा बाह्यभिघातैरतिपीडनैर्वा||४||
रूक्षान्नपानैरतिसेवितैर्वा शोकेन मिथ्याप्रतिकर्मणा वा|
विचेष्टितैर्वा विषमातिमात्रैः कोष्ठे प्रकोपं समुपैति वायुः||५||
Vata Dosha gets aggravated in the Koshta (Gastro-intestinal tract) because of the following factors:
1. Ati parisrava of vit, Sleshma and Pitta: Excessive production / excretion of faeces, Kapha and Pitta
2. Paripeedana.i. e pressure on or obstruction of Vayu by the increase in the quantity of feces, Kapha and Pitta
3. Suppression of Vegas (manifested natural urges) moving downwards (like urine, flatus and feces)
4. Shoka: Affliction by grief
5. Improper administration of elimination therapies and
6. Excessive or abnormal physical activities [4-5]

Gulma Samprapti – Pathogenesis:
कफं च पित्तं च स दुष्टवायुरुद्धूय मार्गान् विनिबध्य ताभ्याम्|
हृन्नाभिपार्श्वोदर बस्तिशूलं करोत्यथो याति न बद्धमार्गः||६||
पक्वाशये पित्तकफाशये वा स्थितः स्वतन्त्रः परसंश्रयो वा|
स्पर्शोपलभ्यः परिपिण्डितत्वाद्गुल्मो यथादोषमुपैति नाम||७||

The vitiated Vayu provokes either Kapha or Pitta or both. They obstruct the channels of circulation to cause pain in the regions of heart, umbilicus, and sides of the chest, abdomen and urinary bladder. Doshas do not get eliminated and are confined to Pakvashaya (colon) Pittashaya (small intestine) or Kaphashaya (Stomach) either independently (Svatantra) or in association with other Doshas (paratantra). It becomes palpable because of its round shape for which it is called Gulma. Depending upon the Doshas involved in the manifestation of this ailment, it is classified into several categories [6-7]

Gulma Sthana – Locations:
बस्तौ च नाभ्यां हृदि पार्श्वयोर्वा स्थानानि गुल्मस्य भवन्ति पञ्च|
पञ्चात्मकस्य प्रभवं तु तस्य वक्ष्यामि लिङ्गानि चिकित्सितं च||८||
The 5 sites of manifestation of Gulma are:
Basti – Urinary bladder,
Nabhi – umbilicus,
Hridi- heart and
Parshva sthana – 2 sides of the abdomen (parsva)
Now signs, symptoms and treatment of the 5 categories of Gulma, viz
Vatika,
Paittika
Kaphaja
Sannipatika and
Raktaja will be explained [8]

Causes Signs, and Symptoms of Vatika Gulma:
रूक्षान्नपानं विषमातिमात्रं विचेष्टितं वेग विनिग्रहश्च|
शोकोऽभिघातोऽतिमलक्षयश्च निरन्नता चानिलगुल्महेतुः||९||
यः स्थान संस्थानरुजां विकल्पं विड्वातसङ्गं गलवक्त्रशोषम्|
श्यावारुणत्वं शिशिरज्वरं च हृत्कुक्षिपार्श्वांस शिरोरुजं च||१०||
करोति जीर्णेऽभ्यधिकं प्रकोपं भुक्ते मृदुत्वं समुपैति यश्च|
वातात् स गुल्मो न च तत्र रूक्षं कषायतिक्तं कटु चोपशेते||११||
Causes for Vataj Gulma are –
1. Rooksha annapanam: Intake of dry diet and drinks
2. Ati matra vichestitam: Excessive and abnormal physical behaviour
3. Vega vinigraha: Suppression of manifested natural urges
4. Shoka: Affliction by grief
5. Abhighata: Affliction by external injury
6. Ati mala: Excessive elimination of excreta and
7. Nirannata: Fasting for a long time.
Signs symptoms as well as characteristic features of Vatika Gulma are:
1. Momentary changes in the location, shape and intensity of pain
2. Vit vata sanga: Obstruction to the passage of the faeces and flatus
3. Gala vaktra shosham: Dryness in the throat and mouth,
4. Shyava aruna shareera: grey and reddish coloration of body
5. Shishira jvara: Fever with cold
6. Hrut, kukshi, Parshva, Shiro rujam: Pain in the region of heart, abdomen, sides of the abdomen (parshva), scapula and head
7. Aggravation of the disease after food is digested and alleviation of ailment by the intake of food
8. In Vataja Gulma, dry, astringent, bitter and pungent types of food are not wholesome. [10-11]

Causes, Signs and Symptoms of Paittika Gulma:

कट्वम्लतीक्ष्णोष्ण विदाहि रूक्ष क्रोधातिमद्यार्कहुताशसेवा|
आमाभिघातो रुधिरं च दुष्टं पैत्तस्य गुल्मस्य निमित्तमुक्तम्||१२||
ज्वरः पिपासा वदनाङ्गरागः शूलं महज्जीर्यति भोजने च|
स्वेदो विदाहो व्रणवच्च गुल्मः स्पर्शासहः पैत्तिकगुल्मरूपम्||१३||

The causative factors of Paitika Gulma:

1. Katu, amla, tikshna, ushna, vidahi anna sevana: Intake of pungent, sour, sharp, hot, Vidahi (which cause acidity or stomach burning sensation) and dry articles of diet

2. Krodha – anger

3. Ama abhighata: Affliction by Ama (Product of improper digestion and metabolism) and

4. Madya sevana: Excessive intake of alcohol and

5. Arka Hutasha Seva - exposure to sun as well as fire.

6. Rudhira dushtam: Vitiation of blood.

Signs and symptoms and characteristic features of Paittaika Gulma:

1. Jwara and pipasa: Fever and excessive thirst

2. Anga raga: Redness of face and limbs

3. Shulam mahat jeeryate bhojanam: Excruciating pain during digestion of food

4. Sveda and vidaha: Sweating and burning sensation and

5. Vrana vaccha gulma: Tenderness of the affected part as if it is wounded. [12-13]

Causes for Kaphaja and Sannipatika Gulma

शीतं गुरु स्निग्धमचेष्टनं च सम्पूरणं प्रस्वपनं दिवा च|
गुल्मस्य हेतुः कफसम्भवस्य सर्वस्तु दिष्टो निचयात्मकस्य||१४||

The causative factors of Kaphaja Gulma are –

1. Sheeta, guru snigdha: Indulgence in cold, heavy and unctuous foods

2. Achesta: Lack of exercise

3. Sampoorana – Over-nourishment and

4. Diva swapna: Sleep during day time

The Sannipatika type of Gulma is produced by all causative factors of Vatika, Paittika and Kaphaja Gulma [14]

Signs and symptoms of Kaphaja Gulma:

स्तैमित्य शीतज्वर गात्रसाद हृल्लास कासारुचि गौरवाणि|
शैत्यं रुगल्पा कठिनोन्नतत्वं गुल्मस्य रूपाणि कफात्मकस्य||१५||

Signs and symptoms of Kaphaja Gulma:

1. Staimitya – numbness or a feeling as if covered with a wet-cloth

2. Sheeta Jvara: Fever associated with feelings of cold

3. Gatra sada, Hrullasa, Kasa, Aruchi, Gaurava: Body stiffness, Nausea, cough, anorexia and heaviness and

4. Kathina unnatam: The affected part of the body is hard to touch and is elevated. It is cold in touch and there is less pain.[15]

Dvi-Doshaja Gulma:

निमित्तलिङ्गान्युपलभ्य गुल्मे द्विदोषजे दोषबलाबलं च|
व्यामिश्रलिङ्गानपरांस्तु गुल्मांस्त्रीनादिशेदौषधकल्पनार्थम्||१६||

Because of the combination of etiological factors of 2 or 3 Doshas, other varieties of Gulma, having signs and symptoms of the respective Doshas are manifested. These are called DviDoshaja (2 Doshas are simultaneously vitiated). [16]

Signs and Symptoms of Sannipatika Gulma:

महारुजं दाहपरीतमश्मवद्घनोन्नतं शीघ्रविदाहि दारुणम्।
मनःशरीराग्निबलापहारिणं त्रिदोषजं गुल्ममसाध्यमादिशेत्॥१७॥

Features of Sannipatika Gulma are as follows;

1. Maha rujam: Excruciating pain

2. Daha: Excessive burning sensation

3. Ashma vad: Stone-like compact elevation of the affected part;

4. Vidahi: Quick sloughing

5. Darunam: Seriousness of the condition and

6. Disappearance of the strength of the mind, body and digestion as well as metabolism. This variety of Gulma is incurable.[17]

Causes, Samprapti, Signs and Symptoms of Raktaja Gulma:

ऋतावनाहारतया भयेन विरूक्षणैर्वेगविनिग्रहैश्च।
संस्तम्भनोल्लेखनयोनिदोषैर्गुल्मः स्त्रियं रक्तभवोऽभ्युपैति॥१८॥
यः स्पन्दते पिण्डित एव नाङ्गैश्चिरात् सशूलः समगर्भलिङ्गः।
स रौधिरः स्त्रीभव एव गुल्मो मासे व्यतीते दशमे चिकित्स्यः॥१९॥

Causes for Raktaja Gulma in ladies:

1. Rutau Anahara – Avoiding food during menstruation

2. Bhaya, Rooksha, Vega Vinigraha: Fear, intake of excessively dry food and suppression of manifested natural urges:

3. Improper administration of Stambhana treatment (astringent, blocking treatment) and emetic therapies

4. Yoni dosha: Gynecological disorder

Raktaja Gulma Lakshana:

Spandate – palpitates / pulsates

Pindita – round mass

Sashoola – associated with colic-pain and

signs and symptoms suggestive of pregnancy.

This Rakthaja Gulma occurs only in women and is treated only after the passage of 10 months. [18- 19]

Line of Treatment – Gulma Chikitsa Sutra:

क्रियाक्रममतः सिद्धं गुल्मिनां गुल्मनाशनम्।
प्रवक्ष्याम्यत ऊर्ध्वं च योगान् गुल्मनिबर्हणान्॥२०॥
रूक्षव्यायामजं गुल्मं वातिकं तीव्रवेदनम्।
बद्धविण्मारुतं स्नेहैरादितः समुपाचरेत्॥२१॥
भोजनाभ्यञ्जनैः पानैर्निरूहैः सानुवासनैः।
स्निग्धस्य भिषजा स्वेदः कर्तव्यो गुल्मशान्तये॥२२॥
स्रोतसां मार्दवं कृत्वा जित्वा मारुतमुल्बणम्।
भित्त्वा विबन्धं स्निग्धस्य स्वेदो गुल्ममपोहति॥२३॥
स्नेहपानं हितं गुल्मे विशेषेणोर्ध्वनाभिजे।
पक्वाशयगते बस्तिरुभयं जठराश्रये॥२४॥
दीप्तेऽग्नौ वातिके गुल्मे विबन्धेऽनिलवर्चसोः।
बृंहणान्यन्नपानानि स्निग्धोष्णानि प्रयोजयेत्॥२५॥
पुनः पुनः स्नेहपानं निरूहाः सानुवासनाः।
प्रयोज्या वातगुल्मेषु कफपित्तानुरक्षिणा॥२६॥

Line of Treatment – Gulma Chikitsa Sutra:

Now the line of treatment is explained, followed by recipes for eradication of these diseases.

Vataja Gulma Chikitsa Sutra:

A patient suffering from Vataja Gulma, caused by dry food and excessive physical activities, associated with excruciating pain and obstruction to faeces and flatus should, in the beginning be administered with

Snehakarma – Oleation,

oil massage,

Oily foods and drinks,

Niruha (decoction enema) and

Anuvasana – Oil enema.

After this, Swedana – sweating treatment is adopted.

Sweating therapy causes

Srotasam Mardava – softness of channels of circulation,

Jitva Marutam ulbanam – alleviates aggravated Vata Dosha

Bhitva Vibandham – relieves constipation,

as a result of which Gulma gets cured.

Administration of Snehapana (unctuous liquid) is useful in Gulma, especially when this disease is located above the umbilical region.

If Gulma is manifested either in Pakvashaya – colon or in Jatara, (other part of abdomen), then Niruha (decoction enema) and Anuvasana (fat enema) is useful.

The Vataja Gulma patient accompanied with constipation and bloating is given unctuous, hot and nourishing diet and drinks after his digestive-power is stimulated;

In Vata Gulma, SnehaPana (oral administration of Sneha), Niruha (a type of medicated enema) and Anuvasana (another type of medicated enema) is administered very frequently. But care is taken against Kapha and Pitta. That is, it is ensured that these therapies do not aggravate Kapha and Pitta in any way. [20-26]

Management of other Doshas:

कफो वाते जितप्राये पित्तं शोणितमेव वा।

यदि कुप्यति वा तस्य क्रियमाणे चिकित्सिते॥२७॥

यथोल्बणस्य दोषस्य तत्र कार्यं भिषग्जितम्।

आदावन्ते च मध्ये च मारुतं परिरक्षता॥२८॥

If, by the therapies for alleviation of Vayu, other Doshas – Pitta, Kapha and Rakta get vitiated, then carefully, treatment is done to pacify the aggravated Dosha, while taking extra precautions for Vata Dosha balance. [27-28]

Line of Treatment of Dvandvaja Gulma:

वातगुल्मे कफो वृद्धो हत्वाऽग्निमरुचिं यदि।

हल्लासं गौरवं तन्द्रां जनयेदुल्लिखेतु तम्॥२९॥

शूलानाह विबन्धेषु गुल्मे वातकफोल्बणे।

वर्तयो गुटिकाश्चूर्णं कफवातहरं हितम्॥३०॥

पित्तं वा यदि संवृद्धं सन्तापं वातगुल्मिनः।

कुर्यादिवरेच्यः स भवेत् सस्नेहैरानुलोमिकैः॥३१॥

Dwandwaja Gulma Chikitsa:

If in a patient of Vataja Gulma, Kapha is aggravated, leading to

Agnisada – low digestion strength

Aruchi – anorexia, Hrullasa – nausea, Gaurava – heaviness, Tandra – drowsiness, fatigue, then he is administered Vamana – emetic therapy.

If Gulma is caused by the predominance of Vata and Kapha, and if it is associated with colic pain, Anaha (distension of the abdomen) and constipation, then the patient is given Varti (rectal suppository), pills and powders which alleviate both Kapha and Vata. [29-31]

Gulme Raktamokshana:

गुल्मो यद्यनिलादीनां कृते सम्यग्भिषग्जिते।
न प्रशाम्यति रक्तस्य सोऽवसेकात् प्रशाम्यति॥३२॥

Bloodletting:

In spite of administration of appropriate therapies for the alleviation of Vata, etc, if Gulma is not cured, then bloodletting is done to eradicate the disease. [32]

Pittajagulma Chikitsasutra:

स्निग्धोष्णेनोदिते गुल्मे पैत्तिके संसनं हितम्।
रूक्षोष्णेन तु सम्भूते सर्पिः प्रशमनं परम्॥३३॥
पित्तं वा पित्तगुल्मं वा ज्ञात्वा पक्वाशयस्थितम्।
कालविन्निर्हरेत् सद्यः सतिक्तैः क्षीरबस्तिभिः॥३४॥
पयसा वा सुखोष्णेन सतिक्तेन विरेचयेत्।
भिषगग्निबलापेक्षी सर्पिषा तैल्वकेन वा॥३५॥

If Paitika Gulma is caused by unctuous and hot things, then administration of Sramsana is useful. (Mild – moderate laxative) If it is caused by dry and hot things, then administration of ghee is best. If Pitta or Paittika Gulma gets lodged in Pakvasaya (colon), then keeping in view the appropriateness of time, the patient should immediately be given Tikta Ksheera basti. (Enema with milk processed with bitter herbs). Alternatively the patient can be given Virechana treatment with milk, warm milk processed with bitter herbs or with Tilvaka ghrita depending upon his digestive power and strength [33-35]

Utility of bloodletting:

तृष्णा ज्वर परीदाह शूलस्वेदाग्निमार्दवे।
गुल्मिनामरुचौ चापि रक्तमेवावसेचयेत्॥३६॥
छिन्नमूला विदह्यन्ते न गुल्मा यान्ति च क्षयम्।
रक्तं हि व्यम्लतां याति, तच्च नास्ति न चास्ति रुक्॥३७॥

If a patient of Gulma is associated with

Trushna – morbid thirst

Jvara – fever

Paridaha – excessive burning sensation

Shula – colic pain, Sweda – sweating

Agni mardava – suppression of the power of digestion and

Aruchi – anorexia, then this is treated by bloodletting.

In Gulma, blood gets vitiated and becomes sour. By bloodletting, this does not happen and the patient remains free from pain [36-37]

Removal of Residual Doshas:

हतदोषं परिम्लानं जाङ्गलैस्तर्पितं रसैः।
समाश्वस्तं सशेषार्तिं सर्पिरभ्यासयेत् पुनः॥३८॥

After removal of vitiated blood, the patient becomes emaciated. He is given Jangala mamsarasa – soup of meat of animals of arid land. He is consoled, and for relieving the residual pain, he is regularly given ghee again. [38]

Surgery:

रक्तपित्तातिवृद्धत्वात् क्रियामनुपलभ्य च।

यदि गुल्मो विदह्येत शस्त्रं तत्र भिषग्जितम्||३९||

If Rakta and Pitta are aggravated in excess in a patient suffering from Gulma, and if bloodletting therapy is not administered, then Gulma may get suppurated. To cure this ailment surgery has to be performed [39]

Apakva or Un-suppurated Gulma:

गुरुः कठिनसंस्थानो गूढमांसान्तराश्रयः|
अविवर्णः स्थिरश्चैव ह्यपक्वो गुल्म उच्यते||४०||

Following signs and symptoms indicate that the Gulma has not undergone suppuration:

1. Guru Kathina: Heaviness and hardness in form
2. Gudha mamsa antarashaya: Located deep inside the muscle tissue
3. Avivarna: No change in the colour of the skin and
4. Sthira: Remaining firmly fixed and elevated

Pachyamana Gulma:

दाहशूलार्तिसङ्क्षोभ स्वप्ननाशारतिज्वरैः|
विदह्यमानं जानीयाद्गुल्मं तमुपनाहयेत्||४१||

Signs and symptoms occur when the Gulma is in the process of suppuration:

Daha: Burning sensation

Shoola: colic pain

Arti: sawing pain

Sankshoba: irritation,

Swapna nasha – insomnia,

disliking for everything and

Jwara – fever.

Treatment: Upanaha – Poultice, hot ointment is applied over it [41]

Pakvagulma Lakshana, Chikitsa:

विदाहलक्षणे गुल्मे बहिस्तुङ्गे समुन्नते|
श्यावे सरक्तपर्यन्ते संस्पर्शे बस्तिसन्निभे||४२||
निपीडितोन्नते स्तब्धे सुप्ते तत्पार्श्वपीडनात्|
तत्रैव पिण्डिते शूले सम्पक्वं गुल्ममादिशेत्||४३||
तत्र धान्वन्तरीयाणामधिकारः क्रियाविधौ|
वैद्यानां कृतयोग्यानां व्यधशोधनरोपणे||४४||
अन्तर्भागस्य चाप्येतत् पच्यमानस्य लक्षणम्|
हृत्क्रोडशूनताऽन्तःस्थे बहिःस्थे पार्श्वनिर्गतिः||४५||

Suppuration of Gulma is characterized by:

Vidaha – sloughing

Bahih tunge: outward protrusion

Unnata- elevation

Syava rakta – Greyish colour with a red margin

A feeling as if touching a bladder full of water. It comes back to its original position after pressing.

Localization in a round form

Supti – numbness and

Parshwapeedana – pain in the sides of Gulma – Tumors of the abdomen

Treatment of this condition is done by surgeons (Dhanvantara school) who are well versed in the art of puncturing, purification and pressing through its sides.

When the Gulma is located in the Antarbhaga (interior of the body), the same signs and symptoms of Pachyamana

Gulma are manifested. There will be swelling in the cardiac region (Hrutkroda) and in case of Gulma located in the exterior of the body there will be protuberance towards the sides of the abdomen [42-45]

Management of Svayampravrutta Gulma: (mobile)

पक्वः स्रोतांसि सङ्क्लेद्य व्रजत्यूर्ध्वमधोऽपि वा|

स्वयम्प्रवृत्तं तं दोषमुपेक्षेत हिताशनैः ||४६||

दशाहं द्वादशाहं वा रक्षन् भिषगुपद्रवान्|

अत ऊर्ध्वं हितं पानं सर्पिषः सविशोधनम्||४७||

शुद्धस्य तिक्तं सक्षौद्रं प्रयोगे सर्पिरिष्यते|४८|

At times, the suppurated Gulma, having softened the passage moves upwards or downwards. Like this, if the Doshas are in the process of elimination on their own (Svayampravrutta) then the physician should ignore it and should only pay attention to prevent any complication for 10 – 12 days. Thereafter, the patient should take ghee for the elimination of Doshas. When the body is purified (made free from morbid Doshas) the patient is given ghee boiled with bitter drugs by adding honey [46-47]

Kaphaja Gulma chikitsa:

शीतलैर्गुरुभिः स्निग्धैर्गुल्मे जाते कफात्मके||४८||

अवम्यस्याल्पकायाग्नेः कुर्याल्लङ्घनमादितः|

मन्दोऽग्निर्वेदना मन्दा गुरुस्तिमितकोष्ठता||४९||

सोत्क्लेशा चारुचिर्यस्य स गुल्मी वमनोपगः|

उष्णैरेवोपचर्यश्च कृते वमनलङ्घने||५०||

योज्यश्चाहारसंसर्गो भेषजैः कटुतिक्तकैः|

सानाहं सविबन्धं च गुल्मं कठिनमुन्नतम्||५१||

दृष्ट्वाऽऽदौ स्वेदयेद्युक्त्या स्विन्नं च विलयेद्भिषक्|

लङ्घनोल्लेखने स्वेदे कृतेऽग्नौ सम्प्रधुक्षिते||५२||

कफगुल्मी पिबेत् काले सक्षारकटुकं घृतम्|

स्थानादपसृतं ज्ञात्वा कफगुल्मं विरेचनैः||५३||

सस्नेहैर्बस्तिभिर्वाऽपि शोधयेद्दाशमूलिकैः|

मन्देऽग्नावनिले मूढे ज्ञात्वा सस्नेहमाशयम्||५४||

गुटिकाचूर्णनिर्यूहाः प्रयोज्याः कफगुल्मिनाम्|

कृतमूलं महावास्तुं कठिनं स्तिमितं गुरुम्||५५||

जयेत्कफकृतं गुल्मं क्षारारिष्टाग्निकर्मभिः|५६|

Management of Kaphaja Gulma:

If caused by cold, heavy and unctuous substances – Langhana (Fasting / lightening therapy) is administered. If he is having less power of digestion, less of pain, heaviness, immobility of gastro-intestinal tract, nausea and anorexia – Vamana – emetic therapy should be administered.

After Vamana and Langhana, patients are given hot regimens. Diet is mixed with pungent and bitter drugs.

If the Gulma is hard and elevated and if the patient is also suffering from bloating and constipation, then in the beginning Swedana – fomentation therapy is applied.

By fasting, emetic and fomentation, therapies, Agni (power of digestion) gets stimulated and the patient suffering from Kaphaja Gulma should take ghee boiled with alkalies and pungent herbs, at the appropriate time.

Having ascertained that the Kapha gulma is dislodged from the place of its manifestation, the patient is administered Virechana. He can also be given Snehabasti (oil enema), or Niruha with Dashamoola Kashaya.

If there is Mandagni – low digestion strength and bloating, then Snehana is given followed by medicines in the form of pill, herbal powder or decoction is administered.

If Kaphaja Gulma has a strong foundation and is extensive in size, hard, immobile and heavy, then the patient is treated with alkalies, Aristas (Alcoholic preparations) and by cauterization (agni Karma) [48 ½ +1/2 56]

Gulme Kshara Prayoga – Administration of Alkalies:

दोष प्रकृति गुल्मर्तुयोगं बुद्ध्वा कफोल्बणे||५६||

बलदोषप्रमाणज्ञः क्षारं गुल्मे प्रयोजयेत्|

एकान्तरं द्व्यन्तरं वा त्र्यहं विश्रम्य वा पुनः||५७||

शरीरबलदोषाणां वृद्धिक्षपणकोविदः|

श्लेष्माणं मधुरं स्निग्धं मांसक्षीरघृताशिनः||५८||

छित्वा छित्वाऽऽशयात् क्षारः क्षरत्वात् क्षारयत्यधः|

Administration of Alkalies

In Kaphaja Gulma, after ascertaining the Dosha, Prakruti (body constitution), season, the physician should administer Kshara.

It is repeated at an interval of 1, 2 or 3 days by the physician who is conversant with the science of reducing a particular Dosha by promoting the physical strength of the patient.

Kapha which is sweet and unctuous gets aggravated in a person who indulges in meat, milk and ghee. Kshara (Alkali) has the property of Ksharana (Liquefaction). Thus it gradually erodes Kaphaja Gulma and brings it downwards. [56 ½ – ½ 59]

Arishta Therapy:

मन्देऽग्नावरुचौ सात्म्ये मद्ये सस्नेहमश्नताम्||५९||

प्रयोज्या मार्गशुद्ध्यर्थमरिष्टाः कफगुल्मिनाम्|६०|

In the course of administering Sneha (unctuous substance) to a patient suffering from Kaphaja Gulma, if he suffers from Mandagni – low digestion strength and Aruchi – anorexia and if he is accustomed to alcohol intake, Arishtas (a type of alcoholic medicine) are administered with a view to clearing his channels. [59- ½ 60]

Agni karma – Cauterization Therapy:

लङ्घनोल्लेखनैः स्वेदैः सर्पिःपानैर्विरेचनैः||६०||

बस्तिभिर्गुटिकाचूर्णक्षारारिष्टगणैरपि|

श्लैष्मिकः कृतमूलत्वाद्यस्य गुल्मो न शाम्यति||६१||

तस्य दाहो हृते रक्ते शरलोहादिभिर्हितः|

औष्ण्यातैक्ष्ण्याच्च शमयेदग्निर्गुल्मे कफानिलौ||६२||

तयोः शमाच्च सङ्घातो गुल्मस्य विनिवर्तते|

दाहे धान्वन्तरीयाणामत्रापि भिषजां बलम्||६३||

क्षारप्रयोगे भिषजां क्षारतन्त्रविदां बलम्|६४|

Agni karma – Cauterization Therapy:

If by Langhana, Vamana, Swedana, ghee intake, Virechana, enema, pills, powders, alkalies and various types of Arishta, Kaphaja Gulma does not get alleviated because of its obstinacy, then Agnikarma is done, prepared with the help of arrow, iron rod etc.

After bloodletting therapy because of its heating and sharp effects, cauterization therapy in Gulma alleviates Kapha and Vata as a result of which Gulma loses its compactness.

In Agnikarma, physicians belonging to Dhanvantara School have proficiency. Similarly, for the administration of Kshara (Alkali therapy), services of physicians who are Kshara-Tantra-vidhi (proficient in the administration Of Alkalies) is better utilized. (60 ½ – 1/9 64)

Ayurvedic medicines for Gulma:
Trayushanadi Ghrta:

सिद्धानतः प्रवक्ष्यामि योगान् गुल्मनिबर्हणान्।
त्र्यूषण त्रिफला धान्य विडङ्ग चव्य चित्रकैः॥६५॥
कल्की कृतैर्घृतं सिद्धं सक्षीरं वातगुल्मनुत्।
इति त्र्यूषणादिघृतम्।

Now effective medicines for the successful treatment of Gulma will be described.

Ghee prepared by boiling with the paste of

Trayushana – Trikatu – Pepper, long pepper and ginger

Triphala – Amla, Harad, Baheda

Dhanyaka – Coriander

Vidanga – False black pepper – Embelia ribes,

Chavya – Piper retrofractum and

Chitraka – Plumbago zeylanica and

Milk cures Vata Gulma. [65-1/2 – ½ 66]

Another Trayushanadi Ghrta:

एत एव च कल्काः स्युः कषायः पाञ्चमूलिकः ॥६६॥
द्विपञ्चमूलिको वाऽपि तद्घृतं गुल्मनुत् परम्।
इति त्र्यूषणादिघृतमपरम्।
(षट्पलं वा पिबेत् सर्पिर्यदुक्तं राजयक्ष्मणि) ॥६७॥
प्रसन्नया वा क्षीरार्थे सुरया दाडिमेन वा।
दध्नः सरेण वा कार्यं घृतं मारुतगुल्मनुत्॥६८॥

Ghee is boiled with the paste of drugs mentioned above (verse 65) and the decoction of either PanchaMoola or DashaMoola.

This medicated ghee is the best recipe for curing Gulma.

In this recipe, Prasanna, Sura, juice of Dadima (Pomegranate) or cream of milk is added while processing in place of milk [66-1/2 68]

Hingu Sauvarchaladi Ghrta:

हिङ्गु सौवर्चलाजाजी बिड दाडिम दीप्यकैः।
पुष्कर व्योष धन्याक वेतस क्षार चित्रकैः॥६९॥
शटी वचाजगन्धैलासुरसैश्च विपाचितम्।
शूलानाहहरं सर्पिर्दध्ना चानिलगुल्मिनाम्॥७०॥
इति हिङ्गुसौवर्चलाद्यं घृतम्।

Ghee prepared with

Hingu – Asafoetida

Sauvarchala – Black salt

Ajaji – Cumin – Cuminum cyminum,

Bida salt

Dadima – Pomegranate – Punica granatum

Dipyaka – Ajowan (fruit) – Trachyspermum roxburghianum,

Pushkara – Inula racemosa

Vyosha – pippali, Maricgha, Shunthi

Dhanyaka – Coriander – Coriandrum sativum,

Kshara – Yavakshara

Vetasa,

Chitraka – Plumbago zeylanica

Shati – Hedyium spicatum

Vacha – Acorus calamus
It is useful for patients suffering from Vataja Gulma. [69-70]

Hapushadi Ghrita:
हपुषा व्योष पृथ्वीका चव्य चित्रक सैन्धवैः।
साजाजी पिप्पलीमूल दीप्यकैर्विपचेद्घृतम्॥७१॥
सकोल मूलकरसं सक्षीर दधि दाडिमम्।
तत् परं वातगुल्मघ्नं शूलानाहविमोक्षणम्॥७२॥
योन्यर्शोग्रहणीदोषश्वासकासारुचिज्वरान्।
बस्तिहृत्पार्श्वशूलं च घृतमेतद्व्यपोहति॥७३॥
इति हपुषाद्यं घृतम्।
Hapusha – Juniperus communis
Vyosa
Prithvika
Chavya – Piper retrofractum
Chitraka – Plumbago zeylanica
Saindhava Lavana – Black salt
Ajaji – Cumin – Cuminum cyminum
Pipalimula – Long pepper root and
Dipyaka – Ajowan (fruit) – Trachyspermum roxburghianum along with these herbs, ghee is prepared by adding
Juice of Kola – Ber fruit – Ziziphus jujuba and Mulaka, milk, curd and juice of Dadima – Pomegranate – Punica granatum.
It is an excellent recipe for the treatment of Vata Gulma.
It cures
Shoola – abdominal colic pain
Anaha – abdominal distension of the female genital tract,
Piles
Sprue syndrome – Grahani Dosha
Shwasa – Asthma
Kasa – Cough
Aruchi – Anorexia
Jwara – Fever and
Parshva, hrut, basti shoola: Pain in the region of urinary bladder including kidney, heart as well as sides of the chest [71-73]

Pippalyadya Ghrta:
पिप्पल्या पिचुरध्यर्धो दाडिमादिद्विपलं पलम्।
धान्यात्पञ्च घृताच्छुण्ठ्याः कर्षः क्षीरं चतुर्गुणम्॥७४॥
सिद्धमेतैर्घृतं सद्यो वातगुल्मं व्यपोहति।
योनिशूलं शिरःशूलमर्शांसि विषमज्वरम्॥७५॥
इति पिप्पल्याद्यं घृतम्।
5 Palas of Ghee is processed with
1½ of Pippali – Long pepper fruit
2 Palas of Dadima – Pomegranate – Punica granatum,
1 Pala of Dhanya – Coriander sativum
1 karsha of Sunthi – Ginger and
20 palas of milk

This medicated ghee.

Instantaneously cures:

Vatika- Gulma

Yoni shoolam – Pain in the female genital organ

Shira shoola -Headache

Arshas – Piles and

Vishama Jvara – irregular fever [74-75]

Other Recipes:

घृतानामौषधगणा य एते परिकीर्तिताः|
ते चूर्णयोगा वर्त्यस्ताः कषायास्ते च गुल्मिनाम्||७६||
कोल दाडिम घर्माम्बुसुरामण्डाम्लकाञ्जिकैः|
शूलानाहहरी पेया बीजपूररसेन वा||७७||
चूर्णानि मातुलुङ्गस्य भावितानि रसेन वा|
कुर्याद्वर्तीः सगुटिका गुल्मानाहार्तिशान्तये||७८||

Groups of drugs described in the above verses, for different recipes of herbal Ghee can also be used in different other forms like powder, Varti (Suppository) and decoctions for the treatment of a patient suffering from Gulma.

These recipes in powder form can be used along with the

Juice of Kola – Ber fruit – Ziziphus jujuba and

Dadima – Pomegranate – Punica granatum,

Hot water

Sura Manda (upper portion of an alcoholic preparation),

Sour Kanji or the juice of bija Pura.

They cure:

Colic pain and

Anaha – abdominal distension

These recipes in powder form can be impregnated with the juice of Matulunga and made to a form of suppository or pill.

These are also useful in curing abdominal distension and pain of a patient suffering from Gulma. [76-78]

Hingvadi Churna & Hingvadi Gutika:

हिङ्गु त्रिकटुकं पाठां हपुषामभयां शटीम्|
अजमोदाजगन्धे च तिन्तिडीकाम्लवेतसौ||७९||
दाडिमं पुष्करं धान्यमजाजीं चित्रकं वचाम्|
द्वौ क्षारौ लवणे द्वे च चव्यं चैकत्र चूर्णयेत्||८०||
चूर्णमेतत् प्रयोक्तव्यमन्नपानेष्वनत्ययम्|
प्रागभक्तमथवा पेयं मद्येनोष्णोदकेन वा||८१||
पार्श्वहृद्बस्तिशूलेषु गुल्मे वातकफात्मके|
आनाहे मूत्रकृच्छ्रे च शूले च गुदयोनिजे ||८२||
ग्रहण्यर्शोविकारेषु प्लीहिन पाण्डवामयेऽरुचौ|
उरोविबन्धे हिक्कायां कासे श्वासे गलग्रहे||८३||
भावितं मातुलुङ्गस्य चूर्णमेतद्रसेन वा|
बहुशो गुटिकाः कार्याः कार्मुकाः स्युस्ततोऽधिकम्||८४||
इति हिङ्ग्वादिचूर्णं गुटिका च|

Hingu - Asafoetida

Trikatuka – Pepper, long pepper and ginger

Patha – Cyclea peltata,

Hapusha – Juniperus communis

Abhaya – Chebulic myrobalan fruit rind – Terminalia chebula,

Shati – Hedyium spicatum

Ajamoda – Ajowan (fruit) – Trachyspermum roxburghianum,

Ajagandha

Tintidika –

Amla – Indian gooseberry fruit – Emblica officinalis,

Dadima – Pomegranate – Punica granatum,

Puskara – Inula racemosa

Dhanya – Coriandrum sativum

Ajaji – Cuminum cyminum,

Chitraka – Plumbago zeylanica

Vacha – Acorus calamus

2 types of ksara (alkalies),

2 types of Lavana (salt) and

Chavya – Piper retrofractum all these are made & administered along with food and drinks.

It can be given before food along with alcoholic drinks or hot water.

It cures:

Pain in the sides of the chest, Cardiac region and Basti (urinary bladder including kidneys)

Gulma caused by Vata and Kapha,

Anaha (abdominal distension),

Dysuria

Pain in anus and female genital tract,

Grahani – Sprue syndrome

Piles

Splenic disorders,

Pandu – Anemia

Aruchi – anorexia,

Urovibandha (stiffness of the chest),

Hikka – hiccup

Kasa – cough

Shwasa – asthma and

Obstruction in the throat

If this powder is impregnated for 7 days with the juice of Matulunga and then made into pills, it becomes therapeutically more effective. [79-84]

Hingvadi Yoga:

मातुलुङ्गरसो हिङ्गु दाडिमं बिडसैन्धवे|
सुरामण्डेन पातव्यं वातगुल्मरुजापहम्||८५||

Juice of Matulunga – Citrus medica

Hingu – Asa foetida

Dadima – Pomegranate – Punica granatum

Bida salt

Saindhava Lavana – Black salt- these is administered along with Suramanda (upper portion of an alcoholic preparation) for the cure of the pain of Vata Gulma [85]

Shatyadi Curna and Shatyadi Gutika:

शटी पुष्कर हिङ्ग्वम्लवेतस क्षार चित्रकान्।
धान्यकं च यवानीं च विडङ्गं सैन्धवं वचाम्॥८६॥
सचव्य पिप्पलीमूलामजगन्धां सदाडिमाम्।
अजाजीं चाजमोदां च चूर्ण कृत्वा प्रयोजयेत्॥८७॥
रसेन मातुलुङ्गस्य मधुशुक्तेन वा पुनः।
भावितं गुटिकां कृत्वा सुपिष्टां कोलसम्मिताम्॥८८॥
गुल्मं प्लीहानमानाहं श्वासं कासमरोचकम्।
हिक्कां हृद्रोगमर्शांसि विविधां शिरसो रुजम्॥८९॥
पाण्ड्वामयं कफोत्क्लेशं सर्वजां च प्रवाहिकाम्।
पार्श्वहृद्बस्तिशूलं च गुटिकैषा व्यपोहति॥९०॥

Shati – Hedyium spicatum

Pushkara – Inula racemosa

Hingu – Asafoetida,

AmlaVetasa – Salix tetrasperma,

Kshara – Yavakshara

Chitraka – Plumbago zeylanica

Dhanyaka – Coriander – Coriandrum sativum

Yavani – Trachyspermum roxburghianum

Vidanga – False black pepper – Embelia ribes,

Saindava – Rock Salt

Vacha – Acorus calamus

Chavya – Piper retrofractum

Pippalimula – Long pepper fruit – Piper longum,

Ajagandha – Cleome gynandra

Dadima – Pomegranate – Punica granatum

Ajaji – Cuminum cyminum and

Ajamoda – Ajowan (fruit) – Trachyspermum roxburghianum are made into powder and administered.

This powder may be impregnated with the:

Juice of Matulunga – Citrus medica or

Madhu- Sukta and made into a fine paste.

Then pills the size of Kola – Ziziphus jujuba fruit is made out of it.

This pill cures:

Gulma

Splenic disorders

Anaha – abdominal distension

Shwasa – asthma

Kasa – cough,

Aruchi – Anorexia,

Hikka – hiccup

Hrut pida – heart disease

Shira shoola – headache

Pandu – anemia

Nausea caused by aggravation of Kapha, Sannipatika type of Pravahika and

Parshva, hrd, basti shula: Pain in side of the chest, cardiac region and Basti (urinary bladder including kidneys) [86-90]

Nagaradi Yoga:

नागरार्धपलं पिष्ट्वा द्वे पले लुञ्चितस्य च|
तिलस्यैकं गुडपलं क्षीरेणोष्णेन ना पिबेत्||९१||
वात गुल्ममुदावर्तं योनिशूलं च नाशयेत्|

Ingredients:

1/2 Pala of nagara – Ginger

2 Palas of Tila – Sesamum indicum and

1 Pala of Guda – Jaggery is made into paste and taken along with hot milk.

This potion cures

Vata-Gulma

Udavarta – upward movement of wind) and

Yoni shoola – Pain in female genital organs [91 ½- 92]

Administration of Castor oil:

पिबेदेरण्डजं तैलं वारुणी मण्डमिश्रितम्||९२||
तदेव तैलं पयसा वातगुल्मी पिबेन्नरः|
श्लेष्मण्यनुबले पूर्वं हितं पित्तानुगे परम्||९३||

Erandataila – Castor oil is taken by a patient suffering from Vata Gulma after mixing it with the Manda (upper portion) of Varuni (a type of alcoholic preparation) or milk.

It is taken with Manda of Varuni, if kapha is secondarily aggravated along with Vata Dosha.

It is taken with milk if Pitta is secondarily aggravated. [92-93]

Lashuna Ksheerapaka:

साधयेच्छुद्धशुष्कस्य लशुनस्य चतुष्पलम्|
क्षीरोदकेऽष्टगुणिते क्षीरशेषं च ना पिबेत्||९४||
वातगुल्ममुदावर्तं गृध्रसीं विषमज्वरम्|
हृद्रोगं विद्रधिं शोथं साधयत्याशु तत्पयः||९५||
इति लशुनक्षीरम्|

4 Palas of Dehusked and dried Lasuna is boiled by adding 8 times of milk and water and reduced to the quantity of milk.

This medicated milk immediately cures

Vata- Gulma,

Udavarta – upward movement of wind

Gridhrasi – sciatica

Vishama Jvara – Recurrent fever

Hrid rogam – heart disease,

Vidradhi – Abscess and

Shotha – oedema. [94-95]

Learn how to prepare Lashuna Ksheerapaka

Taila panchaka

तैलं प्रसन्ना गोमूत्रमारनालं यवाग्रजम्|
गुल्मं जठरमानाहं पीतमेकत्र साधयेत्||९६||
इति तैलपञ्चकम्|

Taila (sesame oil), Prasanna (a type of alcoholic drink), cow's urine, aranala (a type of sour drink) and YavaKshara is taken together for the cure of Gulma Jathara and Anaha (abdominal bloating) [96]

Administration of Shilajit:

पञ्चमूलीकषायेण सक्षारेण शिलाजतु।
पिबेत्तस्य प्रयोगेण वातगुल्मात् प्रमुच्यते||९७||
इति शिलाजतुप्रयोगः।

Intake of Shilajatu along with the decoction of Panchamoola added with Kshara (alkali preparation) Yava – Barley – Hordeum vulgare Kshara cures Vataja Gulma. [97]

Administration of Boiled Barley:
वाट्यं पिप्पलीयूषेण मूलकानां रसेन वा।
भुक्त्वा स्निग्धमुदावर्तोद्वातगुल्मादिविमुच्यते||९८||

Intake of Vatya (boiled barley) along with the soup of Pippali – Long pepper fruit – Piper longum or the juice of Mulaka – Radish – Raphanus sativus by adding Sneha (ghee) cures Udavarta (upward movement of Vata) and Vata-Gulma [98]

Swedana – Sweating Therapy:
शूलानाह विबन्धार्तं स्वेदयेद्वातगुल्मिनम्।
स्वेदैः स्वेद विधावुक्तैर्नाडीप्रस्तर सङ्करैः||९९||

If the patient of Vata- Gulma has symptoms like

Shula – colic pain,

Anaha – abdominal distension and

Vibandha – constipation, then he is given fomentation therapy with the help of Nadi, Prastara or Sankara type of fomentation as described in Sutra 14[99]

Basti – Enema Therapy:
बस्तिकर्म परं विद्याद्गुल्मघ्नं तद्धि मारुतम्।
स्वे स्थाने प्रथमं जित्वा सद्यो गुल्ममपोहति||१००||
तस्मादभीक्ष्णशो गुल्मा निरूहैः सानुवासनैः।
प्रयुज्यमानैः शाम्यन्ति वातपित्तकफात्मकाः||१०१||
गुल्मघ्ना विविधा दिष्टाः सिद्धाः सिद्धिषु बस्तयः|१०२|

Medicated enema is the best therapy for curing Gulma.

In the beginning, it overcomes Gulma. Therefore, Niruha and Anuvasana types of medicated enema are administered frequently for the cure. Over dosage or taking this medicine for a longer period than prescribed may cause Vatika, Paittika and Kaphaja type of Gulma.

Different effective recipes of medicated enema for successful treatment of this disease are described in the Siddhi section of this work. [100-101]

Herbal Oils & Ghee:
गुल्मघ्नानि च तैलानि वक्ष्यन्ते वातरोगिके||१०२||
तानि मारुतजे गुल्मे पानाभ्यङ्गानुवासनैः।
प्रयुक्तान्याशु सिध्यन्ति तैलं ह्यनिलजित्परम्||१०३||

Recipes of medicated oils in the chapter dealing with the treatment of Vata-Roga (Chikitsa 28) should be useful for Pana (oral intake), massage and Anuvasana type of medicated enema by a patient suffering from Vataja Gulma. Medicated oil is the best for overcoming Vata. Therefore, these recipes cure Gulma instantaneously.

Ghee for Purification of Body:
नीलिनीचूर्णसंयुक्तं पूर्वोक्तं घृतमेव।
समलाय प्रदातव्यं शोधनं वातगुल्मिने||१०४||

Recipes of medicated ghee described earlier in the chapter is administered along with the powder of Neelini – Indigofera tinctorea to the patient suffering from Vata Gulma for the elimination (Shodhana) of excreta (Mala) from his body.[102- 104]

Nilinyadya Ghrita:

नीलिनी त्रिवृता दन्ती पथ्या कम्पिल्लकैः सह।
शोधनार्थं घृतं देयं सबिडक्षार नागरम्||१०५||

For purification (elimination of waste products from the body), ghee is administered along with

Nilini – Indigofera tinctoria

Trivrit – Operculina turpethum

Danti – Baliospermum montanum,

Pathya – Chebulic Myrobalan fruit rind – Terminalia chebula and

Kampillaka – Mallotus phillippinensis

By adding Bida a (type of salt), Kshara (Alkalies) and Nagara (ginger) [105]

Neelinyadi Ghrita – 2

नीलिनीं त्रिफलां रास्नां बलां कटुकरोहिणीम्।
पचेद्विडङ्गं व्याघ्रीं च पलिकानि जलाढके||१०६||
तेन पादावशेषेण घृतप्रस्थं विपाचयेत्।
दध्नः प्रस्थेन संयोज्य सुधाक्षीरपलेन च||१०७||
ततो घृतपलं दद्याद्यवागूमण्डमिश्रितम्।
जीर्णे सम्यग्विरिक्तं च भोजयेद्रसभोजनम्||१०८||
गुल्मकुष्ठोदरव्यङ्गशोफपाण्डुवामयज्वरान्।
श्वित्रं प्लीहानमुन्मादं घृतमेतद्व्यपोहति||१०९||
इति नीलिन्याद्यं घृतम्।

Neelinyadi Ghrita – 2

1 Pala of each of

Nilini

Triphala – Haritaki, Amalaki and vibhitaki

Rasna – Pluchea lanceolata / Vanda roxburghi,

Bala – Country mallow (root) – Sida cordifolia,

Katuka Rohini – Kutki – Picrorhiza kurroa

Vidanga – False black pepper – Embelia ribes and

Vyaghri – Kantakari

is boiled in 1 Adhaka of water till 1/4th remains.

This is boiled by adding 1 prastha of Ghee, 1 Prastha of curd and 1 Pala of the milky- latex of Sudha (Snuhi).

1 Pala of this medicated ghee is administered to the patient by mixing it with Yavagu (thick gruel) or Manda (a type of thin gruel).

When the recipe is digested and when he is properly purged, he is given food in the form of meat soup.

This medicated ghee cures

Gulma,

Kushta – skin diseases

Udara – obstinate abdominal diseases including ascites

Vyanga – dark spots on the face

Shotha – oedema

Pandu – anemia,

Jwara – fever

Leucoderma,
Splenic disorders and
Insanity [106-109]

Diet for Vata- Gulma

कुक्कुटाश्च मयूराश्च तित्तिरिक्रौञ्चवर्तकाः|
शालयो मदिरा सर्पिर्वातगुल्मभिषग्जितम्||११०||
हितमुष्णं द्रवं स्निग्धं भोजनं वातगुल्मिनाम्|
समण्डवारुणीपानं पक्वं वा धान्यकैर्जलम्||१११||
मन्देऽग्नौ वर्धते गुल्मो दीप्ते चाग्नौ प्रशाम्यति|
तस्मान्ना नातिसौहित्यं कुर्यान्नातिविलङ्घनम्||११२||
सर्वत्र गुल्मे प्रथमं स्नेहस्वेदोपपादिते|
या क्रिया क्रियते सिद्धिं सा याति न विरूक्षिते||११३||

Meat of cock, peacock, Tittiri, Kraunca and Vartaka, Different types of Sali Rice, Madira (alcoholic drink) and ghee - these are to be used in the treatment of Vata- Gulma. Hot, liquid and unctuous foods and drinks like Varuni (a type of alcoholic drink) along with its Manda (upper portion) or water boiled by adding Dhanyaka – Coriander – Coriandrum sativum are useful for a patient suffering from Vata- Gulma.

If there is suppression of the power of digestion then Gulma gets aggravated, and if the power of digestion is stimulated then Gulma gets alleviated. Therefore, the patient should not eat in excess nor should he fast in excess. [110-112]

Medicines for Pittaja Gulma Chikitsa:
Trayamanadi Ghurta:

जले दशगुणे साध्यं त्रायमाणाचतुष्पलम्|
पञ्चभागस्थितं पूतं कल्कैः संयोज्य कार्षिकैः||११८||
रोहिणी कटुका मुस्ता त्रायमाणा दुरालभा|
कल्कैस्तामलकीवीरा जीवन्ती चन्दनोत्पलैः||११९||
रसस्यामलकानां च क्षीरस्य च घृतस्य च|
पलानि पृथगष्टाष्टौ दत्त्वा सम्यग्विपाचयेत्||१२०||
पितरक्तभवं गुल्मं वीसर्पं पैत्तिकं ज्वरम्|
हृद्रोगं कामलां कुष्ठं हन्यादेतद्घृतोत्तमम्||१२१||
इति त्रायमाणाद्यं घृतम्|

Trayamanadya Ghurta:

4 Palas of Trayamana – Gentiana kurroo is boiled with 10 times of water and reduced to 1/5th.

To this decoction, the paste of 1 Karsha – 12 g each of

Katurohini – Kutki

Musta – Nut grass (root) – Cyperus rotundus,

Trayamana – Gentiana kurroa

Duralabha – Alhagi camelorum

Tamalaki – Phyllanthus niruri

Veera

Jivanti – Leptadenia reticulata,

Chandana – Santalum album and

Utpala – Nymphaea stellata and

8 Palas each of the juice of Amalaka,

Milk and

Ghee is added and cooked properly.

This excellent recipe of medicated ghee cures:

Gulma caused by Pitta and Raktha

Visarpa – erysipelas

Paittika types of fever

Hrd roga – Heart disease

Kamala – Jaundice and

Kushta – skin diseases [118-121]

Amalakadi Ghrta:

रसेनामलकेक्षूणां घृतपादं विपाचयेत्।

पथ्यापदं पिबेत्सर्पिस्तत्सिद्धं पित्तगुल्मनुत्॥१२२॥

इत्यामलकाद्यं घृतम्।

To the juice of Amla and Ikshu, $1/4^{th}$ ghee in quantity is added and cooked. During cooking, $1/4^{th}$ paste of Pathya – Chebulic Myrobalan fruit rind – Terminalia chebula in quantity is added. Intake of this medicated ghee cures Paittika Gulma. [122]

Drakshadya Ghrita:

द्राक्षां मधूकं खर्जूरं विदारीं सशतावरीम्।

परूषकाणि त्रिफलां साधयेत्पलसम्मितम्॥१२३॥

जलाढके पादशेषे रसमामलकस्य च।

घृतमिक्षुरसं क्षीरमभयाकल्कपादिकम्॥१२४॥

साधयेत्तद्घृतं सिद्धं शर्कराक्षौद्रपादिकम्।

प्रयोगात् पित्तगुल्मघ्नं सर्वपित्तविकारनुत्॥१२५॥

इति द्राक्षाद्यं घृतम्।

1 Pala each of Draksha – Raisin – Vitis vinifera,

Madhuka –Madhuca longifolia

Vidari – Pueraria tuberosa,

Shatavari – Asparagus racemosus

Parushaka – Falsa Fruit – Grewia asiatica and

Triphala is boiled with 1 Adhaka of water and reduced to fourth.

To this, juice of Amalaki, ghee, sugarcane juice, milk and $1/4^{th}$ in quantity of the paste of Abhaya – Terminalia chebula is added.

After it is cooked, $1/4^{th}$ of the quantity of sugar and honey is added.

This recipes cures Paittika Gulma and other diseases caused by Pitta [123-125]

Vasa Ghrutha for Pittaja Gulma

वृषं समूलमापोथ्य पचेदष्टगुणे जले।

शेषेऽष्टभागे तस्यैव पुष्पकल्कं प्रदापयेत्॥१२६॥

तेन सिद्धं घृतं शीतं सक्षौद्रं पित्तगुल्मनुत्।

रक्तपित्त ज्वर श्वास कास हृद्रोग नाशनम्॥१२७॥

इति वासाघृतम्।

Vasa Ghrutha:

Vasa – Adhathoda vasica along with its root is crushed and boiled in 8 times of water till $1/8^{th}$ remains. To this the paste of the flower of Vata and ghee is added and it is cooked. After it is cooled, honey is added and given to the patient.

This ghee cures:

Pitta-gulma

Rakta Pitta – a disease characterized by bleeding from different parts of the body,

Jvara – fever

Shwasa – Asthma

Kasa – coughing and

Hrd roga – cardiac ailments [126-127]

Trayamana Ksheera Yoga for Pitta Gulma

दिवपलं त्रायमाणाया जल दिव प्रस्थ साधितम्।

अष्टभाग स्थितं पूतं कोष्णं क्षीरसमं पिबेत्||१२८||

पिबेदुपरि तस्योष्णं क्षीरमेव यथाबलम्।

तेन निर्हतदोषस्य गुल्मः शाम्यति पैत्तिकः||१२९||

2 Palas of Trayamana are to be boiled in 2 Prasthas of water and reduced to 1/8th.

When lukewarm, this decoction is mixed with equal quantities of milk and given to the patient. Thereafter, the patient is taking more milk depending upon his power of digestion.

This eliminates morbid Doshas, and thus, cures Paittika type of Gulma [128-129]

Recipes for purgation:

द्राक्षाभयारसं गुल्मे पैत्तिके सगुडं पिबेत्।

लिह्यात्कम्पिल्लकं वाऽपि विरेकार्थं मधु द्रवम्||१३०||

For purgation, the patient suffering from Paittika Gulma should take the juice or decoction of Draksha – Raisin – Vitis vinifera and Abhaya – Terminalia chebula mixed with jaggery.

He may also take Kampillaka in the form of linctus by mixing it with honey. [130]

Massage therapy:

दाह प्रशमनोऽभ्यङ्गः सर्पिषा पित्तगुल्मिनाम्।

चन्दनाद्येन तैलेन तैलेन मधुकस्य वा||१३१||

Burning sensation in a patient of pitta- Gulma can be alleviated by using ghee or Chandanadya Taila – Sesame (Sesamum indicum) or Madhuka– Licorice – Glycyrrhiza glabra Taila for massage [131]

Medicated Enema:

ये च पित्तज्वरहराः सतिक्ताः क्षीरबस्तयः|

हितास्ते पित्तगुल्मिभ्यो वक्ष्यन्ते ये च सिद्धिषु||१३२||

Recipes of Ksira- basti (medicated enema made of milk and other drugs) prepared by boiling milk with bitter drugs, which alleviate Pitta- Jvara, are also useful for Pitta- Gulma. Such recipes are also described in Siddhi Sthana. [132]

Diet and Drinks for Pitta- Gulma

शालयो जाङ्गलं मांसं गव्याजे पयसी घृतम्।

खर्जूरामलकं द्राक्षां दाडिमं सपरूषकम्||१३३||

आहारार्थं प्रयोक्तव्यं पानार्थं सलिलं शृतम्।

बला विदारीगन्धाद्यैः पित्तगुल्म चिकित्सितम्||१३४||

Different types of Sali rice, meat of animals inhabiting arid land, cow milk, goat milk, ghee Kharjura – Dates – Phoenix dactylifera, amalaka, draksa, Dadima – Pomegranate – Punica granatum and Parusaka - these are given as diet to the patient suffering from Pitta Gulma. To such patients, water boiled withBala – Country mallow (root) – Sida cordifolia, Vidarigandha etc, is given for drinking [134]

Stimulation of Digestive power:

आमान्वये पित्तगुल्मे सामे वा कफवातिके।
यवागूभिः खडैर्यूषैः सन्धुक्ष्योऽग्निर्विलङ्घिते॥१३५॥

After administration of fasting therapy in Pitta- Gulma, Vata- Gulma or Kapha-Gulma when these are associated with Ama, the patient is given Yavagu (gruel), Khada and Yusha (soup) for stimulating his power of digestion. [135]

Importance of Agni:

शमप्रकोपौ दोषाणां सर्वेषामग्निसंश्रितौ।
तस्मादग्निं सदा रक्षेन्निदानानि च वर्जयेत्॥१३६॥

Alleviation and aggravation of all Doshas is dependent upon Agni (power of digestion and metabolism). Therefore, it is always necessary to maintain Agni and to avoid factors responsible for the vitiation of Agni. [136]

Medicine and treatment for Kaphaja gulma:
Surgical Management of Kapha- Gulma:

वमनं वमनार्हाय प्रदद्यात् कफगुल्मिने।
स्निग्धस्विन्नशरीराय गुल्मे शैथिल्यमागते॥१३७॥
परिवेष्ट्य प्रदीप्तांस्तु बल्वजानथवा कुशान्।
भिषक्कुम्भे समावाप्य गुल्मं घटमुखे न्यसेत्॥१३८॥
सङ्गृहीतो यदा गुल्मस्तदा घटमथोद्धरेत्।
वस्त्रान्तरं ततः कृत्वा भिन्द्याद्गुल्मं प्रमाणवित्॥१३९॥
विमार्गाजपदादर्शैर्यथालाभं प्रपीडयेत्।
मृद्नीयाद्गुल्ममेवैकं न त्वन्त्रहृदयं स्पृशेत्॥१४०॥
तिलैरण्डातसीबीजसर्षपैः परिलिप्य च।
श्लेष्मगुल्ममयःपात्रैः सुखोष्णैः स्वेदयेद्भिषक्॥१४१॥

The patient of Kapha Gulma is administered Snehana and Swedana, thereafter, Vamana therapy is administered if needed.

After the mass of Gulma has become soft by the administration of these therapies, at the brim, it is covered with a piece of cloth and made to enter the mouth of a jar containing ignited Balvaja or Kusha.

When because of the negative pressure created inside the jar, the mouth of the jar becomes strongly adhered to brim of the mass of Gulma, the jar is pulled. Then though another piece of cloth, the mass of Gulma is tied at its Root (peduncle) and punctured by a physician well versed in this technique. Thereafter, with the help of implements like Vimarga, Ajapada and Adarsha, whatever is available, the mass of Gulma is squeezed.

Thereafter with the paste of Tila – Sesamum indicum, Eranda – Castor, seeds of Atasi – Linseed – Linum usitatissimum and sarshapa it is fomented with the help of an iron pan made tolerably warm. [137-141]

Dashamuli Ghrita:

सव्योष क्षार लवणं दशमूलीशृतं घृतम्।
कफगुल्मं जयत्याशु सहिङ्गुबिडदाडिमम्॥१४२॥
इति दशमूलीघृतम्।

Ghee boiled with the decoction of DashaMula along with the paste of Vyosa, ksara (Alkali) Lavana (rock Salt), Hingu, bida and Dadima cures Kapha- Gulma immediately. [142]

Bhallatakadya Ghrta:

भल्लातकानां द्विपलं पञ्चमूलं पलोन्मितम्।
साध्यं विदारीगन्धाद्यमापोथ्य सलिलाढके॥१४३॥
पादशेषे रसे तस्मिन् पिप्पली नागरं वचाम्।
विडङ्गं सैन्धवं हिङ्गु यावशूकं बिडं शटीम्॥१४४॥

चित्रकं मधुकं रास्नां पिष्ट्वा कर्षसमं भिषक्|
प्रस्थं च पयसो दत्वा घृतप्रस्थं विपाचयेत्||१४५||
एतद्भल्लातकघृतं कफगुल्महरं परम्|
प्लीह पाण्ड्वामय श्वास ग्रहणी रोग कासनुत्||१४६||
इति भल्लातकाद्यं घृतम्|

2 Palas of Bhallataka – Purified Semecarpus anacardium and 1 Pala of each of the drugs belonging to Kusdra Pancha-Mula group is boiled in 1 Adhaka of water till 1/4th remains.

To this decoction the paste of 1 Karsa of each of

Pippali – Long pepper fruit – Piper longum

Nagara – Ginger Rhizome – Zingiber officinalis

Vacha – Acorus calamus

Vidanga – False black pepper – Embelia ribes

Saindhava Lavana – Black salt

Hingu – Asa foetida

Yavakshara – Alkali of Barley

Bida salt

Shati – Hedyium spicatum

Chitraka – Plumbago zeylanica

Madhuka – Licorice – Glycyrrhiza glabra and

Rasna – Pluchea lanceolata / Vanda roxburghi

1 Prastha of milk and

1 Prastha of Ghee is added and cooked

This is called Bhallatak Ghrta.

It is an excellent recipe for the cure of Kapha Gulma.

It also cures

Pliha – Splenic disorders

Pandu – anemia

Shwasa – asthma

Grahani – sprue syndrome and

Kasa – cough [143-146]

Ksheera shatpala Ghruta:

पिप्पली पिप्पलीमूल चव्य चित्रक नागरैः|
पलिकैः सयवक्षारैर्घृतप्रस्थं विपाचयेत्||१४७||
क्षीरप्रस्थं च तत् सर्पिहन्ति गुल्मं कफात्मकम्|
ग्रहणी पाण्डुरोगघ्नं प्लीह कास ज्वरापहम्||१४८||
इति क्षीरषट्पलकं घृतम्|

1 Prastha of ghee is boiled with 1 Prastha of milk and the paste of 1 Pala of each of

Pippali – Long pepper fruit – Piper longum,

Pippalimula

Chavya

Chitraka – Plumbago zeylanica

Nagara – Ginger

and

YavaKshara – Alkali

It cures

Kapha- Gulma

Grahani – sprue syndrome
Pandu – anemia
Pliha – splenic disorders
Kasa – cough and
Jwara – fever [147-148]

Mishraka Sneha:
त्रिवृतां त्रिफलां दन्तीं दशमूलं पलोन्मितम्‌|
जले चतुर्गुणे पक्त्वा चतुर्भागस्थितं रसम्‌||१४९||
सर्पिरेरण्डजं तैलं क्षीरं चैकत्र साधयेत्‌|
स सिद्धो मिश्रकस्नेहः सक्षौद्रः कफगुल्मनुत्‌||१५०||
कफवातविबन्धेषु कुष्ठप्लीहोदरेषु च|
प्रयोज्यो मिश्रकः स्नेहो योनिशूलेषु चाधिकम्‌||१५१||
इति मिश्रकः स्नेहः|
1 Pala each of Trivrt, Triphala, Danti – Baliospermum montanum and Dashamoola is boiled with 4 times of water till
$1/4^{th}$ remains.
To this decoction, ghee, castor oil and milk are added and cooked.
This Misraka Sneha (mixture of ghee and oil) is administered along with honey.
It cures
Kapha- gulma
Constipation caused by Kapha and Vata,
Kustha – skin diseases and
Pliha – splenic disorders.
This is used specially for the cure of Yoni- sula (pain in the female genital tract). [149-151]

Purgation Therapy:
यदुक्तं वातगुल्मघ्नं स्रंसनं नीलिनीघृतम्‌|
द्विगुणं तद्विरेकार्थे प्रयोज्यं कफगुल्मिनाम्‌||१५२||
सुधाक्षीरद्रवे चूर्णं त्रिवृतायाः सुभावितम्‌|
कार्षिकं मधुसर्पिभ्यां लीढ्वा साधु विरिच्यते||१५३||
The recipe of Nilini Ghrta which is prescribed for Sramsana (mild purgation) in the treatment of Vata –Gulma (wide
verses 106-109) can also be used in double dose (2 Palas) for purgation in the treatment of Kapha- Gulma.
1 Karsa of the powder of Trivrt well impregnated with the milky latex of Sudha is given to this patient by mixing
with honey and ghee for proper purgation. [152-153]

Danti Haritaki :
जलद्रोणे विपक्तव्या विंशतिः पञ्च चाभयाः|
दन्त्याः पलानि तावन्ति चित्रकस्य तथैव च||१५४||
अष्टभागावशेषं तु रसं पूतमधिक्षिपेत्‌|
दन्तीसमं गुडं पूतं क्षिपेत्रत्राभयाश्च ताः||१५५||
तैलार्धकुडवं चैव त्रिवृतायाश्चतुष्पलम्‌|
चूर्णितं पलमेकं तु पिप्पलीविश्वभेषजम्‌||१५६||
तत्‌ साध्यं लेहवच्छीते तस्मिंस्तैलसमं मधु|
क्षिपेच्चूर्णपलं चैकं त्वगेलापत्रकेशरात्‌||१५७||
ततो लेहपलं लीढ्वा जग्ध्वा चैकां हरीतकीम्‌|
सुखं विरिच्यते स्निग्धो दोषप्रस्थमनामयम्‌||१५८||

गुल्मं श्वयथुमर्शांसि पाण्डुरोगमरोचकम्|
हृद्रोगं ग्रहणीदोषं कामलां विषमज्वरम्||१५९||
कुष्ठं प्लीहानमानाहमेषा हन्त्युपसेविता|
निरत्ययः क्रमश्चास्या द्रवो मांसरसौदनः||१६०||
इति दन्तीहरीतकी|

In 1 Drona of water 25 fruits of Haritaki – Chebulic Myrobalan fruit rind – Terminalia chebula and 25 Palas of each Danti – Baliospermum montanum and Chitraka and boiled till 1/8th remains.

In this decoction, 25 fruits of Haritaki (boiled earlier), ½ Kudava of oil, 4 Palas of Trivrit and 1 Pala of the lines suggested for the powder of Tvak, Ela, Patra – Cinnamomum tamala Nees and Eberum and Kesara is added.

The patient is given 1 Pala of this linctus along with 1 fruit of Haritaki (added to this recipe). This, when administered to an oleated patient, causes painless purgation.

It eliminates 1 Prastha of waste- product from the body without any difficulty.

It cures

Gulma

Svayathu – oedema

Arshas: piles

Pandu: anemia

Aruchi: anorexia

Hrd roga: heart diseases

Grahani: sprue syndrome

Kamala: Jaundice

Visama Jvara – irregular fever

Kushta – skin diseases

Pliha – splenic disorders and

Anaha – abdominal distension

After the administration of this recipe, the patient is given liquid food including meat soup and rice which constitute the safe regimen. [154-160]

Other Recipes and Therapies for Kaphaja Gulma:

Effective recipes of Niruha (decoction enema) for the successful treatment of Kapha- Gulma will be described in the Siddhi section. Similarly, effective recipes of Arista (a type of alchoholic preparation) for the effective treatment of this ailment will be described in chapters dealing with the treatment of sprue syndrome (Cikitsa 15) and piles (Cikitsa 14).

Powders and pills described in this chapter for the treatment of Kapha-Gulma provide Ksara (alkalies), Hingu – Asa foetida and Amala- Vetasa are taken in double the prescribed quantity.

Recipes of Alkalies (Ksharas) prescribed for the treatment of sprue syndrome (in Cikitsa 15) are also effective and safe for the treatment of Kapha- Gulma. In the end Daha (cauterisation) therapy is useful in this condition. [161-163]

Diet and Drinks for Kaphaja gulma

प्रपुराणानि धान्यानि जाङ्गला मृगपक्षिणः|
कौलत्थो मुद्गयूषश्च पिप्पल्या नागरस्य च||१६४||
शुष्कमूलकयूषश्च बिल्वस्य वरुणस्य च|
चिरबिल्वाङ्कुराणां च यवान्याश्चित्रकस्य च||१६५||
बीजपूरक हिङ्ग्वम्लवेतस क्षार दाडिमैः|
तक्रेण तैलसर्पिभ्र्यां व्यञ्जनान्युपकल्पयेत्||१६६||
पञ्चमूलीशृतं तोयं पुराणं वारुणीरसम्|
कफगुल्मी पिबेत्काले जीर्णं माध्वीकमेव वा||१६७||

Diet and drinks useful for a patient suffering from Kapha- Gulma:

1) Old corns and cereals, meat of animals inhabiting arid land and birds, and soups of Kulattha and Mudga

2) Vegetable dishes prepared of Pippali, Nagara, Soup of dried Radish, Bilva, Varuna, tender (leaves) of Cirabilva, Yavani and Chitraka prepared by adding Beejapuraka, Hingu, Amlavestasa, Ksara, Dadima, Butter- milk , oil and Ghee;

3) Water boiled with Panca- Mula and

4) Old Varuni (a type of alchoholic drink) is taken by the patient at the appropriate time. After the digestion of food Madhvika (another type of alcoholic drink) is taken. [164-167]

Digestive Stimulants:

यवानीचूर्णितं तक्रं बिडेन लवणीकृतम्|

पिबेत् सन्दीपनं वातकफमूत्रानुलोमनम् ||१६८||

Butter- milk sprinkled with the powder of Yavani and made saline by adding Lavana (rock- salt) is given to the patient to drink. This potion stimulates the power of digestion and helps in the downward movement of Vata, Kapha and urine. [168]

Incurability and Complications:

सञ्चितः क्रमशो गुल्मो महावास्तुपरिग्रहः|

कृतमूलः सिरानद्धो यदा कूर्म इवोन्नतः||१६९||

दौर्बल्यारुचिहृल्लासकासवम्यरतिज्वरैः |

तृष्णातन्द्राप्रतिश्यायैर्युज्यते न स सिध्यति||१७०||

गृहीत्वा सज्वरश्वासं वम्यतीसारपीडितम्|

हृन्नाभिहस्तपादेषु शोफः कर्षति गुल्मिनम्||१७१||

When Gulma, gradually accumulated, surrounds a large area, deep-rooted, when it is engrossed with veins, when it is elevated like a tortoise and when it is associated with weakness, anorexia, Nausea, Cough, vomiting, Arati (Disliking for everything), fever, morbid thirst, drowsiness as well as coryza, it becomes incurable. Oedema in cardiac region, umbilical region and upper as well as lower limbs in a patient of Gulma who is afflicted with fever, dyspnoea, vomiting and diarrhea drags him towards death.

Management of Raktaja Gulma:

रौधिरस्य तु गुल्मस्य गर्भकाल व्यतिक्रमे|

स्निग्ध स्विन्नशरीरायै दद्यात् स्नेह विरेचनम्||१७२||

पलाश क्षारपात्रे द्वे द्वे पात्रे तैलसर्पिषोः|

गुल्म शैथिल्य जननीं पक्त्वा मात्रां प्रयोजयेत्||१७३||

प्रभिद्येत न यद्येवं दद्याद्योनिविशोधनम् |

क्षारेण युक्तं पललं सुधाक्षीरेण वा पुनः||१७४||

आभ्यां वा भावितान् दद्याद्योनौ कटुकमत्स्यकान्|

वराहमत्स्यपित्ताभ्यां लक्तकान् वा सुभावितान्||१७५||

अधोहरैश्चोर्ध्वहरैर्भावितान् वा समाक्षिकैः|

किण्वं वा सगुडक्षारं दद्याद्योनिविशोधनम्||१७६||

रक्तपित्तहरं क्षारं लेहयेन्मधुसर्पिषा|

लशुनं मदिरां तीक्ष्णां मत्स्यांश्चास्यै प्रदापयेत्||१७७||

बस्तिं सक्षीरगोमूत्रं सक्षारं दाशमूलिकम्|

अदृश्यमाने रुधिरे दद्याद्गुल्मप्रभेदनम्||१७८||

प्रवर्तमाने रुधिरे दद्यान्मांसरसौदनम्|

घृततैलेन चाभ्यङ्गं पानार्थं तरुणीं सुराम्||१७९||

रुधिरेऽतिप्रवृत्ते तु रक्तपित्तहरीः क्रियाः|

कार्या वातरुगार्तायाः सर्वा वातहरीः पुनः||१८०||
घृततैलावसेकांश्च तित्तिरींश्चरणायुधान्|
सुरां समण्डां पूर्वं च पानमम्लस्य सर्पिषः||१८१||
प्रयोजयेदुत्तरं वा जीवनीयेन सर्पिषा|
अतिप्रवृत्ते रुधिरे सतिक्तेनानुवासनम्||१८२||

The patient suffering from Rakta- Gulma, after 10th month, is given oleation and fomentation therapies followed by Sneha Virechana (purgation therapy with unctuous ingredients).

Two Patras of Palasha-Ksara (Alkali preparation of Palasa tree) and two Patras of oil and ghee are boiled together and administered to the patient in appropriate dose with a view to suppressing (loosening) the Gulma. If the mass of Gulma does not break by the administration of this recipe, 1 of the following recipes is inserted into the vagina for the cleansing of Yoni (female genital tract)

1) Oil cake mixed with alkalies

2) Oil cake mixed with the milky latex of Sudha

3) Katuka- Maaatsya (small fish called Saphari which is pungent in taste) impregnated with alkalies and milky later of Sudha

4) A peace of cloth well impregnated with the bile of Varaha or Matsya

5) A peace of cloth well impregnated with the drugs which cause vomiting or purgation and smeared with honey; and

6) Kinva (Yeast which is used for fermentation, Asavas and Aristas) mixed with Jaggery and Alkalies

If inspite of it, if bleeding does not occur, then for breaking the Rakta Gulma,the patient may be given alkalies prescribed for the treatment of Raktha-Pitta (A disease characterized by bleeding from different parts of the body) along with honey and ghee in the form of a linctus. She is given Lasuna, a sharp type of Madira (a variety of alcoholic drink) and fish. She may also be given medicated enema (uttara basti – enema given through the vaginal route) prepared with the decoction of Dasa-Mula mixed with milk, Cow's urine and Alkalies.

After the bleeding, the patient is given rice mixed with meat soup.

Ghee and oil is used for massage of her body, and for drinking; she is given freshly prepared Sura (a type of Alcoholic drink).

If there is excessive bleeding, then therapies prescribed for excessive pain is given, then she is given all therapies Avaseka (sprinkling of water), Tittiri, Charanayudha (cock), Sura along with its Manda (upper portion of the fermented liquid) and ghee prepared with sour drugs as food, drinks and regimens.

Ghee boiled with drugs belonging to the Jivaniya group is used for Uttara Basti (douching the vaginal tract). If there is excessive bleeding then anuvasana type of medicated enema is administered by boiling with bitter – drugs [172-182]

Summary:

तत्र श्लोकाः-

स्नेहः स्वेदः सर्पिर्बस्तिश्चूर्णानि बृंहणं गुडिकाः|
वमनविरेकौ मोक्षः क्षतजस्य च वातगुल्मवताम्||१८३||
सर्पिः सतिक्तसिद्धं क्षीरं प्रशंसनं निरूहाश्च|
रक्तस्य चावसेचनमाश्वासनसंशमनयोगाः||१८४||
उपनाहनं सशस्त्रं पक्वस्याभ्यन्तरप्रभिन्नस्य|
संशोधनसंशमने पित्तप्रभवस्य गुल्मस्य||१८५||
स्नेहः स्वेदो भेदो लङ्घनमुल्लेखनं विरेकश्च|
सर्पिर्बस्तिर्गुटिकाश्चूर्णमरिष्टाश्च सक्षाराः||१८६||
गुल्मस्यान्ते दाहः कफजस्याग्रेऽपनीतरक्तस्य|
गुल्मस्य रौधिरस्य क्रियाक्रमः स्त्रीभवस्योक्तः||१८७||
पथ्यान्नपानसेवा हेतूनां वर्जनं यथास्वं च|

नित्यं चाग्निसमाधिः स्निग्धस्य च सर्वकर्माणि||१८८||
हेतुर्लिङ्गं सिदि्धः क्रियाक्रमः साध्यता न योगाश्च|
गुल्मचिकित्सितसङ्ग्रह एतावान् व्याहृतोऽग्निवेशस्य||१८९||

Agnivesa has described the following topics in this chapter dealing with the treatment of Gulma

1) Oleation and formenation therapies, recipes of Ghee enema, powder, nourishing pills, emetic, purgation and oleation therapies for the treatment of Vata- Gulma

2) Medicated ghee prepared by boiling it with bitter drugs milk, laxatives, recipes for Niruha type of medicated enema, blood- letting, Ashvasana (consolation), recipes for alleviation, application of hot ointment, surgical management of suppurated and internally ruptured ailment, elimination and alleviation therapies for the treatment of Paittika Gulma;

3) Oleation, formentation, puncturing, fasting, emetic and purgative therapies, recipes for medicated ghee, medicated enema, pills, powders, aristas (type of alcoholic drink), Alkalies, cauterization as the terminal therapy after blood-letting for the treatment of Kapha- Gulma

4) Management of Raktaja Gulma occurring in women and

5) Use of wholesome food and drinks, prevention of the very productive grounds of various types liable to bring about morbid conditions, need for regularly maintaining the power of digestion and metabolism (Agni), need for oleation therapy before all types of treatment, etiology, signs and symptoms, management, line of treatment, curability and incurability and recipes in respect of different types of Gulma.

इत्यग्निवेशकृते तन्त्रे चरकप्रतिसंस्कृते चिकित्सितस्थाने गुल्मचिकित्सितं नाम पञ्चमोऽध्यायः||५||

Thus, ends the fifth chapter dealing with the treatment of Gulma in the section of Chikitsa sthana of the work by Agnivesha and redacted by Charaka.

12

Chikitsasthana Chapter 6 Prameha Chikitsitam

6th Chapter of Charaka Samhita Chikitsasthana deals with treatment of Prameha – causes, symptoms, types, treatment and diet for urinary disorders and diabetes.

Treatment of Urinary Disorders Including Diabetes

अथातः प्रमेहचिकित्सितं व्याख्यास्यामः||१||

इति ह स्माह भगवानात्रेयः||२||

We shall now expound the chapter on the treatment or Prameha (urinary disorders including diabetes).

Thus, said Lord Atreya [1-2]

निर्मोहमानानुशयो निराशः पुनर्वसुर्ज्ञानतपोविशालः|

कालेऽग्निवेशाय सहेतुलिङ्गानुवाच मेहाञ्शमनं च तेषाम्||३||

Punarvasu who is free from delusion, ego, anger and attachment, and who has generosity because of his knowledge and penance, spoke to Agnivesha at the appropriate time about the aetiology, signs, symptoms and treatment of Meha [3]

Causes of Prameha:

आस्यासुखं स्वप्नसुखं दधीनि ग्राम्यौदकानूपरसाः पयांसि|

नवान्नपानं गुडवैकृतं च प्रमेहहेतुः कफकृच्च सर्वम्||४||

Asya shuka – eating as per one's will,

Swapna Sukha- Addiction to the pleasure of sedentary habits and sleep

Dadhi- excess intake of curds

Gramya udaka aanupa rasa – soup of meat of domesticated and aquatic animals and animals from marshy land,

Payas- excess intake of milk and its products preparations,

Navanna – freshly harvested grains

Nava pana- freshly prepared alcoholic drinks,

Guda vaikrtam- preparations of jaggery and

All Kapha- aggravating factors [4]

Prameha Samprapti – Pathogenesis:

मेदश्च मांसं च शरीरजं च क्लेदं कफो बस्तिगतं प्रदूष्य|

करोति मेहान् समुदीर्णमुष्णैस्तानेव पित्तं परिदूष्य चापि||५||

क्षीणेषु दोषेष्ववकृष्य बस्तौ धातून् प्रमेहाननिलः करोति|

दोषो हि बस्तिं समुपेत्य मूत्रं सन्दूष्य मेहाञ्जनयेद्यथास्वम्||६||

Kapha vitiates Medas (fat tissue), Mamsa (muscle tissue) and Kleda (liquid elements) of the body located in Basti (urinary tract) and causes different types of meha.

Similarly, Pitta aggravated by hot things, vitiates those elements and causes different types of Pittaja Prameha.

When other 2 Doshas are in a relatively diminished state, the aggravated Vata draws tissue elements, viz, Ojas, Majja and Lasika into the urinary tract and vitiates them to cause the 3rd category of Prameha (Vataja Meha). Different doshas having entered the urinary tract in vitiated conditions give rise to the respective categories of Meha [5-6]

Classification and Prognosis:

साध्याः कफोत्था दश, पित्तजाः षट् याप्या, न साध्यः पवनाच्चतुष्कः|

समक्रियत्वादिविषमक्रियत्वान्महात्ययत्वाच्च यथाक्रमं ते||७||

Kaphaja Prameha are of 10 types and they are curable because of the compatibility of the therapies meant for their cure (Samakriyatvat).

Pittaja Prameha are of 6 types and they are only palliable (Yapya) because of the incompatibility of the therapies meant for their treatment. (Vishama Kriyatvaat)

Vatika prameha are of 4 types they are incurable because of their extremely serious nature. [7]

Prameha Dosha Dushya: Doshas and tissues that get affected by Prameha:

कफः सपित्तः पवनश्च दोषा मेदोऽस्रशुक्राम्बुवसालसीकाः|

मज्जा रसौजः पिशितं च दूष्याः प्रमेहिणां, विंशतिरेव मेहाः||८||

Doshas like Kapha, Pitta and Vayu and

Dusyas like Medas, Raka, Shukra Ambu (body fluid), Vasa (fat), Lasika (Lymph) majja (Marrow), Rasa (end product of digestion), Ojas (Immunity factor) and Mamsa (muscle) are responsible for the causation of Prameha which is of 20 types [8]

Prameha Lakshana – Signs and symptoms:

जलोपमं चेक्षुरसोपमं वा घनं घनं चोपरि विप्रसन्नम्|

शुक्लं सशुक्रं शिशिरं शनैर्वा लालेव वा वालुकया युतं वा||९||

विद्यात् प्रमेहान् कफजान् दशैतान् क्षारोपमं कालमथापि नीलम्|

हारिद्र माञ्जिष्ठमथापि रक्तमेतान् प्रमेहान् षडुशन्ति पित्तात्||१०||

मज्जौजसा वा वसयाऽन्वितं वा लसीकया वा सततं विबद्धम्|

चतुर्विधं मूत्रयतीह वाताच्छेषेषु धातुष्वपकर्षितेषु||११||

10 types of Kaphaja Meha:

1. Udaka meha – Jalopama – The urine resembling water

2. Ikshumeha – urine resembling sugarcane juice

3. Sandra Meha – The urine having high density (ghana), thick

4. Sandra Prasada Meha – The urine having density in lower layers, transparency in the upper layer (Ghanam cha upari viprassannam)

5. Shukla Meha- The urine having white colour

6. Shukra Meha – The urine containing seminal fluid

7. Sheeta meha- The urine with cold touch

8. Shanaih Meha- The urine passing out slowly

9. Lala Meha – The urine containing slimy material like saliva and

10. Sikata Meha- The urine containing sand- like substance, gravels. Read more – Ayurvedic treatment of gravels in urine

6 types of Pittaja Meha:

1. Kshara Meha- The urine resembling the solution of alkali

2. Kala Meha – The urine having black colour

3. Neela Meha – The urine having blue, indigo –colour

4. Haridra meha – The urine having yellow colour like turmeric and

5. Manjistha Meha – The urine having reddish colour like that of Manjishta and

6. Rakta Meha – The urine having blood in it

4 types of Vataja Meha

1. Majja Meha- The urine mixed with Majja or bone- marrow

2. Ojas Meha or Madhu Meha – The urine mixed with Ojas

3. Vasa Meha – The urine mixed with Vasa or Muscle fat

4. Lasika Meha or Hasti Meha- The urine mixed with Lasika or Lymph

Decrease of other Dhatus or Tissue elements is responsible for the causation of the above mentioned 4 varieties of Vataja Prameha [9-11]

Characteristic Feature:

वर्णं रसं स्पर्शमथापि गन्धं यथास्वदोषं भजते प्रमेहः|

श्यावारुणो वातकृतः सशूलो मज्जादिसाद्गुण्यमुपैत्यसाध्यः||१२||

Different categories of Prameha described in verses 9-11 above are characterized by the colour; taste, touch and smell of the respective Dosha.

Vata types of Prameha are characterized by:

Shyava aruna varna mutra- greyish – red discoloration of urine,

Shoola – pain and

Majjadi sadgunya – attributes of Majja etc.

These varieties are incurable. [12]

Prameha Poorvaroopa:

स्वेदोऽङ्गगन्धः शिथिलाङ्गता च शय्यासन स्वप्नसुखे रतिश्च|

हृन्नेत्रजिह्वाश्रवणोपदेहो घनाङ्गता केशनखातिवृद्धिः||१३||

शीतप्रियत्वं गलतालुशोषो माधुर्यमास्ये करपाददाहः|

भविष्यतो मेहगदस्य रूपं मूत्रेऽभिधावन्ति पिपीलिकाश्च||१४||

Premonitory Signs and Symptoms:

Sweda – Sweating

Anga gandha – bad body odour

Shithilangata – flabbiness of body

Shayyasana – liking for constantly lying on the bed, feeling sedentary

Rati – sleeping and leading an easy life

Hrut Upadeha – a feeling as if the heart region is covered with some paste / coating

Netra, Jihva, Shravana Srava – exudation of excreta from eyes, tongue and ears

Ghana angata – bulkiness of the body

Kesha, kha, nakha ati vriddhi- excessive growth of hair and nails

Sheeta priyata – liking for cold things

Gala, talu shosha – dryness of the throat and palate

Madhura aasya – sweet taste in the mouth

Kara pada daha – burning sensation in hands and legs and

Mutre pipilika – swarming of ants on the urine [13-14]

Prameha Chikitsa Sutra – Line of treatment:

स्थूलः प्रमेही बलवानिहैकः कृशस्तथैकः परिदुर्बलश्च|

सम्बृंहणं तत्र कृशस्य कार्यं संशोधनं दोषबलाधिकस्य||१५||

स्निग्धस्य योगा विविधाः प्रयोज्याः कल्पोपदिष्टा मलशोधनाय |
ऊर्ध्वं तथाऽधश्च मलेऽपनीते मेहेषु सन्तर्पणमेव कार्यम्||१६||
गुल्मः क्षयो मेहनबस्तिशूलं मूत्रग्रहश्चाप्यपतर्पणेन|
प्रमेहिणः स्युः, परितर्पणानि कार्याणि तस्य प्रसमीक्ष्य वह्निम्||१७||

Prameha Chikitsa Sutra – Line of treatment:
Patients suffering from Prameha can be classified into 2 categories viz,
1) Sthula Pramehi – Those who are obese and strong. They are given Shodhana (cleansing, purification treatment).
2) Krusha Pramehi – Those that is emaciated and weak. They are given nourishing treatment – Brumhana therapy (Read more about Brumhana treatment)
In both the above cases, patient is administered Snehana – oleation treatment. Then, Vamana, Virechana recipes, described in KalpaSthana are administered. After Dosha is eliminated, the patient is given Santarpana or nourishing therapy because Apatarpana (fasting) therapy in this condition may produce
Gulma (cystic tumor), Kshaya (chronic respiratory disorder),
Meha – chroni urinary tract disorder
Bastishoola – bladder pain
Mutragraha – urinary retention
Hence, based on the state of Agni (digestion strength), Prameha patient should be given Santarpana (nourishing therapy), after Shodhana. [15-17]
Shamana – alleviation Therapy:
If the patient of Prameha who needs Shodhana or elimination therapy is not eligible for it, he is given Shamana treatment (with oral medicines) [18 1/2]

Pathya for Prameha:
संशोधनं नार्हति यः प्रमेही तस्य क्रिया संशमनी प्रयोज्या|
मन्थाः कषाया यवचूर्णलेहाः प्रमेहशान्त्यै लघवश्च भक्ष्याः||१८||
ये विष्किरा ये प्रतुदा विहङ्गास्तेषां रसैर्जाङ्गलजैर्मनोज्ञैः|
यवौदनं रूक्षमथापि वाट्यमद्यात् ससक्तूनपि चाप्यपूपान्||१९||
मुद्गादियूषैरथ तिक्तशाकैः पुराणशाल्योदनमाददीत|
दन्तीङ्गुदीतैलयुतं प्रमेही तथाऽतसीसर्षपतैलयुक्तम्||२०||
सषष्टिकं स्यात्तृणधान्यमन्नं यवप्रधानस्तु भवेत् प्रमेही|

The patient suffering from Prameha is given the following food:
Mantha (flour of different types of corn mixed with water), Kashaya (herbal decoctions), barley powder, Avaleha prepared of barely and such other light-to-digest eatables.
Mamsarasa prepared from Vishkira, Pratuda and Vihanga such Jangala animals.
Yavaudana (cooked barley) without adding any dry articles, Vatya (barley porridge) Saktu (roasted corn flour) and Apupa (Pan- cakes) mixed with the meat- soup of gallinaceous (Vishkira) and pecker birds (Pratuda) and animals inhabiting arid land (Jangala);
Purana Shali – old rice cooked and mixed with the soup of green gram etc. and preparations of bitter vegetables
4. Cooked Shashtika rice and Truna Dhanyas mixed with oil of Danti, Ingudi, Atasi and Sarshapa. [18-21]

Importance of Barley:
यवस्य भक्ष्यान् विविधांस्तथाऽद्यात् कफप्रमेही मधुसम्प्रयुक्तान्||२१||
निशिस्थितानां त्रिफलाकषाये स्युस्तर्पणाः क्षौद्रयुता यवानाम्|
तान् सीधुयुक्तान् प्रपिबेत् प्रमेही प्रायोगिकान्मेहवधार्थमेव||२२||
ये श्लेष्ममेहे विहिताः कषायास्तैर्भावितानां च पृथग्यवानाम्|
सक्तूनपूपान् सगुडान् सधानान् भक्ष्यांस्तथाऽन्यान् विविधांश्च खादेत्||२३||

खराश्वगोहंसपृषद्भृतानां तथा यवानां विविधाश्च भक्ष्याः|
देयास्तथा वेणुयवा यवानां कल्पेन गोधूममयाश्च भक्ष्याः||२४||

Barley should constitute the principal ingredient of food of the patient suffering from Prameha.

The patient suffering from Kaphaja Prameha should take eatables prepared of barley mixed with honey.

Barley soaked in Triphala Kashaya and is kept overnight. It is mixed with honey. It is a nourishing (Tarpana) diet.

It is taken by the patient suffering from Prameha regularly to overcome the disease.

Barley is soaked separately with each of the decoctions prescribed for the treatment of Kaphaja Prameha and taken by the Patient in form of Saktu (Roasted flour), Apupa (pan-cake), Dhana (fried barely) and other types of eatables along with jaggery.

Various eatables prepared from barley or bamboo seed or wheat previously eaten by asses, horse, cows, swans and deer and collected from their Dung – is given to the patient suffering from Prameha. [21-24]

Specific Therapies:

संशोधनोल्लेखनलङ्घनानि काले प्रयुक्तानि कफप्रमेहान्|
जयन्ति पित्तप्रभवान् विरेकः सन्तर्पणः संशमनो विधिश्च||२५||

Purification therapies including Vamana and Langhana – fasting therapies, administered at appropriate time, cure Kaphaja types of Prameha.

Similarly, Pittaja Pramehas are overcome by Virechana, Santarpana (nourishing therapy) and Shamana – alleviation therapies. [25]

Recipes for Pramehas in General:

दार्वीं सुराह्वां त्रिफलां समुस्तां कषायमुत्क्वाथ्य पिबेत् प्रमेही|
क्षौद्रेण युक्तामथवा हरिद्रां पिबेद्रसेनामलकीफलानाम्||२६||

The Patient suffering from Prameha should take the decoction of

Darvi – Berberis aristata

Triphala and

Musta – Cyperus rotundus, mixed with honey

He may also take turmeric, along with the juice of Amalaki [26]

Recipes for Kaphaja Prameha –

हरीतकी कट्फल मुस्त लोध्रं पाठा विडङ्गगार्जुन धन्वनाश्च|
उभे हरिद्रे तगरं विडङ्गं कदम्बशालार्जुनदीप्यकाश्च||२७||
दार्वी विडङ्गं खदिरो धवश्च सुराह्वकुष्ठागुरुचन्दनानि|
दार्व्यग्निमन्थौ त्रिफला सपाठा पाठा च मूर्वा च तथा श्वदंष्ट्रा||२८||
यवान्युशीराण्यभयागुडूचीचव्याभयाचित्रकसप्तपर्णाः|
पादैः कषायाः कफमेहिनां ते दशोपदिष्टा मधुसम्प्रयुक्ताः||२९||

The following 10 decoctions, mixed with honey and can be given to patients suffering from Kaphaja Prameha

1) Decoction of

Haritaki – Terminalia chebula

Katphala – Myrica nagi

Musta – Cyperus rotundus and

Lodhra – Symplocos racemosa

2) Decoction of

Patha – Cissampelos parieta

Vidanga – Embelia ribes

Arjuna—Terminalia arjuna and

Dhanvana – Grewia tiliaefolia

3) Decoction of
Haridra – Curcuma longa
Daru haridra – Berberis aristata
Tagara – Valeriana walichii and
Vidanga – Embelia ribes
4) Decoction of
Kadamba
Shala –Shorea robusta
Arjuna- Terminalia arjuna and
Deepyaka – Trachyspermum ammi
5) Decoction of
Darvi – Berberis aristata
Vidanga – Embelia ribes
Khadira – Acacia catechu and
Dhava
6) Decoction of
Surahva – Devadaru – Cedrus deodara
Kustha – Saussarea lappa
Aguru – Aquilaria agallocha and
Chandana – Santalum album
7) Decoction of
Darvi – Berberis aristata
Agnimantha
Triphala and
Patha – Cissampelos pariera
8) Decoction of
Patha – Cissampelos pariera
Murva and
Svadamshtra – Tribulus terrestris
9) Decoction of
Yavani – Hyoscyamus niger
Usheera – Vetiveria zizanoides
Abhaya – Terminalia chebula and
Guduchi – Tinospora cordifolia and
10) Decoction of
Chavya – Piper retrofractum
Abhaya – Terminalia chebula
Citraka – Plumbago zeylanica and
Saptaparna –Alstonia scholaris [27-29]

Recipes for Pittaja Prameha
उशीर लोध्राञ्जन चन्दनानामुशीर मुस्तामलकाभयानाम्‌।
पटोल निम्बामलकामृतानां मुस्ताभया पद्मकवृक्षकाणाम्‌॥३०॥
लोध्राम्बु कालीयक धातकीनां निम्बार्जुनाम्रातनिशोत्पलानाम्‌।
शिरीष सर्जार्जुनकेशराणां प्रियङ्गुपद्मोत्पल किंशुकानाम्‌॥३१॥
अश्वत्थ पाठासनवेतसानां कटङ्कटेर्युत्पलमुस्तकानाम्‌।
पैतेषु मेहेषु दश प्रदिष्टाः पादैः कषाया मधुसम्प्रयुक्ताः॥३२॥

The following 10 decoctions is mixed with honey and given to patient suffering from Pittaja Prameha.

1. Decoction of
Usheera – Vetiveria zizanioides
Lodhra – Symplocos racemosa
Anjana – aqueous extract of Berberis aristata
Chandana – Sandalwood – Santalum album

2. Decoction of
Ushira – Vetiver – Vetiveria zizanioides
Musta – Cyperus rotundus
Amalaka – Amla and
Abhaya – Terminalia chebula

3. Decoction of
Patola – Pointed Gourd – Trichosanthes dioica
Nimba – Neem – Azadirachta indica
Amalaka and
Amruta – Giloy – Tinospora cordifolia

4. Decoction of
Musta – Cyperus rotundus,
Abhaya – Terminalia chebula,
Padmaka – Prunus cerasoides and
Vrukshaka – Kutaja – Holarrhena antidysenterica

5. Decoction of
Lodhra – Symplocos racemosa,
Ambu,
Kaliyaka,
Dhataki – Woodfordia fruticosa

6. Decoction of
Nimba – Neem – Azadirachta indica
Arjuna – Terminalia arjuna
Amruta – Tinospora cordifolia
Nisha – Turmeric and
Utpala – Nymphaea alba

7. Decoction of
Sirisa – Albizia lebbeck
Sarja – Copal tree resin,
Arjuna (terminalia arjuna) and
Kesara – Mesua ferrea

8. Decoction of
Priyangu –Callicarpa macrophylla
Padma – Lotus – Nelumbo nucifera,
Utpala –Nymphaea alba and
Kimshuka – Butea monosperma

9. Decoction of
Ashvattha – Peepal, Buddha tree – Ficus religiosa
Patha – Cyclea peltata
Asana – Indian Kino tree - Pterocarpus marsupium
and
Amlavetasa – Garcinia pedunculata Roxb. / Rheum emodi Wall.

and
10. Decoction of
Katankateri – Daru Haridra – Berberis aristata
Utpala –Nymphaea alba and
Musta – Cyperus rotundus . [30-32]

Treatment of Vataja Prameha:
सर्वेषु मेहेषु मतौ तु पूर्वौ कषाययोगौ विहितास्तु सर्वे|
मन्थस्य पाने यवभावनायां स्युर्भोजने पानविधौ पृथक् च||३३||
सिद्धानि तैलानि घृतानि चैव देयानि मेहेष्वनिलात्मकेषु|
मेदः कफश्चैव कषाययोगैः स्नेहैश्च वायुः शममेति तेषाम्||३४||
The two recipes of decoction described in verse- 26 are meant for the treatment of all varieties of Prameha.
These decoctions can be used for the preparation of Mantha (a drink prepared of roasted corn flour mixed with water), for the impregnation of barley and for the preparation of different kinds of food and drinks.
Medicated oils and medicated ghee are prepared by cooking with these decoctions is administered to patients sufferings from Vatika Prameha. These Kashayas correct the vitiated Medas and Kapha, and the aggravated Vata in these patients gets alleviated by the unctuous ingredients (viz, oil and ghee) included in these recipes. [33-34]

Recipes for Kaphaja and Paittika Prameha
कम्पिल्ल सप्तच्छद शालजानि बैभीत रौहीतक कौटजानि|
कपित्थपुष्पाणि च चूर्णितानि क्षौद्रेण लिह्यात् कफपित्तमेही||३५||
पिबेद्रसेनामलकस्य चापि कल्कीकृतान्यक्षसमानि काले|
जीर्णे च भुञ्जीत पुराणमन्नं मेही रसैर्जाङ्गलजैर्मनोज्ञैः||३६||
Powder of
Kampillaka,
Barks of Saptacchada (Saptaparna) – Alstonia scholaris – Stem bark, Shala – Shorea robusta,
Bibhitaka – Terminalia bellirica,
Rohitaka and
Kutaja – Connessi bark (Holarrhena antidysenterica Wall.) and
Flower of Kapittha is added with honey, made to linctus (leha) and taken by patients suffering from Kaphaja and Pittaja Prameha.
One Aksha (12 g) of the paste of above mentioned herbs is mixed with the juice of Amalaki (Gooseberry) and given at the appropriate time to patients suffering from Kaphaja and Pittaja types of Prameha.
After the digestion of this medicine, the patient is given to eat old rice cooked and mixed with the delicious soup of the meat of animals living in arid land. [35-36]

Taila and Ghrita medicines for Prameha:
दृष्ट्वाऽनुबन्धं पवनात् कफस्य पित्तस्य वा स्नेहविधिर्विकल्प्यः|
तैलं कफे स्यात् स्वकषायसिद्धं पित्ते घृतं पित्तहरैः कषायैः||३७||
त्रिकण्टकाश्मन्तकसोमवल्कैर्भल्लातकैः सातिविषैः सलोधैः|
वचापटोलार्जुननिम्बमुस्तैर्हरिद्रया पद्मकदीप्यकैश्च||३८||
मञ्जिष्ठया चागुरुचन्दनैश्च सर्वैः समस्तैः कफवातजेषु|
मेहेषु तैलं विपचेद्, घृतं तु पैत्तेषु, मिश्रं त्रिषु लक्षणेषु||३९||
If Vata is secondarily aggravated along with Kapha or Pitta, then the patient is administered medicated oil or medicated ghee.
If Vata is associated with Kapha, medicated oil is prepared by boiling oil with the decoction of herbs which alleviate Kapha and

For Vata, associated with Pitta, medicated ghee is prepared by cooking ghee with the decoction of herbs which alleviate Pitta.

Trikantaka– Tribulus terrestris

Ashmantaka

Somavalka

Bhallataka – Semecarpus anacardium Linn.

Ativisha – Aconitum heterophyllum

Lodhra – Symplocos racemosa,

Vacha –Acorus calamus Linn.)

Patola – Pointed Gourd – Trichosanthes dioica

Arjuna – Terminalia arjuna

Nimba – Neem

Musta – Cyperus rotundus

Haridra – turmeric – Curcuma longa

Padmaka – Prunus cerasoides,

Deepyaka – Trachyspermum ammi ,

Manjishta – Rubia cordifolia

Agaru – Aquilaria agallocha and

Chandana – Sandalwood – Santalum album

All these herbs together are used in the preparation of medicated oil for the treatment of Kaphaja Prameha, associated with Vata. If symptoms of Pitta are also associated, then these herbs are processed with oil and ghee together to prepare Yamaka.

Medicine for All Types of Prameha

फलत्रिकं दारुनिशां विशालां मुस्तां च निःक्वाथ्य निशां सकल्काम्|
पिबेत् कषायं मधुसम्प्रयुक्तं सर्वप्रमेहेषु समुद्धतेषु||४०||

The decoction of

Triphala,

Daruharidra,

Vishala and

Musta

is mixed with the paste of turmeric and honey.

Intake of this medicine cures all types of Prameha even when these are manifested in acute form. [40]

Madhvasava:

लोध्रं शटीं पुष्करमूलमेलां मूर्वां विडङ्गं त्रिफलां यमानीम्|
चव्यं प्रियङ्गुं क्रमुकं विशालां किराततिक्तं कटुरोहिणीं च||४१||
भाङ्गीं नतं चित्रकपिप्पलीनां मूलं सकुष्ठातिविषं सपाठम्|
कलिङ्गकन् केशरमिन्द्रसाह्वां नखं सपत्रं मरिचं प्लवं च||४२||
द्रोणेऽम्भसः कर्षसमानि पक्त्वा पूते चतुर्भागजलावशेषे|
रसेऽर्धभागं मधुनः प्रदाय पक्षं निधेयो घृतभाजनस्थः||४३||
मध्वासवोऽयं कफपित्तमेहान् क्षिप्रं निहन्यादि्द्विपलप्रयोगात्|
पाण्ड्वामयार्शास्यरुचिं ग्रहण्या दोषं किलासं विविधं च कुष्ठम्||४४||

इति मध्वासवः|

Lodhra – Symplocos racemosa

Shati – Zadoary (root) – Hedychium spicatum / Curcuma zeodaria,

Puskaramoola – Inula racemosa,

Ela – Cardamom,

Murva – Root,

Vidanga – False black pepper – Embelia ribes,

Triphala – Amalaki, Haritaki, Vibhitaki,

Yavani – Hyoscyamus niger,

Chavya,

Priyangu – Callicarpa macrophylla,

Kramuka – Betel nut,

Vishala,

Kiratatikta – Swertia chirata ,

Katurohini – Picrorhiza kurroa,

Bharngi – Clerodendron serratum (root),

Nata – Indian valerian (root) – Valeriana wallichi,

Chitraka – Leadwort – Plumbago zeylanica,

Pippalimoola – Long pepper root – Piper longum,

Kushta – Saussurea lappa,

Ativisha – Aconitum heterophyllum,

Patha – Cyclea peltata,

Kalingaka – Connessi Bark – Holarrhena antidysenterica,

Kesara – Mesua ferrea,

Indrasahva

Nakha,

Patra – Cinnamon leaf – Cinnamomum tamala

Maricha – Black pepper

Plava – Nyctanthes arbor-tristis

– one Karsha (12 g) of each of these herbs is boiled in one Drona (12.288 l) of water till $1/4^{th}$ remains. This decoction along with half part of honey is kept for fermentation in a vessel smeared with ghee for a fort night to prepare Madhvasava.

It instantaneously cures Kaphaja and Paittika types of Meha when administered in a dose of 2 Pala (96 ml)

It also cures

Pandu – anemia

Arshas – piles

Aruchi – anorexia,

Grahani Dosha (sprue syndrome),

Kilasa (a type of leucoderma) and

Different types of Kushta (skin diseases). [41-44]

Dantyasava and Bhallatakasava:

क्वाथः स एवाष्टपलं च दन्त्या भल्लातकानां च चतुष्पलं स्यात्।

सितोपला त्वष्टपला विशेषः क्षौद्रं च तावत् पृथगासवौ तौ||४५||

In the above decoction (wide verses 41-44)

8 Palas of Danti – Baliospermum montanum

8 Palas of Sugar and

The same quantity of honey (as described in verses 41-44) is added and processed.

Similarly, in the above mentioned decoction (wide verses 41-44)

4 Palas of Bhallataka – Semecarpus anacardium

8 Palas of sugar and the same quantity of Honey (as described inverses 41-44) is added and processed.

These 2 Asavas namely Dantyasava and Bhallatokusava are useful in the treatment of Prameha [45]

Food and drinks:

सारोदकं वाऽथ कुशोदकं वा मधूदकं वा त्रिफलारसं वा।
सीधुं पिबेद्वा निगदं प्रमेही माध्वीकमग्र्यं चिरसंस्थितं वा||४६||
मांसानि शूल्यानि मृगद्विजानां खादेद्यवानां विविधांश्च भक्ष्यान्।
संशोधनारिष्टकषायलेहैः सन्तर्पणोत्थाऽ शमयेत् प्रमेहान्||४७||
भृष्टान् यवान् भक्षयतः प्रयोगाच्छुष्कांश्च सक्तून्न भवन्ति मेहाः।
श्वित्रं च कृच्छ्रं कफजं च कुष्ठं तथैव मुद्गामलकप्रयोगान्||४८||

The patient suffering from Prameha should drink

Sarodaka (water boiled with the heart- wood of Khadira (Acacia catechu etc),

Kushodaka (water boiled with Kusha),

Madhudaka (water mixed with honey),

Triphala Rasa (Juice or Kashaya of Triphala) or

Seedhu (a type of wine) which is of superior quality and which is prepared after fermenting for a long time.

Spit –roasted meat of animals and birds and different eatables prepared of barley should be given to the patient to eat.

Different types of Prameha caused by over- nourishment is alleviated by the administration of elimination therapies, Aristas (a type of wine), decoctions and various types of linctus

Persons habitually taking roasted barley, dry corn-flour, Mudga – green gram – Averrhoa carambola and Amalaka do not suffer from Prameha, Svitra (Leucoderma), Krcchra (drysuria) and Kaphaja Kustha (skin diseases caused by Kapha). [46-48]

Recipes:

सन्तर्पणोत्थेषु गदेषु योगा मेदस्विनां ये च मयोपदिष्टाः।
विरूक्षणार्थं कफपित्तजेषु सिद्धाः प्रमेहेष्वपि ते प्रयोज्याः||४९||

Effective recipes suggested by me for producing drying effect on obese patients while describing the management of diseases caused by over- nourishment are useful in the treatment of Pramehas caused by Kapha and Pitta. [49]

Exercise and other Regimens:

व्यायामयोगैर्विविधैः प्रगाढैरुद्वर्तनैः स्नानजलावसेकैः।
सेव्यत्वगेलागुरुचन्दनाद्यैर्विलेपनैश्चाशु न सन्ति मेहाः||५०||

Pramehas get immediately cured by different types of strenuous exercise, unction, bath, sprinkling of water over the body and application of ointment made of Sevya (Usheera), Tvak (Cinnamon) , Ela (cardamom), Aguru, Chandana (Sandalwood) etc. [50]

Apatarpana – Depletion Therapy

क्लेदश्च मेदश्च कफश्च वृद्धः प्रमेहहेतुः प्रसमीक्ष्य तस्मात्।
वैद्येन पूर्वं कफपित्तजेषु मेहेषु कार्याण्यपतर्पणानि||५१||

Aggravated Kleda (Sticky or liquid elements in the body), Medas (fat tissue) and Kapha are responsible for the causation of Prameha.

Keeping this in view, the physician, in the beginning, should administer depletion therapies to patients suffering from Kaphaja and Patittika types of Prameha. [51]

Vatolbana Prameha:

या वातमेहान् प्रति पूर्वमुक्ता वातोल्बणानां विहिता क्रिया सा।
वायुर्हि मेहेष्वतिकर्शितानां कुप्यत्यसाध्यान् प्रति नास्ति चिन्ता||५२||

Medicines described earlier for the Vatika Prameha are actually meant for Vatolbana Prameha where Vayu is secondarily (subsequently) aggravated.

Vata does get secondarily aggravated in Prameha because of excessive depletion of tissue elements.

The Physician need not make efforts to correct irremediable ailments.

If Vata is primarily aggravated to cause Prameha, then this Vatika Prameha is irremediable [52]

Prohibitions:

यैर्हेतुभिर्ये प्रभवन्ति मेहास्तेषु प्रमेहेषु न ते निषेव्याः|

हेतोरसेवा विहिता यथैव जातस्य रोगस्य भवेच्चिकित्सा||५३||

Factors responsible for the causation of different types of Prameha is avoided even after these Pramehas are manifested.

For the prevention of the occurrence of a disease different etiological factors are described to be avoided. These very causative factors are also required to be avoided during the treatment of that particular disease (even after its manifestation). [53]

Differential Diagnosis

हारिद्रवर्णं रुधिरं च मूत्रं विना प्रमेहस्य हि पूर्वरूपैः|

यो मूत्रयेत् न वदेत् प्रमेहं रक्तस्य पित्तस्य हि स प्रकोपः||५४||

If the colour of the urine is yellow or if blood is excreted through the urine without the prior manifestation of premonitory signs and symptoms of Prameha, such a person should on the other hand be diagnosed as a case of Rakta- Pitta (a disease characterized by bleeding from different parts of the body.). [54]

Classification

दृष्ट्वा प्रमेहं मधुरं सपिच्छं मधूपमं स्यादि्द्विविधो विचारः|

क्षीणेषु दोषेष्वनिलात्मकः स्यात् सन्तर्पणाद्वा कफसम्भवः स्यात्||५५||

If the patient suffering from Prameha passes urine which is sweet, slimy and honey- like, then there are two possibilities.

It is caused either by the diminution of Doshas and that case it is Vatika type or by over- nourishment when it is of the Kaphaja type. [55]

Prognosis:

सपूर्वरूपाः कफपित्तमेहाः क्रमेण ये वातकृताश्च मेहाः|

साध्या न ते, पित्तकृतास्तु याप्याः, साध्यास्तु मेदो यदि न प्रदुष्टम्||५६||

Kaphaja and Paittika types of prameha, if preceded by their premonitory signs and symptoms, are incurable.

Similarly, Vatika Prameha, where Vayu is aggravated right from the beginning, is incurable.

Paittika types of Prameha are generally, palliable. But they are curable if Medas (adipose tissue) is not vitiated. [56]

Hereditary Diabetes:

जातः प्रमेही मधुमेहिनो वा न साध्य उक्तः स हि बीजदोषात्|

ये चापि केचित् कुलजा विकारा भवन्ति तांश्च प्रवदन्त्यसाध्यान्||५७||

Patients who are diabetic right from the time of birth (congenital) and those who are born of diabetic parent's genes are incurable.

Similarly, other hereditary (Kulaja= familial) ailments are to be considered as incurable. [57]

Diabetic Carbuncles

प्रमेहिणां याः पिडका मयोक्ता रोगाधिकारे पृथगेव सप्त|

ताः शल्यविद्भिः कुशलैश्चिकित्स्याः शस्त्रेण संशोधनरोपणैश्च||५८||

7 types of Carbuncles of patients suffering from Prameha described by me in the quadrate on diseases (Rogadhikara)

are to be treated by expert surgeons with the help of Sastras (surgical operations.), samsodhaka (cleansing) and Ropana (healing) therapies.[58]

तत्र श्लोकाः-
हेतुर्दोषो दूष्यं मेहानां साध्यतानुरूपश्च।
मेही द्विविधस्त्रिविधं भिषग्जितमतिक्षपणदोषः॥५९॥
आद्या यवान्नविकृतिर्मन्था मेहापहाः कषायाश्च।
तैलघृतलेहयोगा भक्ष्याः प्रवरासवाः सिद्धाः॥६०॥
व्यायामविधिर्विविधः स्नानान्युद्वर्तनानि गन्धाश्च।
मेहानां प्रशमार्थं चिकित्सिते दिष्टमेतावत्॥६१॥
Summary:
In the chapter dealing with the treatment for alleviation of Prameha following topics have been discussed
1. Etiology of the Disease
2. Doshas and Dusyas (tissue elements) involved in the pathogenesis of the disease
3. Curability and other wise of the disease
4. Signs and symptoms of the disease
5. 2 types of Prameha
6. 3 categories of therapy. Viz Samsodhana (elimination therapy), Samsamana(alleviation therapy) and Nidana Parivarjana (avoiding the causeative factors)
7. Disadvantages of over depletion
8. Eatables prepared of barley, Mantha, (thin gruel) and decoctions for the cure of Prameha.
9. Medicated oils, medicated ghee, various recipes of linctus, food preparations, good quality Asavas (alcoholic drinks) having known therapeutic utility. And
10. Different methods of exercise, baths, unctions and frangrant applications for the treatment of Prameha.[59 -61]

इत्यग्निवेशकृते तन्त्रे चरकप्रतिसंस्कृते चिकित्सितस्थाने प्रमेहचिकित्सितं नाम षष्ठोऽध्यायः॥६॥
Thus, ends the 6th chapter dealing with the treatment of Prameha (urinary disorders including diabetes) of Chikitsa section of Agnivesha's work as redacted by Charaka.

13

Chikitsasthana Chapter 7
KushthaChikitsitam

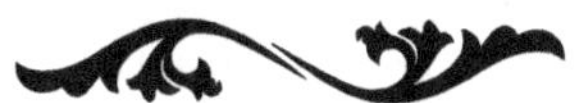

The 7th chapter of Charaka Samhita Chikitsa Sthana is Kushta Chikitsa. It deals with causes, types, symptoms and treatment of skin diseases.

अथातः कुष्ठचिकित्सितं व्याख्यास्यामः||१||
इति ह स्माह भगवानात्रेयः||२||
We shall now expound the chapter on the treatment of Kushta (skin diseases).
Thus said Lord Atreya.[1-2]

Contents:
हेतुं द्रव्यं लिङ्गं कुष्ठानामाश्रयं प्रशमनं च|
शृण्वग्निवेश! सम्यग्विशेषतः स्पर्शनघ्नानाम्||३||
Listen, Oh! Agnivesha, to my explanation about the causes, Dravya (Doshas and Dusyas), sign and symptoms, Ashraya (substratum) and Prashamana (remedies) of Kushta (skin diseases) having Sparshaghnata – impairment of touch sensation as its specific feature. [3]

Kusta Nidana – Causes for skin diseases as per Ayurveda:
विरोधीन्यन्नपानानि द्रवस्निग्धगुरूणि च|
भजतामागतां छर्दिं वेगांश्चान्यान्प्रतिघ्नताम्||४||
व्यायाममतिसन्तापमतिभुक्त्वोपसेविनाम्|
शीतोष्णलङ्घनाहारान् क्रमं मुक्त्वा निषेविणाम्||५||
घर्मश्रमभयार्तानां द्रुतं शीताम्बुसेविनाम्|
अजीर्णाध्यशिनां चैव पञ्चकर्मापचारिणाम्||६||
नवान्न दधि मत्स्यातिलवणाम्ल निषेविणाम्|
माष मूलक पिष्टान्नतिलक्षीरगुडाशिनाम्||७||
व्यवायं चाप्यजीर्णेऽन्ने निद्रां च भजतां दिवा|
विप्रान् गुरून् धर्षयतां पापं कर्म च कुर्वताम्||८||
Kushta (skin diseases) is caused by the vitiation of Doshas etc, in persons indulging in unwholesome regimens as follows:
1. Virodhi anna pana and Snigdha guru pana: Intake of wrong food combinations such as milk with fish. Read more about such bad food combinations.
Drinks which are unctuous and heavy to digest
2. Suppression of the urge for vomiting and other natural urges
3. Physical exercise in excessive heat and after taking heavy meal

4. Haphazard intake of foods with hot and cold properties and fasting.

5. Use of cold water immediately after exposure to scorching sun heat, exertion or exposure to frightening situation;

6. Intake of excess food, uncooked food and intake of food before the previous meal is digested.

7. Improper administration of Panchakarma therapies

8. Excessive intake of foods of freshly harvested grains, curd, fish, salt and sour substances

9. Excessive intake of Masha (black gram), Mulaka (radish), Pastry, Tila (Sesame seeds) and Jaggery.

10. Performance of sexual act while suffering with indigestion

11. Sleep during day time and

12. Insult to Brahmins, and preceptors, and getting indulged in other sinful acts.[4-8]

Kushta Samprapti – Pathogenesis:

वातादयस्त्रयो दुष्टास्त्वग्रक्तं मांसमम्बु च|

दूषयन्ति स कुष्ठानां सप्तको द्रव्यसङ्ग्रहः||९||

अतः कुष्ठानि जायन्ते सप्त चैकादशैव च|

न चैकदोषजं किञ्चित् कुष्ठं समुपलभ्यते||१०||

The 3 vitiated Doshas, Viz, Vata, Pitta and Kapha, in turn vitiate the

Tvak – skin or Rasa Dhatu

Rakta – Blood

Mamsa – Muscle tissue and

Ambu – Lymph or plasma part of blood tissue

These taken together, constitute the seven-fold pathogenic substances of Kustha. These are together called – Kushta Dravya Sangraha.

All the 18 types of Kustha (skin diseases) are caused by the above seven factors.

Kushtas are never caused by the vitiation of only one of the above mentioned pathogenic substances, i.e. all of them are necessarily involved in the causation of the disease. [9-10]

Kushta Purvaroopa – Premonitory Signs and Symptoms:

स्पर्शाज्ञत्वमतिस्वेदो न वा वैवर्ण्यमुन्नतिः|

कोठानां लोमहर्षश्च कण्डूस्तोदः श्रमः क्लमः||११||

व्रणानामधिकं शूलं शीघ्रोत्पत्तिश्चिरस्थितिः|

दाहः सुप्ताङ्गता चेति कुष्ठलक्षणमग्रजम्||१२||

Premonitory signs and symptoms of Kustha are as follows

1. Sparsajnatva – lack of touch sensation in the skin lesion area

2. Ati sweda or Na Va – Excessive sweating or absence of sweating

3. Vaivarnyam – discoloration

4. Unnatih – elevation of skin

5. Kotha – skin eruptions

6. Loma harsha – Horripulation

7. Kandu, Toda, Shrama and Klama – itching, pricking pain, physical exhaustion and mental fatigue.

8. Vrana adhikam shoolam – Excessive pain in the ulcerated parts Shigrotpatti chirastithih - Instantaneous appearance and continued persistence of these ulcers and

9. Daha, Suptangata – Burning sensation and numbness. [11-12]

Eighteen Types of Kushtas

अत ऊर्ध्वमष्टादशानां कुष्ठानां कपालोदुम्बरमण्डलऋष्यजिह्व पुण्डरीक सिध्म काकणकैककुष्ठ चर्माख्य- किटिम विपादिकालसक दद्रु चर्मदल पामा विस्फोटक शताारु विचर्चिकानां लक्षणान्युपदेक्ष्यामः||१३||

We shall now describe the signs and symptoms of 18 varieties of Kustha viz

1. Kapala
2. Udumbara
3. Mandala
4. Rsyajihva
5. Pundarika
6. Sidhma
7. Kakanaka
8. Ekakustha
9. Charmakhya
10. Kitiba
11. Vipadika
12. Alasaka
13. Dadru
14. Charmadala
15. Pama
16. Visphota
17. Shataru
18. Vicharchika [13]

Out of these, the first seven are called Mahakushta.
The remaining 11 are called Kshudra Kushta.

Signs and Symptoms of Mahakushta:

कृष्णारुण कपालाभं यद्रूक्षं परुषं तनु|
कापालं तोदबहुलं तत्कुष्ठं विषमं स्मृतम्||१४||

Kapala Kushta
Kapala refers to broken pieces of earthen pot.
Kapala type of Kustha is characterized by:
1. Krishna arunam kapalabham – The patches in the skin look like black and reddish pieces – Kapala (broken pieces of earthen pot)
2. Ruksham parusham tanu – Skin lesions are dry, rough and thick to touch
3. Toda bahulam – These are associated with excessive pain and
4. This ailment is difficult of cure. [14]
It is caused due to Vata Dosha increase.

Udumbara Kushta:

दाह कण्डूरुजारागपरीतं लोमपिञ्जरम्|
उदुम्बरफलाभासं कुष्ठमौदुम्बरं विदुः||१५||

Daha – Burning sensation
Kandu – itching
Ruja – pain
Raga – redness
Loma pinjaram – The hair on the patches turn brown and
It looks like the fruit of Udumbara (fig).[15]
It is caused due to Pitta Dosha increase.

Mandala Kushta:

श्वेतं रक्तं स्थिरं स्त्यानं स्निग्धमुत्सन्नमण्डलम्|

कृच्छ्रमन्योन्यसंसक्तं कुष्ठं मण्डलमुच्यते||१६||

Mandala type of Kustha is characterized by the following

1. Svetham, raktham – white and red in color
2. Sthiram, Styanam, Snigdha, Utsanna, Mandala – It is stable, compact, unctuous and circular with elevated patches
3. Krichra sadhya- it is difficult to cure and
4. Anyonya samsaktam – Patches are matted with each other. [16]

It is caused due to the Kapha Dosha increase.

Rushyajihva Kushta:

कर्कशं रक्तपर्यन्तमन्तः श्यावं सवेदनम्|
यदृष्यजिह्वासंस्थानमृष्यजिह्वं तदुच्यते||१७||

Karkasham – rough

Rakta paryanta – red edges

Antaha Shyava – brown inside

Sa vedana – painful

Rushyajihva yadrushya – It resembles the tongue of Rushya (a type of antelop with blue testicles). [17]

It is caused due to Vata and Pitta Dosha increase.

Pundareeka Kushta:

सश्वेतं रक्तपर्यन्तं पुण्डरीकदलोपमम्|
सोत्सेधं च सदाहं च पुण्डरीकं तदुच्यते||१८||

Pundarika types of Kustha is characterized by the following

Sa shvetam rakta paryanta – white in color with red edges

Pundarika dala upamam – It resembles the leaf of lotus and

Utseda – elevated

Daha – Burning sensation [18]

It is caused due to the increase of Kapha and Pitta Dosha.

Sidhma Kustha

श्वेतं ताम्रं तनु च यद्रजो घृष्टं विमुञ्चति|
अलाबूपुष्पवर्णं तत् सिध्मं प्रायेण चोरसि||१९||

Svetam, Tamram – White and coppery in color

Tanu, Ghrustam vimunchati – Thin, and when rubbed, it emits small particles of the skin in the form of dust

Alabu pushpa varnam – It resembles the flower of alabu (Lagenaria siceraia) and

Prayena Cha Urasi – It is generally located in the chest. [19]

It is caused due to Vata and Kapha Dosha increase.

G) Kakana Kusta

यत् काकणन्तिकावर्णमपाकं तीव्रवेदनम्|
त्रिदोषलिङ्गं तत् कुष्ठं काकणं नैव सिध्यति||२०||
इति सप्त महाकुष्ठानि|

Kakanantika varna – Red in color like the seed of Gunja (Abrus preccatorius Linn)

Apakam – Does not get suppurated

Teevra vedanam – extremely painful

Signs and symptoms of the vitiation of all the 3 Doshas are manifested and

Asadhya – incurable. [20]

11 Kshudra- Kustha

Eka Kushta
अस्वेदनं महावास्तु यन्मत्स्यशकलोपमम्|
तदेककुष्टं,
Asvedana – Absence of sweating
Extensive localization and
Yat matsya shakalopamam – Resembles the scales of fish.
It occurs due to increase of Vata and Kapha Dosha

Charmakhya –
चर्माख्यं बहलं हस्तिचर्मवत्||२१||
In Charma Kushta, the skin over the patch becomes thick like the skin of the elephant (Hasti charmavat)
It occurs due to increase of Vata and Kapha Dosha

Kitibha:
श्यावं किणखरस्पर्शं परुषं किटिमं स्मृतम् |
Shyavam- It is blackish brown in color
Kina khara sparsham – It is rough in touch like a scar tissue and
Parusham – It is hard to touch
It occurs due to increase of Vata and Kapha Dosha

Vaipadika / Vipadika
वैपादिकं पाणिपादस्फुटनं तीव्रवेदनम्||२२||
Pani pada sphutanam and Tivra vedanam – cracks in palms and soles of feet as well as excruciating pain.
It occurs due to increase of Vata and Kapha Dosha

Alasaka:
कण्डूमद्भिः सरागैश्च गण्डैरलसकं चितम् |
Ganda – nodular growth associated with
Kandu – excessive itching sensation, and
Saraga – redness
It occurs due to increase of Vata and Kapha Dosha

Dadru:
सकण्डू राग पिडकं दद्रु मण्डलमुद्गतम्||२३||
Dadru is characterized by
Sa kandu – itching sensation,
Raga – redness
Pidaka – pimples and
Mandala udgatam – circular patches with elevated edges.

Charmadala
रक्तं सकण्डु सस्फोटं सरुग्दलति चापि यत्|
तच्चर्मदलमाख्यातं संस्पर्शासहमुच्यते||२४||
Raktam – redness,
Kandu – itching,

Sasphotam – Pustules, boils
Sa ruk dala – pain, cracks in the skin and
Sam sparsha asaha – tenderness, very painful to touch
It occurs due to increase of Pitta and Kapha Dosha

Pama

पामाश्वेतारुणश्यावाः कण्डूलाः पिडका भृशम् |

Pama is characterized by
Kandu – excessive itching,
Sveta, aruna, shyava pidaka – eruptions which are white, reddish or blackish brown in color
It occurs due to increase of Pitta and Kapha Dosha

Sphota

स्फोटाः श्वेतारुणाभासो विस्फोटाः स्युस्तनुत्वचः||२५||

Sphota – boils
Shveta – white
Arunabhasa – reddish
Tanu tvacha – skin over the rash will become thin.
It occurs due to increase of Pitta and Kapha Dosha

Shataru

रक्तं श्यावं सदाहार्तिं शतारुः स्याद्बहुव्रणम् |

Raktam – red
Shyava – brown
Daha – Burning sensation
Arti – painful
Bahuvrana – covers a large skin area.
It occurs due to increase of Pitta and Kapha Dosha

Vicharchika

सकण्डूः पिडका श्यावा बहुस्रावा विचर्चिका||२६||
इत्येकादश क्षुद्रकुष्ठानि|

Shyava pidaka – blackish brown eruptions
Kandu – itching sensation and
Bahu srava – excessive exudation [21-26]
It occurs due to increase of Kapha Dosha
Vicharchika is correlated with eczema.

Dosha Dominance in different skin diseases:

वातेऽधिकतरे कुष्ठं कापालं मण्डलं कफे|
पित्ते त्वौदुम्बरं विद्यात् काकणं तु त्रिदोषजम्||२७||
वातपित्ते श्लेष्मपित्ते वातश्लेष्मणि चाधिके|
ऋष्यजिह्वं पुण्डरीकं सिध्मकुष्ठं च जायते||२८||
चर्माख्यमेककुष्ठं च किटिमं सविपादिकम्|
कुष्ठं चालसकं ज्ञेयं प्रायो वातकफाधिकम्||२९||
पामा शतारुर्विस्फोटं ददुश्चर्मदलं तथा|
पित्तश्लेष्माधिकं प्रायः कफप्राया विचर्चिका||३०||

1) Kapala – Vata Dosha increase
2) Mandala – Kapha
3) Audumbara – Pitta
4) Kakana – Vata, Pitta and Kapha
5) Rushya Jihva – Vata and Pitta
6) Pundarika – Kapha and Pitta
7) Sidhma – Vata and Kapha
8) Charmakhya, Ekakhya, Kitibha, Vipadika and Alasaka Vata and Kapha
9) Pama, Shataru, Visphota, Dadru and Charmadala Pitta and Kapha
10) Vicharchika – Kapha [27-30]

Line of treatment:

सर्वं त्रिदोषजं कुष्ठं दोषाणां तु बलाबलम् |
यथास्वैर्लक्षणैर्बुद्ध्वा कुष्ठानां क्रियते क्रिया||३१||
दोषस्य यस्य पश्येत् कुष्ठेषु विशेषलिङ्गमद्रिक्तम्|
तस्यैव शमं कुर्यात्ततः परं चानुबन्धस्य||३२||

All varieties of Kushta are caused by the simultaneous vitiation of all the 3 Doshas. However, some Doshas are predominant and others are not. Keeping this in view and after ascertaining this from manifested signs and symptoms, the physician should decide the line of treatment.

In the beginning, the dominant Dosha(s) should be treated followed by the secondary vitiated Doshas. [31-32]

Varieties of Diseases and Doshas

कुष्ठविशेषैर्दोषा दोषविशेषैः पुनश्च कुष्ठानि|
ज्ञायन्ते तैर्हेतुर्हेतुस्तांश्च प्रकाशयति||३३||

One can determine the nature of the predominant Dosha from the specific variety of Kustha and vice versa.

The causative factors are determined on the basis of specific manifestation. One can also determine the cause for Kushta by looking at the imbalanced Doshas [33]

Skin symptoms of vitiated Doshas

रौक्ष्यं शोषस्तोदः शूलं सङ्कोचनं तथाऽऽयामः|
पारुष्यं खरभावो हर्षः श्यावारुणत्वं च||३४||
कुष्ठेषु वातलिङ्गं,

Following are the signs and symptoms of vitiated Vata Dohsa in Kustha:

Raukshyam -Roughness, dryness
Parushya – hardness
Khara – coarseness
Harsha – horripilation and
Shyava aruna – brown as well as reddish coloration

Pitta skin symptom:

दाहो रागः परिस्रवः पाकः|
विस्रो गन्धः क्लेदस्तथाऽङ्गपतनं च पित्तकृतम्||३५||

Following are the signs and symptoms of vitiated Pitta in Kustha

Daha – Burning sensation
Raga – redness
exudation,
Srava – suppuration

Visra gandha – smell like raw meat, stickness and

Anga Patana – sloughing of limbs

Kapha symptoms:

श्वैत्यं शैत्यं कण्डू: स्थैर्यं चोत्सेधगौरवस्नेहा:।

कुष्ठेषु तु कफलिङ्गं जन्तुभिरभिभक्षणं क्लेद:॥३६॥

Following are the signs and symptoms of vitiated kapha in Kustha:

Shvaityam – White coloration,

Shaityam – cold in touch,

Kandu – itching,

localization,

Utsedha – elevation,

Gaurava – heaviness,

Jantu bhirabhikshnam - maggot formation and

Kleda – Stickness [34-36]

Prognosis:

सर्वैर्लिङ्गैर्युक्तं मतिमान् विवर्जयेदबलम्।

तृष्णा दाहपरीतं शान्ताग्निं जन्तुभिर्जग्धम्॥३७॥

वातकफप्रबलं यद्यदेकदोषोल्बणं न तत् कृच्छ्रम्।

कफपित्त-वातपित्तप्रबलानि तु कृच्छ्रसाध्यानि॥३८॥

A wise physician must not undertake the treatment of following types of patients suffering from Kustha:

1) The patient of Kusta with the signs and symptoms of all the 3 vitiated Doshas

2) The patient who is weak

3) The patient who is suffering from morbid thirst, burning sensation

4) The patient having no digestion strength and

5) The patient having maggots in the patches of Kustha. [37- 38]

Kushta Chikitsa Sutra – Line of treatment:

वातोत्तरेषु सर्पिर्वमनं श्लेष्मोत्तरेषु कुष्ठेषु।

पित्तोत्तरेषु मोक्षो रक्तस्य विरेचनं चाग्रे॥३९॥

वमन विरेचनयोगाः कल्पोक्ताः कुष्ठिनां प्रयोक्तव्याः।

प्रच्छन्नमल्पे कुष्ठे महति च शस्तं सिराव्यधनम्॥४०॥

बहुदोषः संशोध्यः कुष्ठी बहुशोऽनुरक्षता प्राणान्।

दोषे ह्यतिमात्रह्रते वायुर्हन्यादबलमाशु॥४१॥

स्नेहस्य पानमिष्टं शुद्धे कोष्ठे प्रवाहिते रक्ते।

वायुर्हि शुद्धकोष्ठं कुष्ठिनमबलं विशति शीघ्रम्॥४२॥

Patients suffering from Kustha dominated by Vata are administered with herbal ghee internally.

Patients suffering from Kustha dominated by Kapha are administered Vamana – emetic therapy.

Patients suffering from Kustha dominated by pitta are given Virechana – purgation therapy.

For Vamana and Virechana in a patient suffering from Kustha, the recipes described in the Kalpa sthana section are employed.

Rakotamokshana – bloodletting:

Pracchanna Raktamokshana Blood- letting is done with a coarse device in case of Kusht with mild symptoms.

Sira Vyadha Raktamokshana – vein puncture – is administered in a more acute stage.

Multiple Shodhana therapies:

Kushta patients with more vitiated Doshas (Bahudosha) are given Shodhana therapies several times, with a lot of care.

Excessive elimination of Doshas (morbid factors) might weaken the patient and the aggravated Vata might endanger the patient's life instantaneously.

After the elimination of Doshas from the gastro- intestinal tract (by Vamana and Virechana) and Raktamokshana from blood, the patient is given Sneha (oil, ghee etc) to drink.

This is because Vayu gets aggravated and the patient becomes weak soon after the elimination therapies. This condition shall be treated by the administration of the Snehapana – oleation therapy.

After administration of above therapies, the patient suffering from Kushta is given treatment as described hereafter. These therapies are to be repeated again and again. The physician should not administer therapies to eliminate large quantities of morbid Doshas at a time. If that is done, then it might weaken the patient and endanger his life. This applies to vitiation of one or more Doshas.

Oleation therapy is given only after the morbid Doshas are eliminated from the body. Without that, administration of oleation therapy might aggravate the disease [39-42]

Selection of medicines for Elimination (Panchakarma) Therapies:

Herbs for Vamana treatment for Kushta treatment:

दोषोत्क्लिष्टे हृदये वाम्यः कुष्ठेषु चोर्ध्वभागेषु|

कुटजफल मदन मधुकैः सपटोलैर्निम्बरसयुक्तैः||४३||

शीतरसः पक्वरसो मधूनि मधुकं च वमनानि|

When Doshas are located in Hrudaya (heart) or the centre of the body, are in a state of Utklesha (increase), then the patient is given Vamana therapy with the help of

For the treatment of different types of Kustha herbs like –

Kutaja – Holarrhena antidysenterica (fruit),

Madanaphala and

Madhuka – Licorice

mixed with the juice / decoction of

Patola – Pointed Gourd – Trichosanthes dioica and

Nimba – Neem is administered.

Shitarasa (sheeta kalpana) Pakvarasa, different types of honey and Madhuka are useful for Vamana.

Virechana herbs for Pitta dominant Kushta:

कुष्ठेषु त्रिवृता दन्ती त्रिफला च विरेचने शस्ता||४४||

सौवीरकं तुषोदकमालोडनमासवाश्च सीधूनि|

शंसन्त्यधोहराणां यथाविरेकं क्रमश्चेष्टः||४५||

Trivrit – Operculina turpethum

Danti – Baliospermum montanum

and Triphala – Amla, Haritaki, Vibhitaki are useful in purgation therapy.

The recipe can be prepared by dissolving them in –

Sauviraka - a type of alcohol

Tushodaka – a sour drink prepared of corns and cereals

Alodana – a kind of liquefied preparation

Asava – alcoholic preparation and

Different types of Sidhu – Vinegar prepared with unboiled sugar cane juice.

After Virechana, Samsarjana can be administered depending upon the extent of success of Virechana.

Herbs for Asthapana (decoction enema) for Kushta:

दार्वी बृहतीसेव्यैः पटोल पिचुमर्द मदन कृतमालैः|

सस्नेहैरास्थाप्यः कुष्ठी सकलिङ्गयवमुस्तैः ||४६||

Decoction enema can be prepared with herbs like

Darvi – Berberis aristata

Brihati – Solanum indicum,

Sevya – Vetiver – Vetiveria zizanioides

Patola – Tricosanthes dioca

Pichumarda – Neem

Madana – Randia dumetorum

Krutamala – Cassia fistula

Kalinga – Holarrhena antidysenterica

Yava – Barley (Hordeum vulgare) and

Musta – Cyperus rotundus

The decoction enema is administered along with oil or fat.

Anuvasana Basti (fat enema) for Kushta

वातोल्बणं विरिक्तं निरूढमनुवासनार्हमालक्ष्य|

फलमधुक निम्ब कुटजैः सपटोलैः साधयेत्स्नेहम्||४७||

After Virechana, if there is Vata increase, then the doctor should decide if the patient is eligible for Basti treatment.

If eligible, Anuvasana basti is administered with fat processed with

Madana Phala – Randia dumetorum

Madhuka– Licorice – Glycyrrhiza glabra,

Nimba – Neem (Azadirachta indica),

Kutaja – Connessi (Holarrhena antidysenterica Wall.) and

Patola -Tricosanthes dioca.

Nasya herbs for Kushta:

सैन्धव दन्ती मरिचं फणिज्झकः पिप्पली करञ्जफलम्|

नस्यं स्यात्सविडङ्गं क्रिमिकुष्ठकफप्रकोपघ्नम् ||४८||

For Nasya medicine preparation, following ingredients are used;

Saindhava – Rock salt

Danti – Baliospermum montanum

Maricha – Black pepper fruit – Piper nigrum,

Phanijjaka – Ocimum basilicum,

Pippali – Long pepper fruit – Piper longum and

Fruit of karanja – Pongamia pinnata

These drugs cure diseases caused by

Krimi – parasitic infestation

Kushta – skin disease and diseases caused by the aggravation of Kapha. [43 -48]

Herbs for Dhumapana for Kushta:

वैरेचनिकैर्धूमैः श्लोकस्थानेरितैः प्रशाम्यन्ति|

कृमयः कुष्ठ किलासाः प्रयोजितैरुत्तमाङ्गस्थाः ||४९||

Administration of the recipes of Vairechanika Dhumapana (eliminative type of smoking therapy) herbs described in Sutrasthana 5/26-27 are used. It is useful in

Krumi (Parasitic infection),

Kilas affecting the head.[49]

Raktamokshana – Bloodletting therapy for skin diseases:

स्थिर कठिन मण्डलानां स्विन्नानां प्रस्तरप्रणाडीभिः।
कूर्चैर्विघट्टितानां रक्तोत्क्लेशोऽपनेतव्यः॥५०॥
आनूपवारिजानां मांसानां पोट्टलैः सुखोष्णैश्च।
स्विन्नोत्सन्नं विलिखेत् कुष्ठं तीक्ष्णेन शस्त्रेण॥५१॥
रुधिरागमार्थमथवा शृङ्गालाबूनि योजयेत् कुष्ठे।
प्रच्छितमल्पं कुष्ठं विरेचयेद्वा जलौकोभिः॥५२॥
ये लेपाः कुष्ठानां युज्यन्ते निर्हृतासृदोषाणाम्।
संशोधिताशयानां सद्यः सिद्धिर्भवेत्तेषाम्॥५३॥

The patches of Kustha which are stable, hard and rounded, are subjected to Prastara and Nadi type of Svedana (Refer Charaka chapter Sweda Sutra 14/42- 43) and rubbed with Kurcha (a surgical brush with hard fibres). The blood oozing out through this process should thereafter be eliminated.

The elevated patches of Kustha are fomented with lukewarm Pottalis (A cloth bundle pack with hot fomenting paste of ingredients) containing meat of semi- aquatic and aquatic animals. Thereafter, blood is eliminated by incising with a sharp edged scalped.

In Kaphaja Kushta with a limited number of patches, blood is eliminated by scratching patch and by applying Shrunga (horn), Alabu (ground) and Jalaukas (Leech therapy).

It is only after the elimination of impurities in the blood (through bloodletting therapy) and elimination of Doshas from the gastrointestinal tract through elimination therapies, that the ointment prescribed Kushta become instantaneously efficacious. [50-53]

Kshara Prayoga for Kushta – Application of Alkalis and other Therapies:

येषु न शस्त्रं क्रमते स्पर्शेन्द्रियनाशनानि यानि स्युः।
तेषु निपात्यः क्षारो रक्तं दोषं च विस्राव्य॥५४॥
पाषाणकठिनपरुषे सुप्ते कुष्ठे स्थिरे पुराणे च।
पीतागदस्य कार्यो विषैः प्रदेहोऽगदैश्चानु॥५५॥
स्तब्धानि सुप्तसुप्तान्यस्वेदनकण्डूलानि कुष्ठानि।
कूर्चैर्दन्तीत्रिवृताकरवीरकरञ्जकुटजानाम्॥५६॥
जात्यर्ककनिम्बजैर्वा पत्रैः शस्त्रैः समुद्रफेनैर्वा।
घृष्टानि गोमयैर्वा ततः प्रदेहैः प्रदेह्यानि॥५७॥

In such conditions where the patches are anesthetic and in which application of surgical instruments is contraindicated, Kshara (alkali preparation) is used.

Pashana Kathina – If the patches of Kushta are hard and rough like stone, if there is numbness and stability and if the condition is chronic, then the patient is given agada – anti poisonous medication internally, and thereafter, ointment containing Visha (Vatsanabha or any poisonous ingredient) is applied.

If the patches of Kushta are numb and absolutely anesthetic, and if there is absence of sweating and itching, then they are rubbed with the Kurcha (brush) made of the stems of

Danti – Baliospermum motanum

Trivrit – Operculina turpethum

Karanja – Pongamia pinnata and

Kutaja – Connessi (Holarrhena antidysenterica)

Or with the

Leaves of

Jati – Jasminum grandiflorum

Arka – Calotropis procera and

Nimba – Neem (Azadirachta indica) or

With sharp instruments, or

With Samudra Phena (cuttle fish bone) or with (dried) cow dung following which the ointments are applied. [54-57]

Treatment of Paittik Kusta:

मारुत कफ कुष्ठघ्नं कर्मोक्तं पित्तकुष्ठिनां कार्यम्|

कफ पित्त रक्तहरणं तिक्तकषायैः प्रशमनं च||५८||

सर्पींषि तिक्तकानि च यच्चान्यद्रक्तपित्तनुत् कर्म|

बाह्याभ्यन्तरमग्र्यं तत् कार्यं पित्तकुष्ठेषु||५९||

Pittaja Kusta is treated on the lines prescribed for the treatment of Vatika and Kaphaja types of Kusthas (skin diseases caused by Vayu and Kapha).

In addition, Kapha, Pitta and Rakta (blood) is eliminated (by Vamana, Virechana and Raktamokshana) and alleviated by recipes containing bitter – astringent herbs.

Similarly, medicated ghee and such other efficacious therapies for the alleviation of Pitta and Rakta are administered both externally and internally for the treatment of Pittaja Kusta [58-59]

Shamana treatment for Kushta – Palliative measures:

दोषाधिक्यविभागादित्येतत् कर्म कुष्ठनुत् प्रोक्तम्|

वक्ष्यामि कुष्ठशमनं प्रायस्त्वग्दोषसामान्यात्||६०||

The remedies for cure of different types of Kusta, categorized on the basis of aggravation of Doshas are described above.

I shall now expound therapies for the cure of Kustha in general as characterized by the affliction of the skin. [60]

Medicines:

दार्वी रसाञ्जनं वा गोमूत्रेण प्रबाधते कुष्ठम्|

अभया प्रयोजिता वा मासं सव्योषगुडतैला||६१||

Intake of Rasanjana (solid extract prepared of the decoction of Daruharidra) along with cow urine cures Kushta (skin diseases).

Intake of Abhaya along with Trikatu (Ginger, pepper and long pepper), Guda (Jaggery) and sesame oil for 1 month cures Kustha. [61]

Patolamuladi Kashaya:

मूलं पटोलस्य तथा गवाक्ष्याः पृथक् पलांशं त्रिफलात्वचश्च |

स्यात्त्रायमाणा कटुरोहिणी च भागाधिका नागरपादयुक्ता||६२||

पलं तथैषां सह चूर्णितानां जले शृतं दोषहरं पिबेन्ना|

जीर्णे रसैर्धन्वमृगद्विजानां पुराणशाल्योदनमाददीत||६३||

कुष्ठानि शोफं ग्रहणीप्रदोषमर्शांसि कृच्छ्राणि हलीमकं च|

षड्ग्रात्रयोगेन निहन्ति चैष हृद्बस्तिशूलं विषमज्वरं च||६४||

Root of Patola – Pointed Gourd – Trichosanthes dioica – 1 Pala- 48 g

Root of Gavakshi (1 Pala)

Triphala – Amla, Haritaki, Vibhitaki – 1 Pala each

Trayamana – 6 Sana and

Nagara – Ginger (4 Sana) is made to a powder.

One Pala of this powder is to be boiled in water.

Intake of this Kashaya alleviates Doshas (causing Kustha) of the patient.

After this potion is digested, the patient is given old rice along with meat soup of animals and birds inhabiting arid land. (Jangala Mamsa)

This recipe when administered for 6 nights (days) cures

Kustha,

Shopha (oedema),

Grahani Dosha (sprue syndrome),

Arsas (piles),

Mutra Krichra (dysuria),

Halimaka (serious type of Jaundice),

Pain in cardiac and urinary bladder region and

Vishamajvara (Recurrent fever) {62- 64}

Mustadi Churna:

मुस्तं व्योषं त्रिफला मञ्जिष्ठा दारु पञ्चमूल्यौ द्वे|

सप्तच्छदनिम्बत्वक् सविशालश्चित्रको मूर्वा||६५||

चूर्णं तर्पणभागैर्नवभिः संयोजितं समध्वाज्यम्] |

सिद्धं कुष्ठनिबर्हणमेतत् प्रायोगिकं भक्ष्यम्||६६||

श्वयथुं सपाण्डुरोगं श्वित्रं ग्रहणी प्रदोषमर्शांसि|

ब्रध्न भगन्दर पिडका कण्डू कोठांश्च विनिहन्ति||६७||

इति मुस्तादिचूर्णम्|

These drugs taken in equal quantites is made of a powder

Musta – Nut grass (root) – Cyperus rotundus

Trikatu – Ginger, black pepper, long pepper,

Triphala (Haritaki, Bibhitaki and Amalaki),

Manjistha – Rubia cordifolia

Devadaru – Cedrus deodara,

Dashamoola (bilva, syonaka, Gambhari, Patali, Ganikarika, Salaparni, Prsniparni, Brhati, Kantakari and Goksura)

Bark of Saptacchada (Saptaparna) – Alstonia scholaris – Stem bark

Bark of Nimba – Neem

Vishala

Chitraka – Leadwort – Plumbago zeylanica and

Murva – Root

This powder is mixed with 9 times of Saktu (roasted corn flour) and be taken by the patient mixed with honey and ghee every day.

This is an infallible remedy for the treatment of Kustha (skin diseases).

It is also useful in treating

Shotha – oedema

Pandu – Anemia

Leucoderma

Grahani – Sprue syndrome,

Bradhna – enlarged inguinal gland,

Fistula in ano

Pimples, Scabies and

Kotha – urticarial rashes [65-67]

Triphaladi Churna:

त्रिफलातिविषाकटुका निम्ब कलिङ्गक वचा पटोलानाम्|

मागधिकारजनीद्वयपद्मकमूर्वाविशालानाम्||६८||

भूनिम्ब पलाशानां दद्यादिवपलं ततस्त्रिवृद्दिद्वगुणा|

तस्याश्च पुनर्ब्राह्मी तच्चूर्णं सुप्तिनुत् परमम्||६९||

Powders of each of these: 2 Palas (96 g) of each of
Triphala (haritaki, Bibhitaki and Amalaki)
Ativisha – Aconitum heterophyllum
Katuki – Picrorhiza kurroa – Root
Nimba – Neem
Kalingaka – Connessi Bark – Holarrhena antidysenterica
Vacha – Acorus calamus
Patola – Pointed Gourd – Trichosanthes dioica
Pippali – Piper longum
Haridra – Turmeric – Curcuma longa
Daruharidra – Berberis aristata
Padmaka
Murva – Root
Vishala
Bhunimba – Andrographis paniculata – Whole plant and
Palash – Butea monosperma
Trivrut – Operculina turpethum – 4 Pala – 192 g
This is an excellent recipe for the cure of Supti (numbness). [68-69]

Use of Sulphur:

लेलीतकप्रयोगो रसेन जात्याः समाक्षिकः परमः|
सप्तदशकुष्ठघाती माक्षिकधातुश्च मूत्रेण||७०||

Administration of Lelitaka (Sulphur) with the juice of (Amalaki) together with honey is the remedy par excellence
for the cure of 17 types of Kustha (skin diseases).
Similar is the therapeutic efficacy of Makshika Dhatu (copper pyrite) taken together with Cow's urine [70]

Use of Mercury:

श्रेष्ठं गन्धकयोगात् सुवर्ण माक्षिक प्रयोगाद्वा|
सर्वव्याधिनिबर्हणमद्यात् कुष्ठी रसं च निगृहीतम्||७१||
वज्रशिलाजतुसहितं सहितं वा योगराजेन|
सर्वव्याधि प्रशमनमद्यात्कुष्ठी निगृह्य नित्यं च||७२||

(copper Pyrtite), the Bhasma so prepared, would be a remedy par excellence for curing all ailments. The patient
suffering from Kustha should take this recipe.
Similarly, Mercury processed with Diamond and Shilajatu, or Yogaraja cures all ailments.
The patient suffering from Kushta should take this recipe every day [71-72]

Madhvasava:

खदिर सुरदारुसारं श्रपयित्वा तद्रसेन तोयार्थः|
क्षौद्रप्रस्थे कार्यः कार्ये ते चाष्टपलिके च||७३||
तत्राश्चूर्णानामष्टपलं प्रक्षिपेत्तथाऽमूनि|
त्रिफलैले त्वङ्मरिचं पत्रं कनकं च कर्षांशम्||७४||
मत्स्यण्डिका मधुसमा तन्मासं जातमायसे भाण्डे|
मध्वासवमाचरतः कुष्ठ किलासे शमं यातः||७५||
इति मध्वासवः|

8 Palas each of these is boiled in water:
Heart- wood of Khadira – Acacia catechu and

Devadaru – Cedrus deodara

To this decoction, 1 Prastha (768 ml) of honey + 8 Palas of the powder (Bhasma or calcined powder) of iron is added.

1 Karsha of each of

Triphala (Haritaki, Bibhitaki and Amalaki) ,

Ela – Elettaria cardamomum

Tvak – Cinnamomum zeylanica

Maricha – Piper nigrum

Patra- Cinnamomum tamala and

Kanaka (Nagakesara) – Messua ferrea

1 Prastha of Matsyandika (Sugar) is added.

This mixture is kept in an iron jar for one month underground for fermentation according to the prescribed procedure. Thereafter, it is administered for curing

Kustha (skin diseases) and

Kilasa (Leucoderma). This formulation is called Madhvasava. [73-75]

Kanakabindvarista:

खदिर कषाय द्रोणं कुम्भे घृतभाविते समावाप्य।

द्रव्याणि चूर्णितानि च षट्पलिकान्यत्र देयानि॥७६॥

त्रिफला व्योष विडङ्ग रजनी मुस्ताटरूषकेन्द्रयवाः।

सौवर्णी च तथा त्वक् छिन्नरुहा चेति तन्मासम्॥७७॥

निदधीत धान्यमध्ये प्रातः प्रातः पिबेत्ततो युक्त्या।

मासेन महाकुष्ठं हन्त्येवाल्पं तु पक्षेण॥७८॥

अर्शःश्वासभगन्दरकासकिलासप्रमेहशोषांश्च।

ना भवति कनकवर्णः पीत्वाऽरिष्टं कनकबिन्दुम्॥७९॥

इति कनकबिन्द्वरिष्टम्।

कुष्ठेष्वनिलकफकृतेष्वेवं पेयस्तथाऽपि पैत्तेषु।

कृतमालक्वाथश्चाप्येष विशेषात् कफकृतेषु॥८०॥

1 Drona (12.288 liters) of the decoction of Khadira is kept in a ghee smeared jar.

To this, 6 Palas of the powder of

Triphala (Haritaki, Bibhitaki and Amalaki),

Trikatu (Sunthi, Pippali, and Maricha),

Vidanga – Embelia ribes

Rajani – Turmeric

Musta – Cyperus rotundus

Atarushaka – Adhatoda vasica

Indrayava – Connessi (seed) – Holarrhena antidysenterica

Bark of Sauvarni – Cassia fistula and

Chinnaruha – Giloy – each taken in equal quantity is added.

The jar containing the recipe is kept inside a heap of grains for a month.

Intake of this every morning in appropriate Dosage for 1 month certainly cures MahaKustha (major types of Kustha).

Kshudra Kustha (minor types of Kustha) can however, be cured by this recipe in 15 days.

It also cures all types of

Arsha – Piles

Shvasa – Asthma

Bhagandara – fistula-in-ano

Kasa – bronchitis,

Kilasa – leucoderma and

Prameha – urinary disorders

The person taking this recipe becomes golden in complexion.

This is called Kanakabindu.

Intake of this recipe is useful in Kusthas caused by Vayu, Kapha and Pitta.

However, use of the decoction of Krtamala (in the place of Khadira) in this recipe will make it separately useful in curing Kaphaja Kustha. [76-80]

Triphalasava:

त्रिफलासवश्च गौडः सचित्रकः कुष्ठरोगविनिहन्ता।

क्रमुक दशमूल दन्ती वराङ्ग मधुयोगसंयुक्तः॥८१॥

Triphalasava prepared with Jaggery together with

Chitraka – Plumbago zeylanica

Kramuka

Dashamula (bilva, Syonaka, Gambhari, Patali, ganikarika, shalaparni, Prsniparni, Brhati, Kantikari and Goksura)

Danti – Baliospermum montanum

Varanga and honey

Cures Kustha (skin diseases) [81]

Kushta Pathya – Diet:

लघूनि चान्नानि हितानि विद्यात् कुष्ठेषु शाकनि च तिक्तकानि।

भल्लातकैः सत्रिफलैः सनिम्बैर्युक्तानि चान्नानि घृतानि चैव॥८२॥

पुराणधान्यान्यथ जाङ्गलानि मांसानि मुद्गाश्च पटोलयुक्ताः।

शस्ता, न गुर्वम्लपयोदधीनि नानूपमत्स्या न गुडस्तिलाश्च॥८३॥

The patient suffering from Kustha (skin diseases) should take following types of diet:

(1) Laghu ahara – Light and wholesome food

(2) Tikta shaka – Vegetables (leafy) having bitter taste

(3) Food preparations and medicated ghee prepared by boiling with Bhallalaka, Triphala and Nimba

(4) Old (not freshly harvested) cereals and

(5) Meat of animals inhabiting arid land (Jangala Mamsa) and preparations of Mudga (green gram) mixed with Patola – Pointed gourd.

Intake of heavy and sour food, milk, curd, meat of animals inhabiting marshy land, fish, Guda (Jaggery) and Tila are prohibited for Patients of Kusta [82-83]

Ointments and Pastes for External Use:

एला कुष्ठं दार्वी शतपुष्पा चित्रको विडङ्गश्च।

कुष्ठा लेपनमिष्टं रसाञ्जनं चाभया चैव॥८४॥

Application of the paste of

Ela –Elettaria cardamomum

Kustha – Saussurea lappa

Darvi – Berberis aristata

Shatapuspa – Anethum sowa

Chitraka – Plumbago zeylanica

Vidanga – Embelia ribes

Rasanjana Aqueous extract of Daruharidra (Berberis aristata) and

Abhaya (Harad) is very effective in curing Kustha (skin diseases). [84]

Chitrakadi lepa for Mandala Kushta

चित्रकमेलां बिम्बीं वृषकं त्रिवृद्र्कनागरकम्|
चूर्णीकृतमष्टाहं भावयितव्यं पलाशस्य||८५||
क्षारेण गवां मूत्रसुतेन तेनास्य मण्डलान्याशु|
भिद्यन्ते विलयन्ति च लिप्तान्यर्काभितप्तानि||८६||

Powder of
Chitraka – Plumbago zeylanica
Ela – Elettaria cardamomum
Bimbi – Coccinia indica
Vishala
Trivrit – Operculina turpethum
Arka – Calotropis procera and
Nagara – Ginger
This is impregnated with the Palasha Kshara and boiled with cow's urine for 8 days.
Application of this paste followed by exposure to the heat of the sun soon leads to the bursting as well as dissolution of Mandala type of Kustha. [85-86]

Mamsyadi Lepa:
मांसी मरिचं लवणं रजनी तगरं सुधा गृहाद्धूमः|
मूत्रं पित्तं क्षारः पालाशः कुष्ठहा लेपः||८७||
The paste of
Mamsi – Nardostachys jatamansi
Maricha – Piper nigrum
Saindhava Rock-salt
Rajani -Turmeric
Tagara – Valeriana wallichii
Sudha – Arka – Calotropis procera
Gruhadhuma (house shoot)
Cow urine
Pitta – bile and
Palasha Kshara (alkali preparation) is used externally for the Kustha (skin diseases). [87]

Trapu adi Lepa for Mandala Kushta
त्रपु सीसमयश्चूर्णं मण्डलनुत् फल्गुचित्रकौ बृहती|
गोधारसः सलवणो दारु च मूत्रं च मण्डलनुत्||८८||
Application of the powder (bhasma or calcined powder) of Trapu (tin) Seesa (Lead) and Ayas (iron) cures Mandala type of Kusht.
Similarly, application of the powder of
Phalgu
Chitraka – Plumbago zeylanica
Brhati – Solanum indicum
Godharasa – liquid extract of the meat of Laguna together with
Saindhava – Rock salt
Devadaru – Cedrus deodara and
Cow-urine cures Mandala type of Kustha. [88]

Kadali adi Lepa:
कदली पलाश पाटलि निचुल क्षाराम्भसा प्रसन्नेन|

मांसेषु तोयकार्यं कार्यं पिष्टे च किण्वे च||८९||
तैर्मेदकः सुजातः किण्वैर्जनितं प्रलेपनं शस्तम्|
मण्डलकुष्ठ विनाशनमातपसंस्थं कृमिघ्नं च||९०||

Kshara (alkali preparation) is prepared of

Kadali – Musa paradisiaca

Palasha – Butea monosperma

Patali and

Nichula

From this Ksara, alkaline water is prepared which is to be made transparent (free from suspended particles).

This liquid is added to meat of animals for the preparation of meat extract.

The same alkaline water is also to be used in the preparation of paste (of drugs) and Kinva (fermenting enzyme).

From the above mentioned meat extract, paste and Kinva, medaka (a type of alcoholic preparation) is prepared.

When this is well fermented, the Kinva (Paste of drugs) is to be taken out and exposed to the heat of the sun.

Application of this paste cures Mandala type of Kustha and Parasitic infestations. [89-90]

Siddharthaka Snana:

मुस्तं मदनं त्रिफला करञ्ज आरग्वध कलिङ्ग यवाः|
दार्वी ससप्तपर्णा स्नानं सिद्धार्थकं नाम||९१||
एष कषायो वमनं विरेचनं वर्णकस्तथोद्घर्षः|
त्वग्दोषकुष्ठशोफप्रबाधनः पाण्डुरोगघ्नः||९२||

The water boiled with

Musta – Cyperus rotundus

Madana – Randia dumetorum

Triphala (Haritaki, Bibhitaki and Amalaki),

Karanja – Pongamia pinnata

Aragvadha – Cassia fistula

Indrayava – Seeds of Kutaja

Darvi – Tree turmeric

Saptaparna – Alstonia scholaris is used for bath.

This bath is called Siddhartha Snana

This term implies the accomplishment of the objective of curing Kustha.

The decoction of the above mentioned drugs is also useful in emetic and purgation therapies.

The powder or paste of these drugs is useful for unction which promotes the color of the skin.

These recipes are useful in the treatment of

Skin disorders

Kustha (skin diseases),

Shotha – oedema and

Pandu – Anemia [91-92]

Kushtadi Lepa:

कुष्ठं करञ्जबीजान्येडगजः कुष्ठसूदनो लेपः|
प्रपुन्नाडबीजसैन्धव रसाञ्जन कपित्थ लोध्राश्च||९३||
श्वेतकरवीरमूलं कुटजकरञ्जयोः फलं त्वचो दाव्याः|
सुमनःप्रवालयुक्तो लेपः कुष्ठापहः सिद्धः||९४||

Kustha – Sausserea lappa

Seeds of Karanja and Edagaja are made to a paste by adding water which cures Kustha (skin diseases).

Similarly, the paste of the

Seeds of Prapunnada
Saindhava – Rock salt
Rasanjana (solid extract of Berberis Arista)
Kapittha – Feronia limonia / Limonia acidissima
Lodhra – Symplococs aristata
Root of white variety of Karaveera – Nerium indicum
Fruits of Kutaja – Holarrhena antidysenterica and
Karanja – Pongamia pinnata and the
Bark of Daruharidra – Berberis aristata along with the
Tender leaves of Jati is applied for curing Kustha [93-94]

लोध्रस्य धातकीनां वत्सकबीजस्य नक्तमालस्य|
कल्कश्च मालतीनां कुष्ठेषून्मर्दनालेपौ||९५||
The paste of
Lodhra – Symplocos racemosa
Dhataki – Woodfordia floribunda
Seed of Karanja – Pongamia pinnata
Naktamala – Pongamia pinnata and
Malati – Jasminum grandiflorum- is to be used externally as unction (Udvartana) and ointment [95]
Shireesha twadagi Lepa:

शैरीषी त्वक् पुष्पं कार्पास्या राजवृक्षपत्राणि|
पिष्टा च काकमाची चतुर्विधः कुष्ठनुल्लेपः||९६||
इति लेपाः|
Application of the paste of either the
Bark of Sirisha – Albizia lebbeck or
The flower of Karpasa – Gossypium herbaceum or
The leaves of Rajavrksa or
Kakamachi – Solanum nigrum cures Kustha (skin diseases). [96]

Kashayas for Kushta for oral and external use:
दार्व्या रसाञ्जनस्य च निम्बपटोलस्य खदिरसारस्य|
आरग्वधवृक्षकयोस्त्रिफलायाः सप्तपर्णस्य||९७||
इति षट् कषाययोगाः कुष्ठघ्नाः सप्तमश्च तिनिशस्य|
स्नाने पाने च हितास्तथाऽष्टमश्चाश्वमारस्य||९८||
आलेपनं प्रघर्षणमवचूर्णनमेत एव च कषायाः|
तैलघृतपाकयोगे चेष्यन्ते कुष्ठशान्त्यर्थम्||९९||
Decoctions of the following 8 recipes are useful in the treatment of Kustha (skin diseases)
1) Rasanjana (solid extract) which is collected from Daruharidra – Berberis aristata
2) Nimba – Azadirachta indica and Patola – Trichosanthes dioica
3) Heart-wood (or solid extract) of Khadira – Acacia catechu
4) Aragvadha and Vrksaka (Kutaja) – Hollarhena dysentrica
5) Triphala(Haritaki, Bibhitaka and Amalaki)
6) Saptaparna – Alstonia scholaris
7) Tinisha and
8) Ashvamara – Nerium indicum
The decoction of the above mentioned recipes are used in bath, as drink, as alepana (external application) for

Pragharsana (rubbing) and Avachurnana (dusting).

These decoctions may be used in the preparation of medicated oil and medicated ghee. [97-99]

Triphaladi Kashaya:

त्रिफला निम्ब पटोलं मञ्जिष्ठा रोहिणी वचा रजनी|

एष कषायोऽभ्यस्तो निहन्ति कफपित्तजं कुष्ठम्||१००||

एतैरेव च सर्पिः सिद्धं वातोल्बणं जयति कुष्ठम्|

एष च कल्पो दिष्टः खदिरासनदारुनिम्बानाम्||१०१||

Habitual intake of

Triphala (Haritaki, Bibhitaki and Amalaki),

Nimba – Azadirachta indica

Patola –Tricosanthes dioica

Manjistha – Rubia cordifolia

Rohini – Picrorhiza kurroa

Vacha – Acorus calamus and

Rajani – Turmeric cures Kustha caused by Kapha and Pitta.

Medicated ghee prepared by boiling with the decoction of the above mentioned drugs cures Vatika type of Kustha (skin diseases)

The decoction prepared of

Khadira – Acacia catechu

Asana –

Devadaru – Cedrus deodara and

Nimba – Azadirachta indica used in the above mentioned manner serves the same therapeutic purpose. [100-101]

Kushtadi taila / Lepa / Udvartana:

कुष्ठार्कतुत्थकट्फलमूलकबीजानि रोहिणी कटुका|

कुटजफलोत्पलमुस्तं बृहतीकरवीरकासीसम्||१०२||

एडगजनिम्बपाठा दुरालभा चित्रको विडङ्गश्च|

तिक्तालाबुकबीजं कम्पिल्लकसर्षपौ वचा दार्वी||१०३||

एतैस्तैलं सिद्धं कुष्ठघ्नं योग एष चालेपः|

उद्वर्तनं प्रघर्षणमवचूर्णनमेष एवेष्टः||१०४||

Medicated oil prepared of

Kustha – Sausserea lappa

Arka – Calotropis procera

Tuttha – Copper sulphate

Katphala – Myrica nagi

Seeds of Mulaka – Raphanus sativus

Katuka rohini – Picrorhiza kurroa

Fruit of Kutaja – Holarrhena antidysenterica

Utpala – Water lily

Musta – Cyperus rotundus

Brhati – Solanum indicum

Karavira – Nerium indicum

Kasisa – Purified green vitriol

Edagaja (Chakramarda) – Cassia tora

Nimba – Azadirachta indica

Patha – Cissampelos pareira

Duralabha – Tragia involucrata
Chitraka – Plumbago zeylanica
Vidanga – Embelia ribes
Seeds of Tiktalabu
Kampillaka – Mallotus phillippinensis
Sarshapa – Mustard
Vacha – Acorus calamus and
Daruharidra – Berberis aristata cures Kustha (skin diseases).
This medicated oil can be used as
Alepa (external Smearing)
Udvartana (Unction),
Pragharsana (rubbing) and
Avacurnana (dusting) [102-104]

Shveta karaviradya Taila:
श्वेत करवीरकरसो गोमूत्रं चित्रको विडङ्गश्च|
कुष्ठेषु तैलयोगः सिद्धोऽयं सम्मतो भिषजाम्||१०५||
इति श्वेतकरवीराद्यं तैलम्|
Medicated oil prepared of the
Juice of the white variety of Karavira – Nerium indicum
Cow- urine
Citraka – Plumbago zeylanica and
Vidanga – Embelia ribes is a well established recipe for the cure of Kustha (skin diseases) among the physicians.
[105]

Shveta Karavirapallavadya Taila:
श्वेतकरवीरपल्लवमूलत्वग्वत्सको विडङ्गश्च|
कुष्ठार्कमूलसर्षपशिग्रुत्वग्रोहिणी कटुका||१०६||
एतैस्तैलं सिद्धं कल्कैः पादांशिकैर्गवां मूत्रम्|
दत्वा तैलचतुर्गुणमभ्यङ्गात् कुष्ठकण्डूघ्नम्||१०७||
इति श्वेतकरवीरपल्लवाद्यं तैलम्|
Medicated oil is prepared of the following
1) Oil (one Part)
2) Cow- urine(four parts)
3) Paste of the
Leaf and root- bark of the white variety of Karavira –Nerium indicum
Vatsaka – Kutaja
Vidanga – Embelia ribes
Kustha – Saussurea lappa
Root of Arka – Calotropis procera
Sarshapa – Mustard
Bark of sigru – Moringa oliefera
Katukarohini – Picrorhiza kurroa (all taken in equal quantities and 1/4th part of the oil in quantity)
Massage of this medicated oil eradicates
Kustha (skin diseases) and Kandu (itching) [106-107]

Tiktekshvadi Taila:

तिक्तालाबुकबीजं द्वे तुत्थे रोचना हरिद्रे द्वे।
बृहतीफलमेरण्डः सविशालश्चित्रको मूर्वा॥१०८॥
कासीस हिङ्गु शिग्रु त्र्यूषण सुरदारु तुम्बुरु विडङ्गम्।
लाङ्गालकं कुटजत्वक् कटुकाख्या रोहिणी चैव॥१०९॥
सर्षपतैलं कल्कैरेतैर्मूत्रे चतुर्गुणे साध्यम्।
कण्डू कुष्ठविनाशनमभ्यङ्गान्मारुतकफहन्तृ॥११०॥
इति तिक्तेक्ष्वाक्वादितैलम्।

Mustard oil is boiled with the

Paste of seeds of Tiktalabu

Both the varieties of Tuttha (Copper sulphate)

Gorochana (cow's bile)

Haridra — Curcuma longa

Daruharidra – Berberis aristata

Fruits of Brhati – Solanum indicum

Eranda – Ricinus communis

Vishala – Citrullus colocynthis

Chitraka – Plumbago zeylanica

Murva—Marsdenia tenacissima

Kasisa (Iron sulphate)

Hingu – Asafoetida

Shigru – Moringa oliefera

Trayushana (Sunthi, Pippali and Maricha)

Suradaru – Cedrus deodara

Tumburu

Vidanga – Embelia ribes

Langalaka –

Bark of Kutaja – Holarrhena antidysenterica and

Katurohini – Picrorhiza kurroa

By adding cow- urine, four times in quantity of the oil.

Massage of this medicated oil cures

Kandu (itches)

Kustha (skin diseases) and

Diseases caused by Vayu as well as Kapha. [108- 110]

Kanakaksheeri Taila:

कनकक्षीरी शैला भार्गी दन्त्याः फलानि मूलं च।
जाती प्रवाल सर्षप लशुन विडङ्गं करञ्जत्वक्॥१११॥
सप्तच्छदार्कपल्लवमूलत्वङ्निम्ब चित्रकास्फोताः।
गुञ्जैरण्डं बृहतीमूलकसुरसार्जकफलानि॥११२॥
कुष्ठं पाठा मुस्तं तुम्बुरुमूर्वावचाः सषड्ग्रन्थाः।
एडगज कुटज शिग्रु त्र्यूषण भल्लातक क्षवकाः॥११३॥
हरितालमवाक्पुष्पी तुत्थं कम्पिल्लकोऽमृतासञ्ज्ञः।
सौराष्ट्री कासीसं दार्वीत्वक् सर्जिकालवणम्॥११४॥
कल्कैरेतैस्तैलं करवीरकमूलपल्लवकषाये।
सार्षपमथवा तैलं गोमूत्रचतुर्गुणं साध्यम्॥११५॥
स्थाप्यं कटुकालाबुनि तत्सिद्धं तेन मण्डलान्याशु।

भिन्द्यादिभिषगभ्यङ्गात्कृमींश्च कण्डूं च विनिहन्यात्||११६||
इति कनकक्षीरीतैलम्|

Sesame oil or mustard oil is added to the decoction of

The roots and leaves of Karaviraka

The paste of Kanakaksiri (Kankustha)

Salia (Manothila)

Bhargi

Fruits and roots of Danti

Tender leaves of Jati – Jasminum grandiflorum

Sarsapa

Lasuna – Allium sativum

Vidanga – Embelia ribes

Bark of Karanja – Pongamia pinnata

Saptacchada

Root- barks and leaves of arka – Calotropis procera

Nimba – Azadirachta indica

Chitraka – Plumbago zeylanica

Asphota

Gunja – Abrus precatorius

Eranda – Ricinus communis

Brhati – Solanum indicum

Mulaka – Raphanus sativus

Seeds of Surasa – Holy basil

Seeds of Arjaka

Kutaja – Holarrhena antidysenterica

Shigru – Moringa oleifera

Trayushana (Sunthi, Pippali and Marica)

Bhallataka – Semecarpus anacardium

Kshavaka

Haritala – Orpiment

Avakpuspi (Apamarga) – Achyranthes aspera

Tuttha – Copper sulphate

Kampillaka

Amrtasanjna (Kharparika Tuttha)

Saurastri – Sphatila

Kasisa – Green vitriole

Bark of Daruharidra – Berberis aristata and

Sarjika lavana

Cow-urine, 4 time in quantity of oil.

This medicated oil is stored in a container of Katukalabu.

Massage of this oil immediately helps in the bursting of the Mandala type of Kustha (skin diseases), cures Krimi (parasitic infestation) and Kandu (itches). [111-116]

Recipe for sidhma:

कुष्ठं तमालपत्रं मरिचं समनःशिलं सकासीसम्|
तैलेन युक्तमुषितं सप्ताहं भाजने ताम्रे||११७||
तेनालिप्तं सिध्मं सप्ताहाह्येति तिष्ठतो घर्मे|

मासान्नवं किलासं स्नानं मुक्त्वा विशुद्धतनोः||११८||
इति सिध्मे लेपः|

The paste of
Kustha – Sausserea lappa
Tamala patra – Cinnamonum tamala
Maricha – Piper nigrum
Manahsila and
Kasisa is mixed with oil and stored for 7 days in a copper vessel.
This paste is applied and the patient should expose himself to the heat of the sun.
This cures:
Sidhma (a type of leucoderma) within a week
Freshly occuring Kilasa (another type of leucoderma) within a month provided the patient does not take bath and his body is cleaned of impurities (by the admistration of elimination therapies) [117-118]

Oil for Kustha:
सर्षप करञ्ज कोषातकीनां तैलान्यथैङ्गुदीनां च|
कुष्ठेषु हितान्याहुस्तैलं यच्चापि खदिरसारस्य||११९||
The oil extracted from the
Seeds of Sarsapa
Karanja
Kosataki and
Ingudi and
The oil boiled with the heart- wood of Khadira – Acacia catechu
Are useful in the treatment of Kustha (skin diseases) [119]

Vipadikahara Ghrta and Taila:
जीवन्ती मञ्जिष्ठा दार्वी कम्पिल्लकः पयस्तुत्थम्|
एष घृततैलपाकः सिद्धः सिद्धे च सर्जरसः||१२०||
देयः समधूच्छिष्टो विपादिका तेन शाम्यतेऽभ्यक्ता|
चर्मैककुष्ठकिटिमं कुष्ठं शाम्यत्यलसकं च||१२१||
इति विपादिकाहरघृततैले|
Medicated ghee and oil is prepared by boiling ghee and or/ oil with the paste of Jivanti
Manjistha – Rubia cordifolia
Daruharidra –Berberis aristata
Kampillaka
Payas (milk) and
Tuttha
When cooking of this is over, Sarjarasa and Madhucchista (bee's wax) is added.
Massage with this oil cures Carmakustha, Ekakustha, and Kitibha and Alasaka varieties of Kustha. [120-121]

Recipes for Mandala Kustha:
किण्वं वराहरुधिरं पृथ्वीका सैन्धवं च लेपः स्यात्|
लेपो योज्यः कुस्तुम्बुरूणि कुष्ठं च मण्डलनुत्||१२२||
Application of the
Paste of Kinva (enzyme used for fermenting Aasavas and Aristas),
Varaha rudhira – Blood of boar,
Prthvika and

Rock salt – Saindhava or

The paste of Kustumburu

Cures Mandala type of Kustha (skin diseases) [122]

Pootikadi Lepa:

पूतीकदारुजटिलाः पक्वसुरा क्षौद्रमुद्गपण्यौं च|

लेपः सकाकनासो मण्डलकुष्ठापहः सिद्धः||१२३||

Application of the paste of

Putika

Devadaru – Cedrus deodara

Jatila

Pakvasura (goraksakarkati)

Kshaudra – honey

Mudgaparni – Phaseolus trilobus and

Kakanasa cures Mandala type of Kustha.

This is a well established recipe [123]

Chitrakadi lepa:

चित्रक शोभाञ्जनकौ गुड्र्च्यपामार्गदेवदारूणि|

खदिरो धवश्च लेपः श्यामा दन्ती द्रवन्ती च||१२४||

लाक्षा रसाञ्जनैलाः पुनर्नवा चेति कुष्ठिनो लेपाः|

दधिमण्डयुताः सर्वे देयाः षण्मारुतकफकुष्ठघ्नाः||१२५||

Paste of the following 6 recipes prepared by adding Dadhimanda (thin butter-milk) cures Kustha (skin diseases) caused by Vayu and Kapha:

1. Chitraka – Plumbago zeylanica and Sobhanjana

2. Guduchi – Tinospora cordifolia, Apamarga – Achyranthes aspera and Devadaru – Cedrus deodara

3. Khadira –Acacia catechu

4. Dhava

5. Syama, Danti, Dravanti, and

6. Laksa, Rasanjana, Ela and Punarnava [124-125]

Edagajadi Udvartana:

एडगज कुष्ठ सैन्धव सौवीरक सर्षपैः कृमिघ्नैश्च|

कृमि कुष्ठमण्डलाख्यं दद्रूकुष्ठं च शममुपैति||१२६||

Application of the paste prepared of

Edagaja

Kustha – Saussurea lappa

Saindhava – salt

Sauviraka

Sarsapa and

Krmighna (Vidanga) – Embelia ribes

Cures

Krmi (Parastic infestation),

Mandala type of Kustha and

Dadru – ring worm [126]

एडगजः सर्जरसो मूलकबीजं च सिध्मकुष्ठानाम्|

काञ्जिकयुक्तं तु पृथङ्मतमिदमुद्वर्तनं लेपाः॥१२७॥

The paste of edagaja or sarjarasa or the seeds of Mulaka prepared by adding Kanji (sour Vinegar) is used as Udavartan (unction) which cures Sidhma (a type of Leucoderma). [127]

Useful herbs for Bath:

वासा तिफला पाने स्नाने चोद्वर्तने प्रलेपे च|
बृहती सेव्य पटोलाः ससारिवा रोहिणी चैव॥१२८॥
खदिरावघात ककुभ रोहीतक लोध्र कुटज धव निम्बाः|
सप्तच्छद करवीराः शस्यन्ते स्नानपानेषु॥१२९॥

The paste or decoction of
Vasa – Adhathoda vasica
Triphala (Haritaki, Bibhitaki and Amalaki)
Brhati – Solanum indicum
Sevya is used for Udvartana (Unction) and Pralepa (external application) by a patient suffering from Kustha.
Similarly, the decoction of
Khadira – Acacia catechu
Avaghata (Karnikara)
Kakubha – Terminalia arjuna
Rohitaka
Lodhra – Symplocos racemosa
Kutaja – Holarrhena antidysentericaica
Dhava
Nimba – Azadirachta indica
Saptacchada (Saptaparna) – Alstonia scholaris – Stem bark
And Karvira – Nerium indicum is useful for bath and drink by a patient suffering from Kustha [128-129]

Pralepa:

जलवाप्य लोह केशर पत्र प्लव चन्दनं मृणालानि|
भागोत्तराणि सिद्धं प्रलेपनं पित्तकफकुष्ठे॥१३०॥

Application of the paste of
Jala (1 part)
Vapya or Kustha (2 parts)
Loha or Agaru (3 Parts)
Kesara (4 parts)
Patra (5 parts) and
Mrunala (8 Parts) is useful in the treatment of Paittika and Kaphaja types of Kustha [130]

यष्ट्याह्व लोध्र पद्मक पटोल पिचुमर्द चन्दनरसाश्च|
स्नाने पाने च हिताः सुशीतलाः पित्तकुष्ठिभ्यः॥१३१॥

The decoction of
Yastyahva – Licorice
Lodhra – Symplocos racemosa
Padmaka – Wild Himalayan Cherry – Prunus cerasoides
Patola – Pointed gourd
Pichumarda – Neem and
Chandana – Santalum album is exceedingly cooling and it is useful for bath and drink of patients suffering from Paittika type of Kustha (skin diseases). [131]

Alepana:
आलेपनं प्रियङ्गु हरेणुका वत्सकस्य च फलानि|
सातिविषा च ससेव्या सचन्दना रोहिणी कटुका||१३२||

Application of the paste of

Priyangu

Harenuka

Fruits of Vatsaka

Ativisa

Sevya

Chandana – Santalum album and

Katurohini is similarly useful in the treatment of Paittika type of Kustha. [132]

तिक्त घृतैर्धौतघृतैरभ्यङ्गो दह्यमानकुष्ठेषु|
तैलैश्चन्दन मधुक प्रपौण्डरीकोत्पलयुतैश्च||१३३||

If there is burning sensation over the patches of Kustha, then area is massaged with

Tiktaghrta (vide- verses 140-143 and 144-150),

Dhautaghrta (Ghee washed with water for 100 or 1000 times, vide-Vrhat nighantu Ratnakara: Visarpa cikitsa) or with the oil boiled with

Chandana – Santalum album

Madhuka – Madhuca longifolia

Prapaundarika and

Utpala [133]

क्लेदे प्रपतति चाङ्गे दाहे विस्फोटके सचर्मदले|
शीता: प्रदेहसेका व्यधो विरेको घृतं तिक्तम्||१३४||

If there is Kleda (stickness or sloughing) falling out of the body (like finger etc) or burning sensation, and in Visphotaka, (pustular eruption) as well as charmadala types of Kustha, application of cooling ointments, sprinkling of cooking Liquids' venesection, purgation and use of Tiktakaghrta (vide- Verses 140-143 and 144-150 are useful. [134]

खदिरघृतं निम्बघृतं दार्वीघृतमुत्तमं पटोलघृतम्|
कुष्ठेषु रक्तपित्त प्रबलेषु भिषग्जितं सिद्धम्||१३५||

If Kustha (skin diseases) is dominated by Rakta and Pitta, then for its treatment,

Khadiraghrta

Nimbaghrta

Darvighrta and

Patolaghrta is used.

These are the well established and excellent recipes [135]

त्रिफलात्वचोऽर्धपलिका: पटोलपत्रं च कार्षिका: शेषा:|
कटुरोहिणी सनिम्बा यष्ट्याह्वा त्रायमाणा च||१३६||
एष कषाय: साध्यो दत्वा द्विपलं मसूरविदलानाम्|
सलिलाढकेऽष्टभागे शेषे पूतो रसो ग्राह्य:||१३७||
ते च कषायेऽष्टपले चतुष्पलं सर्पिषश्च पक्तव्यम्|
यावत्स्यादष्टपलं शेषं पेयं तत: कोष्णम्||१३८||
तद्वातपित्तकुष्ठं वीसर्पं वातशोणितं प्रबलम्|

ज्वर दाहगुल्म विद्रधि विभ्रमविस्फोटकान् हन्ति॥१३९॥

1/2 Pala of each of

Haritaki (fruits- Pulp)

Bibhitaki (fruits Pulp)

Amalaki (fruits-pulp) and

Patola

1 Karsa of Each of

Katurohini

Nimba

Yasti and

Trayamana, and

2 Palas of

Dehusked seeds of Masura is boiled into 1 Adhaka of water and reduced to 1/8th.

The decoction should then be collected by straining through a cloth.

In this decoction (8 palas), 4 Palas of ghee is added and cooked till 1/4th remains.

This medicated ghee is given internally while it is luke-warm.

It cures

Kustha (skin diseases) caused by Vayu ad Pitta,

Visarpa (erysipelas)

Serious type of Vatarakta (gout),

Jwara – fever,

Daha – burning sensation,

Gulma – phantom tumor

Abscess

Giddiness and

Visphotaka – pustlar eruptions [136- 139]

Tikta shatpala ghrita

निम्ब पटोलं दार्वीं दुरालभां तिक्तरोहिणीं त्रिफलाम्।
कुर्यादर्धदलांशं पर्पटकं त्रायमाणां च॥१४०॥
सलिलाढकसिद्धानां रसेऽष्टभागस्थिते क्षिपेत् पूते।
चन्दन किराततिक्तक मागधिकास्त्रायमाणां च॥१४१॥
मुस्तं वत्सकबीजं कल्कीकृत्यार्धकार्षिकान् भागान्।
नवसर्पिषश्च षट्पलमेतत्सिद्धं घृतं पेयम्॥१४२॥
कुष्ठ ज्वर गुल्मार्शो ग्रहणी पाण्ड्वामयश्वयथुहारि।
पामा विसर्प पिडका कण्डूमदगण्डनुत्सिद्धम्॥१४३॥
इति तिक्तषट्पलकं घृतम्।

1/2 Palas of

Nimba – Azadirachta indica

Patola – Trichosanthes dioica

Daruharidra – Berberis aristata

Duralabha –

Tiktarohini –

Triphala (Haritaki, Bhibitaki and amalaki),

Parpataka and

Trayamana is boiled with 2 Adhakas of water till 1/8th remains.

The decoction is strained out, and to this, the paste of 1/2 Karsa of each of

Chandana – Santalum album
Kiratatikta – Swertia chirata
Pippali – Piper longum
Trayamana – Gentiana kurroa
Musta – Cyperus rotundus and
Seeds of Vatsaka – and
6 Palas of freshly collected ghee is added and cooked
This medicated ghee is useful in the treatment of
Kustha (obstinate skin diseases including leprosy)
Jwara – fever
Gulma – phantom tumour
Arshas – piles
Scabies
Visarpa – Erysipelas
Pidaka -Pimples
Kandu – itching
Mada or Unmada – insanity and
Ganda (scrofula) [140-143]

Mahatiktaka ghrita:

सप्तच्छदं प्रतिविषां शम्पाकं तिक्तरोहिणीं पाठाम्।
मुस्तमुशीरं त्रिफलां पटोल पिचुमर्द पर्पटकम्॥१४४॥
धन्वयवासं चन्दनमुपकुल्यां पद्मकं हरिद्रे द्वे।
षड्ग्रन्थां सविशालां शतावरीं सारिवे चोभे॥१४५॥
वत्सकबीजं यासं मूर्वाममृतां किराततिक्तं च।
कल्कान् कुर्यान्मतिमान्यष्ट्याह्वं त्रायमाणां च॥१४६॥
कल्कश्चातुर्भागो जलमष्टगुणं रसोऽमृतफलानाम्।
द्विगुणो घृतात्प्रदेयस्तत्सर्पिः पाययेत्सिद्धम्॥१४७॥
कुष्ठानि रक्तपित्त प्रबलान्यर्शांसि रक्तवाहीनि।
वीसर्पमम्लपित्तं वातासृक् पाण्डुरोगं च॥१४८॥
विस्फोटकान्सपामानुन्मादं कामलां ज्वरं कण्डूम्।
हृद्रोग गुल्म पिडका असृग्दरं गण्दमालां च॥१४९॥
हन्यादेतत् सर्पिः पीतं काले यथाबलं सद्यः।
योगशतैरप्यजितान्महाविकारान्महातिक्तम्॥१५०॥
इति महातिक्तकं घृतम्।

The paste of all these drugs is taken in the quantity of 1/4th part of ghee:
Saptacchada
Prativisa
Sampaka (Aragvadha) –Cassia fistula
Tiktarohini
Patha – Cyclea peltata
Musta – Cyperus rotundus
Usira – Vetiveria zizanioides
Triphala (haritaki, Bibitaki and amalaka)
Patola – Tricosanthes dioica
Pichumarda
Parpataka

Dhanvayavasa
Chandana – Santalum album
Upakulya (Pippali) – Piper nigrum
Padmaka
Haridra – Curcuma longa
Daruharidra – Berberis aristata
Sadgrantha
Visala
Shatavari – Asparagus racemosus
2 varieties of sariva (Krsna and Sveta) – Hemidesmus indicus
Seeds of vatsaka
Yasa
Murva – Marsedenia tenacissima
Amrta – Tinospora cordifolia
Kiratatikta – Swertia chirata
Yastimadhu – Glycyrrhiza glabra and
Trayamana – Gentiana kurroa
To this,
Ghee (1 part)
Water (8 parts) and
The juice of Amrtaphala or amalaki (2 Palas) is added and cooked
Administration of this medicated ghee cures
Kustha (skin diseases)
Raktapitta (an ailment characterized by bleeding from different parts of the body)
Serious types of piles with bleeding
Visarpa (erysipelas)
Amlapitta (acidity in the stomach)
Vatarakta – gout
Pandu – Anemia
Visphotaka – Pustular eruption
Pama – Scabies
Unmada – insanity
Kamala –Jaundice
Jwara – fever
Kandu – itching
Hrdroga- heart disease
Gulma – Phantom tumor
Pidaka – pimples
Asrgdara – menorrhagia
Gandamala – Scrofula
This ghee is administered in appropriate time and suitable time in accordance with the strength of the patient.
It immediately cures the above mentioned illness even if they are not cured by hundreds of other recipes. This is called Mahatiktakagrta [144-150]

दोषे हृतेऽपनीते रक्ते बाह्यान्तरे कृते शमने ।
स्नेहे च कालयुक्ते न कुष्ठमनुवर्तते साध्यम्।।१५१।।

By the elimination of vitiated Doshas, bloodletting, external and internal administration of alleviation therapies and administration of medicated ghee in appropriate time, the curable types of Kustha (skin diseases) get (finally) cured.

[151]

Mahakhadira Ghrita:

खदिरस्य तुलाः पञ्च शिंशपासनयोस्तुले।
तुलार्धाः सर्व एवैते करञ्जारिष्टवेतसाः॥१५२॥
पर्पटः कुटजश्चैव वृषः कृमिहरस्तथा।
हरिद्रे कृतमालश्च गुडूची त्रिफला त्रिवृत्॥१५३॥
सप्तपर्णश्च सङ्क्षुण्णा दशद्रोणेषु वारिणः।
अष्टभागावशेषं तु कषायमवतारयेत्॥१५४॥
धात्रीरसं च तुल्यांशं सर्पिषश्चाढकं पचेत्।
महातिक्तक कल्कैस्तु यथोक्तैः पलसम्मितैः॥१५५॥
निहन्ति सर्वकुष्ठानि पानाभ्यङ्गनिषेवणात्।
महाखदिरमित्येतत् परं कुष्ठविकारनुत्॥१५६॥
इति महाखदिरं घृतम्।

5 Tulas of Khadira – Acacia catechu

1 Tula of Simsapa – Dalbergia sissoo

1 Tula of Asana and

1/2 Tula of each of

Karanja – Nerium indicum

Arista (nimbi)

Vetasa

Parpata

Kutaja – Holarrhena antidysenterica

Vrsa

Krimihara (Vidanga) – Embelia ribes

Haridra – Curcuma longa

Daruharidra – Berberis aristata

Krtamala

Guduchi – Tinospora cordifolia

Triphala (Haritakai, Bibhitaki, and amalaki)

Trivrt – Operculina turpethum and

Saptaparna – Alstonia scholaris is made to a coarse powder and

Boiled by adding 10 Dronas of water till 1/8th remains.

To this decoction,

1 Adhaka juice of Dhatri

1 adhaka ghee and

1 Pala paste of each of

Saptaparna – Alstonia schloris

Prativisa

Sampaka (Aragvadha) – Cassia fistula

Tiktarohini

Patha – Cyclea peltata

Musta – Cyperus rotundus

Usira – Vetiveria zizanoides

Triphala (Haritaki, Bibhitaki and Amalaki)

Patola – Tricosanthes dioica

Pichumarda

Parpataka
Dhanvayavasaka
Chandana – Santalum album
Upakulya (Pippali) – Piper longum
Padmaka
Haridra – Curcuma longa
Daruharidra – Berberis aristata
Sadgrantha
Visala
Shatavari – Asparagus racemosus
Both the varieties of Sariva (Krsna and Sveta) – Hemidesmus indicus
Seeds of Vatsaka
Yasa
Murva
Amrta – Tinospora cordifolia
Kiratatika – Swertia chirata
Yastimadhu – Glycyyrhiza glabra and
Trayamana is added and cooked
This medicated ghee, know as Mahakhadiraghrta, cures all types of
Kustha (skin diseases) by internal intake and massage [152-156]

Recipe for bath etc:

प्रपतत्सु लसीका प्रसुतेषु गात्रेषु जन्तुजग्धेषु|
मूत्रं निम्बविडङ्गे स्नानं पानं प्रदेहश्च||१५७||

If the fingers etc., of the patient get separated by sloughing, if there is serous exudation and if maggots are formed in the ulcers, then the patient suffering from Kustha is give cow urine, nimbi and Vidanga [in appropriate form] for bath, pana (internal intake) and Pradeha (external application of thick ointment). [157]

वृष कुटज सप्तपर्णाः करवीर करञ्ज निम्ब खदिराश्च|
स्नाने पाने लेपे क्रिमिकुष्ठनुदः सगोमूत्राः||१५८||

Vrusha (Vasa), Kutaja, Saptaparna, Karvira, Karanja, Nimba and Khadira along with cow- urine is used for bath, Pana (internal intake), and Lepa (external application).
This cures Krmi (parasitic infestion) and Kustha (skin diseases). [158]

Use of Vidanga and Khadira:

पानाहार विधाने प्रसेचने धूपने प्रदेहे च|
कृमिनाशनं विडङ्गं विशिष्यते कुष्ठहा खदिरः||१५९||

Vidanga which is effective in destroying Krmi (Parasites) and Khadira which cures Kustha (skin diseases) are useful for the patient of Kustha.
These 2 drugs are to be used [in suitable form] for the preparation of food and drinks, Prasecana (sprinkling), Dhupana (fumination) and Pradeha (application of thick ointment).
The latter, viz Khadira is especially useful in the treatment of Kustha. [159]

Recipe:

एडगजः सविडङ्गो मूलान्यारग्वधस्य कुष्ठानाम्|
उद्दालनं श्वदन्ता गोश्ववराहोष्ट्रदन्ताश्च||१६०||

Edagaja

Vidanga – Embelia ribes
Roots of Aragvadha – Cassia fistula and
Teeth of dog, cow, horse, boar and camel
Are useful in curing Kustha (skin diseases) [160]

Recipe:

एदगजः सविडङ्गो द्वे च निशे राजवृक्षमूलं च।
कुष्ठोद्दालनमग्र्यं सपिप्पलीपाकलं योज्यम्||१६१||

Use of
Edagaja,
Vidanga,
Haridra,
Daruharidra,
root of Rajavrksa,
Pippali and
Pakala (Kustha) are exceedingly useful in the treatment of Kustha (obstinate skin disease including leprosy). [161]

Treatment of Leucoderma
Use of Udumbara for Purgation:

श्वित्राणां सविशेषं योक्तव्यं सर्वतो विशुद्धानाम्।
श्वित्रे संसनमग्र्यं मलपूरस इष्यते सगुडः||१६२||
तं पीत्वा सुस्निग्धो यथाबलं सूर्यपादसन्तापम्।
संसेवेत विरिक्तस्त्र्यहं पिपासुः पिबेत् पेयाम्||१६३||

The patient of Svitra (Leucoderma) is cleansed by the administration of elimination therapies, and thereafter, the following therapy is employed:
The jucie of Malapu (Kakodumbarika) along with Jaggery is excellent for causing Sramsana (a type of purgation) for a patient suffering from leucoderma.
The patient should first of all take oleation therapy, therafter; this recipe is given according to the strength of the patient.
After the administration of this recipe, the patient should expose himself to the heat of the sun.
This will cause purgation.
Pathya: After this purgation therapy, the patient will feel thirsty for which he is given Peya (thin Gruel) for three days. [162- 163]

Treatment of Pustular eruptions in Leucoderma:

श्वित्रेऽङ्गे ये स्फोटा जायन्ते कण्टकेन तान्भिन्द्यात्।
स्फोटेषु विस्रुतेषु प्रातः प्रातः पिबेत् पक्षम्||१६४||
मलपूमसनं प्रियङ्गुं शतपुष्पां चाम्भसा समुत्क्वाथ्य।
पालाशं वा क्षारं यथाबलं फाणितोपेतम्||१६५||

Pustular eruptions over the patches of leucoderma are punctuered with the help of a thorn for the removal of serous fluid from these pustules.
After the exudation of the fluid, the patient should take every morning, contionuously for 15 days, the decoction of Malapya (kakodumbarika), Asana, Priyangu and Satapuspa prepared by boiling with water.
Alternatively, he may take the Ksara (alkali preparation) of Palasa along with Phanita (a type of sugar) in a dose appropriate to his strength. [164-165]

Use of Khadira:

यच्चान्यत् कुष्ठघ्नं श्वित्राणां सर्वमेव तच्छस्तम्|
खदिरोदक संयुक्तं खदिरोदकपानग्र्यं वा||१६६||

All the recipes prescribed for the treatment of Kustha (skin diseases) are also useful for the treatment of Leucoderma.

Among them, drinks prepared of Khadira or mixed with the decoction of Khadira are excellent for the cure of leucoderma. [166]

Recipes for external Application:

समनःशिलं विडङ्गं कासीसं रोचनां कनकपुष्पीम्|
श्वित्राणां प्रशमार्थं ससैन्धवं लेपनं दद्यात्||१६७||

Manashila

Vidanga – Embelia ribes

Kasisa

Gorochana

Kanakapuspi (Svarnaksiri) and

Rock salt is used for external applkication in the treatment of Leucoderma [167]

Medicine for external application:

कदलीक्षारयुतं वा खरास्थि दग्धं गवां रुधिरयुक्तम्|
हस्तिमदाध्युषितं वा मालत्याः कोरकक्षारम्||१६८||
नीलोत्पलं सकुष्ठं ससैन्धवं हस्तिमूत्रपिष्टं वा|
मूलकबीजावल्गुजलेपः पिष्टो गवां मूत्रे||१६९||
काकोदुम्बरिका वा सावल्गुजचित्रका गवां मूत्रे|
पिष्टा मनःशिला वा संयुक्ता बर्हिपित्तेन||१७०||
लेपः किलासहन्ता बीजान्यावल्गुजानि लाक्षा च|
गोपित्तमञ्जने द्वे पिप्पल्यः काललोहरजः||१७१||

The following recipe is used for external application in the treatment of Leucoderma:

1. the ashes of the bone of ass mixed with the Ksara (alkali prepared) of Kadali and the blood of cattle,

2. Ksara (alkali preparation) of the bud of Malati mixed with Hastimada (rut of elephant)

3. Nilotpala, Kustha and Saindava made to a paste by adding urine of elephant

4. seeds of Mulaka and Avalguja made to a paste by adding cow-urine

5. Kakodumbara, Avalguja and Citraka made to a paste by adding cow-urine

6. Manahsila made to a paste by adding pea-cock bile and

7. Seeds of Avalguja, Laksa, cow-bile, both the type of Anjana (Sauviranjana and Rasanjana), Pippali and the powder (bhasma) of Kalaloha (black iron). [168- 171]

शुद्ध्या शोणितमोक्षैर्विरूक्षणैर्भक्षणैश्च सक्तूनाम्|
श्वित्रं कस्यचिदेव प्रणश्यति क्षीणपापस्य||१७२||

In very rare cases, patients of Leucoderma, who are free from the effects of their sinful acts get cured by the administration of elimination therapies, bloodletting and intake of unctuous food like Saktu (roasted corn flour) [172]

Varieties:

दारुणं चारुणं श्वित्रं किलासं नामभिस्त्रिभिः|
विज्ञेयं त्रिविधं तच्च त्रिदोषं प्रायशश्च तत्||१७३||
दोषे रक्ताश्रिते रक्तं ताम्रं मांससमाश्रिते|

श्वेतं मेदःश्रिते शिवत्रं गुरु तच्चोतरोतरम्||१७४||

Svitra (Leucodernma) is of 3 varieties, namely,

• Daruna,

• Charuna, and

• Kilasa.

All of them are generally caused by the simultaneous vitiations of all the 3 Doshas.

If located in Rakta (blood) it is red in colour,

If in Mamsa (muscle tissue), it is of coppery colour, and

If located in medas (fat) it is white in color.

The subsequent ones are more serious than the previous ones. [173-174]

Prognosis:

यत् परस्परतोऽभिन्नं बहु यद्रक्तलोमवत्|

यच्च वर्षगणोत्पन्नं तच्छिवत्रं नैव सिध्यति||१७५||

अरक्तलोम तनु यत् पाण्डु नातिचिरोत्थितम्|

मध्यावकाशे चोच्छूनं शिवत्रं तत्साध्यमुच्यते||१७६||

If the patches of Svitra (leucoderma) are matted together, if there are several patches, if the small hair over the patches are red in color and if the patient is suffering from this disease for several years, then this is incurable.

If the small hairs over the patches are not red, if the skin is thin white, if the disease is of recent origin and if the space between two patches is elevated, then the disease is curable. [175-176]

Causative Factors

वचांस्यतथ्यानि कृतघ्नभावो निन्दा सुराणां गुरुधर्षणं च|

पापक्रिया पूर्वकृतं च कर्म हेतुः किलासस्य विरोधि चान्नम्||१७७||

Untruthfulness, Ungratefulness, Disrespect for the Gods, insult of the preceptors, sinful acts, misdeeds of past lives and intake of mutually contradictory food are the causative factors of Kilasa (Leucoderma). [177]

तत्र श्लोकाः:-

हेतुर्द्रव्यं लिङ्गं विविधं ये येषु चाधिका दोषाः|

कुष्ठेषु दोषलिङ्गं समासतो दोषनिर्देशः||१७८||

साध्यमसाध्यं कृच्छ्रं कुष्ठं कुष्ठापहाश्च ये योगाः|

सिद्धाः किलासहेतुर्लिङ्गं गुरुलाघवं तथा शान्तिः||१७९||

इति सङ्ग्रहः प्रणीतो महर्षिणा कुष्ठनाशनेऽध्याये|

स्मृतिबुद्धिवर्धनार्थं शिष्याय हुताशवेशाय||१८०||

Summary:

The sage (Lord Punarvasu), in this chapter has explained various details on the treatment of Kustha (skin diseases) with a view to sharpening the memory and intellect of the disciple Agnivesa. These details are as follows:

1. Hetu (Etiology)

2. Dravya(pathogenic substance)

3. Various signs and symptoms

4. Predominace of Various Doshas in different types of Kustha

5. signs and symptoms manifested in different types of Kustha

6. a brief description of the aggravated Doshas

7. curability and incurability of Kustha

8. cases of Kustha which are difficult of cure

9. various well established recipes for the cure of Kustha

10. etiology and signs as well as symptoms of Kilasa

11. incurability and curability of Kilasa and

12. therapies for the treatment of Kilasa [178- 180]

इत्यग्निवेशकृते तन्त्रे चरकप्रतिसंस्कृते चिकित्सितस्थाने कुष्ठचिकित्सितं नाम सप्तमोऽध्यायः||७||

Thu ends the seventh chapter on the treatment of Kustha (skin diseases) of the Chikitsa section of Agnivesa's work as redacted by Charaka

14

Chikitsasthana Chapter 8
Rajayakshma Chikitsitam

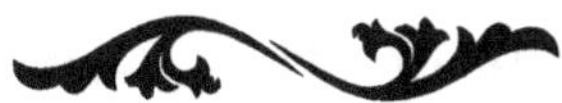

The 8th chapter of Charaka Samhita Chikitsa Sthana is called Rajayakshma Chikitsa Adhyaya. Rajayaksma refers to a set of chronic respiratory disorders including tuberculosis.

Treatment of Rajayakshma – Tuberculosis

अथातो राजयक्ष्म चिकित्सितं व्याख्यास्यामः||१||

इति ह स्माह भगवानात्रेयः||२||

Let us expound the chapter on the treatment of Rajayakshma.Thus, said Lord Atreya [1-2]

Mythological Origin of Rajyaksma:

दिवौकसां कथयतामृषिभिर्वै श्रुता कथा|

काम व्यसन संयुक्ता पौराणी शशिनं प्रति||३||

रोहिण्यामतिसक्तस्य शरीरं नानुरक्षतः|

आजगामाल्पतामिन्दोर्देहः स्नेहपरिक्षयात्||४||

दुहितृणामसम्भोगाच्छेषाणां च प्रजापतेः|

क्रोधो निःश्वासरूपेण मूर्तिमान् निःसृतो मुखात्||५||

प्रजापतेर्हि दुहितृरष्टाविंशतिमंशुमान्|

भार्यार्थं प्रतिजग्राह न च सर्वास्ववर्तत||६||

गुरुणा तमवध्यातं भार्यास्वसमवर्तिनम्|

रजःपरीतमबलं यक्ष्मा शशिनमाविशत्||७||

सोऽभिभूतोऽतिमहता गुरुक्रोधेन निष्प्रभः|

देवदेवर्षिसहितो जगाम शरणं गुरुम्||८||

अथ चन्द्रमसः शुद्धां मतिं बुद्ध्वा प्रजापतिः|

प्रसादं कृतवान् सोमस्ततोऽश्विभ्यां चिकित्सितः||९||

स विमुक्तग्रहश्चन्द्रो विरराज विशेषतः|

ओजसा वर्धितोऽश्विभ्यां शुद्धं सत्त्वमवाप च||१०||

क्रोधो यक्ष्मा ज्वरो रोग एकार्थो दुःखसञ्ज्ञकः|

यस्मात् स राज्ञः प्रागासीद्राजयक्ष्मा ततो मतः||११||

स यक्ष्मा हुङ्कृतोऽश्विभ्यां मानुष लोकमागतः|

लब्ध्वा चतुर्विधं हेतुं समाविशति मानवान्||१२||

The mythological story narrated by the Gods to the sages regarding origin of Rajayakshma relates to the habitual sex indulgence of Chandra (the moon). The moon being exceedingly attached to Rohini – nakshtra (the star Aldebaram) did not care for his health. He became emaciated due to the depletion of unctuousness. He was, therefore, not able to satisfy the sexual urge of the rest of the daughters of Daksha Prajapati. Therefore, Daksha's anger came out of his mouth in the form of breath and took a physical form.

The moon had earlier been married to the 28 daughters of Prajapati but failed sexually. So, the moon was afflicted by Rajayakshma as a result of Daksha's expression of anger. Moon's discriminatory treatment with his wives and the resultant preponderance of Rajas (the second Guna representing passionate disposition) as well as weakness, being subdued by the excessive anger of Daksha, the moon was depleted of his complexion.

Accompanied by the gods and godly sages, Daksha was treated with the twin doctors of Gods – Ashwini Kumaras. Moon's vitality (Ojas) was enhanced, he became free from ailments, became gifted with complexion and attained purity of mind (Shuddha Sattva)

क्रोधो यक्ष्मा ज्वरो रोग एकार्थो दुःखसञ्ज्ञकः।

The words Krodha, Yakshma, Jvara and Roga are all synonymous, and they connote Duhkha (misery).

Since it inflicted misery (Yakshma) upon the Rajan or the king [of stars], the ailment is known as Raja- Yakshma. This Rajayakshma, being ousted [from the heaven] by the 2 Asvins, came down to the world of human beings. Thus, this disease afflicts human beings activated by the 4- fold causative factors. [3-12]

Rajayakshma Nidana – Four fold causative factors:

अयथाबलमारम्भं वेगसन्धारणं क्षयम्।
यक्ष्मणः कारणं विद्याच्चतुर्थं विषमाशनम्॥१३॥

The causative factors of the Rajayakshma are of 4 categories, namely

1. Ayatha balam aarambham – Over excretion (exceeding one's own capacity)
2. Vega sandharana – Suppression of natural urges
3. Kshaya – Depletion of tissue elements'
4. Vishamashanam – Irregular dieting [13]

Etiology of Rajayakshma caused by Over- exertion:

युद्धाध्ययनभाराध्वलङ्घनप्लवनादिभिः।
पतनैरभिघातैर्वा साहसैर्वा तथापरैः॥१४॥
अयथाबलमारम्भैर्जन्तोरुरसि विक्षते।
वायुः प्रकुपितो दोषावुदीर्योभौ प्रधावति॥१५॥

Vata gets aggravated due to chest injury caused by

Yuddha – fighting,

Adhyayana – reading (reciting Mantras) loudly,

Bhara – carrying excessive weight,

Adhva – walking long distance,

Langhana – observing fast for a long time,

Plavana – excess swimming,

Patana – falls,

Abhighata – assault and other forms of over exertion exceeding one's own capacity.

The above activities aggravate Vata dosha. Vata in turn stimulates Pitta and Kapha and rapidly circulates all over the body (Pradhavati).[14 - 15]

11 Symptoms of Rajayakshma caused due to excess physical exertion:

स शिरःस्थः शिरःशूलं करोति गलमाश्रितः।
कण्ठोद्ध्वंसं च कासं च स्वरभेदमरोचकम्॥१६॥
पार्श्वशूलं च पार्श्वस्थो वर्चोभेदं गुदे स्थितः।
जृम्भां ज्वरं च सन्धिस्थ उरःस्थश्चोरसो रुजम्॥१७॥

क्षणनादुरसः कासात् कफं ष्ठीवेत् सशोणितम्|
जर्जरेणोरसा कृच्छ्रमुरःशूलातिपीडितः||१८||
इति साहसिको यक्ष्मा रूपैरेतैः प्रपद्यते|
एकादशभिरात्मज्ञो भजेतस्मान्न साहसम्||१९||

When the aggravated Vata Dosha is located in head, it causes –

1. Shiro ruja – Headache

When located in the throat it causes

2. Kantho dvamsa – Irritation in the throat, loss of voice

3. Kasa – Cough

4. Svara bhedam- Hoarseness of voice and

5. Aruchi – Anorexia

When located in the sides of the chest, it causes

6. Parsvasula (pain in the sides of the chest)

When located in the anus, it causes

7. Atisara – Diarrhea

When located in the joints, it causes

8. Yawning and

9. Jwara – Fever and

When located in the chest, it causes

10. Ura shoola – Pain in the chest.

Because of the injury to the chest, as well as coughing,

11. The patient spits out phlegm along with blood

Thus the patient suffers from unbearable pain in his chest die to the pulmonary damage (Jarjarena Urasa).

These 11 symptoms mentioned above are manifested in the patients suffering from Yakshma (tuberculosis) caused by over- exertion. Therefore, a wise person should not indulge in over- exertion. [16 -19]

Causes of Rajayakshma caused by suppression of natural urges:

ह्रीमत्त्वाद्वा घृणित्वाद्वा भयाद्वा वेगमागतम्|
वातमूत्रपुरीषाणां निगृह्णाति यदा नरः||२०||
तदा वेगप्रतीघातात् कफपित्ते समीरयन्|
ऊर्ध्वं तिर्यगधश्चैव विकारान् कुरुतेऽनिलः||२१||

When a person suppresses the manifested natural urges of flatus, urine and stool because of bashfulness, aversion and fear, the Vata gets aggravated due to obstruction to its movement, and it aggravates Kapha, Pitta along with Vata Dosha.

This aggravated Vayu, moving upwards, downwards and side wards, causes 11 symptoms or disorders as below.[20-21]

11 symptoms of Rajayakshma caused due to suppression of natural urges:

प्रतिश्यायं च कासं च स्वरभेदमरोचकम्|
पार्श्वशूलं शिरःशूलं ज्वरमंसावमर्दनम्||२२||
अङ्गमर्दं मुहुश्छर्दिं वर्चोभेदं त्रिलक्षणम्|
रूपाण्येकादशैतानि यक्ष्मा यैरुच्यते महान्||२३||

namely

1. Pratishyaya - Coryza

2. Kasa – Cough

3. Svara bheda – Hoarseness of voice

4. Aruchi – Anorexia

5. Parshva shula – Pain in the sides of the chest

6. Shiro ruja – Headache

7. Jwara – Fever

8. Amsa avamardanam – Kneading pain in the shoulder region

9. Anga mardam – Malaise

10. Muhur chardi – Frequent vomiting and

11. Varcho bhedam – Diarrhoea having the signs and symptoms of all the 3 Doshas. [22-23]

Causes of Rajayakshma caused by Kshaya (Diminution of Tissues):

ईर्ष्योत्कण्ठाभय त्रास क्रोध शोकातिकर्शनात्।

अतिव्यवायानशनाच्छुक्रमोजश्च हीयते॥२४॥

ततः स्नेहक्षयाद्वायुवृद्धो दोषावुदीरयन्॥

Shukra (semen) and Ojas (immune system) get diminished because of excessive emaciation as a result of jealousy, anxiety, fear, apprehension, anger, grief, excessive indulgence in sex, fasting and intake of less nourishing food and aggravation of Vata Dosha.

This aggravated Pitta and Kapha, and produced 11 signs and symptoms as below.[24 - 25 1/2]

11 Symptoms of Rajayakshma caused due to Kshaya – tissue depletion:

प्रतिश्यायं ज्वरं कासमङ्गमर्दं शिरोरुजम्॥२५॥

श्वासं विड्भेदमरुचिं पार्श्वशूलं स्वरक्षयम्।

करोति चांससन्तापमेकादशगदानिमान् ॥२६॥

लिङ्गान्यावेदयन्त्येतान्येकादश महागदम्।

सम्प्राप्तं राजयक्ष्माणं क्षयात् प्राणक्षयप्रदम्॥२७॥

1. Pratishyaya (coryza)

2. Jwara – Fever

3. Kasa – Cough

4. Anga marda – Malaise

5. Shiro ruja – Headache

6. Shwasa – Dyspnoea

7. Vit bheda – Diarrhea

8. Aruchi – Anorexia

9. Parshva shula -Pain in the chest

10. Svara kshayam – Aphasia

11. Burning sensation in the shoulder region. [25 1/2 -27]

Causes of Rajayakshma caused by Vishamashana (Diet irregularities):

विविधान्यन्नपानानि वैषम्येण समश्नतः।

जनयन्त्यामयान् घोरान्विषमान्मारुतादयः॥२८॥

स्रोतांसि रुधिरादीनां वैषम्यादिविषमं गताः।

रुद्ध्वा रोगाय कल्पन्ते पुष्यन्ति च न धातवः॥२९॥

Irregularity in intake of foods and drinks leads to Vata aggravation, resulting in the manifestation of acute diseases with irregular increase of Doshas.

The aggravated Doshas caused due to food irregularities obstruct Srotas – channels of tissues like blood channels. This causes obstruction to flow of nutrition from one Dhatu (tissue) to the other leading to tissue depletion. This leads to manifestation of below 11 symptoms:[28 -29]

11 symptoms of Rajayakshma caused due to Vishamashana – irregular diet:

प्रतिश्यायं प्रसेकं च कासं छर्दिमरोचकम्।
ज्वरमंसाभितापं च छर्दनं रुधिरस्य च॥३०॥
पार्श्वशूलं शिरःशूलं स्वरभेदमथापि च।
कफपित्तानिलकृतं लिङ्गं विद्याद्यथाक्रमम्॥३१॥
इति व्याधिसमूहस्य रोगराजस्य हेतुजम्।
रूपमेकादशविधं हेतुश्चोक्तश्चतुर्विधः॥३२॥

(1) Pratishyaya – coryza

(2) Praseka – excessive salivation

(3) Kasa – Cough

(4) Chardi – Vomiting and

(5) Aruchi – Anorexia the aggravated Pitta causes

(6) Jwara – Fever

(7) Mamsa abhitapa – Burning sensation in the shoulders and

(8) Rudhira Chardi – Hemoptysis and the aggravated Vayu causes

(9) Parshva shula – Pain in the sides of the chest

(10) Shira shula – Headache and

(11) Svara bheda – Hoarseness of voice

Thus, Rajayakshma being a conglomeration of several diseases is manifested in 11 forms depending upon 4 fold causative factors. [28-32]

Rajayaksma Purvaroopa- Premonitory Signs and symptoms:

पूर्वरूपं प्रतिश्यायो दौर्बल्यं दोषदर्शनम्।
अदोषेष्वपि भावेषु काये बीभत्सदर्शनम्॥३३॥
घृणित्वमशनतश्चापि बलमांसपरिक्षयः।
स्त्रीमद्यमांसप्रियता प्रियता चावगुण्ठने॥३४॥
मक्षिकाघुणकेशानां तृणानां पतनानि च।
प्रायोऽन्नपाने केशानां नखानां चाभिवर्धनम्॥३५॥
पतत्रिभिः पतङ्गैश्च श्वापदैश्चाभिधर्षणम्।
स्वप्ने केशास्थिराशीनां भस्मनश्चाधिरोहणम्॥३६॥
जलाशयानां शैलानां वनानां ज्योतिषामपि।
शुष्यतां क्षीयमाणानां पततां यच्च दर्शनम्॥३७॥
प्रागूपं बहुरूपस्य तज्ज्ञेयं राजयक्ष्मणः॥३८॥

The following are the premonitory signs and symptoms of Rajayakshma having several varieties.

1. Pratishyaya (Coryza) and Daurbalyam – weakness

2. Dosha darshanam – Finding fault with right things

3. Beebhatsa darshanam – Appearance of ugly signs and symptoms in the body

4. Ghrunitvam Ashnataha – Feeling of disgust towards food

5. Bala mamsa kshaya – Diminution of strength and muscle tissue

6. Stri madya mamsa priyata – Liking towards women, alcohol and meat

7. Priyata avaghuntane – Liking for isolation

8. His food and drinks are infested with the fall of flies insects, hair and nails

9. Assault by birds, wasps and animals

10. Climbing of heaps of hair, bones and ashes in dreams and

11. Dreams of ponds, mountains and forests, which are already dried, or getting dried and the fall of planets. [33-38]

Rajayakshma Samprapti – Patho-physiology:

रूपं त्वस्य यथोद्देशं निर्देक्ष्यामि सभेषजम्॥३८॥
यथास्वेनोष्मणा पाकं शारीरा यान्ति धातवः|
स्रोतसा च यथास्वेन धातुः पुष्यति धातुतः॥३९॥
स्रोतसां सन्निरोधाच्च रक्तादीनां च सङ्क्षयात्|
धातूष्मणां चापचयाद्राजयक्ष्मा प्रवर्तते॥४०॥
तस्मिन् काले पचत्यग्निर्यदन्नं कोष्ठसंश्रितम्|
मलीभवति तत् प्रायः कल्पते किञ्चिदोजसे॥४१॥
तस्मात् पुरीषं संरक्ष्यं विशेषाद्राजयक्ष्मिणः|
सर्वधातुक्षयार्तस्य बलं तस्य हि विड्बलम्॥४२॥
रसः स्रोतःसु रुद्धेषु स्वस्थानस्थो विदह्यते |
स ऊर्ध्वं कासवेगेन बहुरूपः प्रवर्तते॥४३॥

Patho-physiology:

Now we shall describe details of signs and symptoms along with remedies of this disease.

The Dhatus (tissues) get nourished with the help of their own Dhatu agni. Rasa dhatu digests food to nourish Rasa Dhatu by means of Rasa Dhatu agni, Rakta gets nourished with the help of Rakta Dhatu agni and so on.

Read related: Understanding Digestion Process From An Ayurveda View

But when there is obstruction of Rasavaha srotas, the rest of the Dhatus lack nourishment (Viz Rakta, Mamsa, Meda, Asthi, Majja and Shukra). Read here to understand Dhatu – tissues)

When Dhatus lack nourishment, they undergo Kshaya – depletion and Dhatu agni (digestion and metabolism strength also depletes).

Hence, the food fails to nourish all the tissues and gets converted to stools. All the nourishment and Ojas gets wasted in the form of stool (Pureesha). Hence, in the case of Rajayakshma, the patient's stool should be protected. (Measures should be taken to channelize nutrition from the stools containing the nutritious part).

Due to obstruction to channels carrying nutritious parts of food (Rasavaha Srotas), Rasa dhatu (end product- nutritious part of food) is struck, leading to symptoms like Kasa – cough etc, in the disease Rajyakshma. This leads to manifestation of 6 or 11 symptoms as explained below. The syndrome that manifests with 6 or 11 symptoms is together called Rajyakshma.

11 Laskhanas (Features) of Rajayakshma:
जायन्ते व्याधयश्चातः षडेकादश वा पुनः|
येषां सङ्घातयोगेन राजयक्ष्मेति कथ्यते॥४४॥
कासोंऽसतापो वैस्वर्यं ज्वरः पार्श्वशिरोरुजा|
छर्दनं रक्तकफयोः श्वासवर्चोगदोऽरुचिः॥४५॥
रूपाण्येकादशैतानि यक्ष्मणः

Thereafter, 6 or 11 forms of diseases are manifested. Their conglomeration is called Rajayakshma.

1. Kasa – Cough
2. Amsa abhitapa – Burning sensation in the shoulders
3. Svara bheda – Impairment of the voice
4. Jwara – Fever
5. Parshva shoola – Pain in the sides of the chest
6. Shiro ruja – Headache
7. Rudhira chardi – Hemoptysis
8. Spitting of phlegm
9. Shvasa – Dyspnoea
10. Varcha -Diarrhea and
11. Aruchi – Anorexia

These are the 11 forms of diseases which constitute Rajayakma (tuberculosis)

6 symptoms of Rajayakshma:
षडिमानि वा|
कासो ज्वरः पार्श्वशूलं स्वरवर्चोगदोऽरुचिः||४६||
सर्वैरर्धैस्त्रिभिर्वाऽपि लिङ्गैर्मांसबलक्षये|
युक्तो वर्ज्यश्चिकित्स्यस्तु सर्वरूपोऽप्यतोऽन्यथा||४७||
1. Kasa – Cough
2. Jwara – Fever
3. Parshva shoola -Pain in the sides of the chest
4. Svara bheda – Impairment of the voice
5. Atisara – Diarrhea and
6. Aruchi – Anorexia-
These 6 ailments also constitute Rajayakshma.
If there is diminution of muscle tissue and strength then the patient of Rajayakshma having all the 11 or 6 or any of the 3 signs and symptoms should not be treated. (He will die soon)
If there is no diminution of muscle tissue or strength, then the patient of Rajayakshma is treated even if all the signs and symptoms are manifested. [38-47]

Pratishyaya (Coryza)- running nose
घ्राणमूले स्थितः श्लेष्मा रुधिरं पित्तमेव वा|
मारुताध्मातशिरसो मारुतं श्यायते प्रति||४८||
प्रतिश्यायस्ततो घोरो जायते देहकर्शनः|
तस्य रूपं शिरःशूलं गौरवं घ्राणविप्लवः||४९||
ज्वरः कासः कफोत्क्लेशः स्वरभेदोऽरुचिः क्लमः|
इन्द्रियाणामसामर्थ्यं यक्ष्मा चातः प्रजायते||५०||
Vata Dosha obstructs Kapha, Rakta (blood) and Pitta at the root of the nose, leading to Pratishyaya – running nose.
Body tissue gets depleted leading to below symptoms –
Shira shula – headache
Gauravam – heaviness
Ghrana viplavah – stuffy nose
Jwara – fever
Kasa – cough
Kaphotklesa – mucous nausea
Svara bheda – Hoarseness of voice
Aruchi – Anorexia,
Klama – fatigue and
Indriyanam Asamarthya – Inability of sensory and motor organs to perform their functions [48-50]

Characteristics of Cough:
पिच्छिलं बहलं विस्रं हरितं श्वेतपीतकम्|
कासमानो रसं यक्ष्मी निष्ठीवति कफानुगम्||५१||
The patient of Rajayakshma, while coughing, spits out
Rasa (Plasma or mucoid secretion) mixed with Phlegm
Pichila – slimy
Bahalam – Thick
Visra – Putrid in odor and

Harita, sweta peeta – green, white or yellow in colour [51]

Characteristics of fever:

अंसपार्श्वाभितापश्च सन्तापः करपादयोः|
ज्वरः सर्वाङ्गगश्चेति लक्षणं राजयक्ष्मणः||५२||

The characteristic features of Jvara in Rajayakshma:

Amsa parshva abhitapa – Burning sensation in the shoulders sides of the chest

Kara pada daha – burning sensation in the hands and feet and

Jwara – increased temperature all over the body [52]

Svarabheda (Hoarseness of Voice):

वातात्पित्तात्कफाद्रक्तात् कासवेगात् सपीनसात्|
स्वरभेदो भवेद्वाताद्रूक्षः क्षामश्चलः स्वरः||५३||
तालुकण्ठ परिप्लोषः पित्ताद्वक्तुमसूयते|
कफाद्भेदो विबद्धश्च स्वरः खुरखुरायते ||५४||
सन्नो रक्तविबद्धत्वात् स्वरः कृच्छ्रात् प्रवर्तते|
कासातिवेगात् कषणः पीनसात्कफवातिकः||५५||

If caused by Vata, Pitta, Kapha, and Raktha, then the symptoms will be –

Svarabheda (Hoarseness of voice)

Kasavega (Strain of coughing) or

Pinasa (Chronic rhinitis) occurs.

If it is caused by Pitta, then there will be

Burning sensation in the palate and throat, and

The patient will refrain from speaking

If it is caused by Kapha,

The voice becomes Vibaddha (obstructed or choked) and

Khurakhura (rubbing noise)

If it is caused by Rakta, then the voice becomes low and because of obstruction, the voice comes out with difficulty.

If the hoarseness of the voice is caused by strain of excessive coughing, then it is associated with injury to the throat.

If it is caused by Pinasa (chronic rhinitis) then the signs and symptoms of Kaphaja and Vatika types (mentioned above) are manifested. [53-55]

Pain in the sides of the chest and head:

पार्श्वशूलं त्वनियतं सङ्कोचायामलक्षणम्|
शिरःशूलं ससन्तापं यक्ष्मिणः स्यात्सगौरवम्||५६||

In a patient of Rajayakshma, pain in the sides of the chest is indeterminate, it is associated with the contraction of chest and sometimes it is associated with the expansion of the chest.

In the patient of Rajayakshma, headache is associated with burning sensation and heaviness. [56]

Spitting of blood:

अभिसन्ने शरीरे तु यक्ष्मिणो विषमाशनात्|
कण्ठात्प्रवर्तते रक्तं श्लेष्मा चोत्क्लिष्टसञ्चितः||५७||

When the body of the patient suffering from Rajayakshma becomes emaciated, the accumulated and excited blood and phlegm comes out from the throat. [57]

Cause of Bleeding

रक्तं विबद्धमार्गत्वान्मांसादीन्नानुपद्यते |

आमाशयस्थमुत्क्लिष्टं बहुत्वात् कण्ठमेति च||५८||

Because of obstruction to the channels of the blood, it becomes incapable of getting converted into Mamsadhatu (Muscle tissue) etc. This gets accumulated in excess in Amasaya (stomach) and being excited, it comes out (Eti= to come) through the throat. [58]

Dyspnoea and Diarrhoea:

वात श्लेष्म विबद्धत्वादुरसः श्वासमृच्छति|
दोषैरुपहते चाग्नौ सपिच्छमतिसार्यते||५९||

The patient of Rajayakshma suffers from Shwasa by Vata and Kapha.

This patient passes the quantity of stool along with mucus because of the suppression of Agni (enzymes) by the vitiated Doshas. [59]

Aruchi (Anorexia or Aversion for food)

पृथग्दोषैः समस्तैर्वा जिह्वाहृदयसंश्रितैः|
जायतेऽरुचिराहारे द्विष्टैरर्थैश्च मानसैः||६०||
कषाय तिक्त मधुरैर्विद्यान्मुखरसैः क्रमात्|
वातादयैररुचिं जातां मानसीं दोषदर्शनात्||६१||

Arochaka (aversion towards food) is caused by individual Doshas and by all the Doshas simultaneously vitiated.

These vitiated Doshas are located in the tongue as well as heart.

In Vata aggravation, the mouth will have astringent taste, in Pitta, bitter taste and in Kapha, it gets sweet taste. [60-61]

Chardi (vomiting):

अरोचकात् कासवेगाद्दोषोत्क्लेशादभयादपि|
छर्दिर्या सा विकाराणामन्येषामप्युपद्रवः||६२||

Chardi (vomiting) is caused due to Arochaka (anorexia), strain of coughing, excitation of Doshas and fear. This vomiting might also occur as a complication in other diseases. [62]

Rajayakshma Chikitsa – treatment:

सर्वस्त्रिदोषजो यक्ष्मा दोषाणां तु बलाबलम्|
परीक्ष्यावस्थिकं वैद्यः शोषिणं समुपाचरेत्||६३||
प्रतिश्याये शिरःशूले कासे श्वासे स्वरक्षये|
पार्श्वशूले च विविधाः क्रियाः साधारणीः शृणु||६४||

All varieties of Rajayakshma are caused by simultaneous vitiation of all the 3 Doshas. After ascertaining the proportionate dominance of Doshas, the physician should treat the patient suffering from these diseases, on the basis of the stage of the ailment.

Various treatments for Pratishyaya (Coryza), headache, cough, dyspnoea, Svarakshaya (Aphasia) and pain in the sides of the chest, in general, will now be described. [63-64]

Chikitsa Sutra – Line of treatment

पीनसे स्वेदमभ्यङ्गं धूममालेपनानि च|
परिषेकावगाहांश्च यावकं वाट्यमेव च||६५||
लवणाम्ल कटूष्णांश्च रसान् स्नेहोपबृंहितान्|
लाव तितिरि दक्षाणां वर्तकानां च कल्पयेत्||६६||
सपिप्पलीकं सयवं सकुलत्थं सनागरम्|
दाडिमामलकोपेतं स्निग्धमाजं रसं पिबेत्||६७||
तेन षड्विनिवर्तन्ते विकाराः पीनसादयः|

मूलकानां कुलत्थानां यूषैर्वा सूपकल्पितैः ||६८||
यव गोधूम शाल्यन्नैर्यथासात्म्यमुपाचरेत्|
पिबेत्प्रसादं वारुण्या जलं वा पाञ्चमूलिकम्||६९||
धान्य नागरसिद्धं वा तामलक्याऽथवा शृतम्|
पर्णिनीभिश्चतसृभिस्तेन चान्नानि कल्पयेत्||७०||

The hot soup of the meat of Lava, Tittiri – Partridge, Daksha and Vartaka, added with Salt, sour as well as pungent herbs and Sneha (oil, ghee etc.) is used for preparing thick gruel. It is used for Swedana, Abhyanga, Dhuma (herbal smoking), Alepana (external application), Parisheka (sprinkling of liquids), Avagaha (dipping, bath). Yavaka Vatya (preparation of barley water) is used in the treatment of Pinasa (Coryza).

The patient should take the soup of the goat added with barley, horse gram, ginger, pomegranate (Dadima), Amalaka and ghee. By this, the ailments like Pinasa (Coryza) etc. get cured.

The soup of radish (Mulaka) and horse gram (Kulattha) is properly prepared. Along with this soup, the patient should take food preparations made of barley, wheat and rice depending on suitability.

The patient should drink the upper portion of Varuni (a type of alcoholic drink) or water boiled with Panchamoola (Bilva, Shyonaka, Gambhari, Paatala and Agnimantha).

For food preparations, the water boiled with coriander and ginger or tamalaki or Parni chatustaya (Shalaparni, Prishnaparni, Mashaparni and Mudgaparni) is used [65-70]

Different types of Swedana for Rajayakshma

कृशरोत्कारिका माष कुलत्थयवपायसैः|
सङ्कर स्वेदविधिना कण्ठं पार्श्वमुरः शिरः||७१||
स्वेदयेत् पत्रभङ्गेण शिरश्च परिषेचयेत्|
बला गुडूची मधुक शृतैर्वा वारिभिः सुखैः||७२||
बस्तमत्स्यशिरोभिर्वा नाडीस्वेदं प्रयोजयेत्|
कण्ठे शिरसि पार्श्वे च पयोभिर्वा सवातिकैः||७३||
औदकानूप मांसानि सलिलं पाञ्चमूलिकम्|
सस्नेहमारनालं वा नाडीस्वेदे प्रयोजयेत्||७४||
जीवन्त्याः शतपुष्पाया बलाया मधुकस्य च|
वचाया वेशवारस्य विदार्या मूलकस्य च||७५||
औदकानूप मांसानामुपनाहाः सुसंस्कृताः|
शस्यन्ते सचतुःस्नेहाः शिरःपार्श्वासशूलिनाम्||७६||

Different types of sweating treatments for Rajayakshma:

Below, different types of Swedana – sweating treatments are explained. To learn in detail about each of these sweating methods, visit Charaka Sutrasthana 14th chapter

Sankara type of Swedana is administered over throat, sides of the chest, chest and head

(vide) and for this purpose,

Krushara – thick gruel,

Utkarika – pudding and

Payasa (milk preparation boiled with black gram, horse gram and barley) is used.

Parisheka (sprinkling) type of Swedana is administered with

Patrabhanga (decoction of leaves having Vata alleviating properties) or

The lukewarm decoction of

Bala – Country mallow (root) – Sida cordifolia,

Guduchi – Tinospora cordifloia and

Madhuka– Licorice – Glycyrrhiza glabra.

Nadisveda is done on throat, head and sides of chest with

The head of the goat and fish or

The decoction of Vata balancing herbs.

For Nadi sveda these may also be used:

The meat of aquatic and semi- aquatic animals,

The decoction of Panchamula (bilva, Syonaka, Gambhari, Patali and Ganikarika),

Sneha (oil, ghee etc.) and

Aranala (sour Gruel)

Upanaha (hot ointment) is done if there is

Shiro ruja – headache,

Parshva shoola – pain in the sides of the chest and

Amsa shoola – shoulder pain

The following ingredients are used:

Jivanti – Leptadenia reticulata,

Shatapushpa – Anethum sowa

Bala – Country mallow (root) – Sida cordifolia,

Madhuka– Licorice – Glycyrrhiza glabra,

Vacha – Acorus calamus Linn

Veshavara – a non veg soup recipe

Vidari- Pueraria tuberosa

Mulaka – Raphanus sativus and

Meat of aquatic as well as semi- aquatic animals sizzled and mixed with 4 types of Sneha (oil, ghee, muscle fat and bone marrow) is useful. [71-76]

Recipes for external application:

शतपुष्पा समधुकं कुष्ठं तगर चन्दने|

आलेपनं स्यात् सघृतं शिरःपार्श्वांसशूलनुत्||७७||

बला रास्ना तिलाः सर्पिर्मधुकं नीलमुत्पलम्|

पलङ्कषा देवदारु चन्दनं केशरं घृतम्||७८||

वीरा बला विदारी च कृष्णगन्धा पुनर्नवा|

शतावरी पयस्या च कतृणं मधुकं घृतम्||७९||

चत्वार एते श्लोकार्धैः प्रदेहाः परिकीर्तिताः|

शस्ताः संसृष्टदोषाणां शिरःपार्श्वांसशूलिनाम्||८०||

नावनं धूमपानानि स्नेहाश्चौत्तरभक्तिकाः|

तैलान्यभ्यङ्गयोगीनि बस्तिकर्म तथा परम्||८१||

External application (Alepana):

The ingredients used: Paste of

Shatapushpa – Anethum sowa

Madhuka– Licorice – Glycyrrhiza glabra,

Kushta – Saussurea lappa,

Tagara – Valeriana wallichii and

Chandana (Sandalwood – Santalum album) along with ghee

Cures:

Shiro ruja – headache and

Parshva amsa shoola – pain in the sides of the chest as well as shoulders

Praseka (external application of thick ointment):

Useful in the treatment of-

Shiro ruja – headache and

Parshva amsa shoola – pain in the sides of the chest as well as shoulders caused by the simultaneous vitiations of 2 Doshas.

Other combinations for paste application for headache, chest and shoulder pain –

1. Bala – Country mallow (root) – Sida cordifolia,

Rasna – Alpinia galanga, sesame seeds, ghee, Yashtimadhu and Blue Lily (Neelotpala)

2. Palankasha (Guggulu - Commiphora mukul Engl.),

Devadaru (Cedrus deodara),

Chandana (Sandalwood – Santalum album),

Kesara and Ghee

3. Veera,

Bala – Country mallow (root) – Sida cordifolia,

Vidari (Ipomoea paniculata / Pueraria tuberosa),

Krsnagandha and

Punarnava – Boerhaavia diffusa and

4. Shatavari – Asparagus racemosus

Payasya – Ipomoea paniculata,

Ksheerakakoli – Lilium polyphyllum

Kattrna,

Madhuka– Licorice – Glycyrrhiza glabra and

Ghee

For these patients, Navana (Inhalation therapy), Dhumapana (smoking therapy), administration of Sneha (Ghee, etc) after the intake of food, massage with medicated oils and medicated enema (Basti) are useful. [77 - 81]

Raktamokshana – Blood-letting Therapy, etc

शृङ्गालाबुजलौकोभिः प्रदुष्टं व्यधनेन वा|

शिरःपार्श्वांसशूलेषु रुधिरं तस्य निर्हरेत्||८२||

प्रदेहः सघृतश्चेष्टः पद्मकोशीरचन्दनैः|

दूर्वा मधुक मञ्जिष्ठाकेशरैर्वा घृताप्लुतैः||८३||

प्रपौण्डरीक निर्गुण्डी पद्म केशरमुत्पलम्|

कशेरुकाः पयस्या च ससर्पिष्कं प्रलेपनम्||८४||

चन्दनाद्येन तैलेन शतधौतेन सर्पिषा|

अभ्यङ्गः, पयसा सेकः शस्तश्च मधुकाम्बुना||८५||

माहेन्द्रेण सुशीतेन चन्दनादिशृतेन वा|

परिषेकः प्रयोक्तव्य इति संशमनी क्रिया||८६||

The patient suffering from headache and pain in the sides of the chest as well as shoulders is administered bloodletting therapy with:

Srunga (Horn)

Alabu (gourd) and

Jalauka (leeches) or

Siravyadha – venesection

For such patients, Pradeha (external application of thick ointment) with the paste of

Padmaka – Prunus cerasoides

Ushira – Vetiver – Vetiveria zizanioides and

Chandana (Sandalwood – Santalum album) added with ghee or

The paste of

Durva (Cynodon dactylon),

Madhuka– Licorice – Glycyrrhiza glabra,

Manjistha – Rubia cordifolia and

Kesara mixed with ghee is useful.

Pralepana (application of ointment) of:

Prapaundarika (Nymphaea lotus) – red variety,

Nirgundi (Vitex negundo),

Padmakesara,

Utpala (Nymphaea alba),

Kaseruka and

Payasya – Impomoea paniculata with ghee is useful in this condition.

Massage with the help of:

Chandanandi taila and

Satadhauta ghrita is useful in this condition.

Pariseka (sprinkling of liquids) with:

Milk,

Decoction of Madhuka– Licorice – Glycyrrhiza glabra,

Cold rain- water or

The decoction of

Chandana (Sandalwood – Santalum album), etc. is useful in this condition.

Thus the alleviation therapies are described. [82-86]

Panchakarma treatment for Rajayakshma

दोषाधिकानां वमनं शस्यते सविरेचनम्|

स्नेहस्वेदोपपन्नानां सस्नेहं यन्न कर्शनम्||८७||

शोषी मुञ्चति गात्राणि पुरीषस्रंसनादपि|

अबलापेक्षिणीं मात्रां किं पुनर्यो विरिच्यते||८८||

The patient suffering from Rajayakshma having excessively vitiated Doshas is given Snehana and Swedana therapies and thereafter, Vamana (emetic therapy) and virecana (purgation therapy) is administered.

The recipe for these therapies should contain Sneha (ghee, oil etc), and these recipes should not have a depleting (Karsana) effect.

The patient of Rajayakshma will die if there are loose bowels. Therefore, the dose of these recipes is such, which a weak person can stand, and he should never be given a strong purgation. [87-88]

Medicines and treatments for Rajayakshma:

योगान् संशुद्ध कोष्ठानां कासे श्वासे स्वरक्षये|

शिरःपार्श्वसशूलेषु सिद्धानेतान्प्रयोजयेत्||८९||

After the Koshta (Gut) is cleaned of impurities by Vamana and Virechana, for the treatment of Kasa (cough), Svasa (Dyspnoea), headache and pain in the sides of the chest as well as shoulders, the following medicines are administered. (89)

Nasya treatment to improve voice:

बला विदारिगन्धाद्यैर्विदार्या मधुकेन वा|

सिद्धं सलवणं सर्पिर्नस्यं स्यात्स्वर्यमुतमम्||९०||

प्रपौण्डरीकं मधुकं पिप्पली बृहती बला|

क्षीरं सर्पिश्च तत्सिद्धं स्वर्यं स्यान्नावनं परम्||९१||

शिरःपार्श्वसशूलघ्नं कासश्वासनिबर्हणम्|

प्रयुज्यमानं बहुशो घृतं चौतरभक्तिकम्||९२||

1. Nasya (nasal drops therapy) with the ghee boiled with
Bala – Country mallow (root) – Sida cordifolia
Vidari (Pueraria tuberosa),
Ashwagandha – Winter Cherry / Indian ginseng (root) – Withania somnifera etc,
or
Vidari (Pueraria tuberosa) and
Madhuka– Licorice – Glycyrrhiza glabra along with salt is excellent for the promotion of voice.
2. Navana (a type of Nasya) of ghee boiled with
Prapaundarika (Nymphaea alba) – red variety,
Madhuka– Licorice – Glycyrrhiza glabra,
Pippali – Long pepper fruit – Piper longum,
Brihati – Solanum indicum,
Bala – Country mallow (root) – Sida cordifolia and
Milk is excellent for the promotion of voice.
The above herbal ghee administered after food, relieves
Shirashoola – headache
Parshwashoola – flank pain
Amsashoola – upper back pain
Kasa – cough
Shwasa – asthma, dyspnoea (90-92)

Dashamoola Ghrita, Bala ghrita, Rasna Ghrita
दशमूलेन पयसा सिद्धं मांसरसेन च।
बलागर्भं घृतं सद्यो रोगानेतान् प्रबाधते॥९३॥
भक्तस्योपरि मध्ये वा यथाग्न्यभ्यवचारितम्।
रास्नाघृतं वा सक्षीरं सक्षीरं वा बलाघृतम्॥९४॥
Dashamoola Ghrita, Bala ghrita, Rasna Ghrita
Medicated ghee prepared by boiling with
Bala – Country mallow (root) – Sida cordifolia,
Decoction of Dashamula(Bilva, Syonaka, Gambhari, Patali, Ganikarika, Salaparni, Prishnaparni – Uraria picta, Brihati – Solanum indicum, Kantakari – Solanum xanthocarpum and Goksura)
Milk and Meat soup is useful in the instantaneous cure of the above mentioned ailments (headache, flanks pain, upper back pain, cough and asthma)
5. Besides, the intake of Rasna ghrita or Bala ghrita along with milk after food or during the course of food in a dose proportionate with the power of digestion of patient is also useful in the treatment of the above mentioned ailments.

Linctus preparation (Leha) for cough, voice hoarseness, asthma etc.
लेहान् कासापहान् स्वर्यांश् श्वास हिक्का निबर्हणान्।
शिरःपार्श्वांसशूलघ्नान् स्नेहांश्चातः परं शृणु॥९५॥
घृतं खर्जूर मृद्वीका शर्करा क्षौद्र संयुतम्।
सपिप्पलीकं वैस्वर्य कास श्वास ज्वरापहम्॥९६॥
दशमूलशृतात् क्षीरात् सर्पिर्यदुदियान्नवम्।
सपिप्पलीकं सक्षौद्रं तत् परं स्वरबोधनम्॥९७॥
शिरःपार्श्वांसशूलघ्नं कासश्वासज्वरापहम्।
पञ्चभिः पञ्चमूलैर्वा शृताद्यदुदियाद्घृतम्॥९८॥
पञ्चानां पञ्चमूलानां रसे क्षीरचतुर्गुणे।
सिद्धं सर्पिर्जयत्येतद्यक्ष्मणः सप्तकं बलम्॥९९॥

खर्जूरं पिप्पली द्राक्षा पथ्या शृङ्गी दुरालभा|
त्रिफला पिप्पली मुस्तं शृङ्गाटगुडशर्कराः||१००||
वीरा शटी पुष्कराख्यं सुरसः शर्करा गुडः|
नागरं चित्रको लाजाः पिप्पल्यामलकं गुडः||१०१||
श्लोकार्धविहितानेतांल्लिह्यान्ना मधुसर्पिषा|
कास श्वासापहान्स्वर्यान्पार्श्वशूलापहांस्तथा||१०२||

Linctus (Leha) for cough, voice hoarseness, asthma etc.
Intake of ghee added with
Kharjura – dates,
Mrudvika – Vitis vinifera
Sharkara – sugar
Honey and Pippali – Long pepper fruit – Piper longum
Cures:
Vaisvarya – Hoarseness of voice
Kasa – cough
Svasa – dyspnoea and
Jvara – fever
The ghee which is collected freshly from the milk boiled with the
Decoction of Dashamula is mixed with Pippali and honey.
This is an excellent recipe for the promotion of voice.
It also cures:
Shiro ruja – headache,
Parshva shoola and amsa shoola – pain in the sides of the chest as well as shoulders,
Kasa – cough,
Svasa – dyspnoea and
Jwara – fever.
Ghee is collected from the milk boiled with 5 varieties of Panchamool;
Brhat Panchamula (Bilva – Aegle marmelos, Syonaka, Gambhari –Gmelina arborea, Patali and Ganikarika),
Ksudrapanchamula (Shalaparni, Prishnaparni – Uraria picta, Brihati – Solanum indicum, Kantakari – Solanum xanthocarpum and Goksura – Tribulus terrestris),
Trnapanchamula (Saraiksu, Darbha, Kasa and Sali),
Kantakapanchamula (Jivaka Rishabhaka – Manilkara hexandra, meda, Jivanti – Leptadenia reticulata and Shatavari – Asparagus racemosus) and
Vallipancamula (Punarnava – Boerhaavia diffusa, Shalaparni, Prishnaparni – Uraria picta, Bala – Country mallow (root) – Sida cordifolia and Eranda –Ricinus communis) [wide Charaka Chikitsa 1:1 :41-44.
This ghee (one part) is cooked by adding the decoction of 5 varieties of Panchamula (3 parts) and milk (1 part). This recipe cures all the 7 ailments of Rajayakshma.
The following 4 recipes, when taken in the form of linctus along with honey cures Kasa (cough), Svasa (Dyspnoea) and pain in the sides of the chest. They also promote voice.
1. Kharjura – Phoenix dactylifera
Pippali – Long pepper fruit – Piper longum,
Draksha – Raisin – Vitis vinifera,
Pathya – Haritaki
Karkatashrungi and
Duralabha – Fagonia cretica
2.Triphala (Haritaki, Bibhitaki and Amalaki)
Pippali – Long pepper fruit – Piper longum

3. Veera,
Shati – Hedychium spicatum
Puskaramula – Inula racemosa, Basil, jaggery and sugar
4. Nagara –
Chitraka – Leadwort – Plumbago zeylanica,
Laja,
Pippali – Long pepper fruit – Piper longum,
Amalaki – Phyllanthus emblica and
Jaggery [89-102]

Sitopaladi Churna

सितोपलां तुगाक्षीरीं पिप्पलीं बहुलां त्वचम्|
अन्त्यादूर्ध्वं द्विगुणितं लेहयेन्मधुसर्पिषा||१०३||
चूर्णितं प्राशयेद्वा तच्छ्वासकासकफातुरम्|
सुप्तजिह्वारोचकिनमल्पाग्निं पार्श्वशूलिनम्||१०४||

Ingredients:
16 parts of Sitopala (misri or sugar with big crystals),
8 parts of Tugaksheeri (bamboo salt)
4 parts of Pippali – Long pepper fruit – Piper longum,
2 parts of Bahula (Bruhadela) Greater cardamom and
1 part of Tvak is made of powder.
This is mixed with honey and ghee, and given to the patient to lick.
Indicated in –
Svasa – dyspnoea
Kasa – cough
Kapha – phlegm
Suptajihva – numbness of the tongue
Arocaka – anorexia
Alpagni – low power of digestion and
Parsvasula – pain in the sides of the chest [103- 104]
Read more about side effects, usage, safety of Sitopaladi Choornam

Treatment of Burning Sensation:

हस्त पादाङ्गदाहेषु ज्वरे रक्ते तथोर्ध्वगे|
वासाघृतं शतावर्या सिद्धं वा परमं हितम्||१०५||

If there is burning sensation in hands, feet or in the body, and if there is fever and bleeding from the upper channels of the body, then the patient is given Vasaghirta or Shatavari ghrita. [105]

Duralabhadi Ghrita:

दुरालभां श्वदंष्ट्रां च चतस्रः पर्णिनीर्बलाम्|
भागान्पलोन्मितान् कृत्वा पलं पर्पटकस्य च||१०६||
पचेद्दशगुणे तोये दशभागावशेषिते|
रसे सुपूते द्रव्याणामेषां कल्कान् समावपेत्||१०७||
शट्याः पुष्करमूलस्य पिप्पली त्रायमाणयोः|
तामलक्याः किरातानां तिक्तस्य कुटजस्य च||१०८||
फलानां सारिवायाश्च सुपिष्टान् कर्षसम्मितान्|
ततस्तेन घृतप्रस्थं क्षीरद्विगुणितं पचेत्||१०९||

ज्वरं दाहं भ्रमं कासमंसपार्श्वशिरोरुजम्।
तृष्णां छर्दिमतीसारमेतत् सर्पिर्व्यपोहति॥११०॥

1 pala of each of

Duralabha – Fagonia cretica

Svadamstra – Tribulus terristeris

4 varieties of Parni (Salaparni, Prishnaparni – Uraria picta, Mashaparni – Teramnus labialis and Mudgaparni – Phaseolus trilobus),

Bala – Country mallow (root) – Sida cordifolia and

Parpataka – Fumaria parviflora is boiled by adding

10 times of ghee, i.e. the Prasthas of water and reduced to 1/10th.

Thereafter, the decoction is properly strained out.

To this fine paste of

1 Karsha of each of

Sati – Hedychium spicatum

Puskaramula – Inula racemosa

Pippali – Long pepper fruit – Piper longum,

Trayamana – Gentiana kurroa

Tamalaki – Bhumi Amla

Kiratatikta – Swertia chirata

Fruits of Kutaja – Holarrhena antidysenterica Wall. and

Sariva – Indian Sarsaparilla – Hemidesmus indicus is added.

Thereafter, 1 prastha of ghee and 2 Prasthas of milk are added and cooked.

This medicated ghee cures

Jvara – fever

Daha – burning sensation

Bhrama – Giddiness

Kasa – cough

Amsa ruja; Parshva ruja; shiro ruja – Pain in shoulders, sides of the chest and head

Trsna – morbid thirst),

Chardi – Vomiting and

Atisara – Diarrhea [106-110]

Jivantyadi ghruta:

जीवन्तीं मधुकं द्राक्षां फलानि कुटजस्य च।
शटीं पुष्करमूलं च व्याघ्रीं गोक्षुरकं बलाम्॥१११॥
नीलोत्पलं तामलकीं त्रायमाणां दुरालभाम्।
पिप्पलीं च समं पिष्ट्वा घृतं वैद्यो विपाचयेत्॥११२॥
एतद्व्याधिसमूहस्य रोगेशस्य समुत्थितम्।
रूपमेकादशविधं सर्पिरग्र्यं व्यपोहति॥११३॥

All these drugs are taken in equal quantities and made into a paste. Ghee is cooked along with this paste:

Jivanti – Leptadenia reticulata

Madhuka– Licorice – Glycyrrhiza glabra

Draksha – Raisin – Vitis vinifera,

Fruits of Kutaja – Holarrhena antidysenterica Wall.

Shati – Hedychium spicatum

Puskaramula – Inula racemosa

Vyaghri

Goksura – Tribulus terrestris
Bala
Nilopala – Water lily
Tamalaki – Phyllanthus niruri
Tryamana – Gentiana kurroo
Duralabha and
Pippali – Long pepper fruit – Piper longum
This excellent recipe of medicated ghee cures all the 11 signs and symptoms of this serious disease (tuberculosis) which is a conglomeration of several ailments. [111-113]

Baladi Ksheera –
बलां स्थिरां पृश्निपर्णीं बृहतीं सनिदिग्धिकाम्|
साधयित्वा रसे तस्मिन्पयो गव्यं सनागरम्||११४||
द्राक्षा खर्जूर सर्पिर्भिः पिप्पल्या च शृतं सह|
सक्षौद्रं ज्वर कासघ्नं स्वर्यं चैतत् प्रयोजयेत्||११५||
आजस्य पयसश्चैवं प्रयोगो जाङ्गला रसाः|
यूषार्थं चणका मुद्गा मकुष्ठाश्चोपकल्पिताः||११६||
Bala – Sida cordifolia
Sthira – Desmodium gangeticum
Prishnaparni – Uraria picta
Brihati – Solanum indicum and
Nidigdhika – Solanum surattense is boiled, and decoction is prepared.
To this decoction,
Cow's milk,
Nagara
Draksha – Raisin – Vitis vinifera,
Kharjura – Phoenix dactylifera
Ghee and
Pippali – Long pepper fruit – Piper longum is added and cooked.
Intake of this recipe along with honey cures
Jwara – fever and
Kasa – cough, and is
Svaryam – promotes voice.
While using this recipe, the patient should take goat- milk and the soup of meat of animals inhabiting arid zone. He should also take the Yusa (vegetable soup) of Canaka, mudga and Makustha [114- 116]

Treatment of different Stages of Tuberculosis:
ज्वराणां शमनीयो यः पूर्वमुक्तः क्रियाविधिः|
यक्ष्मिणां ज्वरदाहेषु ससर्पिष्कः प्रशस्यते||११७||
Therapeutic measure described earlier for the treatment of different types of Jvara (vide Charaka Jwara Chikitsa – 3rd chapter) Cikitsa 3) is employed along with ghee for the treatment of fever and burning sensation of the patient suffering from tuberculosis. [117]

Treatment of Excessive Phlegm:
कफप्रसेके बलवान् श्लैष्मिकश्छर्दयेन्नरः|
पयसा फलयुक्तेन माधुकेन रसेन वा||११८||
सर्पिष्मत्या यवाग्वा वा वमनीयोपसिद्धया|

वान्तोऽन्नकाले लघ्वन्नमाददीत सदीपनम्॥११९॥

If there is excessive expectoration of phlegm, if the patient is strong (i.e. not too weak) and if is of Kapha Prakrti (constitution dominated by Kapha), then he is given emetic therapy with the following recipes:

1. Milk boiled with Madanaphala
2. Milk boiled with the decoction of Madhuyasti (Licorice) and
3. Yavagu (thick gruel) prepared by boiling with emetic drugs and added with ghee.

After the administration of the emetic therapy, and during the meal- time, the patient is given light diet which is prepared with such drugs as are stimulant of digestion like Sunthi. [118-119]

Diet and Drinks for excessive Phlegm:

यव गोधूम माध्वीक सिध्वरिष्टसुरासवान्।
जाङ्गलानि च शूल्यानि सेवमानः कफं जयेत्॥१२०॥

Intake of yava, Godhuma – wheat – Triticum sativum, Madhvika, Sidhu, Arista, Sura, Asava, meat of animals inhabiting arid zone and Shoolya type of Meat (meat roasted on a spike preparation overcomes kapha). [120]

Role of Vata in Expectoration:

श्लेष्मणोऽतिप्रसेकेन वायुः श्लेष्माणमस्यति।
कफप्रसेकं तं विद्वान् स्निग्धोष्णेनैव निर्जयेत्॥१२१॥

During excessive expectoration of Phlegm, it is Vata which stimulates the phlegm to come out. Therefore, a wise physician should treat such a condition (of expectation of phlegm) with the help of unctuous and hot remedies. [121]

Treatment of vomiting:

क्रिया कफप्रसेके या वम्यां सैव प्रशस्यते।
हृद्यानि चान्नपानानि वातघ्नानि लघूनि च॥१२२॥

Therapeutic measures described for the treatment of expectoration of phlegm is employed if there is vomiting [in the patient of tuberculosis]. To such a patient, diet and drinks which are Hrudya (useful for the heart), which alleviate Vata and which are light are given. [122]

Treatment of Diarrhoea:

प्रायेणोपहताग्नित्वात् सपिच्छमतिसार्यते।
प्राप्नोति चास्यवैरस्यं न चान्नमभिनन्दति॥१२३॥
तस्याग्निदीपनान् योगानतीसारनिबर्हणान्।
वक्त्रशुद्धिकरान् कुर्यादरुचिप्रतिबाधकान्॥१२४॥
सनागरानिन्द्रयवान् पाययेत्तण्डुलाम्बुना।
सिद्धां यवागूं जीर्णे च चाङ्गेरीतक्रदादिमैः॥१२५॥
पाठा बिल्वं यमानी च पातव्यं तक्रसंयुतम्।
दुरालभा शृङ्गवेरं पाठा च सुरया सह॥१२६॥
जम्ब्वाम्रमध्यं बिल्वं च सकपित्थं सनागरम्।
पेयामण्डेन पातव्यमतीसारनिवृत्तये॥१२७॥

In the patient of tuberculosis, generally Agni (enzymes responsible for digestion and metabolism) is afflicted. This causes diarrhoea accompanied with mucus and Asyavairasa (distaste in the mouth). Such a patient does not relish any food.

To such a patient, the following recipes, which stimulate the power of digestion, which stops diarrhoea, which cleanses the mouth and which counteracts anorexia is administered:

1. Indrayava – Wrightia tinctoria with Nagara is mixed with Tandulambu (rice- wash) and the patient is given Yavagu (thick gruel) cooked along with Changeri – Oxalis corniculata, butter- milk and Dadima – Pomegranate – Punica

granatum.

2. Patha – Cyclea peltata, Bilva – Aegle marmelos and Yavani – Carum copticum is mixed with butter milk. The patient should drink this potion.

3. Duralabha – Fagonia cretica, srngavera – Zingiber officinale and Patha – Cyclea peltata is taken along with Sura (a type of alcoholic drink) and

4. Pulp of the seeds of jambu – Syzygium cumini and Amra – mango – Mangifera indica, Bilva – Aegle marmelos, Kapittha – Limonia acidissima and Nagara are mixed with the Manda (upper portion) of Peya (thin gruel).

The above mentioned recipes cure diarrhea. [123-127]

Preparations of Khada

एतानेव च योगांस्त्रीन् पाठादीन् कारयेत् खडान्।
ससूप्यधान्यान्सस्नेहान् साम्लान्सङ्ग्रहणान् परम्||१२८||

The recipes described in verses 126-127 can also be prepared in the form of Khada (a type of sour drink) by adding pulses, fats and sour ingredients. Such Khada preparations are useful in stopping diarrhea. [128]

Recipes of Khada

वेतसार्जुनजम्बूनां मृणालीकृष्णगन्धयोः।
श्रीपर्ण्या मदयन्त्याश्च यूथिकायाश्च पल्लवान्||१२९||
मातुलुङ्गस्य धातक्या दाडिमस्य च कारयेत्।
स्नेहाम्ललवणोपेतान् खडान् साङ्ग्राहिकान् परम्||१३०||
चाङ्गेर्याश्चुक्रिकायाश्च दुग्धिकायाश्च कारयेत्।
खडान्दधिसरोपेतान् ससर्पिष्कान्सदाडिमान्||१३१||

Leaves of Vetasa – Garcinia pedunculata, Arjuna (Terminalia arjuna), Jambu – Syzygium cumini, Mrnali, Krsnagandha, Sriparni – Gmelina arborea, Madayanti – Lawsonia inermis and Yuthika – Jasminum auriculatum is mixed with Matulunga – Citrus medica , Dhataki – Woodfordia fruticosa, Dadima – Pomegranate – Punica granatum, fats, sour ingredients and salt for preparing Khadas which are excellent for counteracting diarrhea.

Similarly, Khadas can be prepared of Changeri – Oxalis corniculata, Chukrika – Rumex vesicarius and Dugdhika –Euphorbia thymifolia mixed with cream of curd, ghee and Dadima – Pomegranate – Punica granatum. [129-131]

Diet and Drinks for Diarrhoea

मांसानां लघुपाकानां रसाः साङ्ग्राहिकैर्युताः।
व्यञ्जनार्थं प्रशस्यन्ते भोज्यार्थं रक्तशालयः||१३२||
स्थिरादिपञ्चमूलेन पाने शस्तं शृतं जलम्।
तक्रं सुरा सचुक्रीका दाडिमस्याथवा रसः||१३३||
इत्युक्तं भिन्नशकृतां दीपनं ग्राहि भेषजम्|१३४|

The soup of different types of meat which are light for digestion is mixed with astringent ingredients. These Vyanjanas (non- cereal side Dishes) along with a red variety of Sali rice is useful in diarrhea.

The patient should drink water boiled with

Laghupanchamula (Shalaparni, Prishnaparni – Uraria picta, Brihati – Solanum indicum, Kantakari – Solanum xanthocarpum and Goksura – Tribulus terrestris),

Butter

Sura

Chukrika – Rumex vesicarius and

the juice of Dadima – Pomegranate – Punica granatum.

Thus medicines which are digestive stimulants and Grahi (constipative) for the patient of tuberculosis having Diarrhoea are described. [132- 134]

Regime to remove Distaste in Mouth:

परं मुखस्य वैरस्यनाशनं रोचनं शृणु ||१३४||

द्वौ कालौ दन्तपवनं भक्षयेन्मुखधावनम्|

तद्वत् प्रक्षालयेदास्यं धारयेत् कवलग्रहान्||१३५||

पिबेद्धूमं ततो मृष्टमद्याद्दीपनपाचनम्|

भेषजं पानमन्नं च हितमिष्टोपकल्पितम्||१३६||

Now, hear the excellent measures for the removal of distaste in the mouth and for the promotion of the liking for food. These are as follows:

1. One should brush his teeth both the times (morning and evening) with the help of tooth- twigs and use Mukhadhavana (drugs to be chewed for correcting the aggravated Doshas in the mouth);

Read more about Ayurvedic way of teeth brushing and tongue scraping

2. Similarly, he should wash the mouth and use Kavala Graha (keeping mouthful of drugs in thin paste in the oral cavity) and

3. One should smoke (medicated cigars) and thereafter, take such drugs, food and drinks which are stimulants of digestion as well as carminative, which are useful and which are deliciously prepared. [134- 136]

Recipes for Mukha dhavana: Chewing:

त्वङ्मुस्तमेला धान्यानि मुस्तमामलकं त्वचम्|

दार्वीत्वचो यवानी च तेजोह्वा पिप्पली तथा||१३७||

यवानी तिन्तिडीकं च पञ्चैते मुखधावनाः|

श्लोकपादेष्वभिहिता रोचना मुखशोधनाः||१३८||

गुटिकां धारयेदास्ये चूर्णैर्वा शोधयेन्मुखम्|

एषामालोडितानां वा धारयेत् कवलग्रहान्||१३९||

The following 5 recipes are useful for Mukhadhavana (drugs to be chewed) for correcting the aggravated Doshas in the mouth:

1. Tvak – Cinnamomum zeylanica ,

Musta (Cyperus rotundus)

Ela (Elettaria cardamomum Maton) and

Dhanya

2. Musta – Cyperus rotundus,

Amalaka – Emblica officinalis, and

Tvak- Cinnamomum zeylanica

3. Darvi – Berberis aristata,

Tvak – Cinnamomum zeylanica and

Yavani – Carum copticum

4. Tejohva (Cavika) and

Pippali – Long pepper fruit – Piper longum

5. Yavani – Carum copticum and

Tintidika – Rhus parviflora

The above mentioned recipes can be prepared in the form of pills to be kept in mouth and sucked.

In the form of powder, these recipes can be used for the massage of gums and teeth for cleaning the mouth.

Mixed with water, the powder or paste of these recipes can be used as Kavalagraha (keeping a mouthful of drugs in thin paste from in the oral cavity). [137-139]

Other recipes for Kavalagraha- Oral rinse:

सुरा माध्वीक सीधूनां तैलस्य मधुसर्पिषोः|

कवलान् धारयेदिष्टान् क्षीरस्येक्षुरसस्य च||१४०||

Ingredients to be used for Kavalagraha (keeping mouthful of drugs in thin paste form in the oral cavity) as per the liking of patient:

Sura – Alcohol

Madhvika,

Sidhu,

Oil,

Honey,

Ghee,

Milk and

Sugar cane juice [140]

Yavani Shadava Churna:

यवानीं तिन्तिडीकं च नागरं साम्लवेतसम्|
दाडिमं बदरं चाम्लं कार्षिकं चोपकल्पयेत्||१४१||
धान्य सौवर्चलाजाजी वराङ्गं चार्धकार्षिकम्|
पिप्पलीनां शतं चैकं द्वे शते मरिचस्य च||१४२||
शर्करायाश्च चत्वारि पलान्येकत्र चूर्णयेत्|
जिह्वा विशोधनं हृद्यं तच्चूर्णं भक्तरोचनम्||१४३||
हृत्प्लीह पार्श्वशूलघ्नं विबन्धानाहनाशनम्|
कास श्वासहरं ग्राहि ग्रहण्यर्शोविकारनुत्||१४४||
इति यवानीषाडवम्|

1 Karsha of each of

Yavani – Carum copticum,

Tintidika -Rhus parviflora,

Amlavetasa – Garcinia pedunculata Roxb,

Dadima — Punica granatum and

Badara – Zizyphus jujuba (sour variety),

1/2 Karsa of each of

Dhanya – Oryza sativa

Sauvaracala

Ajaji – Nigella sativa and

Varanga (Tvak),

100 Pippalis – Piper longum

200 fruits of Maricha – Black pepper fruit – Piper nigrum and

4 Palas of Sarkara are made into powder.

This recipe, when administered, cleanses the tongue.

It is a cardiac tonic and it promotes relish for food.

It cures heart diseases, spleen disorders, pain in the sides of the chest, constipation, Anaha (flatulence) cough, Svasa (asthma), Grahani (Sprue syndrome) and Arsas (piles).

It is Grahi i.e it works as a constipative in a patient suffering from diarrhea. [141-144]

Talisadi churna and Talisadi Gutika

तालीशपत्रं मरिचं नागरं पिप्पली शुभा|
यथोतरं भागवृद्ध्या त्वगेले चार्धभागिके||१४५||
पिप्पल्यष्टगुणा चात्र प्रदेया सितशर्करा|
कास श्वासारुचिहरं तच्चूर्णं दीपनं परम्||१४६||
हृत्पाण्डु ग्रहणीदोष शोष प्लीह ज्वरापहम्|

वम्यतीसारशूलघ्नं मूढवातानुलोमनम्||१४७||
कल्पयेद्गुटिकां चैतच्चूर्णं पक्त्वा सितोपलाम्|
गुटिका ह्यग्निसंयोगाच्चूर्णाल्लघुतराः स्मृताः||१४८||
इति तालीशाद्यं चूर्णं गुटिकाश्च|

Ingredients:

1 part Talisapatra – Taxus baccata,

2 parts Maricha – Black pepper fruit – Piper nigrum

3 parts Nagara – Zingiber officinale

4 parts Pippali – Long pepper fruit – Piper longum

1/2 Part Tvak – Cinnamomum zeylanica

1/2part Ela (Elettaria cardamomum Maton) and

32parts white sugar is made to a powder.

This powder, when administered, cures

Kasa – cough,

Svasa – Asthma and

Aruchi – Anorexia

Hrdroga – heart diseases

Pandu – Anemia

Grahanidosa – sprue syndrome

Shosha—depletion of body tissues.

Splenic disorders

Jwara – fever

Chardi – vomiting

Atisara – diarrhea

Colic pain

It is an excellent stimulant of digestion;

It causes downward movement of obstructed Vayu in the abdomen.

Read more about uses, side effects and research about Talisadi Churna.[145 -148]

Administration of Meat

शुष्यतां क्षीणमांसानां कल्पितानि विधानवित्|
दद्यान्मांसादमांसानि बृंहणानि विशेषतः||१४९||

If the patient is emaciated and reducton of muscle, tissues, then he is given meat of carnivorous animals which are especially nourishing. This meat is suitably prepared by an expert acquainted with the method of such preparations. [149]

Giving Carnivorous Meat in Disguise:

शोषिणे बार्हिणं दद्याद्बर्हिशब्देन चापरान्|
गृध्रानुलूकांश्चाषांश्च विधिवत् सूपकल्पितान्||१५०||
काकांस्तित्तिरिशब्देन वर्मिशब्देन चोरगान्|
भृष्टान् मत्स्यान्त्रशब्देन दद्याद्गण्डूपदानपि||१५१||
लोपाकान् स्थूलनकुलान् बिडालांश्चोपकल्पितान्|
शृगालशावांश्च भिषक् शशशब्देन दापयेत्||१५२||
सिंहानृक्षांस्तरक्षूंश्च व्याघ्रानेवंविधांस्तथा|
मांसादान् मृगशब्देन दद्यान्मांसाभिवृद्धये||१५३||
गजखड्गितुरङ्गाणां वेशवारीकृतं भिषक्|

दद्यान्महिषशब्देन मांसं मांसाभिवृद्धये||१५४||

To the patient suffering from Shosha – wasting of body tissues, following types of meat is given to eat:

1. Meat of peacock

2. The meat of vultures, owls and blue- joys in the disguise of peacock meat, after preparing in a suitable manner according to the prescribed methods

3. The meat of crow in the disguise of the meat of partridge.

4. The meat of snakes in disguise of the meat of Varmi (an edible fish which is round and long in shape like a snake)

5. The fried meat of earth- worm in the disguise of the intestine of fish.

6. The meat of Lopaka (fox), Sthula Nakula (large mongoose), cat and cubs of jackal, properly dressed, in the disguise of the meat of rabbit

7. Similarly, the meat of lion, bear, hyena, tiger and such other carnivorous animals is given in the disguise of the meat of deer to promote the muscle tissues of the meat of deer to promote the muscle tissues of such patients and

8. The meat of elephant, rhinoceros and horse, well seasoned with spices is given in the disguise of buffalo meat for the promotion of muscle tissues of the patient [150-154]

Therapeutic Utility of Meat:

मांसेनोपचिताङ्गानां मांसं मांसकरं परम्|

तीक्ष्णोष्णलाघवाच्छस्तं विशेषान्मृगपक्षिणाम्||१५५||

The meat of carnivorous animals, exceedingly promotes the muscle tissues of the patient.

Similarly, the meat of different types of deer and birds is useful for such patients because of its sharpness, heating effects and lightness [155]

Need for Disguising the Identity of Meat:

मांसानि यान्यनभ्यासादनिष्टानि प्रयोजयेत्|

तेषूपधा, सुखं भोक्तुं तथा शक्यानि तानि हि||१५६||

जानञ्जुगुप्सन्नैवाद्याज्जग्धं वा पुनरुल्लिखेत्|

तस्माच्छद्मोपसिद्धानि मांसान्येतानि दापयेत्||१५७||

The meat of some animals, not withstanding its utility for patients, is not considered edible in tradition. To enable the patient to take such meat without any reservation or hatred, such meats are administered in disguise.

If the patient comes to know the exact identity of such meat, then out of hatred he may not eat it. Even if he eats such meat out of complication, he may vomit it out. Therefore, the meat of such animals is cooked properly and given to the patient in disguise, in the name of the meat which is traditionally edible. [156-157]

Wholesome Meat:

बर्हितित्तिरिदक्षाणां हंसानां शूकरोष्ट्रयोः|

खरगोमहिषाणां च मांसं मांसकरं परम्||१५८||

The meat of peacock, partridge, cock, swan, hog, camel, ass, bull and buffalo is excellent for the promotion of muscle tissue. [158]

Meat of different Groups of Animals:

योनिरष्टविधा चोक्ता मांसानामन्नपानिके|

तां परीक्ष्य भिषग्विद्वान् दद्यान्मांसानि शोषिणे||१५९||

प्रसहा भूशयानूपवारिजा वारिचारिणः|

आहारार्थं प्रदातव्या मात्रया वातशोषिणे||१६०||

प्रतुदा विष्किराश्चैव धन्वजाश्च मृगद्विजाः|

कफपित्तपरीतानां प्रयोज्याः शोषरोगिणाम्||१६१||

विधिवत्सूपसिद्धानि मनोज्ञानि मृदूनि च|
रसवन्ति सुगन्धीनि मांसान्येतानि भक्षयेत्||१६२||

In the chapter on "Annapana vidhi" dealing with the properties of ingredients of food and drinks (Read here – Charaka Sutrasthana 27/87) meat of 8 groups of animals is described. The learned physician should examine the meat keeping the description made there in view and administer suitable meat to the patient suffering from depletion of body tissues.

To the patient, suffering from depletion of tissues caused by aggravated Vata, the meat of birds and animals belonging to the categories of Prasaha (animals and birds who eat by snatching), Bhusaya (animals who live in burrows on the earth) Anupa (animals inhabiting marshy land), Varija (aquatic animals) and Varicara (birds moving in the water) should be given in appropriate quantity to eat.

To the patient, suffering from depletion of tissues caused by aggravated Kapha and Pitta, the meat of birds and animals belonging to the categories of Pratuda (pecker birds), Viskira (Gallinacious birds) and Dhanvaja (animals dwelling in arid (zone) is administered.[159-162]

Specific Utility of Meat and Alcohol:

मांसमेवाश्नतः शोषो माध्वीकं पिबतोऽपि च|
नियतानल्पचितस्य चिरं काये न तिष्ठति||१६३||

Depletion of tissues does not remain for a long time in the patient who eats meat, who drinks Madhvika (a type of alcoholic drink) and who is strong minded. [163]

Prevention of Tuberculosis:

वारुणीमण्डनित्यस्य बहिर्मार्जनसेविनः|
अविधारितवेगस्य यक्ष्मा न लभतेऽन्तरम्||१६४||

Tuberculosis will not be able to find entry into the body of a person who regularly takes Varunimanda (upper portion of the Varuni type of alcoholic drink) and who attends to the manifested natural urges (of defecation, urination, etc). [164]

Alcoholic drinks as Anupana:

प्रसन्नां वारुणीं सीधुमरिष्टानासवान्मधु|
यथार्हमनुपानार्थं पिबेन्मांसानि भक्षयन्||१६५||

After taking meat, Anupana (postprandial drink) used are

Prasanna

Varuni

Sidhu

Arista

Asava or

Madhvika type's alcoholic drinks, depending upon their suitability [165]

Therapeutic Utility of Alcoholic Drinks

मद्यं तैक्ष्ण्यौष्ण्यवैशद्यसूक्ष्मत्वात् स्रोतसां मुखम्|
प्रमथ्य विवृणोत्याशु तन्मोक्षात् सप्त धातवः||१६६||
पुष्यन्ति धातुपोषाच्च शीघ्रं शोषः प्रशाम्यति|

Madya (alcoholic drinks) is Teekshna (sharp), Ushna (hot) Vishada (non- slimy) and Sooksma (which can penetrate subtle channels) in its property. Therefore, it is capable of forcefully and quickly opening the orifices of srotas (channels of circulation) as a result of which 7 categories of tissue elements get proper nourishment. [166-167]

Recipes of Medicated Ghee:

मांसादमांसस्वरसे सिद्धं सर्पिः प्रयोजयेत्||१६७||
सक्षौद्रं, पयसा सिद्धं सर्पिर्दशगुणेन वा|
सिद्धं मधुरकैर्द्रव्यैर्दशमूलकषायकैः||१६८||
क्षीर मांस रसोपेतैर्घृतं शोषहरं परम्|
पिप्पली पिप्पलीमूल चव्य चित्रक नागरैः||१६९||
सयावशूकैः सक्षीरैः स्रोतसां शोधनं घृतम्|
रास्नाबलागोक्षुरकस्थिरावर्षाभुसाधितम्||१७०||
जीवन्ती पिप्पली गर्भे सक्षीरं शोषनुद्घृतम्|
यवाग्वा वा पिबेन्मात्रां लिह्याद्वा मधुना सह||१७१||
सिद्धानां सर्पिषामेषामद्यादन्नेन वा सह|
शुष्यतामेष निर्दिष्टो विधिराभ्यवहारिकः||१७२||

The following recipes are administered to the patient suffering from muscle wasting:

1. Ghee, boiled with the soup of the meat of carnivoros animals, is given along with honey

2. Ghee boiled with 10 times of milk

3. Ghee, cooked with the decoction of Dashamula (bilva –Aegle marmelos, syonaka, Gambhari—Gmelina arborea, Patali, Ganikarika, salaparni, Prsniparni, Brihati – Solanum indicum, Kantakari – Solanum surratense and Goksura—Tribulus terrestris), milk, meat soup and the paste of drugs belonging to Madhura gana (Jivaniya Gana), is excellent in depletion of body tissues.

4. Ghee, cooked with milk (4 times of ghee) and the paste of Pippali – Long pepper fruit – Piper longum, Pippalimula, Chavya – Piper retrofractum, Chitraka – Leadword – Plumbago zeylanica, Nagara and Yavaksara, is excellent for cleansing the channels of circulation and

5. Ghee cooked with milk and the paste of Rasna, Bala, Goksura, Sthira – Desmodium gangeticum and Varsabhu and added with Jivanti – Leptadenia reticulata as well as Pippali – Long pepper fruit – Piper longum cures depletion of body tissues.

All the above-mentioned recipes of medicated ghee are given in appropriate dose along with Yavagu (thick gruel) or these are to be mixed with honey and administered in the form of a linctus or these are to be given to the patient along with food. Thus the food and drinks for the patient suffering from depletion of body tissues are described [167-172]

External Therapies:

बहिःस्पर्शनमाश्रित्य वक्ष्यतेऽतः परं विधिः|
स्नेहक्षीराम्बुकोष्ठेषु स्वभ्यक्तमवगाहयेत्||१७३||
स्रोतो विबन्धमोक्षार्थं बलपुष्ट्यर्थमेव च|
उत्तीर्णं मिश्रकैःस्नेहैः पुनराक्तैः सुखैः करैः||१७४||

Hereafter, remedies for external use will be described. The patient should take a bath in a tub (Kostha) containing Sneha (oil, ghee, etc), milk or water. These medicated baths help in the opening up of the obstructed channels of circulation and promote strength. After finishing the bath, the patient is given a gentle massage after smearing his body with ghee and oil, mixed together. Thereafter, the patient should sit leisurely and unction (Utsadana) is applied all over his body] [173-174]

Recipes for Unction – Utsadana

मृद्नीयात् सुखमासीनं सुखं चोत्सादयेन्नरम्|
जीवन्तीं शतवीर्यां च विकसां सपुनर्नवाम्||१७५||
अश्वगन्धामपामार्गं तर्कारीं मधुकं बलाम्|
विदारीं सर्षपं कुष्ठं तण्डुलानतसीफलम्||१७६||
माषांस्तिलांश्च किण्वं च सर्वमेकत्र चूर्णयेत्|

यवचूर्णत्रिगुणितं दध्ना युक्तं समाक्षिकम्||१७७||
एतदुत्सादनं कार्यं पुष्टिवर्णबलप्रदम्|

All these drugs are made to a powder, and to this, three times of the powder of barley is added:

Jivanti – Leptadenia reticulata,

Satavirya - Asparagus racemosus

Vikasa (manjistha) – Rubia cordifolia

Punarnava – Boerhavia diffusa

Ashwagandha – Winter Cherry / Indian ginseng (root) – Withania somnifera,

Apamarga – Achyranthes aspera

Tarkari (Jaya) - Clerodendrum phlomidis

Madhuka– Licorice – Glycyrrhiza glabra

Bala – Country mallow (root) – Sida cordifolia

Vidari (Pueraria tuberosa),

Sarsapa – Brassica campestris

Kushta – Saussurea lappa,

Tandula

Fruits of atasi – Linum usitatissimum

Masha

Tila – Sesame (Sesamum indicum) and

Kina (material used for fermenting)

This should then be mixed with curd and honey in small quantities and used for unction which promotes nourishment, complexion and strength. [175- 178]

Recipe for Medicated bath:

गौर सर्षप कल्केन कल्कैश्चापि सुगन्धिभिः||१७८||
स्नायाद्‌ऋतुसुखैस्तोयैर्जीवनीयौषधैः शृतैः|१७९|

The patient of depletion of tissues is bathed with warm or cold water depending upon the nature of the season. This water is boiled with drugs belonging to Jivaniya gana. Before taking bath, his body is rubbed with the paste of white mustard seed or fragrant drugs [178-179]

Regime:

गन्धैः समाल्यैर्वासोभिर्भूषणैश्च विभूषितः||१७९||
स्पृश्यान् संस्पृश्य सम्पूज्य देवताः सभिषग्द्विजाः|
इष्ट वर्ण रस स्पर्श गन्धवत् पानभोजनम्||१८०||
इष्टमिष्टैरुपहितं सुखमद्यात् सुखप्रदम्|

The patient of depletion of tissues should apply perfume, wear garlands, [beautiful] garments and ornaments, touch auspicious objects, offer prayer to the Gods, physicians and Brahmins, and thereafter, he should take food and drinks which are of agreeable colour, taste, touch and smell. The food and drinks are consumed leisurely. These ingredients of food and drinks are agreeable or is mixed with other agreeable articles [179-181]

Wholesome Corns and Cereals

समातीतानि धान्यानि कल्पनीयानि शुष्यताम्||१८१||
लघून्यहीनवीर्याणि स्वादूनि गन्धवन्ति च|
यानि प्रहर्षकारीणि तानि पथ्यतमानि हि||१८२||
यच्चोपदेक्ष्यते पथ्यं क्षतक्षीणचिकित्सिते|
यक्ष्मिणस्तत् प्रयोक्तव्यं बलमांसाभिवृद्धये||१८३||

The patients suffering from depletion of body tissues should take corn and cereals which were harvested before one year, which are appropriately cooked, which are light, which are not devoid of potency, which are tasteful and which are of good smell.

Such ingredients of food and drinks, which are invigorating, are wholesome for the patient. Wholesome diet and drinks which are to be described in the chapter dealing with the treatment of Ksatasina (Chikitsa 11) is given and muscle tissue. [181-183]

Useful Regime:

अभ्यङ्गोत्सादनैश्चैव वासोभिरहतैः प्रियैः|
यथर्तुविहितैः स्नानैरवगाहैर्विमार्जनैः||१८४||
बस्तिभिः क्षीरसर्पिर्भिर्मांसैर्मांसरसौदनैः|
इष्टैर्मद्यैर्मनोज्ञानां गन्धानामुपसेवनैः||१८५||
सुहृदां रमणीयानां प्रमदानां च दर्शनैः|
गीतवादित्रशब्दैश्च प्रियश्रुतिभिरेव च||१८६||
हर्षणाश्वासनैर्नित्यं गुरूणां समुपासनैः|
ब्रह्मचर्येण दानेन तपसा देवतार्चनैः||१८७||
सत्येनाचारयोगेन मङ्गल्यैरप्यहिंसया|
वैद्यविप्रार्चनाच्चैव रोगराजो निवर्तते||१८८||

Rajayakshma – the king diseases, gets cured by Abhyanga, Utsadana, wearing of new and pleasant garments, taking medicated bath in consonance with the temperature of the season, external cleansing, using medicated enema, taking milk, ghee, meat and food mixed with meat soup, drinking agreeable alcoholic preparations, applying pleasing perfumes, observing friendly and beautiful ladies, hearing vocal and instrumental music, hearing invigorating and consulting talks, paying regular prayers to preceptors, observing celibacy, giving donations, performing penance, offering prayers to the Gods, speaking the truth, maintaining good conduct, performing auspicious and non-violent activities and showing respect to physicians and learned Brahmins [184-188]

Performance of Yajna:

यया प्रयुक्तया चेष्ट्या राजयक्ष्मा पुरा जितः|
तां वेदविहितामिष्टिमारोग्यार्थी प्रयोजयेत्||१८९||

The patient desirous of regaining his health should perform the Yajna (Sacrificial ceremony) enjoined by the Vedas, by the performance of which the disease tuberculosis was cured in the days of the yore. [189]

To sum up
तत्र श्लोकौ-
प्रागुत्पत्तिर्निमित्तानि प्रागूपं रूपसङ्ग्रहः|
समासाद् व्यासतश्चोक्तं भेषजं राजयक्ष्मणः||१९०||
नामहेतुरसाध्यत्वं साध्यत्वं कृच्छ्रसाध्यता|
इत्युक्तः सङ्ग्रहः कृत्स्नो राजयक्ष्मचिकित्सिते||१९१||

Origin of the disease in the days of Yore, etiology, premonitory signs and symptoms, various categories of manifested signs and symptoms, medicaments, described in brief and in detail, derivation of the term Rajayakshma, incurability, curability, curability with difficulty- all these in respect of Rajayakshma are described fully in this chapter on Rajayakshma Chikitsa. [190-191]

इत्यग्निवेशकृते तन्त्रे चरकप्रतिसंस्कृते चिकित्सास्थाने राजयक्ष्मचिकित्सितं नामाष्टमोऽध्यायः||८||

Thus, ends the 8th chapters dealing with the treatment of Rajayaksma (tuberculosis) in the Chikitsa sthana of work of Agnivesha, as redacted by Charaka.

15

Chikitsasthana Chapter 9 Unmada Chikitsitam

The 9th chapter of Charaka Samhita Chikitsa Sthana deals with Unmada – symptoms, types, treatment, therapies and medicines for insanity or psychosis. It also explains the importance of old ghee – Purana ghritham in the treatment of neurological and psychiatric disorders.

Chapter 9
Unmad Chikitsa – Treatment of psychosis, insanity

अथात उन्माद चिकित्सितं व्याख्यास्यामः||१||
इति ह स्माह भगवानात्रेयः||२||
We shall now expound the chapter on the treatment of Unmada (insanity).
Thus, said Lord Atreya. [1-2]

बुद्धि स्मृति ज्ञानतपोनिवासः पुनर्वसुः प्राणभृतां शरण्यः|
उन्मादहेत्वाकृतिभेषजानि कालेऽग्निवेशाय शशंस पृष्टः||३||
Punarvasu, the abode of intellect, memory, knowledge and penance and the protector (Sharanya) of living beings while replying to questions, explained to Agnivesha the aetiology, signs, symptoms, and treatment of Unmada [3]

Causes – Unmada Nidana:
विरुद्ध दुष्टाशुचि भोजनानि प्रधर्षणं देव गुरु द्विजानाम्|
उन्माद हेतुर्भय हर्ष पूर्वो मनोऽभिघातो विषमाश्च चेष्टाः||४||
The causative factors of Unmada (insanity) are as follows:
1) Intake of Viruddha (mutually contradictory), Dushta (polluted) and Ashuchi (impure) foods and drinks
2) Pradharsana (insult) to the gods, Guru and Dvijas (people belonging to the families of Brahmanas, Ksatriyas and Vaishyas)
3) Affliction of the mind because of fear and sudden happiness and
4) Unwholesome physical and mental activities.[4]

Unmada Samprapti – Pathogenesis:
तैरल्प सत्त्वस्य मलाः प्रदुष्टा बुद्धेर्निवासं हृदयं प्रदूष्य|
स्रोतांस्यधिष्ठाय मनोवहानि प्रमोहयन्त्याशु नरस्य चेतः||५||
The causative factors described above vitiate the Doshas of a person having less of Sattva (intellect), which afflict Hrudaya (heart), which is the abode of intellect and while being located in the Manovaha srotas (Channels carrying Psychic impulses), they afflict the mind. [5]

Unmada Lakshana – Signs and Symptoms

धी विभ्रमः सत्त्व परिप्लवश्च पर्याकुला दृष्टिरधीरता च|
अबद्धवाक्त्वं हृदयं च शून्यं सामान्यमुन्मादगदस्य लिङ्गम्||६||
स मूढचेता न सुखं न दुःखं नाचारधर्मौ कुत एव शान्तिम्|
विन्दत्यपास्तस्मृतिबुद्धिसङ्गो भ्रमत्ययं चेत इतस्ततश्च||७||

General signs and symptoms of Unmada:

Dhee Vibhrama – Intellectual confusion,

Satva pariplava – Fickleness of mind,

Paryakula – impatience,

Drushti adhirta – unsteadiness of eyes

Abaddha vaktavam – irrelevant speech and

Hrudaya Shunya – a sensation of vacuum in the heart (Vacant mindedness)

Other symptoms include:

He will have a bewildered mind & becomes incapable of experiencing pleasure and sorrow.

He becomes incapable of conducting himself appropriately.

Therefore, he loses peace of mind altogether and becomes devoid of memory, intellect and recognition.

His mind wavers here and there. [6-7]

Unmada – definition:

समुद्भ्रमं बुद्धिमनःस्मृतीनामुन्मादमागन्तुनिजोत्थमाहुः|८|

The term Unmada stands for Samudbhrama i.e perversion because in this ailment, the intellect, mind and memory get perverted.

It is of 2 types, viz,

Agantu (exogenous) and

Nijottha (Endogenous) [8]

Unmada Bheda – types:

तस्योद्भवं पञ्चविधं पृथक् तु वक्ष्यामि लिङ्गानि चिकित्सितं च||८||

Now, the signs, symptoms and treatment of the 5 varieties of Unmada will be described separately. [1/2]

Vataja,

Pittaja

Kaphaja

Sannipatika – combined vitiation of all the three Doshas

Agantuja – due to exogenous causes

Causes, signs and Symptoms of Vatika Unmada:

रूक्षाल्प शीतान्न विरेक धातु क्षयोपवासैरनिलोऽतिवृद्धः|
चिन्तादि जुष्टं हृदयं प्रदूष्य बुद्धिं स्मृतिं चाप्युपहन्ति शीघ्रम्||९||
अस्थानहासस्मितनृत्यगीतवागङ्गविक्षेपणरोदनानि|
पारुष्यकार्श्यारुण वर्णताश्च जीर्णे बलं चानिलजस्य रूपम्||१०||

Nidana: Vata gets exceedingly aggravated by

Ruksha ahara – The intake of unctuous food,

Alpa ahara and Shitanna – less of food and cold food,

Dhatu vireka – excessive elimination of Doshas by excess Panchakarma treatment

Dhatu kshaya – depletion of tissue elements and

And

Upavasa – fasting.

The aggravated Vata adversely affects the heart afflicted with mental agony (including worry, passion and anger) and instantaneously afflicts intellect and memory.

Signs and symptoms of Vatika Unmada:

1. Laughing, smiling, dancing, singer, speaking, moving limbs of the body and weeping in inappropriate place and

2. Parushya, Karshya and Aruna Varna skin – Roughness of skin, emaciation and reddish coloration of the skin.

These signs and symptoms become more conspicuous after the digestion of food (when normally Vayu gets aggravated). [9-10]

Pittaja Unmada Nidana, Lakshana

अजीर्ण कट्वम्ल विदाह्यशीतैर्भोज्यैश्चितं पित्तमुदीर्णवेगम्।

उन्मादमत्युग्रमनात्मकस्य हृदि श्रितं पूर्ववदाशु कुर्यात्॥११॥

अमर्ष संरम्भ विनग्नभावाः सन्तर्जनातिद्रवणौष्ण्यरोषाः ।

प्रच्छायशीतान्नजलाभिलाषाः पीता च भाः पित्तकृतस्य लिङ्गम्॥१२॥

The pitta gets aggravated by

Ajirna – indigestion,

Katu, amla ahara – intake of pungent, sour foods

Vidahi (which causes burning sensation) and hot food

This aggravated Pitta afflicts the heart of a patient devoid of self-control and leads to serious type of Unmada.

Paittik Unmada lakshana – symptoms:

1. Intolerance, over daring, nakedness, intimidation, running about, excessive heat in the body and anger,

2. Desire for shady place, cold food and cold water and anger

3. Yellow complexion [11-12]

Kaphaja Unmada Nidan Lakshan:

सम्पूरणैर्मन्द विचेष्टितस्य सोष्मा कफो मर्मणि सम्प्रवृद्धः।

बुद्धिं स्मृतिं चाप्युपहत्य चित्तं प्रमोहयन् सञ्जनयेद्विकारम्॥१३॥

वाक्चेष्टितं मन्दमरोचकश्च नारीविविक्तप्रियताऽतिनिद्रा।

छर्दिश्च लाला च बलं च भुङ्क्ते नखादिशौक्ल्यं च कफात्मकस्य॥१४॥

Kapha, along with Ushma (Pitta) gets aggravated because of Sampurna (over nourishment) and lethargy.

This aggravated Kapha afflicts the vital organ (heart), adversely affects intellect and memory, and vitiates the mind leading to morbidity (Kaphaja Unmada).

Signs and symptoms of Kaphaja Unmada

1. Manda vak chestitam – Sluggishness in speech and activities

2. Aruchi – Anorexia

3. Nari vivikta priyata – Liking for women and lonely places

4. Ati nidra – Excessive sleep

5. Chardi – vomiting and

6. Lala srava – excessive salivation

7. Aggravation of the condition immediately after taking food (when Kapha gets normally aggravated) and

8. Nakhadi shauklam – Whitening of nails etc. [13-14]

Sannipatika Type of Unmada – Schizophrenia:

यः सन्निपात प्रभवोऽतिघोरः सर्वैः समस्तैः स च हेतुभिः स्यात्।

सर्वाणि रूपाणि बिभर्ति ताद्ग्विरुद्धभैषज्यविधिर्विवर्ज्यः॥१५॥

Sannipatika type of Unmada (where all the 3 Doshas, Viz. Vata, Pitta and Kapha get simultaneously aggravated) is a serious ailment.

It is caused by the (simultaneous) vitiation of all the 3 Doshas by their (respective) causative factors (as listed above) In this condition, signs and symptoms of all 3 Doshas are manifested. Such a condition needs therapeutic measures which are mutually contradictory. Therefore, the physician should not attend to such a patient since this condition will be incurable. [15]

Agantuja Unmada – due to exogenous causes:

देवर्षि गन्धर्व पिशाच यक्ष रक्षःपितृणामभिधर्षणानि।
आगन्तु हेतुर्नियमव्रतादि मिथ्याकृतं कर्म च पूर्वदेहे।।१६।।

Exogenous types of Unmada are caused by improper observance of Niyama (spiritual disciplines) in the present life and improper conduct of the past life which leads to seizures by the Gods, Rishis (Sages), Gandharvas, Pisachas, Yakshas, Rakshas (demons) and Pitrus (manes) [16]

Agantu Unmada Lakshana:

अमर्त्यवाग्विक्रम वीर्यचेष्टो ज्ञानादिविज्ञानबलादिभिर्यः।
उन्माद कालोऽनियतश्च यस्य भूतोत्थमुन्मादमुदाहरेत्तम्।।१७।।

Bhutonmada (Seizures by supernatural being), in general is characterized by the following
1. Supernatural speech, valour, potency and activities manifested as a result of Supernatural knowledge (Jnana) and intellectual excellence (Vijnana) as well as strength etc, and
2. Time of occurrence being not determined [17]

Modes of Seizure

अदूषयन्तः पुरुषस्य देहं देवादयः स्वैस्तु गुणप्रभावैः।
विशन्त्यदृश्यास्तरसा यथैव च्छायातपौ दर्पणसूर्यकान्तौ।।१८।।

The Gods, etc, because of their own qualities and powers, cause seizures of the individual without afflicting his physique
Like one can see his reflection instantaneously in Suryakanta mani (a gem), these supernatural beings are invisible and they afflict the human being instantaneously.[18]

आघातकालो हि स पूर्वरूपः प्रोक्तो निदानेऽथ सुरादिभिश्च।
उन्माद रूपाणि पृथङ्निबोध कालं च गम्यान् पुरुषांश्च तेषाम्।।१९।।

The time of seizure, premonitory signs and actual signs and symptoms of Bhutonmada are already described, in general, in Nidana Sthana. Now, the signs and symptoms of seizures by the gods etc are being specially described in respect to each of these varieties. [19]
Specific Signs and Symptoms of Agantuja Unmada

Devonmada – Insanity Caused by the Gods:

तद्यथा- सौम्यदृष्टिं गम्भीरमधृष्यम कोपनम स्वप्न भोजनाभिलाषिणमल्प स्वेद मूत्र पुरीष वातं शुभगन्धं फुल्ल पद्मवदनमिति देवोन्मत्तं विद्यात्;

The patient is of gentle look, earnest, invincible, free from anger, sleep and desire for food, having less of sweat, urine, stool and flatus. He emits a good aroma from the body and has a face like a blooming lotus.

Guru unmada:

गुरुवृद्धसिद्धर्षीणामभिशापाभिचाराभिध्यानानुरूपचेष्टाहारव्याहारं तैरुन्मत्तं विद्यात्;

A person having the activities and speech as ordained by the Abhisapa (cure), Abhichara (spell) and Abhidhyana (desire to transform on the basis of will- power) of preceptors, senior persons, Siddhas (those who have obtained spiritual perfection) and Rshis (Sages) is to be diagnosed as suffering from Unmada (insanity) caused by the seizure of preceptors etc.

Pitru Unmada: Caused by Manes:
अप्रसन्न दृष्टिमपश्यन्तं निद्रालुं प्रतिहत वाचमनन्नाभिलाषमरोचकाविपाकपरीतं च पितृभिरुन्मत्तं विद्यात्;
Characterized by unhappy look, inability to see, sleepiness, interrupted speech, lack of desire for food, anorexia and indigestion.

Gandharva Unmada: by Gandharva (celestial musicians)
(चण्डं साहसिकं तीक्ष्णं गम्भीरमधृष्यं) मुखवाद्य नृत्य गीतान्नपानस्नानमाल्यधूपगन्धरतिं रक्तवस्त्रबलिकर्महास्यकथानुयोगप्रियं शुभगन्धं च गन्धर्वोन्मत्तं विद्यात्;
Characterised by violent acts, over bravery, sharpness, seriousness, invincibility and liking for Mukhavadya (Vocal music or musical instruments played with mouth), dancing, singing, good food, good drinks, Garlands, incense, perfume, red apparel, Bali (offering of Sacrifices), laughing and talking (engagement in humorous talks). Pleasuring aroma comes out from his body.

Yakshonmada – semi-divine celestial beings, attendants of Kubera, the god of wealth:
असकृत्स्वप्नरोदनहास्यं नृत्य गीत वाद्य पाठ कथान्नपानस्नानमाल्यधूपगन्धरतिं रक्तविप्लुताक्षं द्विजातिवैद्यपरिवादिनं रहस्यभाषिणं च यक्षोन्मत्तं विद्यात्;
Characterized by frequent sleep, cry and laugh, liking for dancing, singing, playing musical instruments, reciting sacred scriptures, telling stories, good food, drinks, bath, garlands, incense and perfumes. His eyes are red and tearful. He despises dvija (persons belonging to the families of Brahmanas, Ksatriyas and Vaisyas) and Physicians. He discloses the secrets of others.

Rakshasonmada Caused by Demons
नष्टनिद्रमन्नपानद्वेषिणमनाहारमप्यतिबलिनं शस्त्र शोणित मांस रक्तमाल्याभिलाषिणं सन्तर्जकं च राक्षसोन्मत्तं विद्यात्;
It is characterized by sleeplessness, hatred for food and drinks, excessive strength of patient in spite of his aversion for food, liking for weapons, blood, meat and red garlands and ferociousness.

Brahma Rakshasa Unmada: By senior devil
प्रहासनृत्यप्रधानं देवविप्रवैद्यद्वेषाव ज्ञाभिः स्तुतिवेदमन्त्रशास्त्रोदाहरणैः काष्ठादिभिरात्मपीडनेन च ब्रह्मराक्षसोन्मत्तं विद्यात्;
Characterized by excessive laughter, dance, hatred and disobedience to the Gods, Vipras (persons belonging to the family of Brahmins) and Physicians. He recites illustrations from hymns, the Vedas, Mantras and other scriptures. He injures himself by pieces of wood etc.

Pishachonmada – a type of demons
अस्वस्थचित्तं स्थानमलभमानं नृत्यगीतहासिनं बद्धाबद्धप्रलापिनं सङ्करकूटमलिनरथ्याचेलतृणाश्मकाष्ठाधिरोहणरतिं भिन्नरूक्षस्वरं नग्नं विधावन्तं नैकत्र तिष्ठन्तं दुःखान्यावेदयन्तं नष्टस्मृतिं च पिशाचोन्मत्तं विद्यात्||२०||
It is characterized by fickle mindedness. He complains of having / getting a suitable and pleasing place to stay. He engages himself in dancing, singing, laughing and incoherent speech. He likes climbing over uneven places, entering into caves, walking in dirty streets and over dirty clothes, and climbing over heaps of grass, stones and woods. His voice is broken and hoarse. He remains naked and runs here and there. He does not stick to one place. He always complains of his miseries before others do and he suffers from loss of memory. [20]

Time of affliction of Unmada:
तत्र चौक्षाचारं तपःस्वाध्यायकोविदं नरं प्रायः शुक्लप्रतिपदि त्रयोदश्यां च छिद्रमवेक्ष्याभिधर्षयन्ति देवाः, स्नानशुचिविविक्तसेविनं धर्मशास्त्रश्रुतिवाक्यकुशलं प्रायः षष्ठ्यां नवम्यां चर्षयः, मातृपितृगुरुवृद्धसिद्धाचार्योपसेविनं प्रायो दशम्याममावस्यायां च पितरः, गन्धर्वाः स्तुतिगीतवादित्ररतिं परदारगन्धमाल्यप्रियं चौक्षाचारं प्रायो द्वादश्यां चतुर्दश्यां च, सत्त्वबलरूपगर्वशौर्ययुक्तं माल्यानुलेपनहास्यप्रियमतिवाक्करणं प्रायः शुक्लैकादश्यां सप्तम्यां च यक्षाः, स्वाध्यायतपोनियमोपवासब्रह्मचर्यदेवयतिगुरुपूजाऽरतिं

भ्रष्टशौचं ब्राह्मणमब्राह्मणं वा ब्राह्मणवादिनं शूरमानिनं देवागारसलिलक्रीडनरतिं प्रायः शुक्लपञ्चम्यां पूर्णचन्द्रदर्शने च ब्रह्मराक्षसाः, रक्षःपिशाचास्तु हीनसत्त्वं पिशुनं स्त्रैणं लुब्धं शठं प्रायो द्वितीयातृतीयाष्टमीषु; इत्यपरिसङ्ख्येयानां ग्रहाणामाविष्कृततमा ह्यष्टावेते व्याख्याताः॥२१॥

Devonmada: The gods possess a person of purity, good conduct, penance and study of religious scriptures, generally on the 1st and 13th days of the bright fortnight (Shukla Paksha) in an opportune moment (at the sight of some off his weak points).

Rushi Unmada: Rsis possesses a person fond of bath, purity and lonely place, and conversant with the sayings of the religious scriptures and the Vedas, generally on the 6th or 9th day of the fortnight (Paksha) in an opportune moment (at the sight of some of his weak points).

Pitru Unmada: Pitrus (manes) possesses a person devoted to the service of his parents, Gurus, Vruddhas (senior persons), Siddhas (those who have accomplished spiritual perfection) and Acharyas (spiritual teachers), generally on the tenth day of the fortnight (Paksha) or on the new moon day [in an opportune moment, i.e. at the sight of some of his weak points].

Gandharva Unmada: Gandharvas (celestial musicians) possess a person fond of Hymns, perfumes, garlands, purify and good conduct, generally on the twelfth or fourteenth day of a fort- night (Paksha) in an opportune moment.

Yaksha Unmada:n possess a person endowed with mental strength, physical strength, good complexion, ego and valour, having liking for garlands, unction and laughter and who is talkative, generally during the 7th or 11th day of the bright fort- night (Sukla Paksa) [in an opportune moment, i.e. at the sight of some of his weak points]

Brahma rakshasa Unmada:

Brahmaraksasa (a class of evil demons) possess a Brahmin or a non Brahmin claiming to be a Brahmin who has abhorrence for the study of religious scriptures, penance, observance of Scriptural rules, Upavasa (fasting), Brahmacarya (celibacy), respect for the Gods, Yatis (recluses) and Gurus (preceptors), and purify, who claims to be brave and who likes a temple and aquatic games, generally on the fifth day of the bright fort- night (Sukla paksa) or on the full moon day [in an opportune moment, i.e. at the sight of some of his weak points]

Raksasa and Pishacha Unmada:

Raksasa and Pisacas (types of evil demons) possess a person who is devoid of will power, who is a backbiter who is fond of women and who is greedy and a cheat, generally on the 2nd, 3rd or 8th day of the fortnight [in an opportunity moment, i.e. at the sight of some of his weak points]

These Grahas (celestial begins) are innumerable. The seizures by the 8 most conspicuous ones among them are described above. [21]

Asadhya Lakshana- Signs of incurability:

सर्वेष्वपि तु खल्वेषु यो हस्तावुद्यम्य रोषसंरम्भान्निःशङ्कमन्येष्वात्मनि वा निपातयेत् स ह्यसाध्यो ज्ञेयः; तथा यः साश्रुनेत्रो मेढ्रप्रवृत्तरक्तः क्षतजिह्वः प्रसृतनासिकश्छिद्यमानचर्माऽप्रतिहन्यमानवाणिः सततं विकूजन् दुर्वर्णस्तृषार्तः पूतिगन्धश्च स हिंसार्थिनोन्मत्तो ज्ञेयः; तं परिवर्जयेत्॥२२॥

In the above mentioned varieties of Unmada, if the patient has raised his hand in a fit anger, daringly thrashes others or himself, he is considered as incurable. Similarly, if the patient, with tears in the eyes, passes blood from the genitals, if he has injuries in his tongue, running nostrils, excised skin, uninterrupted (long) speech, constant mumbling, discoloration of body, excessive thirst and putrid smell of body, he is to be considered as suffering from Unmada (insanity) as a result of possession of violent spirit, and hence, he should not be treated. [22]

Management of Ratyarthi Unmada:

रत्यर्चनाकामोन्मादिनौ तु भिषगभिप्रायाचाराभ्यां बुद्ध्वा तदङ्गोपहारबलिमिश्रेण।
मन्त्रभैषज्यविधिनोपक्रमेत्॥२३॥

If the Unmada (insanity) is cured by the possession of evil spirits desirous of pleasure or worship, the physician should ascertain the nature of possession through the intentions and behaviour of the patient, and treat him by the administration of appropriate Mantras and medicines along with the requisite presents and sacrifices. [23]

तत्र द्वयोरपि निजागन्तु निमित्तयोरुन्मादयोः
समासविस्तराभ्यां भेषज विधिमनुव्याख्यास्यामः||२४||

Now we shall expound therapeutic measures for both endogenous (nija) and exogenous (Agantuja) types of Unmada in brief as well as in detail [24]

Unmada Chikitsa Sutra – Line of Treatment

उन्मादे वातजे पूर्वं स्नेहपानं विशेषवित्|
कुर्यादावृतमार्गे तु सस्नेहं मृदु शोधनम्||२५||
कफ पित्तोद्भवेऽप्यादौ वमनं सविरेचनम्|
स्निग्ध स्विन्नस्य कर्तव्यं शुद्धे संसर्जन क्रमः||२६||
निरूहं स्नेहबस्तिं च शिरसश्च विरेचनम्|
ततः कुर्याद्यथादोषं तेषां भूयस्त्वमाचरेत्||२७||
हृदिन्द्रिय शिरःकोष्ठे संशुद्धे वमनादिभिः|
मनःप्रसादमाप्नोति स्मृतिं सञ्ज्ञां च विन्दति||२८||
शुद्धस्याचार विभ्रंशे तीक्ष्णं नावनमञ्जनम्|
ताडनं च मनो बुद्धि देह संवेजनं हितम्||२९||
यः सक्तोऽविनये पट्टैः संयम्य सुदृढैः सुखैः|
अपेत लोह काष्ठाद्ये संरोध्यश्च तमोगृहे||३०||
तर्जनं त्रासनं दानं हर्षणं सान्त्वनं भयम्|
विस्मयो विस्मृतेर्हेतोर्नयन्ति प्रकृतिं मनः||३१||
प्रदेहोत्सादनाभ्यङ्गधूमाः पानं च सर्पिषः|
प्रयोक्तव्यं मनोबुद्धिस्मृतिसञ्ज्ञाप्रबोधनम्||३२||
सर्पिःपानादिरागन्तोर्मन्त्रादिश्चेष्यते विधिः|३३|

In Vataja Unmada, the physician should first of all ascertain the nature of Vata, and in the beginning, administer Sneha (oil, Ghee, etc).

If the passage of Vata is obstructed (Avruta Marga), then the patient is given laxative along with Sneha (oil, ghee etc) only in small quantities. – Sasneha Mrudu Shodhana.

If caused by Kapha or Pitta, Vamana and Virechana treatments are given, after Snehana and Swedana. These therapies are followed up with Samsarjana Krama (from lighter to heavier diet gradually according to the prescribed procedure).

Thereafter, he is given Niruha (decoction enema), Sneha Basti (oil / fat enema) and Nasya therapy (therapies for the elimination of Doshas from the head).

Depending upon the predominance of Doshas, these elimination therapies are required to be administered repeatedly.

Benefits of Panchakarma treatment:

By the administration of Vamana etc therapies, the heart, sense organs, head and Koshta (Gastro- intestinal tract) gets cleaned as a result of which, the mind gets refreshed and the patient gains memory as well as consciousness.

If, even after the body is cleansed, the patient exhibits perversion of conduct, then he is given Teekhsna navana Nasya – strong inhalation therapy,

Teekshna Anjana – collyriums and even beatings which are useful for stimulating his mind, intellect and the body.

If the patient has a strong physique, and he is disobedient, then he is tied tightly with pieces of cloth, without hurting his body, and kept confined to a dark room devoid of iron (rods) and wooden pieces.

Shouting with anger, terrorizing (with the help of police men), and donation (presents), exhilaration, consolation, fear and exhibition of surprising acts bring back the natural state of the mind by counteracting the causes of his loss of memory.

The patient suffering from Unmada is administered Pradeha (application of thick ointments), Utsadana (unction), Abhyanga (massage), Dhuma (fumigation) and ghee for taking internally to stimulate his mind, intellect, memory and consciousness.

The patient suffering from Agantuja Unmada (insanity) is given Pana (to be taken internally) etc, and Mantras etc are recited for his benefit. [25-33 1/3]

अतः सिद्धतमान्योगाञ्छृणून्मादविनाशनान्||३३||

Now, we shall describe the most efficacious recipes for the cure of Unmada (insanity) [33 ½]

Kalyanaka ghrita:

हिङ्गु सौवर्चल व्योषैर्दिर्वपलांशैर्घृताढकम्|
चतुर्गुणे गवां मूत्रे सिद्धमुन्मादनाशनम्||३४||
विशाला त्रिफला कौन्ती देवदार्वेलवालुकम्|
स्थिरा नतं रजन्यौ द्वे सारिवे द्वे प्रियङ्गुका||३५||
नीलोत्पलैला मञ्जिष्ठा दन्ती दाडिम केशरम्|
तालीशपत्रं बृहती मालत्याः कुसुमं नवम्||३६||
विडङ्गं पृश्निपर्णी च कुष्ठं चन्दन पद्मकौ|
अष्टाविंशतिभिः कल्कैरेतैरक्षसमन्वितैः||३७||
चतुर्गुणे जले सम्यग्घृतप्रस्थं विपाचयेत्|
अपस्मारे ज्वरे कासे शोषे मन्देऽनले क्षये||३८||
वातरक्ते प्रतिश्याये तृतीयक चतुर्थके|
छर्द्यर्शो मूत्रकृच्छ्रेषु विसर्पोपहतेषु च||३९||
कण्डू पाण्ड्वामयोन्मादविषमेहगदेषु च|
भूतोपहतचित्तानां गद्गदानामचेसाम्||४०||
शस्तं स्त्रीणां च वन्ध्यानां धन्यमायुर्बलप्रदम्|
अलक्ष्मी पाप रक्षोघ्नं सर्वग्रह विनाशनम्||४१||
कल्याणकमिदं सर्पिः श्रेष्ठं पुंसवनेषु च|
इति कल्याणकं घृतम्|

Kalyanaka Ghruta:

2 Palas (96 g) of each of

Hingu – Asa foetida,

Sauvarchala – Sochal salt

Shunthi – Ginger,

Maricha – Black pepper fruit – Piper nigrum and

Pippali – Long pepper fruit – Piper longum is made to a paste and cooked with 1 Adhaka of ghee by adding 4 times (adhakas) of cow's urine. This medicated ghee is efficacious in curing Unmada (insanity) [34]

1 Aksha of each of the 28 herbs, namely

Vishala

Haritaki – Terminalia chebula

Bibhitaki – Terminalia bellerica

Amalaki – Phyllanthus emblica

Kaunti

Devadaru -Cedrus deodara

Elavaluka

Sthira

Ela – Cardamom

Manjistha – Rubia cordifolia

Danti – Baliospermum montanum

Dadima – Pomegranate – Punica granatum

Keshara – Mesua ferrea

Talisapatra

Brihati – Solanum indicum

Fresh Malati flower – Jasminum grandiflorum

Vidanga – Embelia ribes

Prishnaparni – Uraria picta,

Kushta – Saussurea lappa

Chandana – Sandalwood – Santalum album and

Padmaka is made to a paste.

This paste is added to 1 Prastha of ghee and cooked by adding 4 times (Prasthas) of water.

Indications:

Apasmara – epilepsy

Jwara – fever

Kasa – cough

Sosha – consumption

Suppression of the power of digestion

Phthisis

Vata Rakta – gout

Pratisyaya – coryza

Trtiyaka and Caturthaka types of Visama Jvara (irregular fever)

Chardi – vomiting

Arsha – piles

Mutra krcchra – Dysuria

Visarpa – Erysipelas

Kandu – itching

Pandu- Anaemia

Unmada – insanity

poisoning

Meha (obstinate urinary disorders including diabetes),

Seizures by supernatural beings (Bhutas)

Gadgada (lulling speech)

Achetas – unconsciousness and

Female infertility

It endows the individual with wealth, longevity and strength

It removes inauspiciousness, sins, demoniac seizures and afflictions by evil spirits.

It is most useful in Pumsavana (the second sacramental ritual or Samskara for getting a child of desired sex) this recipe is called Kalyanaka Sarpih [35-41 ½]

Mahakalyanaka Ghurta

एभ्य एव स्थिरादीनि जले पक्त्वैकविंशतिम्||४२||

रसे तस्मिन् पचेत् सर्पिर्गृष्टिक्षीरे चतुर्गुणे|

वीरार्द्रमाषकाकोलीस्वयङ्गुप्तर्षभर्धिभिः||४३||

मेदया च समैः कल्कैस्तत् स्यात् कल्याणकं महत्|

बृंहणीयं विशेषेण सन्निपातहरं परम्||४४||
इति महाकल्याणकं घृतम्|

A decoction is prepared of the 21 herbs beginning with Sthira – Desmodium gangeticum, described in the earlier recipe viz,

Sthira – Desmodium gangeticum

Nata

Haridra (turmeric – Curcuma longa),

Daru Haridra – Tree Turmeric (stem) – Berberis aristata,

Sariva – Indian Sarsaparilla – Hemidesmus indicus,

Krsna Sariva

Priyangu (Callicara macrophylla),

Nilotpala,

Ela (Elettaria cardamomum Maton),

Manjistha – Rubia cordifolia

Danti – Baliospermum montanum

Dadima – Pomegranate – Punica granatum,

Kesara,

Talisapatra,

Brihati – Solanum indicum,

fresh flowers of Malati,

Vidanga – Embelia ribes

Prishnaparni – Uraria picta,

Kushta – Saussurea lappa,

Candana (Sandalwood – Santalum album) and

Padmaka – Prunus cerasoides

To this decoction, ghee, 4 times of Grushtiksheera (milk of Vira, green Masa, Rddhi and Meda – Polygonatum cirrhifolium (1/4th in quantity of ghee, all ingredients taken in equal quantities) should be added and cooked.

This is called Mahakalyanaka Ghrta. It is exceedingly nourishing and it cures diseases caused by Sannipata (simultaneous vitiation of all the three Doshas). 42 ½ 44

Mahapaishachika Ghrita

जटिलां पूतनां केशीं चारटीं मर्कटीं वचाम्|
त्रायमाणां जयां वीरां चोरकं कटुरोहिणीम्||४५||
वयःस्थां शूकरीं छत्रामतिच्छत्रां पलङ्कषाम्|
महापुरुषदन्तां च कायस्थां नाकुलीद्वयम्||४६||
कटम्भरां वृश्चिकालीं स्थिरां चाहृत्य तैर्घृतम्|
सिद्धं चातुर्थकोन्मादग्रहापस्मार नाशनम्||४७||
महापैशाचिकं नाम घृतमेतद्यथाऽमृतम्|
बुद्धिस्मृतिकरं चैव बालानां चाङ्गवर्धनम्||४८||
इति महापैशाचिकं घृतम्|

Ghee cooked with [the paste of]

Jatila (Jatamamsi) – Nardostachys jatamansi

Putanam (Haritaki) – Terminalia chebula

Keshi (Bhutakesi) –

Charati (Kumbhi)

Markati (Sukasimbi),

Vacha – Acorus calamus

Trayamana – Gentiana kurroo
Jaya (Jayanti)
Vira (Ksirakakoli or Salaparni),
Choraka (Candalaka)
Katurohini
Vayahstha(Brahmi or Guduci)
Sukari (Varahikanda),
Chatra (Madhurika),
Aticchatra (Satapuspa),
Palankasa (Guggulu)
Maha purushadanta (Shatavari or Visnukranta)
Kayastha (Suksmaila)
Both the types of Nakuli (Rassna),
Katambhara (Katabhi)
Vrscikali (Vrscikapatri) and
Sthira
Indications:
Chaturthaka (a type of Vishama Jvara or recurrent fever)
Unmada (insanity, psychosis)
Graha (Seizures by evil spirits) and
Apasmara (epilepsy)
It works like nectar.
It promotes intellect and memory and helps in the development of the physique of children. [45-48]

Lasunadi Ghrta:
लशुनानां शतं त्रिंशदभयास्त्र्यूषणात् पलम्।
गवां चर्म मसी प्रस्थो द्व्याढकं क्षीरमूत्रयोः॥४९॥
पुराणसर्पिषः प्रस्थ एभिः सिद्धं प्रयोजयेत्।
हिङ्गुचूर्णपलं शीते दत्त्वा च मधुमाणिकाम्॥५०॥
तद्दोषागन्तुसम्भूतानुन्मादान् विषमज्वरान्।
अपस्मारांश्च हन्त्याशु पानाभ्यञ्जननावनैः॥५१॥
इति लशुनाद्यं घृतम्।
Ingredients of Lashunadi Ghrita
100 Dehusked cloves of Lasuna – Garlic
30 fruits of Haritaki – Terminalia chebula
1 Pala (48 g) of Tryushana (Ginger, pepper, long pepper)
1 Prastha (768 ml) of the ash of bovine leather, and
2 Adhakas of each of cow's milk and
Cow's urine is cooked with 2 Prasthas of cow's ghee (ten years old), after it is well cooked and cooled,
1 Pala of the powder of Hingu (asafoetida) and 2 Manikas of honey is added.
Use of this medicated ghee internally and for massage as well as inhalation therapy cures endogenous as well as exogenous types of Unmada (insanity) and Visama Jvara (irregular fever). [49-51]

Lasunadi Ghrta (Second Recipe)
लशुनस्याविनष्टस्य तुलार्धं निस्तुषीकृतम्।
तदर्धं दशमूलस्य द्व्याढकेऽपां विपाचयेत्॥५२॥
पादशेषे घृतप्रस्थं लशुनस्य रसं तथा।

कोलमूलकवृक्षाम्लमातुलुङ्गार्द्रकै रसैः||५३||
दाडिमाम्बुसुरामस्तुकाञ्जिकाम्लैस्तदर्धिकैः|
साधयेत्त्रिफलादारुलवणव्योषदीप्यकैः||५४||
यवानीचव्यहिङ्गुवम्लवेतसैश्च पलाधिकैः|
सिद्धमेतत् पिबेच्छूलगुल्मार्शोजठरापहम्||५५||
ब्रध्नपाण्डुवामयप्लीहयोनिदोषज्वरकृमीन्|
वातश्लेष्मामयान् सर्वानुन्मादांश्चापकर्षति||५६||
इत्यपरं लशुनाद्यं घृतम्|

1/2 Tula (50 Palas) of dehusked and unpolluted cloves of Ganikarika, Salaparni, Prsniparni, Brhati, Kantakari and Goksura) is boiled in 4 Adhakas of water and reduced to ¼ th

To this decoction,

2 Prasthas of ghee,

2 Prasthas of garlic juice,

1 Prastha each of juice of

Kola, Mulaka (radish),

Vrukshamla, Matulunga, Ardraka and Dadima and

1 Prastha of each of Sura, Mastu and sour Kanjika is added.

This is cooked by adding the powder or paste of 1/2 Pala of each of

Triphala (Haritaki, Bibhitaki and Amalaki), Devadaru, Lavana, Amla vetasa

Indicated in –

Shoola – abdominal colic

Gulma – abdominal tumor, distension

Pandu – Anemia, initial stages of liver disorders

Arsha – Hemorrhoids

Bradhna – Prolapsed rectum

Pandu – Anemia, initial stages of liver disorders

Yonidosha – Gynecological disorder

Jwara (fever)

Krumi – worm infestation (in wounds and in intestines)

Diseases caused by Vata and Kapha and all varieties of Unmada [52-56]

Recipes of Medicated Ghee

हिङ्गुना हिङ्गुपर्ण्या च सकायस्थवयःस्थया|
सिद्धं सर्पिर्हितं तद्वद्वयःस्थाहिङ्गुचोरकैः||५७||
केवलं सिद्धमेभिर्वा पुराणं पाययेद्घृतम्|
पाययित्वोत्तमां मात्रां श्वभ्रे रुन्ध्याद्गृहेऽपि वा||५८||

The patient suffering from Unmada is administered the following recipes of medicated ghee:

1. 10 year old ghee, cooked with Hingu and Hinguparni (according to some : Vamshapatrika)

2. 10 year old ghee cooked with Kayastha (Sukshma Ela – Lesser cardamom) and Vayahstha (Brahmi) and

3. 10 year old ghee cooked with Vayastha, Hingu and to such patients,

4. The patient is made to drink the above mentioned recipes of medicated ghee or the unprocessed ghee in a heavy dose and kept confined to an underground cellar or a house. [57-58]

Old Ghee and Its Therapeutic Utility:

विशेषतः पुराणं च घृतं तं पाययेद्भिषक्|
त्रिदोषघ्नं पवित्रत्वादिविशेषाद्ग्रहनाशनम्||५९||
गुण कर्माधिकं पानादास्वादात् कटुतिक्तकम्|

उग्रगन्धं पुराणं स्याद्दशवर्षस्थितं घृतम्||६०||

लाक्षारसनिभं शीतं तद्धि सर्वग्रहापहम्|

मेध्यं विरेचनेष्वग्र्यं प्रपुराणमतः परम्||६१||

नासाध्यं नाम तस्यास्ति यत् स्याद्वर्षशतस्थितम्|

दृष्टं स्पृष्टमथाघ्रातं तद्धि सर्वग्रहापहम्||६२||

अपस्मारग्रहोन्मादवतां शस्तं विशेषतः|६३|

The patient suffering from Unmada is specially given old Ghee by the physician to alleviate all the 3 Doshas, and because of sacred nature, it specially cures demoniac seizures.

When taken internally, it has better properties and therapeutic utilities in comparison to ordinary ghee.

In taste, old ghee is pungent and bitter and it has a sharp pungent smell. Ghee stored for ten years is called Purana (cold in potency and it is like the solution of lac. It is cold in potency and it is this old ghee, which cures all types of demoniac seizures.

It promotes intellect and as a purgative it is excellent.

The ghee which is stored for more than ten years, is called Prapurana (exceedingly old) Ghrita. There is no disease which cannot be cured by the ghee which is one hundred years old.

Even the look, touch and smell of this 100 years old ghee is especially useful in curing Apasmara (epilepsy), Graha (demoniac seizures) and Unmada (insanity). [59-63 ½]

Read more about Purana ghrita – old ghee – how to make, how to use

एतानौषधयोगान् वा विधेयत्वमगच्छति||६३||

अञ्जनोत्सादनालेपनावनादिषु योजयेत्|

It is not possible to administer the above mentioned recipes orally, then these are to be administered in the form of Anjana (collyrium) , Utsadana (unction), Alepa (external use of ointment) and Navana (inhalation therapy). [63 ½- 64 ½]

Recipes for Inhalation and Collyrium:

शिरीषो मधुकं हिङ्गु लशुनं तगरं वचा||६४||

कुष्ठं च बस्तमूत्रेण पिष्टं स्यान्नावनाञ्जनम्|

तद्वद्व्योषं हरिद्रे द्वे मञ्जिष्ठाहिङ्गुसर्षपाः||६५||

शिरीषबीजं चोन्मादग्रहापस्मारनाशनम्|

Shireesha (Albizia lebbeck),

Madhuka (licorice), Asafoetida, garlic,

Tagara – Valeriana wallichii

Vacha – Acorus calamus

Kushta – Saussurea lappa

The powder / paste of the above herbs is triturated by adding goat's urine. This paste is used [after dilution] for inhalation therapy and collyrium.

Similarly, the paste of Vyosha (Sunthi, Pippali and Maricha), Haridra (turmeric), Daruharidra (Berberis aristata), Manjistha (Rubia cordifolia), Hingu (asafoetida), Sarshapa (mustard) and the seeds of Shireesha is used in a paste form for curing Unmada (insanity), Graha (demoniac seizures) and apasmara (epilepsy) [64 ½- 66 ½]

Anjana Varti:

पिष्ट्वा तुल्यमपामार्गं हिङ्ग्वालं हिङ्गु पत्रिकाम्||६६||

वार्तिः स्यान्मरिचार्धांशा पिताभ्यां गोशृगालयोः|

तयाऽञ्जयेदपस्मारभूतोन्मादज्वरार्दितान्||६७||

भूतार्तानमरार्तांश्च नरांश्चैव दृगामये|

1 Part each of

Apamarga – Achyranthes aspera

Hingu – asafoetida

Ala (Haritala) and

Hingupatrika, and

1/2 part of Maricha (black pepper) is made into a paste by adding the bile of cow and jackal.

Out of this paste, vartis (enlongated pills) is prepared.

This is used as Collyrium by the patient suffering from Apasmara (epilepsy), Bhutonmada (insanity caused by demoniac seizures) eye- diseases in the patient suffering from the seizures of demons and the Gods, [66 ½ – 68 ½]

Maricha Anjana:

मरिचं चातपे मांसं सपित्तं स्थितमञ्जनम्||६८||

वैकृतं पश्यतः कार्यं दोषभूतहतस्मृतेः|

Maricha – black pepper is impregnated in the bile [of cow and Jackal] and dried in the sun for one month. Application of this as collyrium cures visual perversion of a patient whose memory is lost as a result of vitiated Doshas and Bhutonmada [68 ½ -69 ½]

Siddharthaka Snana, Udvartana:

सिद्धार्थको वचा हिङ्गु करञ्जो देवदारु च||६९||

मञ्जिष्ठा त्रिफला श्वेता कटभीत्वक् कटुत्रिकम्|

समांशानि प्रियङ्गुश्च शिरीषो रजनीद्वयम्||७०||

बस्तमूत्रेण पिष्टोऽयमगदः पानमञ्जनम्|

नस्यमालेपनं चैव स्नानमुद्वर्तनं तथा||७१||

अपस्मारविषोन्मादकृत्यालक्ष्मीज्वरापहः|

भूतेभ्यश्च भयं हन्ति राजद्वारे च शस्यते||७२||

सर्पिरेतेन सिद्धं वा सगोमूत्रं तदर्थकृत्|

These herbs taken in equal quantities are triturated by adding goat's urine and made to a paste:

Siddharthaka – White mustard seed

Vacha – Acorus calamus

Hingu – Asafoetida

Karanja – Pongamia pinnata

Devadaru – Cedrus deodara

Manjistha – Randia dumetorum

Triphala (Haritaka, Bibhitaka and Amalaki) ,

Shveta,

Bark of Katabhi

Trikatu (Ginger, pepper, black pepper),

Priyangu – Callicara macrophylla

Shireesha – Albizia lebbeck

Haridra – Turmeric and

Daruharidra – Berberis aristata

Use of this antitoxic recipe, in the form of drink, collyrium, inhalation, Alepana (external application), bath and Udavartana (unction) cures Apasmara (epilepsy), Visha (Poisoning) unmada (Insanity), Krtya (evil effects of Spells) , alaksmi (inauspiciousness) and fever. It removes the fear of evil spirits. A person using this recipe also earns royal favor.

With the above mentioned herbs, ghee is cooked by adding cow's urine. This medicated ghee also produces the therapeutic effects described above. [69 ½ – 73 ½]

Dhumapana – Smoke inhalation:

प्रसेके पीनसे गन्धैर्धूमवर्तिं कृतां पिबेत्||७३||

वैरेचनिकधूमोक्तैः श्वेताद्यैर्वा सहिङ्गुभिः|

If there is excessive salivation and Peenasa (chronic rhinitis), the patient is given Dhuma Varti (medicated Cigar) prepared with fragrant herbs for smoking.

These fragrant herbs are described in the recipe dealing with "Vairechanika Dhuma" (eliminative type of smoking) (Charaka Sutra Sthana 5:27). Similarly, he is given cigar prepared of Sveta etc. along with Hingu. [73 ½ – 74 ½]

Pradhamana Nasya:

शल्लकोलूक मार्जार जम्बूक वृकबस्तजैः||७४||

मूत्रपित् शकृल्लोमनखैश्चर्मभिरेव च|

सेकाञ्जनं प्रधमनं नस्यं धूमं च कारयेत्||७५||

वातश्लेष्मात्मके प्रायः ...|७६|

If Unmada (insanity) is caused by the predominance of Vata and Kapha, then the patient is given Seka (fomentation), Anjana (Collyrium therapy), Pradhamana (a type of inhalation therapy), Nasya (another type of Inhalation therapy) and Dhuma (fumigation therapy), with the help of urine, bile, faeces, Loma (small hair), nail and skin (as per a availability) of animals and birds like Sallaka, Uluka (owl), Marjara (cat), Jambuka (bear), Vruka and Basta (goat) [74 ½ – 76 ½]

Treatment of Paittika Type of Unmada:

... पैत्तिके तु प्रशस्यते|

तिक्तकं जीवनीयं च सर्पिः स्नेहश्च मिश्रकः||७६||

शीतानि चान्नपानानि मधुराणि मृदूनि च|

In Paittika type of Unmada the patient is given Tiktaka Ghrta (Maha Tiktaka Ghrta- vide Cikitsa 7: 144-150), vide Cikitsa 5:149 -151) and food as well as drinks which are cooling, sweet and light. [57 ¼ -77 1/3]

Raktamokshana – Bloodletting:

शङ्खकेशान्तसन्धौ वा मोक्षयेज्ज्ञो भिषक् सिराम्|

उन्मादे विषमे चैव ज्वरेऽपस्मार एव च||७७||

Blood-letting is administered by Venesection – Sira Vyadha, at the joint of the hair-line and temporal region, which is useful in the treatment of Unmada (insanity), Vishama Jvara (irregular fever) and Apasmara (epilepsy) [77 2/3]

Diet:

घृत मांस वितृप्तं वा निवाते स्थापयेत् सुखम्|

त्यक्त्वा मतिस्मृतिभ्रंशं सञ्ज्ञां लब्ध्वा प्रमुच्यते ||७८||

The patient is made to drink and eat ghee and meat till his satisfaction, and thereafter, made to sleep in a house without cross-ventilation. As a result of this, he overcomes perversion of the mind and loss of memory and regains consciousness. Thus, he becomes free from the ailment. [78]

Regimens:

आश्वासयेत् सुहृद्वा तं वाक्यैर्धर्माथसंहितैः|

ब्रूयादिष्टविनाशं वा दर्शयेदद्भुतानि वा||७९||

बद्धं सर्षपतैलाक्तं न्यसेद्वोतानमातपे|

कपिकच्छ्वाऽथवा तप्तैर्लोहितैलजलैः स्पृशेत्||८०||

कशाभिस्ताडयित्वा वा सुबद्धं विजने गृहे|

रुन्ध्याच्चेतो हि विभ्रान्तं व्रजत्यस्य तथा शमम्||८१||
सर्पणोद्धृतदंष्ट्रेण दान्तैः सिंहैर्गजैश्च तम्|
त्रासयेच्छस्त्रहस्तैर्वा तस्करैः शत्रुभिस्तथा||८२||
अथवा राजपुरुषा बहिर्नीत्वा सुसंयतम्|
त्रासयेयुर्वधेनैनं तर्जयन्तो नृपाज्ञया||८३||
देहदुःखभयेभ्यो हि परं प्राणभयं स्मृतम्|
तेन याति शमं तस्य सर्वतो विप्लुतं मनः||८४||

The patient is consoled by friends with religious and moral statements. They should announce the news of the loss of something which the patient loves or exhibit surprising events. Having smeared his body with mustard oil and tied [with ropes], he is made to lie flat in the sun and his body is rubbed with Kapikacchu or Branded with hot iron rods or burnt with hot oil or water. Having beaten with a hunter and tied properly, he is kept confined to lonely house as a result of which the perturbed mind of the patient regains composure.

He is terrorized by the biting of snakes having their fangs removed, with lions and elephants well tamed or by criminals as well as enemies with weapons in their hands, alternatively by police (royal personnel) having taken him outside and properly arrested with the threat of execution by the order of the king.

The 'danger to life' is taken more seriously than the fear of injury to the body. Therefore, the weak mind of the patient suffering from Unmada gets distracted from all the sides and regains composure through the above mentioned measures.[79- 84]

इष्ट द्रव्य विनाशात्तु मनो यस्योपहन्यते|
तस्य तत्सदृश प्राप्तिसान्त्वाश्वासैः शमं नयेत्||८५||
काम शोक भय क्रोध हर्षेर्ष्यालोभसम्भवान्|
परस्परप्रतिद्वन्द्वैरेभिरेव शमं नयेत्||८६||

If mental derangement is caused because of loss of something which the patient loved, then he is made to regain a similar object. Simultaneously, he is consoled with pleasing assurances [of friends] as a result of which he becomes free from the ailment. If Unmada (insanity) is caused by passion, grief, fear, anger, exhilaration, jealousy and greed then the exposure of the patient to mutually contradictory psychic factors will cure the ailment. [85-86]

बुद्ध्वा देशं वयः सात्म्यं दोषं कालं बलाबले|
चिकित्सितमिदं कुर्यादुन्मादे भूतदोषजे||८७||

Keeping in view, Desha (region or physique), age, wholesomeness, nature of the vitiated Dosha, time of onset and aggravation of the attack and the strength as well as weakness of disease, the physician should apply therapeutic measures described earlier even in case of Unmada caused by Bhutadosha (demoniac seizure). [87]

देवर्षि पितृगन्धर्वैरुन्मतस्य तु बुद्धिमान्|
वर्जयेदञ्जनादीनि तीक्ष्णानि क्रूरकर्म च||८८||
सर्पिष्पानादि तस्येह मृदु भैषज्यमाचरेत्|
पूजां बल्युपहारांश्च मन्त्राञ्जनविधींस्तथा||८९||
शान्तिकर्मेष्टिहोमांश्च जपस्वस्त्ययनानि च|
वेदोक्तान् नियमांश्चापि प्रायश्चितानि चाचरेत्||९०||

If the patient is suffering from Devonmada (caused by Gods), Rishi Unmada (Sages), Pitru Unmada (Manes) and Gandharvas (a group of celestial beings), then a wise physician should avoid Teekshna Anjana (sharp, strong collyrium) etc. and physical violence and torture.

Such a patient is given medicated ghee and other mild remedies. Prayers, sacrifices, presents and application of Collyrium sanctified by the recitation of incantations, propitiating rituals, Ishti Homa (Vedic Sacrifices), Japa (recitation of incantation), Svastyayana (Auspicious rituals), observance of Vedic rules and Prayaschitta (expiation, reconciliation) are useful for such patients. [88-90]

Prevention of Agantuja Unmada – Exogeneous Unmada – Schizophrenia:

भूतानामधिपं देवमीश्वरं जगतः प्रभुम्।
पूजयन् प्रयतो नित्यं जयत्युन्मादजं भयम्||९१||

If one worships Lord Siva, the supreme controller of all Bhutas (supernatural beings) and all the omnipotent master of the universe regularly with devotion, then he becomes free from the attack of unmada (insanity). [91]

Daiva- Vyapashraya Cikitsa:

रुद्रस्य प्रमथा नाम गणा लोके चरन्ति ये।
तेषां पूजां च कुर्वाण उन्मादेभ्यः प्रमुच्यते||९२||
बलिभिर्मङ्गलैर्होमैरोषध्यगदधारणैः।
सत्याचारतपोज्ञानप्रदाननियमव्रतैः||९३||
देवगोब्रह्मणानां च गुरूणां पूजनेन च।
आगन्तुः प्रशमं याति सिद्धैर्मन्त्रौषधैस्तथा||९४||

The worship of Pramathas, the attendants of Lord Rudra, who roam about the universe, makes the patient free from Unmada (insanity). Exogenous type of Unmada gets cured by Bali (Sacrifices), Mangala (Recitation of auspicious Mantras), Homa (offering oblations to the fire), wearing talismans containing anti-toxic herbs, observance of truthfulness, maintenance of good conduct, practice of penance, recourse of knowledge, charity, observance of scriptural rules and religious bows, offering prayer to the Gods, cows, Brahmins and by the application of perfected Mantras and medicines [92-94]

Therapeutic Measures:

यच्चोपदेक्ष्यते किञ्चिदपस्मार चिकित्सिते।
उन्मादे तच्च कर्तव्यं सामान्याद्धेतुदूष्ययोः||९५||

Therapeutic measures, which are to be described in the next Chapter, should also be applied to a suffering from Unmada (insanity) because both Apasmara (epilepsy) and Unmada (insanity) share the same etiological factors as well as pathological process i.e. affliction of tissues elements. [95]

निवृत्तामिषमद्यो यो हिताशी प्रयतः शुचिः।
निजागन्तुभिरुन्मादैः सत्त्ववान् न स युज्यते||९६||

A person who abstains from eating meat and drinking alcohol, and takes only wholesome food, who is disciplined and pure, and who has strong will power doesn't get afflicted by either endogenous or exogenous types of Unmada (insanity) [96]

Vigata Unmada Lakshana – Signs of Cure:

प्रसादश्चेन्द्रियार्थानां बुद्ध्यात्ममनसां तथा।
धातूनां प्रकृतिस्थत्वं विगतोन्मादलक्षणम्||९७||

Clarity of sense faculties in perceiving their objects, clarity of intellect, spirit as well as mind and normalcy of the tissue elements, constitute the signs and the symptoms of the person free from Unmada (insanity) [97]

Summary:

तत्र श्लोकः:-
उन्मादानां समुत्थानं लक्षणं सचिकित्सितम्।
निजागन्तु निमितानामुक्तवान् भिषगुत्तमः||९८||

The etiology, signs and symptoms and treatment of endogenous and exogenous varieties of Unmada (insanity) are physician. [98]

इत्याग्निवेशकृते तन्त्रे चरकप्रतिसंस्कृतेऽप्राप्ते दृढबलपूरिते चिकित्सास्थाने उन्मादचिकित्सितं नाम नवमोऽध्यायः||९||

Thus, ends the ninth chapter dealing with the treatment of Unmada in the Chikitsa section of Agnivesha's work as redacted by Charaka, restored by Dridhabala.

16
Chikitsasthana Chapter 10
Apasmara Chikitsitam

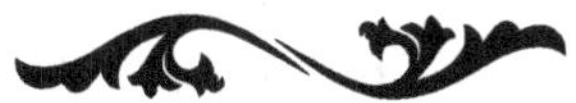

The 10th chapter of Charaka Samhita Chikitsa Sthana is Apasmara Chikitsa Adhyaya. It deals with causes, symptoms, types and Ayurvedic treatment of epilepsy.

अथातोऽपस्मार चिकित्सितं व्याख्यास्यामः||१||
इति ह स्माह भगवानात्रेयः||२||

Let us expound the chapter on the treatment of Apasmara (Epilepsy). Thus said Lord Atreya [1-2]

Definition of Apasmara
स्मृतेरपगमं प्राहुरपस्मारं भिषग्विदः|
तमःप्रवेशं बीभत्स चेष्टं धी सत्त्व सम्प्लवात्||३||

According to the experts in the science of medicine, the term "Apasmara" implies 'loss of memory', characterized by
Tamah pravesha – loss of consciousness (entering into darkness) and
Beebhasta chestam – fearful – disgusting movements of limbs caused by
Dhi sattva samplavat – derangement of intellect and the mind [3]

Apasmara Nidana – Causes:
विभ्रान्त बहुदोषाणामहिताशुचि भोजनात् |
रजस्तमोभ्यां विहते सत्त्वे दोषावृते हृदि||४||
चिन्ता काम भय क्रोध शोकोद्वेगादिभिस्तथा|
मनस्यभिहिते नृणामपस्मारः प्रवर्तते||५||

Causes:

Attacks of epilepsy, in a person, are caused by the upward movement of excessively accumulated Doshas as a result of the following:

1. Habitual intake of unwholesome and unclean food;

2. Suppression of the Sattva (one of the attributes of mind representing purity and consciousness) by Rajas (attribute of the mind representing energy, attraction and dynamism) and Tamas (the third attribute of mind representing passiveness, inaction, darkness and ignorance);

3. Occlusion of the heart by the aggravated Doshas; and

4. Affliction of mind by worry, passion, fear, anger, grief, anxiety etc. [4-5]

Pathogenesis, Signs and Symptoms:
धमनीभिः श्रिता दोषा हृदयं पीडयन्ति हि|
सम्पीड्यमानो व्यथते मूढो भ्रान्तेन चेतसा||६||

पश्यत्यसन्ति रूपाणि पतति प्रस्फुरत्यपि|
जिह्वाक्षिभ्रूः स्रवल्लालो हस्तौ पादौ च विक्षिपन्||७||
दोषवेगे च विगते सुप्तवत् प्रतिबुद्ध्यते|८|

By the above-mentioned factors Doshas located in the Vessels (Dhamani= Artery) afflict the heart and cause disturbances in the functions. The person, thus affected, is afflicted with stupor and malfunctioning of mental activities.

The signs and symptoms:

He visualize non-existent forms, falls down and gets tremors.

Akshi bhru vikshepa – His eyes and eyebrows become distorted

Lala srava – Saliva comes out from his mouth and

Hasta pada vikshepa – His hands and legs become convulsed.

When the fits are over, he regains consciousness as if he were getting up from sleep. [6-8 ½]

Apasmara Bheda – Lakshana:

पृथग्दोषैः समस्तैश्च वक्ष्यते स चतुर्विधः||८||

Types of Apasmara, their Signs & Symptoms

Apasmara (epilepsy) is of 4 types, namely

i) Vatika – Due to Vata Dosha

ii) Paittika – Due to Pitta Dosha

iii) Shlaismika – Due to Kapha Dosha

iv) Sannipatika – Due to simultaneous imbalance of all the three Doshas.[8 ½]

Vataja Apasmara Lakshana:

कम्पते प्रदशेद्दन्तान् फेनोद्वामी श्वसित्यपि|
परुषारुण कृष्णानि पश्येद्रूपाणि चानिलात्||९||

characterized by:

Kampa – trembling

Pradeshad dantan – Gnashing of teeth,

Phenodvami – vomiting froth

Shvasa – panting, rigorous breathing

The patient gets visual aura of forms which are rough, pink or black in colour [9]

Pittaja Apasmara Lakshana:

पीत फेनाङ्गवक्त्राक्षः पीतासृग्रूपदर्शनः|
सतृष्णोष्णानलव्याप्तलोकदर्शी च पैत्तिकः||१०||

Paittika type of epilepsy is characterized by:

Yellowness of the form, limbs, face and eyes

He gets a visual aura of yellow or blood- red objects.

He suffers from morbid thirst and heat

He visualizes the whole world as if set in flames [10]

Kaphaja Apasmara Lakshana:

शुक्ल फेनाङ्ग वक्त्राक्षः शीतो हृष्टाङ्गजो गुरुः|
पश्यञ्छुक्लानि रूपाणि श्लैष्मिको मुच्यते चिरात्||११||
सर्वैरितैः समस्तैस्तु लिङ्गैर्ज्ञेयस्त्रिदोषजः|

The Slaishmika type of epilepsy characterized by:

Shukla Phenanga Vaktra Aksha – White colour of the foam from the mouth, body, face and eyes,

Sheeta – feeling of cold,
Hrushtanga – horripilation
Guru – feeling of heaviness
Pashyan Shuklani Roopani – patient visualizes the aura of white objects.
Muchyate Chiraat – He recovers from the fit after a long time. [11 - 12½]

Apasmara Asadhya Lakshana:
अपस्मारः स चासाध्यो यः क्षीणस्यानवश्च यः||१२||
In the Sannipatika type of epilepsy:
Signs and symptoms of all the above mentioned 3 varieties are manifested. This type of epilepsy is incurable.
Epilepsy, which occurs in emaciated persons or which is of long standing is also incurable. [12½]

Frequency of Fits – Apasmara Vega:
पक्षाद्वा द्वादशाहाद्वा मासाद्वा कुपिता मलाः|
अपस्माराय कुर्वन्ति वेगं किञ्चिदथान्तरम्||१३||
The aggravated Doshas cause attacks of epilepsy once in 15 days, 12 days or a month. The attack may, however, take place even after a shorter period. [13]

Apsmara Chikitsa Sutra –
तैरावृतानां हृत्स्रोतोमनसां सम्प्रबोधनम्|
तीक्ष्णैरादौ भिषक् कुर्यात् कर्मभिर्वमनादिभिः||१४||
वातिकं बस्तिभूयिष्ठैः पैत्तं प्रायो विरेचनैः|
श्लैष्मिकं वमनप्रायैरपस्मारमुपाचरेत्||१५||
Line of Treatment:
The physician should first restore the activities of the heart, channels (vessels) and the mind which are occluded by Doshas by the use of sharp (strong) remedial measures like Vamana (emetic therapy) etc.
The patient suffering from Vatika epilepsy is administered mainly with Basti (medicated enema) therapy;
One suffering from the Paittika type of epilepsy is mainly given Virechana (purgation) therapy and
The one suffering from the Slaismika type of epilepsy is given Vamana (emetic) therapy. [14-15]

Ayurvedic medicines for Epilepsy:
सर्वतः सुविशुद्धस्य सम्यगाश्वासितस्य च|
अपस्मार विमोक्षार्थं योगान् संशमनाञ्छृणु||१६||
After the patient is cleansed of impurities from his body by the administration of emetic therapy, etc and after he is well consoled, he should be given alleviation therapies for the cure of Apasmara (Epilepsy). The recipes for this purpose are furnished in subsequent verses. [16]

Panchagavya Ghruta:
गोशकृद्रसदध्यम्ल क्षीरमूत्रैः समैर्घृतम्|
सिद्धं पिबेदपस्मार कामला ज्वर नाशनम्||१७||
इति पञ्चगव्यं घृतम्|
Cow ghee is cooked by adding the
Juice of cow dung,
Sour curd prepared out of cow milk and cow urine, each of them taken in equal quantities.
The medicated ghee, thus prepared, cures
Apasmara – epilepsy
Kamala – Jaundice and

Jwara – fever [17]
Read more about side effects,

Maha panchagavya Ghritam:

द्वे पञ्चमूल्यौ त्रिफला रजन्यौ कुटज त्वचम्|
सप्तपर्णमपामार्गं नीलिनीं कटुरोहिणीम्||१८||
शम्पाकं फल्गुमूलं च पौष्करं सदुरालभम्|
द्विपलानि जलद्रोणे पक्त्वा पादावशेषिते||१९||
भार्गीं पाठां त्रिकटुकं त्रिवृतां निचुलानि च|
श्रेयसीमाढकीं मूर्वां दन्तीं भूनिम्ब चित्रकौ||२०||
द्वे सारिवे रोहिषं च भूतीकं मदयन्तिकाम्|
क्षिपेत्पिष्ट्वाऽक्षमात्राणि तेन प्रस्थं घृतात् पचेत्||२१||
गोशकृद्रसदध्यम्लक्षीरमूत्रैश्च तत्समैः|
पञ्चगव्यमिति ख्यातं महत्तदमृतोपमम्||२२||
अपस्मारे तथोन्मादे श्वयथावुदरेषु च|
गुल्मार्शःपाण्डुरोगेषु कामलायां हलीमके||२३||
शस्यते घृतमेतत्तु प्रयोक्तव्यं दिने दिने|
अलक्ष्मी ग्रहरोगघ्नं चातुर्थक विनाशनम्||२४||
इति महापञ्चगव्यं घृतम्|

2 Palas of each of
Bilva – Aegle marmelos
Agnimantha – Premna mucronata
Shyonaka – Oroxylum indicum
Gambhari – Gmelina arborea
Patala – Stereospermum suaveolens
Shalaparni – Desmodium gangeticum
Prinshnaparni – Urarica picta
Gokshura – Tribulus terrestris
Brihati – Solanum indicum
Kantakari – Solanum xanthocarpum,
Haritaki – Terminalia chebula
Bibhitaki – Terminalia bellerica
Amalaka – Phyllanthus emblica
Haridra – turmeric – Curcuma longa
Daru Haridra – Tree Turmeric (stem) – Berberis aristata
Bark of kutaja – Holarrhena antidysenterica
Saptaparna – Alstonia scholaris
Apamarga –Achyranthes aspera
Neelini – Indigofera tinctorea
Katurohini – Picrorhiza kurroa
Shampaka (Aragvadha) – Cassia fistula
Root of Phalgu (Kasthodumbarika) – Phalgumoola
Puskaramula – Inula racemosa and
Duralabha – should be added with
1 Drona – 12.288 litres of water, boiled and reduced to 1/4th, filtered.
Along with this decoction, 2 Prasthas (1.536 kg) of cow ghee is cooked by adding 2 Prasthas (1.536 liter) of each of the juice of

Cow dung
Sour curd prepared of cow milk, and cow urine and
The paste of 1 Aksha (12 g) of each of
Bharangi – Clerodendrum serratum
Patha – Cyclea peltata
Shunthi – Zingiber officinale
Maricha – Piper nigrum
Pippali – Long pepper fruit – Piper longum
Trivrta – Operculina turpethum
Nicula [Hijjala] - Barringtonia acutangula
Shreyasi (Hastipippali) – Scindapsus officinalis
Adhaki – Pigeon Pea – Cajanus cajan
Murva – Marsdenia tenacissima
Danti – Baliospermum montanum
Bhunimba – Phyllanthus niruri
Chitraka – Leadword – Plumbago zeylanica
Sveta Sariva – Indian Sarsaparilla – Hemidesmus indicus,
Krsna Sariva – Indian Sarsaparilla – Ichnocarpus frutescens
Rohisha - Cymbopogon martinii
Bhutika
Madayantika – Lawsonia inermis
Indications:
This medicated ghee, known as Maha pancha gavya is like ambrosia in the treatment of
Apasmara – epilepsy
Unmada – insanity
Svayathu – oedema
Udara – obstinate abnormal diseases including ascites
Gulma – Phantom tumour
Arshas – piles
Pandu – Anemia
Kamala – Jaundice and
Halimaka – a serious type of Jaundice
This medicated ghee is used regularly every day to dispel inauspiciousness and evil effects of bad planets.
It also cures Chaturthaka (Quartan) type of Vishama Jvara (Irregular fever) [18-24]

Brahmi Ghritam
ब्राह्मीरस वचा कुष्ठशङ्खपुष्पीभिरेव च|
पुराणं घृतमुन्मादालक्ष्म्यपस्मारपापनुत्||२५||
Old cow ghee (1 part) is cooked with
4 parts of Brahmi Juice (Bacopa monnieri) and
The paste of
Vacha – Acorus calamus Linn.,
Kushta – Saussurea lappa and
Shankhapuspi – (1/4th part in total)
This medicated ghee is indicated in –
Unmada – insanity
Alaksmi – inauspiciousness
Apasmara – epilepsy and

Papa – effects of devil deeds [25]

Hingu Saindhava Ghrita:
घृतं सैन्धव हिङ्गुभ्यां वार्षे बास्ते चतुर्गुणे|
मूत्रे सिद्धमपस्मारहृद्ग्रहामयनाशनम्||२६||
1 part of Cow ghee is cooked by adding [in total] 4 parts of the urine of bull and goat urine and the paste of rock salt and asafoetida (1/4 the part in total).
This medicated ghee cures
Apasmara (epilepsy)
Hrud roga – heart diseases and
Diseases caused by the evil effects of bad planets. [26]

Vachadi Ghritam:
वचा शम्पाक कैटर्यवयःस्थाहिङ्गुचोरकैः|
सिद्धं पलङ्कषायुक्तैर्वातश्लेष्मात्मके घृतम्||२७||
Ghee (1 part) is cooked with the paste of
Vacha – Acoruss calamus
Shampaka – Cassia fistula
Kaitarya – Myrica nagi (Parvata)
Nimba – Neem (Azadirachta indica),
Vayashtha (Guduchi) – Tinospora cordifolia
Hingu – Asa foetida
Choraka and
Palankasha or Guggulu (Commiphora mukul) (1/4th part in total) [4 parts of water is added according to the general rule, because in the present recipe, there is no liquid].
This medicate ghee is useful in the treatment of Vatika and Slaismika type of epilepsy. [27]

Jivaniya yamaka:
तैलप्रस्थं घृतप्रस्थं जीवनीयैः पलोन्मितैः|
क्षीरद्रोणे पचेत् सिद्धमपस्मारविनाशनम्||२८||
1 Prasthas of each oil and cow ghee is added with the paste of 1 Pala (48 g) of each Jeevaneeya Gana herbs
Jeevaka
Rishabhaka
Meda
Mahameda
Kakoli – Fritillaria roylei
Kshira Kakoli Lilium polyphyllum
Mudgaparni – Phaseolus trilobus
Mashaparni – Teramnus labialis,
Jivanti – Leptadenia reticulata and
Madhuka– Licorice – Glycyrrhiza glabra
and 1 Drona (12.288 liters) of milk and cooked.
This medicated ghee is an effective recipe for the cure of Apasmara (epilepsy) [28]

Recipes for medicated Ghee:
कंसे क्षीरेक्षुरसयोः काश्मर्येऽष्टगुणे रसे|
कार्षिकैर्जीवनीयैश्च घृतप्रस्थं विपाचयेत्||२९||

वातपितोद्भवं क्षिप्रमपस्मारं नियच्छति|
तद्वत् काश विदारीक्षुकुश क्वाथ शृतं घृतम्||३०||

2 Prasthas of ghee is added with

1 Kamsa of each of milk and sugarcane juice,

16 Prasthas of the decoction of Kashmarya (Gmelina arborea) and

1 Karsha of each of the 10 drugs belonging to Jeevaniya Group (vide Sutra 4: 9) and cooked.

This medicated ghee instantaneously cures epilepsy caused by Vata and Pitta.

Similarly, ghee cooked by adding

Decoction of Kasha and Kusa (Desmostachya bipinnata) and

Juice of Vidari (Pueraria tuberosa) and sugarcane is useful in the treatment of this ailment. [29-30]

Madhukadi Ghrita:

मधुक द्विपले कल्के द्रोणे चामलकीरसात्|
तद्वत् सिद्धो घृतप्रस्थः पितापस्मारभेषजम्||३१||

2 Prasthas of ghee is cooked by adding

2 Dronas of Juice of Amalaki – Indian gooseberry and

2 palas of the paste of Madhuka– Licorice – Glycyrrhiza glabra

This medicated ghee instantaneously cures the Paittika type of Apasmara (epilepsy). [31]

Recipe of medicated Oil:

अभ्यङ्गः सार्षपं तैलं बस्तमूत्रे चतुर्गुणे|
सिद्धं स्याद्गोशकृन्मूत्रैः स्नानोत्सादनमेव च||३२||

Mustard oil cooked with 4 times of goat urine is useful for massage for a patient suffering from epilepsy.

Such a patient should use cow-dung for the purpose of unction and cow urine for the purpose of Snana (bath) [32]

Katabhyadi Taila:

कटभी निम्ब कट्वङ्ग मधु शिग्रु त्वचां रसे|
सिद्धं मूत्रसमं तैलमभ्यङ्गार्थे प्रशस्यते||३३||

Sesame oil (1 part) is cooked with goat's urine (1 part) and the decoction of the barks of

Katabhi – Celastrus paniculatus

Nimba – Neem (Azadirachta indica)

Katvanga – Oroxylum indicum and

Madhushigru – Acorus calamus (3 parts)

This medicated oil is used for massage, effective in the treatment of epilepsy. [33]

Palankashadi taila:

पलङ्कषा वचा पथ्या वृश्चिकाल्यर्क सर्षपैः|
जटिला पूतना केशीनाकुली हिङ्गु चोरकैः||३४||
लशुनातिरसाचित्रा कुष्ठैर्विड्भिश्च पक्षिणाम्|
मांसाशिनां यथालाभं बस्तमूत्रे चतुर्गुणे||३५||
सिद्धमभ्यञ्जनं तैलमपस्मारविनाशनम्|
एतैश्चैवौषधैः कार्यं धूपं सप्रलेपनम्||३६||

Sesame oil is cooked by adding 4 times of goat's urine and paste (1/4th of oil) of

Palankasa

Vacha – Acorus calamus Linn.,

Pathya – Haritaki

Vrischikali

Arka – Calotropis gigantea

Sarsapa – Brassica campestris

Jatila – Nardostachys jatamansi D C.

Putanakesi –Golomi,

Nakuli

Hingu – Asa foetida,

Coraka

Lasuna – Garlic – Allium sativum Linn.,

Atirasa – Asparagus root – Asparagaus racemosus,

Chitra – Baliospermum montanum,

Kustha – Saussurea lappa and

the stool of meat- eating birds according to their availability

This medicated oil is very effective in curing Apasmara (Epilepsy).

The above mentioned drugs (ingredients prescribed to be used as paste) should also be used for Dhupana (fumigation) and Pralepana (external application in paste form) [for curing patients suffering from epilepsy] [34-36]

Recipe for ointment and Fumigation:

पिप्पलीं लवणं चित्रां हिङ्गु हिङ्गुशिवाटिकाम्|
काकोलीं सर्षपान् काकनासां कैटर्य चन्दने||३७||
शुनःस्कन्धास्थिनखरान् पर्शुकां चेति पेषयेत्|
बस्तमूत्रेण पुष्यर्क्षे प्रदेहः स्यात् सधूपनः||३८||

Pippali – Piper longum

Lavanam – rock-salt,

Chitra – Baliospermum montanum(danti),

Hingu – Asa foetida,

Hingusivatika(Vamsapatrika),

Kakoli – Fritillaria roylei

Sarsapa – Mustard

Kakanasa

Kaitarya – Myrica nagi

Chandana – Sandalwood – Santalum album and

Shoulder bones, nails and ribs of the dog is made to a paste by triturating with goat's urine in the constellation of Pusya (8th naksatra).

Use of this for Pradeha (external application in the form of thick paste) and Dhupana (fumigation) [cures epilepsy]. [37-38]

Recipes for Unction:

अपेतराक्षसी कुष्ठ पूतनाकेशि चोरकैः|
उत्सादनं मूत्रपिष्टैर्मूत्रैरेवावसेचनम्||३९||
जलौकःशकृता तद्वद्दग्धैर्वा बस्तरोमभिः|
खरास्थिभिर्हस्तिनखैस्तथा गोपुच्छलोमभिः||४०||

Apetaraksasi

Kushta – Saussurea lappa

Putanakesii and

Choraka is triturated by adding cow or goat's urine and made to a paste.

This is used as unction for the treatment of epilepsy

The body of the patient is sprinkled with the urine of cow or goat

Similarly, unction is done with the help of the following recipes:

1. Stool of leech
2. Ashes of the small hair of the goat
3. Ashes of the bone of ass
4. Ashes of the nails of elephant and
5. Ashes of the hair in the tail of the cow. [39-40]

Dhumapana – Recipe for Inhalation:

कपिलानां गवां मूत्रं नावनं परमं हितम्|

श्वशृगालबिडालानां सिंहादीनां च शस्यते||४१||

भार्गी वचा नागदन्ती श्वेता श्वेता विषाणिका|

ज्योतिष्मती नागदन्ती पादोक्ता मूत्रपेषिताः||४२||

योगास्त्रयोऽतः षड् बिन्दून् पञ्च वा नावयेदि्भषक्|

Inhalation of the urine of cows having reddish brown (Kapila) colour is exceedingly useful for the cure of epilepsy.

Similarly inhalation of the urine of the dog, jackal, cats etc, is useful in this condition.

Inhalation of 5 or 6 drops of the following 3 recipes is useful in the treatment of epilepsy:

1. Bhargi, Vacha (Acorus calamus Linn.) and Nagadanti (Kasthapatala) triturated with cow urine
2. Sveta (Sveta Aparajita) and veta Visanika (Satavari) triturated with cow urine
3. Jyotismati (Celastrus paniculatus) and Nagadanti triturated with cow urine. [41- 43½]

Medicated Oil for Navana Nasya:

त्रिफला व्योष पीतद्रुयवक्षार फणिज्झकैः||४३||

श्यामापामार्ग कारञ्जफलैर्मूत्रेऽथ बस्तजे|

साधितं नावनं तैलमपस्मारविनाशनम्||४४||

1 part Oil is cooked with 4 parts Goat's urine and the paste of

Haritaki – Terminalia chebula

Bibhitaki –Terminalia bellerica

Amalaki – Phyllanthus emblica

Sunthi – Zingiber officinale

Pippali – Long pepper fruit – Piper longum

Maricha – Black pepper fruit – Piper nigrum,

Pitadru – Devadaru (Cedrus deodara)

Yavaksara

Phanijjhaka

Apamarga – Achyranthes aspera and

Fruits of Karanja (Pongamia pinnata) (1/4th part in total)

By inhalation of this medicated oil Apasmara (epilepsy) is cured [43 1/3 -44]

Pippalyadi Pradhamana Nasya:

पिप्पली वृश्चिकाली च कुष्ठं च लवणानि च|

भार्गी च चूर्णितं नस्तः कार्यं प्रधमनं परम्||४५||

Pippali,

Vrishchikali

Kushta

Lavana

Bharngi

Above mentioned herbs should be powdered and administered in the form of powder nasya[45]

Kayasathadya Varti:

कायस्थां शारदान्मुद्गान्मुस्तोशीरयवांस्तथा|

सव्योषान् बस्तमूत्रेण पिष्ट्वा वर्तीः प्रकल्पयेत्||४६||

अपस्मारे तथोन्मादे सर्पदष्टे गरार्दिते|

विषपीते जलमृते चैताः स्युरमृतोपमाः||४७||

The powder of below mentioned herbs should be administered

Kayastha

Sharada

Mudga

Musta (Cyperus rotundus)

Ushira – Vetiver – Vetiveria zizanioides

Yava – Barley (Hordeum vulgare)

Sunthi – Zingiber officinale

Pippali – Long pepper fruit – Piper longum and

Maricha – Black pepper fruit – Piper nigrum is made to a paste by triturating with Goat's urine.

From this paste Vartis (elongated pills) are prepared.

Application of this thin paste prepared by rubbing with water in the eyes [as collyrium] works like ambrosia in curing

Apsmara – epilepsy

Unmada – insanity

Snake bite

Afflictions by poisons

Maladies caused by taking poisons internally (lying unconscious like a dead person). [46-47]

Mustadya Varti:

मुस्तं वयःस्थां त्रिफलां कायस्थां हिङ्गु शाद्वलम्|

व्योषं माषान् यवान्मूत्रैर्बास्तमैषार्षभैस्त्रिभिः||४८||

पिष्ट्वा कृत्वा च तां वर्तिमपस्मारे प्रयोजयेत्|

किलासे च तथोन्मादे ज्वरेषु विषमेषु च||४९||

These are made to a paste by triturating with the urine of goat, sheep and bull:

Musta – Cyperus rotundus

Vayastha

Daru Haridra – Tree Turmeric (stem) – Berberis aristata

Haritaki – Terminalia chebula

Bibhitaki – Terminalia bellerica

Amalaki – Phyllanthus emblica

Kayastha [ela] – Elettaria cardamomum

Hingu – Asa foetida

Sadvala [Durva (Cynodon dactylon)]

Sunthi – Zingiber officinale

Pippali – Long pepper fruit – Piper longum

Maricha – Black pepper fruit – Piper nigrum

Musa and

Yava – Barley (Hordeum vulgare)

From this paste, Vartis (elongated pills) are prepared.

These Vartis are rubbed over a stone by adding water, and the thin paste, thus obtained, is used as collyrium.

These cures

Apasmara – epilepsy

Kilasa – a type of leucoderma

Unmada – insanity and

Vishama Jvara – irregular fever [48-49]

Dhupana – Recipes for Collyrium and Fumigation:

पुष्योद्धृतं शुनः पित्तमपस्मारघ्नमञ्जनम्|
तदेव सर्पिषा युक्तं धूपनं परमं मतम्||५०||
नकुलोलूक मार्जार गृध्र कीटाहिकाकजैः|
तुण्डैः पक्षैः पुरीषैश्च धूपनं कारयेद्भिषक्||५१||
आभिः क्रियाभिः सिद्धाभिर्हृदयं सम्प्रबुध्यते|
स्रोतांसि चापि शुध्यन्ति ततः सञ्ज्ञां स विन्दति||५२||

Dog-bile, collected during Pusya constellation, is used as a collyrium for the cure of Apasmara (epilepsy).

This bile mixed with ghee is used for fumigation which is excellent for curing epilepsy

For the treatment of epilepsy, the physician gives fumigation therapy with the help of the beaks, feather and stool of mongoose, owl bird, cat, vulture, Kita (scorpion etc) snake and crow.

With the help of these therapies, the heart of the patient gets stimulated and the channels get cleansed as a result of which the patient regains consciousness. [50-52]

Treatment of Exogenous Epilepsy:

यस्यानुबन्धस्त्वागन्तुर्दोषलिङ्गाधिकाकृतिः|
दृश्येत तस्य कार्यं स्यादागन्तून्मादभेषजम्||५३||

In some patients of epilepsy, exogenous factors [like seizures by evil spirits] are secondarily involved and in such cases signs and symptoms [of these exogenous factors] are manifested over and above those of the Doshas (endogenous factors).

Treatment of such patients should be on the lines suggested for exogenous types of Unmada (insanity) vide chapter 9. [53]

Atattvabhinivesha or Psychic Perversions

अनन्तरमुवाचेदमग्निवेशः कृताञ्जलिः|
भगवन्! प्राक् समुद्दिष्टः श्लोकस्थाने महागदः||५४||
अतत्त्वाभिनिवेशो यस्तद्धेत्वाकृतिभेषजम्|
तत्र नोक्तमतः श्रोतुमिच्छामि तदिहोच्यताम्||५५||
शुश्रूषवे वचः श्रुत्वा शिष्यायाह पुनर्वसुः|
महागदं सौम्य! शृणु सहेत्वाकृतिभेषजम्||५६||
मलिनाहारशीलस्य वेगान् प्राप्तान्निगृह्णतः|
शीतोष्ण स्निग्ध रूक्षाद्यैर्हेतुभिश्चातिसेवितैः||५७||
हृदयं समुपाश्रित्य मनोबुद्धिवहाः सिराः|
दोषाः सन्दूष्य तिष्ठन्ति रजोमोहावृतात्मनः||५८||
रजस्तमोभ्यां वृद्धाभ्यां बुद्धौ मनसि चावृते|
हृदये व्याकुले दोषैरथ मूढोऽल्पचेतनः ||५९||
विषमां कुरुते बुद्धिं नित्यानित्ये हिताहिते|
अतत्त्वाभिनिवेशं तमाहुराप्ता महागदम्||६०||
स्नेहस्वेदोपपन्नं तं संशोध्य वमनादिभिः|
कृत संसर्जनं मेध्यैरन्नपानैरुपाचरेत्||६१||

ब्राह्मी स्वरस युक्तं यत् पञ्चगव्यमुदाहृतम्|
तत् सेव्यं शङ्खपुष्पी च यच्च मेध्यं रसायनम्||६२||
सुहृदश्चानुकूलास्तं स्वाप्ता धर्मार्थवादिनः|
संयोजयेयुर्विज्ञानधैर्यस्मृतिसमाधिभिः ||६३||

Thereafter, Agnivesha with folded hands said, 'O Lord! In Sutra section (Charaka Samhita Sutrathana 19/3) you have mentioned in brief Atatvabhinivesha (physic perversion) as Mahagada (serious disease). But its aetiology, signs and symptoms and treatment are not described. I want to hear descriptions. Kindly narrate them in the present context". Having heard this, Lord Punarvasu addressed his disciple "My child, hear about this Mahagada (serious disease) along with its aetiology, signs and symptoms and treatment."

In a person indulging in habitual intake of impure food, suppression of the manifested natural urges, excessively indulging in diet, which are cold, hot, unctuous etc; and having his soul occluded by Rajas (one of the attributes of the mind) and Moha or Tamas (another attribute of mind), the vitiated Doshas afflict the Manobuddivaha Sira (channels carrying the impulses of the mind and intellect) and get lodged in the heart.

With predominant Rajas and Tamas occluding the intellect and the mind and the aggravated Doshas disturbing the functions of the heart, the person who is ignorant and mentally weak, makes perverted judgments regarding eternal and ephemeral events and wholesome and unwholesome objects. This Mahagada (serious disease) according to expert physicians is called Atattvabhinivesha (Perversion of the mind).

Such a patient should be administered with Snehana, Swedana therapies followed by Panchakarma treatments like Vamana and then Samsarjana Krama (gradual administration of lighter to heavier food). Thereafter, diet and drinks which are promoters of intellect should be given to him.

Panchagavya Ghruta and Maha Panchagavya Ghrut described above are given to such a patient along with the juice of Brahmi.

Similarly, other Medhya Rasayanas (promotes of intellect) like Sankhapushpi is given to him

His friends and sympathizers and preceptors preaching religious sermons should instil into him understanding, patience, memory and the power of concentration (Samadhi). [54-63]

Treatment of Chronic Epilepsy

प्रयुञ्ज्यातैललशुनं पयसा वा शतावरीम्|
ब्राह्मीरसं कुष्ठरसं वचां वा मधुसंयुताम्||६४||
दुश्चिकित्स्यो ह्यपस्मारश्चिरकारी कृतास्पदः |
तस्माद्रसायनैरेनं प्रायशः समुपाचरेत्||६५||

If the disease epilepsy is resistant to conventional modes of treatment, if it is chronic and if it has acquired a firm footing, then it is generally treated with the following recipes of elixirs:

1. Garlic with oil
2. Shatavari (Asparagus racemosus) with milk
3. Juice of Brahmi (Bacopa monnieri) with Honey
4. Juice of decoction of Kushta – Saussurea lappa with honey and
5. Powder of Vaca (Acorus calamus Linn.) with honey[64 -65]

Precautions

जलाग्निद्रुमशैलेभ्यो विषमेभ्यश्च तं सदा|
रक्षेदुन्मादिनं चैव सद्यः प्राणहरा हि ते||६६||

The patient suffering from Apasmara (epilepsy) and unmada (insanity) is specially protected from water, fire, trees, mountains and uneven places. These may cause instantaneous death of the patient. [66]

तत्र श्लोकौ-
हेतुं कुर्वन्त्यपस्मारं दोषाः प्रकुपिता यथा|

सामान्यतः पृथक्त्वाच्च लिङ्गं तेषां च भेषजम्||६७||

महागदसमुत्थानं लिङ्गं चोवाच सौषधम्|

मुनिर्व्याससमासाभ्यामपस्मारचिकित्सिते ||६८||

In this chapter on the treatment of Apasmara (epilepsy), the sage has described in brief as well as in detail the following topics:

1. Etiological factors of epilepsy

2. The mode of vitiation of Doshas

3. Signs and symptoms in general and of different varieties of epilepsy

4. Treatment of different types of epilepsy and.

5. Epilepsy, signs and symptoms of Mahagada (serious Disease or Mental Perversion) [67 -68]

इत्यग्निवेशकृते तन्त्रे चरकप्रतिसंस्कृतेऽप्राप्ते दृढबलसम्पूरिते चिकित्सा स्थानेऽपस्मार चिकित्सितं नाम दशमोऽध्यायः||१०||

Thus, ends the 10th chapter dealing with the treatment of Apasmara (epilepsy) in the section on therapeutics of Agnivesha's work as redacted by Charaka, completed by Drudhabala.

17

Chikitsasthana Chapter 11 Kshataksheena Chikitsitam

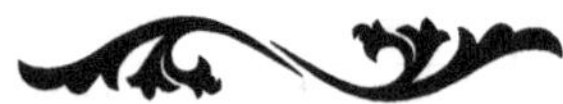

Kshataksheena refers to injury or excessive exertion such as swimming, running, wrestling for long hours, leading to respiratory symptoms and depletion of body tissues. Charaka Sanhita explains this condition in the 11th chapter of Chikitsa Sthana. This condition is correlated to phthisis by a few and even with tuberculosis by few others.

अथातः क्षतक्षीण चिकित्सितं व्याख्यास्यामः||१||
इति ह स्माह भगवानात्रेयः||२||
We shall now expound the chapter on the treatment of Kshata Ksheena (Phthsis)
Thus, said lord Atreya [1-2]

उदार कीर्ति ब्रह्मर्षिरात्रेयः परमार्थवित्|
क्षतक्षीण चिकित्सार्थमिदमाह चिकित्सितम्||३||
Kind and famous sage Atreya herewith started explaining about Kshataksheena.

Ksata Kseena Nidana – causes:
धनुषाऽऽयस्यतोऽत्यर्थं भारमुद्वहतो गुरुम्|
पततो विषमोच्चेभ्यो बलिभिः सह युध्यतः||४||
वृषं हयं वा धावन्तं दम्यं वाऽन्यं निगृह्णतः|
शिला काष्ठाश्म निर्घातान् क्षिपतो निघ्नतः परान्||५||
अधीयानस्य वाऽत्युच्चैर्दूरं वा व्रजतो द्रुतम्|
महानदीं वा तरतो हयैर्वा सह धावतः||६||
सहसोत्पततो दूरं तूर्णं चातिप्रनृत्यतः|
तथाऽन्यैः कर्मभिः क्रूरैर्भृशमभ्याहतस्य च||७||
विक्षते वक्षसि व्याधिर्बलवान् समुदीर्यते|
स्त्रीषु चातिप्रसक्तस्य रूक्षाल्पप्रमिताशिनः||८||
Causes:
1. Straining in excess with a bow, Injury due to continuous use of bow
2. Bhara – Lifting heavy weight.
3. Falling while walking over uneven place or from high altitudes
4. Fighting with stronger persons
5. Stopping an enraged bull, stallion or any other strong animals requiring control
6. Throwing heavy stone, wooden blocks or equipments made of stone
7. Killing powerful animals
8. Reciting scriptures, verses on a very high tone

9. Walking for long distances, walking too fast

10. Crossing a big river by swimming

11. Running along with a running horse

12. Sudden high and long jump

13. Practicing violent dance for a long time and

14. Being excessively injured by other violent and cruel acts.

Kshatakshina is caused because of the above activities by a person who indulges too much in sexual activities, who takes dry food stuffs (causes Vata increase), who takes less food at irregular intervals.

These activities lead to exertion in such a person and leads to injury of the chest and lungs. [4-8]

Kshat Ksheen Samprapti –

उरो विरुज्यते तस्य भिद्यतेऽथ विभज्यते।

प्रपीड्येते ततः पार्श्वे शुष्यत्यङ्गं प्रवेपते॥९॥

क्रमाद्वीर्यं बलं वर्णो रुचिरग्निश्च हीयते।

ज्वरो व्यथा मनोदैन्यं विड्भेदोऽग्निवधादपि॥१०॥

दुष्टः श्यावः सुदुर्गन्धः पीतो विग्रथितो बहुः।

कासमानस्य च श्लेष्मा सरक्तः सम्प्रवर्तते॥११॥

स क्षतः क्षीयतेऽत्यर्थं तथा शुक्रौजसोः क्षयात्।१२।

Pathogenesis

Because of the above mentioned causative factors,

The chest gets broken, punctured and cracked;

Sides of the chest get pressed and

Pravepana -emaciation with tremor in limbs.

Gradually it leads to

Veerya hani – loss of potency, loss of fertility

Balahani – loss of strength and immunity

Varnahani – loss of complexion

Ruchi hani – Loss of taste, anorexia

Agnihani – loss of digestion strength.

The person suffers with

Jwara – fever,

Vyatha – worries

Manodainya – mental debility, depression

Vid bheda – diarrhoea, IBS

Agnivadha – lack of hunger, absence of digestion strength.

While coughing, the patient spits out phlegm which is Dusta (putrid), Shyava (gray colored sputum), Durgandha (foul smelling), Peeta (yellow) and Vigrathita (knotty), in large quantities along with blood.

The person suffering from Kshatakseena becomes excessively emaciated due to further wastage of semen and Ojas (vital essence). [9- ½ 12].

Kshataksheena Poorvaroopa:

अव्यक्तं लक्षणं तस्य पूर्वरूपमिति स्मृतम्॥१२॥

उरोरुक्शोणितच्छर्दिः कासो वैशेषिकः क्षते।

क्षीणे सरक्त मूत्रत्वं पार्श्वपृष्ठकटिग्रहः॥१३॥

Premonitory Signs and symptoms:

Less manifested symptoms constitute premonitory signs and symptoms in Kshataksheena.

If there is Kshata (Injury) patient exhibits the below said symptoms –

Uro ruk – Pain in the chest,

Shonita chardi – Blood- vomiting and

Kasa – Cough are specially manifested, and

If there is Ksaya (diminution of tissue elements), then

Sa rakta mutratva – Heamaturia and

Parshva Prstha kati graha – Stiffness of the sides of chest, back and lumbar region are specially manifested. [12 ½-13]

Sadhya Asadhyatva – Prognosis:

अल्प लिङ्गस्य दीप्ताग्नेः साध्यो बलवतो नवः|

परिसंवत्सरो याप्यः सर्वलिङ्गं तु वर्जयेत्||१४||

If the signs and symptoms are manifested in lesser quantities, if the power of digestion (of the patient) is strong, if the patient has good strength and if the disease is new (freshly occurred), then it is curable.

If the disease lasts for more than a year, then it is Yapya (palliable – Cannot be completely cured).

If all the signs and symptoms of the disease are simultaneously manifested, then such a patient should not be treated, because the condition is incurable. [14]

Treatment based on symptoms:

उरो मत्वा क्षतं लाक्षां पयसा मधु संयुताम्|

सद्य एव पिबेज्जीर्णे पयसाऽद्यात् सशर्करम्||१५||

पार्श्व बस्ति रुजी चाल्प पित्ताग्निस्तां सुरायुताम्|

भिन्न विट्कः समुस्तातिविषा पाठां सवत्सकाम्||१६||

लाक्षां सर्पिर्मधूच्छिष्टं जीवनीय गणं सिताम्|

त्वक्क्षीरीं समितां क्षीरे पक्त्वा दीप्तानलः पिबेत्||१७||

इक्ष्वालिका बिस ग्रन्थि पद्म केशर चन्दनैः|

शृतं पयो मधुयुतं सन्धानार्थं पिबेत् क्षती||१८||

यवानां चूर्णमादाय क्षीर सिद्धं घृत प्लुतम्|

ज्वरे दाहे सिता क्षौद्र सक्तून् वा पयसा पिबेत्||१९||

मधूक मधुक द्राक्षा त्वक्क्षीरी पिप्पली बलाः|

कासी पार्श्वास्थि शूली च लिह्यात्सघृत माक्षिकाः||२०||

If there is fresh injury to the chest, the patient is given:

Laksha (Lac) along with milk and honey

After Laksha is digested, he is given food along with milk and sugar.

If there is Parshva basti ruja (pain in the sides of the chest or in kidney region) and if there is Alpa Pitta, Agni [less of Pitta and digestion strength], then the patient is given Laksa (lac) along with Sura (alcoholic Drink)

If there is diarrhea, then the patient is given Laksha (lac) along with Musta (Cyperus rotundus), Tinisha, Patha (Cissampelos pareira) and Vatsaka (Holarrhena antidysenterica).

If the patient has strong digestion strength, then he is given milk cooked with Laksha (Lac), ghee, bee's wax, drugs belonging to Jeevvaniya group, sugar and Tavakksiri.

For the healing of injury, the patient should take milk boiled with Ikshuvalika, Bisagranthi (lotus stalk knot), Padma Kesara (Lotus stamen) and Chandana (Sandalwood), by adding honey.

If there is fever and burning sensation in the body, then the patient is given

Barley powder cooked with milk and added with ghee

Alternatively, such a patient should take sugar, honey and Saktu (roasted corn- flour) mixed with milk.

If the patient is suffering from cough and pain in the sides of the chest as well as bones, then he should take linctus prepared of the powder of Madhuca– Licorice, Draksha – Raisin, Tavaksheeri, pippali – Piper nigrum and Bala – Country mallow (root) mixed with ghee and honey. [15-20]

Eladi Gutika

एलापत्र त्वचोऽर्धाक्षाः पिप्पल्यर्धपलं तथा।
सिता मधुक खर्जूर मृद्वीकाश्च पलोन्मिताः॥२१॥
सञ्चूर्ण्य मधुना युक्ता गुटिकाः सम्प्रकल्पयेत्।
अक्षमात्रां ततश्चैकां भक्षयेन्ना दिने दिने॥२२॥
कासं श्वासं ज्वरं हिक्कां छर्दिं मूर्च्छां मदं भ्रमम्।
रक्त निष्ठीवनं तृष्णां पार्श्वशूलमरोचकम्॥२३॥
शोष प्लीहाढ्यवातांश्च स्वरभेदं क्षतं क्षयम्।
गुटिका तर्पणी वृष्या रक्तपित्तं च नाशयेत्॥२४॥
इत्येलादिगुटिका।

1/2 Aksha of each of

Ela – Elettaria cardamomum

Patra – Cinnamomum tamala Nees and Eberum

Tvak,

1/2 Pala of Pippali – Piper nigrum,

1 pala each of

Sita – white variety of Cynodon dactylon

Madhuka– Licorice – Glycyrrhiza glabra

Kharjura – Phoenix sylvestris and

Mrudvika – Vitis vinifera is made to a powder.

This powder is added with honey to make a paste.

From out of this paste, pills of 1 Aksa each are prepared. 1 such pill is taken every day.

It is indicated in –

Kasa – cough

Svasa – Asthma

Jvara – fever

Hikka – hiccup

Chardi – vomiting

Murccham – fainting

Rakta nisthivanam – hemoptysis

Trshunam – morbid thirst

Parshva shula – pain in the sides of the chest

Aruchi – anorexia

Sosha – consumption

Pliha – splenic enlargement

Adhyavata – Rheumatic disorders

Svara bhedam – hoarseness of voice

Ksata – Injury to the chest

Ksaya – diminution of tissue elements and

Raktapitta – condition characterized by bleeding from different parts of the body.

This pill improves energy and acts as aphrodisiac. [21-24]

Treatment of Excessive Bleeding

रक्तेऽतिवृत्ते दक्षाण्डं यूषैस्तोयेन वा पिबेत्।
चटकाण्डरसं वाऽपि रक्तं वा छागजाङ्गलम्॥२५॥
चूर्णं पौनर्नवं रक्तशालितण्डुलशर्करम्।

रक्तष्ठीवी पिबेत् सिद्धं द्राक्षारसपयोघृतैः||२६||

If there is excessive bleeding (hemoptysis), then the patient should eat eggs of Daksha (wild hen) along with juice (vegetable soup) or water.

He may also take the soup of the eggs of sparrows or (preparations) of the blood of goats or wild animals (like deer, etc).

The patient having hemoptysis (blood spitting) should take the powder of Punarnava, red variety of Shali rice and sugar cooked along with grape juice, milk and ghee. [25-26]

Symptomatic treatment:

मधूक मधुक क्षीर सिद्धं वा तण्डुलीयकम्|

मूढवातस्त्वजामेदः सुराभृष्टं ससैन्धवम्||२७||

क्षामः क्षीणः क्षतोरस्कस्त्व निद्रः सबलेऽनिले|

शृत क्षीरसरेणाद्यात् सक्षौद्र घृत शर्करम्||२८||

शर्करां यवगोधूमौ जीवकर्षभकौ मधु|

शृतक्षीरानुपानं वा लिह्यात् क्षीणः क्षती कृशः||२९||

क्रव्याद मांस नियूहं घृतभृष्टं पिबेच्च सः|

पिप्पली क्षौद्र संयुक्तं मांस शोणित वर्धनम्||३०||

न्यग्रोधोदुम्बराश्वत्थ प्लक्ष शाल प्रियङ्गुभिः|

ताल मस्तक जम्बूत्वक्प्रियालैश्च सपद्मकैः||३१||

साश्वकर्णैः शृतात् क्षीराददद्याज्जातेन सर्पिषा|

शाल्योदनं क्षतोरस्कः क्षीणशुक्रश्च मानवः||३२||

यष्ट्याह्व नागबलयोः क्वाथे क्षीरसमं घृतम्|

पयस्या पिप्पली वांशी कल्क सिद्धं क्षते शुभम्||३३||

कोल लाक्षा रसे तद्वत् क्षीराष्ट गुण साधितम्|

कल्कैः कट्वङ्ग दार्वीत्वग्वत्सकत्वक्फलैर्घृतम्||३४||

Milk is boiled in the paste of Madhuka– Licorice and madhuka – Madhuca longifolia. With this milk, Tanduliyaka is cooked – useful in hemoptysis – blood spitting from mouth.

If there is Mudhavata, the patient should take the fat of goat fried with Sura type of alcohol and mixed with Saindhava – rock salt.

If the patient is weak, emaciated and has chest injury, sleeplessness and excessive aggravation of Vata, then he should take goat's fat boiled with the cream of milk and added with honey, ghee and sugar.

If the patient is emaciated, having injury in the chest and diminution of body tissues, he is given sugar, barley, wheat, Jivaka, Rishabhaka and honey in a linctus form. This potion promotes muscle tissue and blood.

The patient having injury to the chest and diminution of semen, should eat Shali – rice mixed with ghee prepared with milk boiled with Nyagrodha (Ficus benghalensis), Udumbara (Ficus racemosa), Ashvattha (Ficus religiosa), Plaksa, Sala (Shorea robusta) Priyangu (Callicara macrophylla), Tuft of Tala, Bark of Jambu(Syzygium cumini), Priyala (Buchanania lanzan), Padmaka – Prunus cerasoides and Asvakarna.

Yastvahvadi Ghrita

Ghee is cooked with equal quantity of milk, decoction of Madhuyasti (licorice) and Nagabala [4 times in total of ghee]. This medicated ghee is useful in the treatment of Kshata (injury to the chest).

Koladi Ghrita

Similarly, ghee is cooked with the decoction of Kola (ber fruit) and Laksha [4 times in total of ghee], 8 times of milk, and the paste of the bark of Katvanga, bark of Darvi, bark of Kutaja – Connessi (Holarrhena antidysenterica Wall.) and fruit of Kutaja – Connessi (Holarrhena antidysenterica Wall.) 1/4th fourth in total of ghee. This medicated ghee is useful in the treatment of Ksata (injury to the chest) [27-34]

Amruta Prasha Ghruta

जीवकर्षभकौ वीरां जीवन्तीं नागरं शटीम्।
चतस्रः पर्णिनीर्मेदे काकोल्यौ द्वे निदिग्धिके॥३५॥
पुनर्नवे द्वे मधुकमात्मगुप्तां शतावरीम्।
ऋद्धिं परूषकं भार्गीं मृद्वीकां बृहतीं तथा॥३६॥
शृङ्गाटकं तामलकीं पयस्यां पिप्पलीं बलाम्।
बदराक्षोट खर्जूर वातामाभिषुकाण्यपि॥३७॥
फलानि चैवमादीनि कल्कान् कुर्वीत कार्षिकान्।
धात्री रस विदारीक्षुच्छाग मांस रसं पयः॥३८॥
कुर्यात् प्रस्थोन्मितं तेन घृतप्रस्थं विपाचयेत्।
प्रस्थार्ध मधुनः शीते शर्कराधैतुलां तथा॥३९॥
द्विकार्षिकाणि पत्रैलाहेमत्वङ्मरिचानि च।
विनीय चूर्णितं तस्माल्लिहयान्मात्रां सदा नरः॥४०॥
अमृतप्राशमित्येतन्नराणाममृतं घृतम्।
सुधामृतरसं प्राश्यं क्षीरमांसरसाशिना॥४१॥
नष्टशुक्र क्षतक्षीण दुर्बल व्याधि कर्शितान्।
स्त्री प्रसक्तान् कृशान् वर्ण स्वर हीनांश्च बृंहयेत्॥४२॥
कास हिक्का ज्वर श्वास दाह तृष्णास्र पित्तनुत्।
पुत्रदं वमि मूर्च्छा हृद्योनिमूत्रामयापहम्॥४३॥ इत्यमृतप्राशघृतम्।

2 Prasthas of ghee is cooked with 2 Prasthas each of
Juice of Dhatri
Juice of Vidari (Ipomoea paniculata / Pueraria tuberosa),
Sugarcane juice
Soup of the meat of the goat
Milk and
1 Karsha each of the paste of
Jivaka – Malaxis acuminata,
Rishabhaka
Veera
Jivanti – Leptadenia reticulata,
Nagara – Zingiber officinale
Shati – Hedychium spicatum
Shalaparni – Desmodium gangeticum
Prishniparni – Uraria picta
Mashaparni – Teramnus labialis
Mudgaparni – Vigna trilobata
Meda – Polygonatum cirrhifolium
Mahameda – Polygonatum cirrhifolium
Kakoli – Fritillaria roylei
Ksheerakakoli – Lilium polyphyllum
Kantakari – Solanum xanthocarpum
Brihati – Solanum indicum
Sveta Punarnava
Rakta punarnava — Boerhavia diffusa
Madhuka– Licorice – Glycyrrhiza glabra
Atmagupta – Mucuna pruriens

Shatavari – Asparagus racemosus
Riddhi
Parushaka – Grewia asiatica
Bharngi – Clerodendrum serratum
Mrudvika – Vitis vinifera
Brhati – Solanum indicum
Shringataka – Trapa bispinosa
Tamalaki – Bhumi amla
Payasya (Ksheera vidari)
Pippali – Long pepper fruit – Piper longum,
Badara – Ziziphus jujuba,
Akshota
Kharjura – Phoenix sylvestris
Vatama,
Abhisuka (Pishta) and
Such other fruits (which are alleviators of Vata and Pitta)
After cooking, when the recipe is cooled,
1 Prastha (768 ml) of honey,
1/2 Tula (2.4 kg) of Sugar, and
The powder [2 karsha each] of
Patra – Cinnamomum tamala Nees and Eberum
Ela (Elettaria cardamomum Maton)
Hema (Mesua ferrea)
Tvak – Cinnamon and
Maricha – Black pepper is added to it.
This medicated ghee is taken by a person in appropriate dose regularly.
This is called 'Amruta Prasa ghritam' and it is like ambrosia for human beings. This linctus is like Sudha (ambrosia worth the consumption of wordily creatures) and Amruta (nectar worth the consumption of the gods).
It is taken along with milk and meat soup.
It promotes
Nourishment of persons who had meat soup
Nourishment of persons, who had wasted semen
Who are suffering from phthisis
Who are weak
Who are emaciated because of chronic diseases
Who are cachectic and
Who have lost their complexion and voice
It cures
Kasa – cough
Hikka – hiccup
Jwara – fever
Svasa – Asthma
Daha – burning sensation
Trushna – morbid thirst
Raktapitta – an ailment characterized by bleeding from different parts of the body
Chardi – vomiting,
Bhrama – fainting, and
Hrudi vyadhi – diseases of the heart,

Female genital tract and urinary tract
It helps in the procreation of a male child. [35-43]

Svadamshtradi Ghrita:
श्वदंष्ट्रोशीर मञ्जिष्ठा बला काश्मर्य कतृणम्|
दर्भमूलं पृथक्पर्णी पलाशर्षभकौ स्थिराम्||४४||
पलिकं साधयेतेषां रसे क्षीरचतुर्गुणे|
कल्कः स्वगुप्ता जीवन्ती मेदर्षभक जीवकैः||४५||
शतावर्यृद्धि मृद्वीका शर्करा श्रावणी बिसैः|
प्रस्थः सिद्धो घृताद्वात पित्तहृद्द्र(द्भ)वशूलनुत्||४६||
मूत्रकृच्छ्र प्रमेहार्शःकास शोष क्षयापहः|
धनुःस्त्रीमद्यभाराध्वखिन्नानां बलमांसदः||४७|| इति श्वदंष्ट्रादिघृतम्|
1 Pala of each of
Svadamstra – Tribulus terrestris
Ushira – Vetiver – Vetiveria zizanioides
Manjistha – Rubia cordifolia
Bala – Country mallow (root) – Sida cordifolia
Kashmarya -Gmelina arborea
Katruna
The root of Darbha – Demostachya bipinnata
Pruthak Parni
Palasa – Butea monosperma
Rishabhaka – Manilkara hexandra and
Sthira – Desmodium gangeticum is made to decoction.
2 Prasthas of ghee is mixed with the above mentioned decoction
8 Prasthas of milk, and the paste of
Svagupta – Mucuna pruriens
Jivanti – Leptadenia reticulata
Meda
Rishabhaka
Jivaka
Shatavari – Asparagus racemosus
Riddhi
Mrdvika – Vitis vinfera
Sarkara – unrefined sugar
Shravani and
Bisa (lotus Stalk) [1/2 Prastha in total] and cooked
This medicated ghee cures:
Hruddrava (Palpitation of heart) caused by Vayu and Pitta
Hrudaya Shoola (pain in cardiac region) caused by Vata and Pitta
Mutrakrucchra (dysuria), piles, bronchitis, consumption and phthisis
It promotes strength and muscle tissues of persons emaciated because of indulgence in archery, women, alcoholics,
carrying heavy weight and walking a long distance. [44-47]

Samasaktu Ghruta
मधुकाष्ट पल द्राक्षा प्रस्थ क्वाथे घृतं पचेत्|
पिप्पल्यष्टपले कल्के प्रस्थं सिद्धे च शीतले||४८||

पृथगष्टपलं क्षौद्र शर्कराभ्यां विमिश्रयेत्‌|
समसक्तु क्षतक्षीणे रक्तगुल्मे च तद्दिधतम्‌||४८||

2 Prasthas of ghee is cooked by adding the decoction of

8 Palas Madhuka– Licorice – Glycyrrhiza glabra and

1 Prastha Draksha – Raisin – Vitis vinifera and

8 Palas of paste of Pippali – Long pepper fruit – Piper longum

After it is cooked and cooled, 8 Palas of each of honey and sugar is added and mixed well

This medicated ghee is administered by adding Saktu (roasted barely flour) in equal quantity.

It is useful in the treatment of

Ksataksina (Phthisis) and

Rakta Gulma (Phantom tumor in ladies resembling pregnancy). [48-49]

Sarpirguda (First recipe)

धात्रीफल विदारीक्षु जीवनीय रसै घृतम्‌|
अजागोपयसोश्चैव सप्त प्रस्थान् पचेद्दिभषक्‌||५०||
सिद्धशीते सिता क्षौद्र द्विप्रस्थं विनयेच्च तत्‌|
यक्ष्मापस्मार पितासृक्कास मेह क्षयापहम्‌||५१||
वय:स्थापनमायुष्यं मांस शुक्र बलप्रदम्‌|
घृतं तु पित्तेऽभ्यधिके लिह्याद्वातेऽधिके पिबेत्‌||५२||
लीढं निर्वापयेत् पित्तमल्पत्वाद्दधन्ति नानलम्‌|
आक्रामत्यनिलं पीतमूष्माणं निरुणद्धि च||५३||
क्षाम क्षीण कृशाङ्गानामेतान्येव घृतानि तु|
त्वक्क्षीरी शर्करा लाज चूर्णै: स्त्यानानि योजयेत्‌||५४||
सर्पिर्गुडान् समध्वंशाञ्जग्ध्वा चानु पय: पिबेत्‌|
रेतो वीर्य बलं पुष्टिं तैराशुतरमाप्नुयात्‌||५५|| इति सर्पिर्गुडा:|

Ingredients to be cooked: 2 Prasthas of ghee is added with

2 Prasthas each of

Juice of Amalaki – Phyllanthus emblica

Vidari - Pueraria tuberosa and

Iksu – Sugar cane

Decoction of drugs belonging to Jivaniya group

Goat milk

Cow milk

After the cooking is over and the recipe is cooled

1 Prastha (768 g) of sugar and 2 prasthas of honey is added and mixed well.

This medicated ghee is useful in the treatment of

Tuberculosis,

Epilepsy,

Raktapitta (an ailment characterized by bleeding from different parts of the body),

Prameha (obstinate urinary disorders including diabetes) and

Ksaya (consumption)

It prevents

Aging,

Promotes longevity and

Endows the person with muscle tissue, semen as well as strength

If the diseases are caused by excess pitta, then this recipe is used as linctus.

If however, the diseases are caused by the excess of Vayu, then it should be taken as a drink.

When this medicated ghee is used (licked) in the form of a linctus, it alleviates Pitta. Since it is in small quantity, it however, doesn't suppress the Agni (power of digestion).

When it is used in the form of a drink, it alleviates Vata and obstructs heat.

This and such other medicated ghee is made to a thick paste by adding the powder of Tvakksiri, sugar and Laja (fried paddy) which is then given to persons who are tired, weak and emaciated.

This and such other recipes of Sapirguda [recipes of medicated ghee in which sugar, honey etc, are added] is added with honey (which is equal in quantity with the powder of Tvakksiri, etc) and taken. Thereafter, the patient should drink milk. This instantaneously promotes semen, potency, strength and nourishment. [50-55]

Sarpirguda (Second recipe)

बला विदारी ह्रस्वा च पञ्चमूली पुनर्नवा|
पञ्चानां क्षीरि वृक्षाणां शुङ्गा मुष्ट्यंशका अपि||५६||
एषां कषाये द्विक्षीरे विदार्याजरसांशिके|
जीवनीयैः पचेत् कल्कै रक्ष मात्रैर्घृताढकम्||५७||
सितापलानि पूते च शीते द्वात्रिंशतं क्षिपेत्|
गोधूम पिप्पली वांशी चूर्ण शृङ्गाटकस्य च||५८||
समाक्षिकं कौडविकं तत् सर्वं खजमूच्छितम्|
स्त्यानं सर्पिर्गुडान् कृत्वा भूर्जपत्रेण वेष्टयेत्||५९||
ताञ्जग्ध्वा पलिकान् क्षीरं मद्यं वाऽनुपिबेत् कफे|
शोषे कासे क्षते क्षीणे श्रमस्त्रीभारकर्शिते||६०||
रक्तनिष्ठीवने तापे पीनसे चोरसि स्थिते|
शस्ताः पार्श्वशिरःशूले भेदे च स्वरवर्णयोः||६१||
इति द्विवतीयसर्पिर्गुडाः|

1 Pala of each of these drugs is made to a decoction:

Bala – Country mallow (root) – Sida cordifolia

Vidari (Ipomoea paniculata / Pueraria tuberosa)

Hrsva Panchamula (Shalaparni, Prishnaparni – Uraria picta, Brihati – Solanum indicum, Kavtakari and Goksura – Tribulus terrestris)

Punarnava – Boerhavia diffusa

And the Sungas (terminal buds) of five Ksirivrksha (Nyagarodha – Ficus bengalensis, Udumbara – Ficus racemosa, Asvatha – Ficus religiosa, Madhuka– Licorice – Glycyrrhiza glabra and Plaksa)

To this

2 parts milk

1 part juice of Vidari (Pueraria tuberosa),

1 part soup of goat meat,

2 Adhakas ghee [in the text, actually 1 Adhaka is mentioned. But in practice, it is to be taken double the quantity according to the general rule (Praibhasa)], and

1 Aksa each of paste of drugs belonging to the Jivaniya group is added and cooked.

When it is well cooked and cooled 32 Palas of Sugar is added

Thereafter, 1 Kudava of each of the powder of

Godhuma – wheat – Triticum sativum

Pippali – Long pepper fruit – Piper longum

Vamsa Locana,

Srngataka and

Honey is added

All of them are stirred with the help of a stirrer (Khaja)

When it becomes dense, cakes (Sarpirgudas) are prepared and each of them is wrapped with Bhurjapatra (thin barks of Bhuja tree)

Having taken this cake 1 Pala in weight, the patient should take milk or alcohol as post- prandial drink.

These are useful in the treatment of phthisis.

These are also useful for persons who are

Emaciated because of excessive exertion,

Over – indulgence in sex and

Exhaustion by lifting excessive weight

These cakes are efficacious in the treatment of

Rakta-Nisthivana — Hemoptysis

Daha -Burning sensation

Pinasa – chronic rhinitis having residual infection in the chest

Parshva shoola — pain in the sides of the chest

Shira shoola – headache

Svara bheda – hoarseness of voice and

Varna nasha – loss of complexion [56-61]

Sarpirgudah (Third recipe)

त्वक्क्षीरी श्रावणी द्राक्षामूर्वर्षभक जीवकैः|

वीरर्धि क्षीरकाकोली बृहती कपिकच्छुभिः||६२||

खर्जूर फलमेदाभिः क्षीरपिष्टैः पलोन्मितैः|

धात्री विदारीक्षु रस प्रस्थैः प्रस्थं घृतात् पचेत्||६३||

शर्कराध तुलां शीते क्षौद्राध प्रस्थमेव च|

दत्वा सर्पिर्गुडान् कुर्यात्कास हिक्का ज्वरापहान्||६४||

यक्ष्माणं तमकं श्वासं रक्तपितं हलीमकम्|

शुक्रनिद्राक्षयं तृष्णां हन्युः काश्र्यं सकामलम्||६५||

इति तृतीयाः सर्पिर्गुडाः|

1 Pala of each of

Tavaksheeri

Sravani (Muditika) – Sphaeranthus indicus

Draksha – Raisin – Vitis vinifera

Murva – Marsedenia tenacissima

Rishabhaka

Jivaka

Vira kanda (Vidari (Pueraria tuberosa)

Riddhi

Ksheerakakoli – Lilium polyphyllum

Brihati – Solanum indicum

Kapikacchu – Mucuna pruriens

Fruit of kharjura – Phoenix sylvestris and

Meda is made to a paste by triturating with milk.

To this paste 2 prasthas of each of these are cooked together:

Juice of Dhatri

Juice of Vidari (Pueraria tuberosa)

Sugarcane juice and

Ghee

After the ghee is well cooked and cooled:

1/2 Tula of sugar and

1 Prastha of honey is added, out of which cakes (Sarpirgudas) are prepared.

These cakes cure

Kasa — cough

Hikka – hiccup

Jwara – fever

Yakshma – tuberculosis

Shvasa – bronchial asthma

Rakta Pitta – an ailment characterized by bleeding from different parts of the body

Halimaka – a serious type of jaundice

Shukra Ksaya – diminution of semen, oligospermia

Insomnia

Trushna – morbid thirst

Karshya – emaciation and

Kamala – Jaundice [in translation, liquids, ghee and honey are taken double the prescribed quantity according rules (Paribhasa),] [62-65]

Sarpirgudah (Fourth recipe)

नवमामलकं द्राक्षामात्मगुप्तां पुनर्नवाम्।

शतावरीं विदारीं च समङ्गां पिप्पलीं तथा।।६६।।

पृथग्दशपलान् भागान् पलान्यष्टौ च नागरात्।

यष्ट्याह्व सौवर्चलयो द्विपलं मरिचस्य च।।६७।।

क्षीर तैल घृतानां च त्र्याढके शर्कराशते।

क्वथिते तानि चूर्णानि दत्वा बिल्वसमान् गुडान्।।६८।।

कुर्यात्तान् भक्षयेत् क्षीणः क्षतः शुष्कश्च मानवः।

तेन सद्यो रसादीनां वृद्ध्या पुष्टिं स विन्दति।।६९।।

इति चतुर्थसर्पिर्गुडाः।

All these drugs are made to powders: 10 palas of each of

Freshly collected and dried Amalaki – Phyllanthus emblica

Draksha – Raisin – Vitis vinifera

Atmagupta – Mucuna pruriens

Punarnava – Boerhavia diffusa

Shatavari – Asparagus racemosus

Vidari – Pueraria tuberosa

Samanga – Rubia cordifolia

Pippali – Long pepper fruit – Piper longum

8 Palas of Nagara – Zingiber officinale

1 Pala of Madhuyasti – Licorice

1 Pala sauvarcala

And

2 Palas of Maricha – Black pepper fruit – Piper nigrum

2 Adhakas each of

Milk

Tila Taila – sesame oil

Ghee and

100 Palas of Sugar are cooked together.

Thereafter, the above mentioned powders are added.

These cakes are taken by persons suffering from phthisis and consumption.

Intake of these cakes instantaneously promotes tissue elements like Rasa (Chyle) etc, as a result of which the individual gets nourished. [66-69]

Sarpir modakah (Fifth recipe)

गो क्षीरार्धाढकं सर्पिः प्रस्थमिक्षु रसाढकम्|
विदार्याः स्वरसात्प्रस्थं रसात्प्रस्थं च तैत्तिरात्||७०||
दद्यात् सिध्यति तस्मिंस्तु पिष्टानिक्षु रसैरिमान्|
मधूक पुष्पकुडवं प्रियाल कुडवं तथा||७१||
कुडवार्धं तुगाक्षीर्याः खर्जूराणां च विंशतिम्|
पृथग्विभीतकानां च पिप्पल्याश्च चतुर्थिकाम्||७२||
त्रिंशत्पलानि खण्डाच्च मधुकात् कर्षमेव च|
तथाऽर्ध पलिकान्यत्र जीवनीयानि दापयेत्||७३||
सिद्धेऽस्मिन् कुडवं क्षौद्रं शीते क्षिप्त्वाऽथ मोदकान्|
कारयेन्मरिचाजाजीपलचूर्णावचूर्णितान्||७४||
वातासृक्पित्तरोगेषु क्षत कासक्षयेषु च|
शुष्यतां क्षीणशुक्राणां रक्ते चोरसि संस्थिते||७५||
कृश दुर्बल वृद्धानां पुष्टिवर्णबलार्थिनाम्|
योनि दोष कृतस्रावहतानां चापि योषिताम्||७६||
गर्भार्थिनीनां गर्भश्च स्रवेद्यासां म्रियेत वा|
धन्या बल्या हितास्ताभ्यः शुक्रशोणितवर्धनाः||७७||
इति पञ्चमसर्पिर्मोदकाः|

1 Adhaka of Cow's milk

2 Prasthas ghee

2 Adhakas Sugarcane Juice

2 Prasthas Juice of Vidari and

2 Prasthas soup of the meat of Tittiri is cooked together

During the final stage of cooking

1 Kudava each of

Paste of Madhuka– Licorice – Glycyrrhiza glabra Puspa

Priyala

½ kudava Tugaksiri

20 fruits of kharjura

20 fruits bibhitaki

1 pala Pippali – Long pepper fruit – Piper longum

30 Palas Sugar

1 Karsa Madhuka– Licorice – Glycyrrhiza glabra and

1/2 Pala Drugs belonging to the Jivaniya group are added.

The above mentioned drugs are made to a paste by triturating with sugar cane juice before adding to the recipe.

After the recipe is fully cooked and cooled, 2 kudavas of honey are added.

From this, Modakas 1 Pala of the powder of Maricha – Black pepper fruit and Ajaji (cumin) are sprinkled.

These Modakas cures

Vatasruk (gout)

Diseases caused by Pitta

Phthisis

Cough and

Kshaya – body tissue depletion.

These are useful for persons suffering from emaciation, who are reduced of semen, whose blood is locked up in the chest, who are thin, weak and old, and also for those desirous of having nourishment, complexion and strength.

These Modakas are also useful for ladies suffering from exudations through the vitiated genital tract, who desire conception and who suffer from miscarriages and death of the foetus in womb. By the use of these pills, ladies are endowed with auspicious strength and wholesomeness. These are promoters of Shukra (sperm) and Sonita (ovum) [70-77]

Recipes

बस्तिदेशे विकुर्वाणे स्त्री प्रसक्तस्य मारुते|

वातघ्नान् बृंहणान् वृष्यान् योगांस्तस्य प्रयोजयेत्||७८||

शर्करा पिप्पली चूर्णैः सर्पिषा माक्षिकेण च|

संयुक्तं वा शृतं क्षीरं पिबेत् कास ज्वरापहम्||७९||

फलाम्लं सर्पिषा भृष्टं विदारीक्षुरसे शृतम्|

स्त्रीषु क्षीणः पिबेद्यूषं जीवनं बृंहणं परम्||८०||

सक्तूनां वस्त्रपूतानां मन्थं क्षौद्र घृतान्वितम्|

यवान्न सात्म्यो दीप्ताग्निः क्षतक्षीणः पिबेन्नरः||८१||

जीवनीयोपसिद्धं वा जाङ्गलं घृतभर्जितम्|

रसं प्रयोजयेत् क्षीणे व्यञ्जनार्थं सशर्करम्||८२||

गोमहिष्यश्वनागाजैः क्षीरैर्मांसरसैस्तथा|

यवान्नं भोजयेद्यूषैः फलाम्लैर्घृतसंस्कृतैः||८३||

दीप्तेऽग्नौ विधिरेषः स्यान्मन्दे दीपनपाचनः|

यक्ष्मिणां विहितो ग्राही भिन्ने शकृति चेष्यते||८४||

In persons indulging in women, [vitiated] Vata afflicts Basti desha (Pelvic region). To such patients, recipes which are alleviators of Vayu, prompters of nourishment and aphrodisiacs are to be administered.

Sugar, powder of Pippali – Long pepper fruit , ghee and or honey is added to milk and given to patient to drink for the cure of cough and fever.

These ingredients can be added to milk after or before boiling, appropriately. Whenever honey is to be used, it is added to the milk when it is boiled and cooled.

Phalamla is fried in ghee and boiled with the juice of Vidari (Ipomoea paniculata / Pueraria tuberosa) and sugarcane. The vegetable soup, thus prepared, is useful for a patient who is emaciated because of the excessive indulgence in women. This is an excellent recipe for the promotion of longevity and nourishment.

Roasted barley flour is sieved through a cloth, and Mantha (thin gruel) is prepared out of it. This gruel is added with honey and ghee, and given to a patient suffering from phthisis, provided that he is accustomed to taking barley as one of the ingredients of the food and if he has strong digestion.

Alternatively, meat of animals of arid zone (Jangala) is boiled with drugs belonging to the Jivaniya group. The meat soup, thus prepared, should be sizzled with ghee, added with sugar and used as a dish (Vyanjana) for a patient suffering from phthisis.

Boiled barley is given to a patient suffering from phthisis along with milk of she-buffalo, mare, she – elephant and she goat or with meat soup or with vegetable soup or with Phalamla sizzled with ghee.

The above-mentioned recipes are given to patients having strong digestion. If the power of digestion is suppressed, then the patient should be given recipes which are stimulants of digestion (Dipana) and carminative (Pacana). If there is Diarrhoea in a patient suffering from phthisis, then the bowel binding recipes prescribed for the treatment of tuberculosis (Chapter 8) are used. [78-84]

Saindhavadi Churna

पलिकं सैन्धवं शुण्ठी द्वे च सौवर्चलात् पले|

कुडवांशानि वृक्षाम्लं दाडिमं पत्रमर्जकात्||८५||
एकैकं मरिचाजाज्योर्धान्यकाद्द्वे चतुर्थिके|
शर्कराया: पलान्यत्र दश द्वे च प्रदापयेत्||८६||
कृत्वा चूर्णमतो मात्रामन्नपाने प्रयोजयेत्|
रोचनं दीपनं बल्यं पार्श्वार्तिश्वासकासनुत्||८७||
इति सैन्धवादिचूर्णम्|

1 Pala each of Saindhava and sunthi

2 Palas of Sauvarchala

1 Kudava of Vrksamla (Dadima – Pomegranate)

1 Kuduva of leaf of Arjaka

1 Pala of Maricha – Black pepper fruit

1 Pala of Ajaji – cumin

2 Palas of Dhanyaka – coriander and

12 Palas of sugar are made with powders and mixed together.

In appropriate quantities, this powder is added to food and drinks.

It is an appetizer, stimulant of digestion and promoter of strength; it cures pain in the sides of the chest, asthma and cough. [85-87]

Shadava

एका षोडशिका धान्याद्द्वे द्वेऽजाज्यजमोदयो:|
ताभ्यां दाडिम वृक्षाम्लं द्विद्विर्व: सौवर्चलात्पलम्||८८||
शुण्ठ्या: कर्ष दधित्थस्य मध्यात् पञ्च पलानि च|
तच्चूर्ण षोडशपले शर्कराया विमिश्रयेत्||८९||
षाडवोऽयं प्रदेय: स्यादन्नपानेषु पूर्ववत्|
मन्दानले शकृद्भेदे यक्ष्मिणामग्निवर्धन:||९०||
इति षाडव:|

Powders of

1 Pala Dhanyaka

2 Pala Ajaji

2 Pala of Ajamoda

4 Palas of Dadima – Pomegranate

1 Pala of Sauvarchala (Black salt)

1 karsa of Sunti – Zingiber offcinale

5 Palas of pulp of Kapittha and

16 Palas of sugar are mixed together.

Like the earlier recipe, the present Sadava [delicious recipe having sweet and sour tastes] is administered along with food and drinks for the treatment of mandanala (suppression of the powder of digestion) and diarrhoea

It promotes the digestive power of patients suffering from tuberculosis [88-90]

Nagabala Kalpa

पिबेन्नागबलामूलमर्धकर्षविवर्धितम्|
पलं क्षीरयुतं मासं क्षीरवृत्तिरनन्नभुक्||९१||
एष प्रयोग: पुष्ट्यायुर्बलारोग्यकर: पर:|
मण्डूकपर्ण्या: कल्पोऽयं शुण्ठीमधुकयोस्तथा||९२||

1/2 Karsha of the root (bark) of Nagabala (Grewia populifolia, Sida spinosa, Urena lobata, Grewia hirsuta) is boiled with milk and given to the patient on the first day.

Thereafter, the powder of Nagabala- root- (bark) is increased by 1/2 Karsha every day, and given by boiling with milk.

On the 8th day, the quantity of Nagabala- root will be 1 Pala (48 g).

Thereafter, the patient should continue to take this drug in the dose of 1 Pala for 1 month.

While taking the milk boiled with this drug, the patient should refrain from taking any cereals. Whenever he feels hungry, he should take only milk.

The recipe is excellent for the promotion of nourishment, longevity, strength and immunity to diseases.

In the above mentioned manner, Mandukaparni, Sunthi (ginger) and Madhuka– Licorice is administered for therapeutic effects described above. [91-92]

Diet and drink

यद्यत् सन्तर्पणं शीतमविदाहि हितं लघु|
अन्नपानं निषेव्यं तत्क्षतक्षीणैः सुखार्थिभिः||९३||
यच्चोक्तं यक्ष्मिणां पथ्यं कासिनां रक्तपितिनाम्|
तच्च कुर्यादवेक्ष्याग्निं व्याधिं सात्म्यं बलं तथा||९४||

Food and drinks which are nourishing, cooling, Vidahi (which do not cause burning sensation), wholesome and light, is used by the patient suffering from phthisis and who is desirous of regaining health.

With due regard to the Agni (digestion strength), nature of disease, wholesomeness and strength, the patient of Phthisis should resort to wholesome diet, and regimens prescribed for tuberculosis, Kasa (cough) and Raktapitta (a disease for characterized by bleeding from different parts of the body). [93-94]

Need for Prompt Attention

उपेक्षिते भवेतस्मिन्ननुबन्धो हि यक्ष्मणः|
प्रागेवागमनात्तस्य तस्मात् त्वरया जयेत्||९५||

If the patient suffering from phthisis is not given appropriate treatment on time, then this may lead to Rajayakshma – tuberculosis. Therefore well before the arrival of this ailment (attack of tuberculosis), the phthisis should be treated, subdued (Cured). [95]

तत्र श्लोकौ-
क्षतक्षय समुत्थानं सामान्य पृथगाकृतिम्|
असाध्ययाप्यसाध्यत्वं साध्यानां सिद्धिमेव च||९६||
उक्तवाञ्ज्येष्ठशिष्याय क्षतक्षीणचिकित्सिते|
तत्त्वार्थविद्वीतरजस्तमोदोषः पुनर्वसुः||९७||

In this chapter, on the treatment of phthisis, Lord Punarvasu who is conversant with Truth and is free from Rajas (1 of the 3 attributes representing fickle mindedness including passion) and Tamas (1 of the 3 attributes representing slackness including ignorance) imparted instructions to the senior disciples on the following points:

1. Etiology of Phthisis;
2. Signs and symptoms of phthisis in general and of each variety
3. Incurability, Paliability and curability of phthisis and
4. Successful treatment of curable variety of phthisis. [96-97]

इत्यग्निवेशकृते तन्त्रेऽप्राप्ते दृढबल पूरिते चिकित्सित स्थाने क्षतक्षीण चिकित्सितं नामैकादशोऽध्यायः||११||

Thus, ends the 11th chapter dealing with the treatment of Phthisis (Ksata Ksina) in the section on therapeutics of Agnivesa's work as redacted by Charaka and not being available, restored by Drdhabala.

18

Chikitsasthana Chapter 12 Shotha Chikitsitam

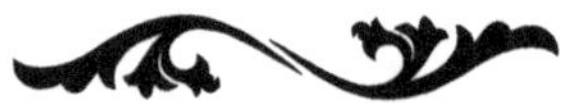

The 12th Chapter of Charaka Samhita Chikitsa Sthana – Shvayathu chikitsa deals with symptoms and treatment of different types of inflammation. The term Shotha, Sotha, Shoth are used as synonyms of Shvayathu.

अथातः श्वयथु चिकित्सितं व्याख्यास्यामः||१||
इति ह स्माह भगवानात्रेयः||२||
Now we shall expound the chapter on the treatment of Svayatu (oedema).
Thus said Lord Atreya [1-2]

भिषग्वरिष्ठं सुर सिद्धजुष्टं मुनीन्द्रमत्र्यात्मजमग्निवेशः|
महागदस्य श्वयथोर्यथावत् प्रकोपरूप प्रशमान पृच्छत्||३||
Agnivesha inquired from the great sage Atreya, the excellent physician and the one respected by the gods and Siddhas (those who have attained special spiritual powers) about a complete description of aetiology, signs and symptoms and treatment. [3]

तस्मै जगादागदवेदसिन्धु प्रवर्तनाद्रिप्रवरोऽत्रिजस्तान्|
वातादि भेदात्त्रिविधस्य सम्यङ्निजानिजैकाङ्गजसर्वजस्य||४||
Lord Atreya, the original source of science of medicine, appropriately explained to Agivesha the Aetiology etc. of the diseases which is classified into 3 categories, namely Vataja, Pittaja and Kaphaja, and also classified differently as exogenous (Agantuja), endogenous (Agantuja), Ekangaja (located in only one limb) and Sarvaja (swelling all over the body). [4]

Nija Shotha Nidana – Causes of Endogenous Variety:
शुद्ध्याम्याभक्तकृशाबलानां क्षाराम्ल तीक्ष्णोष्ण गुरूपसेवा|
दध्याममृच्छाक विरोधि दुष्टगरोपसृष्टान्ननिषेवणं च||५||
अर्शांस्यचेष्टा न च देहशुद्धिर्मर्मोपघातो विषमा प्रसूतिः|
मिथ्योपचारः प्रतिकर्मणां च निजस्य हेतुः श्वयथोः प्रदिष्टः||६||
Following are the causative factors of endogenous type of oedema:
Diseases arising due to the complications occuring due to improper or erroneous administration of cleansing (panchakarma) therapies
Getting emaciated or debilitated due to non-consumption of foods (starvation, fasting)
Intake of Kshara (Alkaline preparation),
Amla (sour food and drinks),
Teekshna (strong, piercing food articles)

Guru (heavy food) by a person who has become emaciated and weak because of Shuddhi (Panchakarma therapies)

Intake of Dadhi (curd), uncooked food, Mrut (Mud), Shaka (leafy vegetable),

Virodhi Anna (wrong food combinations),

Dushta Anna (Polluted food and water)

food afflicted with Gara (artificially prepared poison);

Afflictions with piles and lack of exercise;

Not administering Panchakarma purification therapies in appropriate times;

Marma upaghata – Afflictions of vital organs because of endogenous diseases (such as kidney disorders, heart disorders etc)

Irregular delivery, abortion and miscarriages and

Inappropriate administration of Panchakarma elimination therapies and improper care of the patient after the administration of these therapies [5-6]

Agantuja Shotha Nidana – Etiology of Exogenous Oedema

बाह्यास्त्वचो दूषयिताऽभिघातः काष्ठाश्मशस्त्राग्निविषायसाद्यैः |

आगन्तुहेतुः, ...|७|

Affliction of skin by the impact of wood, stone, weapon, fire, poison and iron gives rise to exogenous type of oedema. [7 ½]

Types of Nija and Agantuja Shotha (endogenous)

... त्रिविधो निजश्च सर्वार्धगात्रावयवाश्रितत्वात्||७||

The endogenous and exogenous oedema are of 3 types, viz,

Sarva Gatra – oedema pervading the whole body,

Ardha Gatra – oedema pervading the half of the body, and

Avayava Ashraya – oedema afflicting only one limb of the body. [7 ½]

Shotha samprapti: Pathogenesis

बाह्याः सिराः प्राप्य यदा कफासृक्पित्तानि सन्दूषयतीह वायुः|

तैर्बद्धधमार्गः स तदा विसर्पन्नुत्सेधलिङ्गं श्वयथुं करोति||८||

Because of the above-mentioned factors, Kapha, Asrik (blood) and Pitta enter the external vessels (Bahya Sira) and afflict Vata Dosha. As a result, the channel of circulation gets obstructed which spreads to the nearby areas, leading to Shotha. Shotha / Shvayatu is characterized by swelling. [8]

Pathogenesis

उरःस्थितैरूर्ध्वमधस्तु वायोः स्थान स्थितैर्मध्यगतैस्तु मध्ये|

सर्वाङ्गगः सर्वगतैः क्वचित्स्थैर्दोषैः क्वचित् स्याच्छ्वयथुस्तदाख्यः||९||

Urdhva Svayathu: If the afflictions take place in the chest, then oedema occurs in the upper part of the body

Adhah Svayathu: If these afflictions take place in the colon or pelvic region, which is the location of Vata, then oedema occurs in the lower part of the body.

Madhya shvayathu: If these afflictions take place in the middle of the body, i.e. between the chest and the pelvic region, then oedema occurs in the middle of the body, and

Sarvaanga Shotha: If these afflictions take place in the whole body, then swelling occurs in the entire body.

If however, these afflictions are located in any particular viscera, such as throat and palate, then oedema takes place in that locality and it is named after the viscera where it occurs (e.g. Gala Shotha) [9]

Shotha Purvaroopa:

ऊष्मा तथा स्याद्दवथुः सिराणामायाम इत्येव च पूर्वरूपम्|१०|

Premonitory signs and symptoms of Sotha Roga

Ushma – Hyperpyrexia, increased temperature

Davathu – burning sensation and

Siranam Ayama – dilatation of the vessels of the locality (10 ½)

सर्वस्त्रिदोषोऽधिक दोष लिङ्गैस्तच्छब्दमभ्येति भिषग्जितं च||१०||

Though all the 3 Doshas are involved in the manifestation of all the types of Shotha, it is on the basis of the predominance of the respective Doshas that

Vatika,

Pattika and

Slaismika (Kaphaja) varieties are determined and therapies are prescribed accordingly. [10]

Shotha Samanya lakshana:

सगौरवं स्यादनवस्थितत्वं सोत्सेधमुष्माऽथ सिरातनुत्वम्|
सलोमहर्षाऽङ्गविवर्णता च सामान्यलिङ्गं श्वयथोः प्रदिष्टम्||११||

The general signs and symptoms of Svayathu:

Sa gauravam – Heaviness

Anavasthitatvam – instability,

Utsedha – swelling

Ushma – rise in temperature,

Sira tanutvam – thinning of vessels,

Loma harsha – horrification and

Anga vivarnata – discoloration of the skin over the limbs [11]

Vataja Shotha Lakshana:

चलस्तनु त्वक्परुषोऽरुणोऽसितः प्रसुप्ति हर्षार्तियुतोऽनिमिततः|
प्रशाम्यति प्रोन्नमति प्रपीडितो दिवाबली च श्वयथुः समीरणात्||१२||

Signs and Symptoms of Vatika Svayathu:

Chala – The nature of the oedema changes very often

Tanu Twak – The skin over the oedematous part becomes thin,

Parusha – rough to touch

Aruna, Asita – red or black in colour;

Prasupti – numbness,

Harsha – tingling sensation, horripilation

Arti – Pain

The oedema gets subsided without any reason

When pressed, the swelling disappears but it appears again after the pressure is withdrawn and

Diva Bali – The swelling is more during day time. [12]

Pittaj Shotha Lakshana:

मृदुः सगन्धोऽसित पीत रागवान् भ्रम ज्वर स्वेद तृषामदान्वितः|
य उष्यते स्पर्शरुगक्षि रागकृत् स पित्तशोथो भृश दाह पाकवान्||१३||

Signs and Symptoms of Paittiks Svayathu:

Mrudu – swelling is soft to touch and

Sagandha – emits odour

Asita Peeta Raagavaan – black, yellow or red in colour

Bhrama, Jwara, Sweda, Trushna, Mada – associated with giddiness, fever, sweating, thirst and intoxication

Ushyate – local rise of temperature

Sparsha Ruk – local tenderness

Akshiragakrut – Eyes of the patient become red and

Brhusha Daha pakavan – Excess and swift burning sensation and suppuration in the affected part. [13]

Kaphaja Shoth Lakshan:

गुरुः स्थिरः पाण्डुररोचकान्वितः प्रसेक निद्रावमि वह्नि मान्द्यकृत्‌|

स कृच्छ्र जन्म प्रशमो निपीडितो न चोन्नमेद्रात्रिबली कफात्मकः||१४||

Signs and Symptoms of Kaphaja Svayathu:

Guru – heaviness in the affected limb / local area

Sthira – oedema remains stable and confined to one area

Pandu, Arochaka – patient suffers from anaemia and anorexia,

Praseka – to excessive salivation,

Nidra – excessive sleep,

Vami – vomiting and

Vahnimandya – suppression of the power of digestion

This type of oedema takes a long time to appear and its cure also takes a long time

Upon pressing and releasing the pressure, the pit doesn't get filled up immediately and

Ratribali – the condition gets aggravated at night. [14]

Asadhyata – Bad prognosis

कृशस्य रोगैरबलस्य यो भवेदुपद्रवैर्वा वमि पूर्वकैर्युतः|

स हन्ति मर्मानुगतोऽथ राजिमान् परिस्रवेद्धीनबलस्य सर्वगः||१५||

Bad prognosis

The patient of Svayathu succumbs to death because of the following:

If oedema occurs in a person who is emaciated and afflicted by other diseases

Vami – If the patient of oedema develops complications, like vomiting, etc

Marmanugata – If the oedema has afflicted the vital organs of the body

Rajiman – If stripes appears over the oedematous part

Parisrava – If there is exudation of fluid from this oedematous part

Heenabalasya Sarvanuga – If there is general oedema all over the body (anasarca) in a weak patient [15]

Sadhyata –

अहीन मांसस्य य एकदोषजो नवो बलस्थस्य सुखः स साधने|१६|

Good prognosis – curability:

Aheena mamsa – if there is no muscle wasting in the patient,

Eka Doshaja – if only one Dosha is involved

Nava – oedema of recent origin

Balasthasya – if the patient has good strength then the condition is curable. [16 ½]

Shotha Chikitsa Sutra: Line of Treatment:

निदान दोषर्तुविपर्यय क्रमैरुपाचरेत्तं बल दोष कालवित्‌||१६||

The physician, after ascertaining –

Bala – strength of the patient,

Dosha – Doshas involved

Kala – time, season, stage of disease, should treat the ailment by administering therapies, contradicting the etiological factors, Doshas and season. [16]

Treatment of Shotha in its different stages:

अथामजं लङ्घन पाचन क्रमै विशोधनैरुल्बण दोषमादितः|

शिरोगतं शीर्ष विरेचनैरधो विरेचनैरूर्ध्वहरैस्तथोर्ध्वजम्||१७||

उपाचरेत् स्नेहभवं विरूक्षणैः प्रकल्पयेत् स्नेहविधिं च रूक्षजे|

विबद्ध विट्केऽनिलजे निरूहणं घृतं तु पितानिलजे सतिक्तकम्||१८||

पयश्च मूच्छोरति दाह तर्षिते विशोधनीये तु समूत्रमिष्यते|

कफोत्थितं क्षार कटूष्ण संयुतैः समूत्र तक्रासव युक्ति भिर्जयेत्||१९||

If Shvayathu is caused by Ama, then the patient is given

Langhana – fasting therapy

Pachana therapy – to get rid of ama, to improve digestion strength

Shodhana – eliminate Panchakarma therapies to alleviate the predominant Dosha involved.

If Sotha is located in the head,

Seersha Virechana (therapies, like inhalation, nasal drops, meant for the elimination of the Doshas from the head) is administered.

If located in the lower body part,

Virechana – Purgation therapy is given, and

If located in the upper part of the body,

Vamana – emetic therapy is administered.

If Shotham is caused by improper administration of the Snehakarma – oleation therapy, then drugs having dryness qualities are administered.

If Svayathu is caused by excessive intake of dry foods and drinks, then Sneha – oleation therapy is given.

If there is constipation and if Svayathu is caused by Vata, then Niruha (decoction enema) is administered.

If Svayathu is caused by the simultaneous aggravation of Pitta and Vata, then Tiktaka Ghrita is administered.

If the patient is suffering from fainting (Murcha), Arati (dislike for everything), burning sensation and morbid thirst, then he is given milk.

If, however, such a patient is to be given elimination therapy, then a suitable recipe along with cow's urine is used.

If Shwayathu is caused by Kapha, then Takrasava mixed with cow's urine and added with Kshara, pungent and hot drugs, is administered. [17-19]

Apathya –

ग्राम्याब्जानूपं पिशितमबलं शुष्कशाकं नवान्नं

गौडं पिष्टान्नं दधि तिलकृतं विज्जलं मद्यमम्लम्|

धाना वल्लूरं समशनमथो गुर्वसात्म्यं विदाहि

स्वप्नं चारात्रौ श्वयथुगदवान् वर्जयेन्मैथुनं च||२०||

Unwholesome diet and regimen:

The Svayathu patient should avoid:

Gramya, Abja, Anupa – Meat of domesticated, aquatic and marsh place animals

Abala – meat that do not promote strength

Shushka shaka: Dried vegetables

Navanna – newly harvested grains

Gauda – Preparations of jaggery,

Pishtanna – pastries, starchy foods

Dadhi – curd,

Tila – sesame, slimy food and drinks, sour alcoholic preparations,

Dhana (germinated barley after frying) and dried meat;

Wrong food combinations

Heavy, unwholesome and Vidahi (which cause burning sensation) food and drink
Sleep during day time and
Sexual intercourse

Treatment of kaphaja Type of Svayathu (Oedema):

व्योषं त्रिवृत्तिक्तक रोहिणी च सायोरजस्का त्रिफला रसेन|
पीतं कफोत्थं शमयेतु शोफं गव्येन मूत्रेण हरीतकी च||२१||

Trikatu (Ginger, black pepper and long pepper),
Trivrt – Operculina turpethum and
Katukarohini – Picrorhiza kurroa
mixed with the powder of Ayoraja – iron is taken along with the
decoction Triphala (haritaki, Vibhitaki, Amalaki) which cures Svayathu caused by Kapha.
Similarly, intake of Haritaki along with Cow's urine cures Kaphaja type of oedema. [21]

Treatment of all the 3 types of Svayatu:

हरीतकी नागर देवदारु सुखाम्बुयुक्तं सपुनर्नवं वा|
सर्वं पिबेत्रिष्वपि मूत्रयुक्तं स्नातश्च जीर्णे पयसाऽन्नमद्यात्||२२||

In all 3 varieties of oedema, viz., Vataja, Pittaja and Kaphaja Svayathu, the Patient is given the paste of
Haritaki – Terminalia chebula
Nagara – Zingiber officinale and
Devadaru – Cedrus deodara along with luke-warm water alternatively.
The patient is given the paste of
Haritaki – Terminalia chebula
Nagara – Zingiber officinale
Devadaru – Cedrus deodara and
Punarnava – Boerhavia diffusa along with cow's urine
After taking these recipes, the patient should take a bath, and after the recipe is digested, he should take food (cereals) along with milk. [22]

Treatment of Vataja Shotha:

पुनर्नवा नागर मुस्त कल्कान् प्रस्थेन धीरः पयसाऽक्षमात्रान्|
मयूरकं मागधिकां समूलां सनागरां वा प्रपिबेत् सवाते||२३||

Punarnava – Boerhavia diffusa
Nagara – Ginger
Musta – Cyperus rotundus
paste of the above, in the dose of 12 grams (Aksha) each, is processed with 1 Prastha (768 ml) of milk, added with
Mayuraka
Magadhika – Long pepper fruit
Pippalimoola – Long pepper root
Nagara – ginger

Treatment of Vata- Pittaja Svayathu:

दन्ती त्रिवृत्त्र्यूषण चित्रकैर्वा पयः शृतं दोषहरं पिबेन्ना|
द्विप्रस्थ मात्रं तु पलार्धिकैस्तैरर्धावशिष्टं पवने सपिते||२४||

1/2 Pala (24 g) of the paste of
Danti – Baliospermum montanum

Trivrut – Operculina turpethum
Trikatu (Ginger, pepper and long pepper fruit) and
Chitraka – Leadword – Plumbago zeylanica is boiled in 2 Prasthas (768 X 2 ml) of milk and reduced to half.
Intake of this liquid is indicated in Vata Paittika type of Svayathu [24]

Recipes:
सशुण्ठि पीतदुरसं प्रयोज्यं श्यामोरुबूकोषणसाधितं वा|
त्वग्दारुवर्षाभुमहौषधैर्वा गुडूचिका नागर दन्तिभिर्वा||२५||
The patient of oedema should take milk boiled with the following recipes.
• Decoction of Sunthi – Zingiber officinale and Pitadaru (Deva Daru or Daru Haridra
• Shyama (Trivrit), castor and black pepper fruit, cinnamon, Devadaru (Cedrus deodara) Varsabhu (Punarnava) and ginger and Danti – Baliospermum montanum [25]

Camel milk:
सप्ताहमौष्ट्रं त्वथवाऽपि मासं पयः पिबेद्भोजनवारिवर्जी|
गव्यं समूत्रं महिषी पयो वा क्षीराशनो मूत्रमथो गवां वा||२६||
The patient should avoid taking food (cereals) and water, but take only camel milk either for a week or for a month [depending upon the strength of the patient and the stage of the disease].
He may also take cow's milk with cow's urine or buffalo milk added with cow's urine. The patient can take either cow's milk or urine alone during this period. [26]

Treatment of Shotha associated with Diarrhoea and Constipation:
तक्रं पिबेद्वा गुरु भिन्न वर्चाः सव्योष सौवर्चल माक्षिकं च|
गुडाभयां वा गुडनागरं वा सदोष भिन्नाम विबद्ध वर्चाः||२७||
If the patient of oedema suffers from diarrhoea, then he should take butter- milk along with Trikatu (Ginger, pepper, Long pepper), black salt and honey.
If he is suffering from constipation or passage of Ama including Doshas with the stool, then he should be given jaggery and Haritaki or Jaggery added with Nagara – Zingiber officinale [27]

Svayathu with Constipation etc:
विड्वात सङ्गे पयसा रसैर्वा प्राग्भक्त मद्यादुरुबूकतैलम् |
स्रोतो विबन्धेऽग्निरुचिप्रणाशे मद्यान्यरिष्टांश्च पिबेत् सुजातान्||२८||
If the patient of oedema suffers from constipation and bloating, he is given castor oil along with milk or meat soup. This recipe is given before taking food.
If there is obstruction to the channels of circulation, if there is suppression of digestion strength with anorexia, then the oedema patient is given well fermented Madyas (a variety of alcoholic preparation containing self- generated alcohol) [28]

Gandiradyarista:
गण्डीर भल्लातक चित्रकांश्च व्योषं विडङ्गं बृहतीद्वयं च|
द्विव प्रस्थिकं गोमय पावकेन द्रोणे पचेत् कूर्चिक मस्तुनस्तु ||२९||
त्रिभागशेषं च सुपूतशीतं द्रोणेन तत् प्राकृत मस्तुना च|
सितोपलायाश्च शतेन युक्तं लिप्ते घटे चित्रक पिप्पलीनाम्||३०||
वैहायसे स्थापितमादशाहात् प्रयोजयंस्तद्विनिहन्ति शोफान्|
भगन्दरार्शःक्रिमि कुष्ठमेहान् वैवर्ण्य कार्श्यानिल हिक्कनं च||३१||
इति गण्डीराद्यरिष्टः|
Gandeeradyarista:

2 Prasthas (768 X 2) of

Gandira

Chitraka – leadwort – Plumbago zeylanica

Vyosa (Ginger, pepper and long pepper),

Vidanga – Embelia ribes

Brhati – Solanum indicum and

Kantakari – Yellow berried nightshade (whole plant) – Solanum xanthocarpum is added with

2 Dronas of Kurchika and cooked over cow dung fuel till 1/3rd remains.

After it is well cooked and cooled, 2 Dronas (2 X12.288 ml) of Prakruta Mastu – Supernatant liquid of curds and 100 Palas of Sitopala (Crystal sugar) is added and be kept in an earthen jar, the inside wall of which is smeared with the powder of Chitraka – Plumbago zeylanica and Pippali – Long pepper fruit – Piper longum.

This Jar is hung from the roof with the help of a net of ropes for 10 days and thereafter, used in medicine.

It is indicated in –

Shopha – oedema,

Bhagandara – Fistula in ano

Arsha – Piles

Krumi – intestinal parasites

Kustha – obstinate skin diseases and

Meha – urinary disorders

Vaivarnya – discoloration of the skin

Karsya – emaciation and

Hikka – Hiccup caused by vayu [29-31]

Astashatarishta

काश्मर्य धात्री मरिचाभयाक्ष द्राक्षा फलानां च स पिप्पलीनाम्|

शतं शतं जीर्णगुडातुलां च सङ्क्षुद्य कुम्भे मधुना प्रलिप्ते||३२||

सप्ताहमुष्णे द्विगुणं तु शीते स्थितं जलद्रोणयुतं पिबेन्ना|

शोफान् विबन्धान् कफवातजांश्च निहन्त्यरिष्टोऽष्टशतोऽग्निकृच्च||३३||

इत्यष्टशतोऽरिष्टः|

Astasatarishta

100 Palas of each of

Kashmarya – Gmelina arborea

Dhatri – Indian gooseberry fruit – Emblica officinalis Gaertn. ,

Maricha – Piper nigrum

Abhaya – haritaki

Aksha – Vibhitaki

Fruits of Draksha – Vitis vinifera and

Pippali – Long pepper fruit – Piper longum is made with coarse powder.

To this, old jaggery and 2 Droni of water is added and kept in a jar, the inside wall of which is smeared with honey.

In the summer season, this Jar is kept sealed for 1 week and in winter for 2 weeks [to facilitate fermentation].

Intake of this cures different types of oedema and constipation caused by Kapha and Vayu.

This is called "Astasata Arista". It promotes the power of digestion. [32-33]

Punarnavadyarista:

पुनर्नवे द्वे च बले सपाठे दन्तीं गुडूचीमथ चित्रकं च|

निदिग्धिकां च त्रिपलानि पक्त्वा द्रोणावशेषे सलिले ततस्तम||३४||

पूत्वा रसं द्वे च गुडात् पुराणातुले मधुप्रस्थयुतं सुशीतम्|

मासं निदध्याद्घृतभाजनस्थं पल्ले यवानां परतस्तु मासात्||३५||
चूर्णीकृतैरर्धपलांशिकैस्तं पत्रत्वगेलामरिचाम्बुलोहैः |
गन्धान्वितं क्षौद्रघृतप्रदिग्धे जीर्णे पिबेद् व्याधिबलं समीक्ष्य||३६||
हृत्पाण्डुरोगं श्वयथुं प्रवृद्धं प्लीहज्वरारोचकमेहगुल्मान्|
भगन्दरं षड्जठराणि कासं श्वासं ग्रहण्यामयकुष्ठकण्डूः||३७||
शाखानिलं बद्धपुरीषतां च हिक्कां किलासं च हलीमकं च|
क्षिप्रं जयेद्वर्णबलायुरोजस्तेजोन्वितो मांस रसान्नभोजी||३८||
इति पुनर्नवाद्यरिष्टः|

Punarnavadyarishtam:

3 Palas of each of

Sveta Punarnava – Spreading Hogweed – Boerhavia diffusa

Rakta Punarnava – Spreading Hogweed – Boerhavia diffusa

Bala – Country mallow (root) – Sida cordifolia

Atibala – Abutilon indicum

Patha – Cyclea peltata

Danti – Baliospermum montanum

Guduchi – Tinospora cordifolia

Chitraka – Plumbago zeylanica and

Nidigdhika – Brinjal Egg plant – Solanum xantocarpum [is made to coarse powder, boiled with 4 Dronas of water] is reduced to 1 Drona.

To this decoction, 2 Tulas of old jaggery is added.

After it is cooled, 2 Prasthas of honey are added.

The recipe is then kept in a jar, and buried inside a heap of barley for over 1 month.

After fermentation, the liquid is strained out, and to this, 1/2 Pala of each of the powder of

Patra – Cinnamomum tamala

Tvak – cinnamon

Ela – Cardamom – Elettaria cardamomum

Maricha – Piper nigrum

Hrivera – Pavonia odorata and

Aguru – Aquilaria agallocha is added.

This liquid is kept in a jar smeared with honey and ghee till it becomes aromatic

This is given to the patient after the digestion of the food, in a suitable dose depending upon the seriousness of the disease.

It immediately cures

Hrud roga – heart disease

Pandu – anaemia

Serious type of oedema

Pliha – splenic enlargement

Jwara – fever

Aruchi – anorexia

Meha – obstinate urinary disorders

Gulma – tumour

Bhagandara – Fistula- in- ano

The six varieties of Jathara Rogas (obstinate abdominal disease)

Kasa – cough

Svasa – Asthma

Grahani – sprue syndrome

Kushta – skin diseases,

Kandu – itching

Aggravation of vayu in the limbs

Constipation

Hikka – hiccup

Kilasa – a type of leucoderma and

Halimaka – a serious type of Jaundice

It endows the patient with complexion, strength, longevity, Ojas (essence of all the 7 Dhatus and Tejas (Lustre).

The patient while using this recipe should take food along with meat soup. [34-38]

Triphaladyarishta [Phalatrikadyarista]

फल त्रिकं दीप्यक चित्रकौ च स पिप्पली लोह रजो विडङ्गम्।

चूर्णीकृतं कौडविकं द्विवरंशं क्षौद्रं पुराणस्य तुलां गुडस्य॥३९॥

मासं निदध्याद्घृतभाजनस्थं यवेषु तानेव निहन्ति रोगान्।

ये चार्शसां पाण्डु विकारिणां च प्रोक्ता हिताः शोफिषु तेऽप्यरिष्टाः॥४०॥

इति त्रिफलाद्यरिष्टः।

1 Kudava (192 g) of each of the powder of

Triphala (Haritaki – Terminalia chebula, Bibhitaki – Terminalia bellerica and Amalaki – Phyllanthus emblica)

Dipyaka – Yavani

Chitraka – Plumbago zeylanica

Pippali – Piper longum

Lauha Bhasma – Iron calx and

Vidanga – Embelia ribes is added with

2 Kudavas of honey and Tula of old Jaggery [to this, 2 Dronas of water is added and fixed well] .This is kept in a jar smeared with ghee [and sealed]. This jar is kept in a heap of barley for a month.

Intake of this recipe cures all the diseases described in Punarnavadyarishta – (see above)

Arishtas (fermented liquids containing self-generated alcohol) prescribed for the treatment of piles and Pandu – anemia (anemia) is also useful in the treatment of Svayathu [39-40]

Krushnadya Churna

कृष्णा स पाठा गजपिप्पली च निदिग्धिका चित्रक नागरे च।

स पिप्पलीमूलरजन्यजाजी मुस्तं च चूर्ण सुखतोयपीतम्॥४१॥

हन्यात्रिदोषं चिरजं च शोफं कल्कश्च भूनिम्ब महौषधस्य।

अयोरजस्त्र्यूषण याव शूक चूर्ण च पीतं त्रिफला रसेन॥४२॥

Krushnadi Churna:

The powder of

Krushna – Long pepper – Pipr longum

Patha – Cyclea peltata

Gaja pippali –

Nidigdhika – Brinjal Egg plant – Solanum xantocarpum

Chitraka – Plumbago zeylanica

Nagara – Zingiber officinale

Pippali mula – Piper nigrum

Haridra – Curcuma longa

Ajaji – Cumin and

Musta – Cyperus rotundus is taken along with luke-warm water.

Cures: Oedema caused by the vitiation of all the 3 Doshas jointly and chronic oedema.

Similar therapeutic effect is obtained by taking the paste of

Bhunimba – Andrographis paniculata and

Shunthi – Zingiber officinale along with the decoction of

Triphala (Haritaki – Terminalia chebula, Bibhitaki – Terminalia bellerica and Amalaki – Phyllanthus emblica) or

By louha Bhasma and the powder of

Sunthi – Zingiber officinale

Pippali – Piper nigrum and

Yavaksara along with

Triphala decoction [41-42]

Kshara Gudika:

क्षार द्वयं स्याल्लवणानि चत्वार्य योरजो व्योष फलत्रिके च|
सपिप्पलीमूल विडङ्ग सारं मुस्ताजमोदामरदारु बिल्वम्||४३||
कलिङ्गकाशिचत्रकमूलपाठे यष्ट्याह्वयं सातिविषं पलांशम्|
सहिङ्गुकर्ष त्वणुशुष्कचूर्णं द्रोणं तथा मूलक शुण्ठकानाम्||४४||
स्याद्भस्मनस्तत् सलिलेन साध्यमालोड्य यावद्घनमप्रदग्धम्|
स्त्यानं ततः कोलसमां तु मात्रां कृत्वा सुशुष्कां विधिनोपयुञ्ज्यात्||४५||
प्लीहोदर श्वित्र हलीमकार्शःपाण्डुवामयारोचक शोष शोफान्|
विसूचिका गुल्मगराश्मरीश्च सश्वास कासाः प्रणुदेत् सकुष्ठाः||४६||
इति क्षारगुडिका|
Kshara Gutika:

1 Pala (48 g) of each of

Yava kshara

Svarji Ksara

sauvarcala – Black salt

Saindhava,

Vida and

Audbhida type of Salt

Lauha Bhasma

Sunthi – Zingiber officinale

Pippali – Piper longum

Marica – Piper nigrum

Haritaki – Terminalia chebula

Bibhitaki – Terminalia bellerica

Amalaki – Phyllanthus emblica

Pippali mula – Piper longum

Dehusked fruits of Vidanga – Embelia ribes

Musta – Cyperus rotundus

Ajamoda – Trachyspermum ammi

Devadaru – Cedrus deodara

Bilva – Aegle marmelos

Kalingaka – Holarrhena antidysenterica

Chitraka mula – Plumbago zeylanica

Patha – Cyclea peltata

Yastimadhu – Glycyrrhiza glabra and

Ativisa – Aconitum heterophyllum and

1 Karsha of Hingu is dried and made to fine powders.

These powders are added to Ksaratoya (alkaline water) prepared from ashes of 1 Drona of Mulaka [For this purpose Mulaka is dried and burnt to ashes]

1 Drona of these ashes is boiled by adding 8 times of water and reduced to $1/4^{th}$. This is then being strained through a cloth for 21 times.

The water, thus obtained, is to be added to the powders of Yava – Barley (Hordeum vulgare) Ksara etc

The recipe is thereafter boiled till it becomes condensed but does not get burnt. From this semi-solid paste, pills of 1 Tola are prepared and dried.

Intake of these pills according to the prescribed procedure, cures

Plihodara – splenic enlargement

Svitra – Leucoderma

Halimaka – a serious type of Jaundice

Arsha – piles

Pandu – anaemia,

Aruchi – anorexia,

Kshya – consumption

Shotha – oedema,

Visucika – chronic Diarrhoea

Gulma – tumour

Poisoning

Asmari – urinary stone

Asthma – cough and

Kushta – skin diseases [43-46]

Gudardaka Yoga:

प्रयोजयेदार्द्रैक नागरं वा तुल्यं गुडेनार्धपलाभिवृद्ध्या।

मात्रा परं पञ्च पलानि मासं जीर्णे पयो यूषरसाश्च भक्तम्।।४७।।

गुल्मोदरार्शःश्वयथु प्रमेहाञ् श्वास प्रतिश्यालसका विपाकान्।

स कामला शोष मनोविकारान् कासं कफं चैव जयेत् प्रयोगः।।४८।।

Jaggery and green ginger taken in equal quantities is given to a patient in a dose of 1/2 Pala on the first day.

On subsequent days, both of the Jaggery and ginger taken together is increased by 1/2 Pala till it reaches the dose of 5 Palas on the 10th day.

In this dose the recipe is given to the patient for 1 month.

After the digestion of this recipe, the patient is given milk, vegetable soup and meat soup to consume.

It cures

Gulma – tumour

Udara – obstinate abdominal diseases including ascites

Arshas – piles

Shotha – oedema

Prameha – obstinate urinary disorders including diabetes

Svasa – Asthma

Pinasa – chronic cold

Alasaka – a type of digestive disorder

Vipaka – indigestion

Kamala – Jaundice

Sosha – consumption

Mano vikara – psychic disorders

Kasa – cough and

Other diseases caused by Kapha Dosha [47-48]

Use of Ginger Juice

रसस्तथैवार्द्रक नागरस्य पेयोऽथ जीर्णे पयसाऽन्नमद्यात्

Similarly, the juice of ginger [mixed with jaggery] is given to the patient [by gradually increasing the dose as described above] for the treatment of the above diseases.

After the liquid is digested, the patient should take food along with milk. [49 ½]

Use of Shilajatu:

जत्वश्मजं च त्रिफलारसेन हन्यात्त्रिदोषं श्वयथुं प्रसह्य||४९||

इति शिलाजतुप्रयोगः|

Intake of Silajatu along with the decoction of Triphala effectively cures oedema caused by the vitiation of all the 3 Doshas. [49 ½]

Kamsa Haritaki

दिवपञ्चमूलस्य पचेत् कषाये कंसेऽभयानां च शतं गुडस्य|

लेहे सुसिद्धेऽथ विनीय चूर्णं व्योषं त्रिसौगन्ध्यमुषास्थिते च||५०||

प्रस्थार्धमात्रं मधुनः सुशीते किञ्चिच्च चूर्णादपि यावशूकात्|

एकाभयां प्राश्य ततश्च लेहाच्छुक्तिं निहन्ति श्वयथुं प्रवृद्धम्||५१||

श्वास ज्वरारोचक मेह गुल्म प्लीह त्रिदोषोदर पाण्डु रोगान्|

काश्यार्मवातावसृगम्लपित्त वैवर्ण्य मूत्रानिलशुक्रदोषान्||५२||

इति कंसहरीतकी|

In 1 Kamsa of the decoction of

Dvipanchamula or

Dashamula (Bilva – Aegle marmelos, Syonaka, Gambhari – Gmelina arborea, Patali – Stereospermum suaveolens, Ganikarika – Clerodendrum phlomidis, Shalaparni – Desmodium gangeticum, Prsniparni, Brhati – Solanum indicum, Kantakari – Solanum xanthocarpum and Goksura – Tribulus terrestris)

100 Palas of jaggery is cooked till linctus is formed.

To this, 4 Palas of the powder of

Trikatu (Ginger, pepper, long pepper) and

2 Palas of the powder of Trisugandhi (Tvak – Cinnamon, ela – cardamom and Patra – Cinnamomum tamala) is added when it is luke- warm.

After it is cooled down, 1/2 Prastha of honey [in actual practice, 1 Prastha is added according to the general rule of Paribhasa] and 2 Palas of yavaksara is added.

The patient should take 1 fruit of Abhaya (Haritaki) and 1 Shukti of the linctus.

This cures aggravated form of

Shotha – oedema

Svasa – Asthma

Jwara – fever

Aruchi – anorexia

Prameha – obstinate urinary disorders including diabetes

Plihodara – enlargement of spleen

Udara – obstinate abdominal diseases caused by the simultaneous vitiation of all the 3 Doshas

Pandu – anemia

Karshya – emaciation

Amavata – rheumatism

Raktapitta – an ailment characterized by bleeding from different parts of the body

Amlapitta – hyperacidity

Vaivarnya – discolouration of the skin and the
Diseases of urine, Vayu as well as semen [50-52]

Patolamuladi Kasaya

पटोलमूलामर दारु दन्तीत्रायन्ति पिप्पल्यभयाविशालाः|
यष्ट्याह्वयं तिक्तकरोहिणी च सचन्दना स्यान्निचुलानि दार्वी||५३||
कर्षोन्मितैस्तैः क्वथितः कषायो घृतेन पेयः कुडवेन युक्तः|
वीसर्प दाह ज्वर सन्निपात तृष्णा विषाणि श्वयथुं च हन्ति||५४||

1 Karsa of each
Patolamula – Trichosanthes dioica
Devadaru – Cedrus deodara
Danti – Baliospermum montanum
Trdyanti
Pippali – Piper nigrum
Abhaya – Terminalia chebula
Visala
Madhuyasti – Licorice
Tiktaka rohini – Picrorhiza kurroa
Chandana – Santalum album
Nichula and
Darvi – Berberis aristata is made to a decoction.
This decoction is added with 1 Kudava of Ghee and given to the patient.
It is indicated in
Visarpa – Erysipelas
Daha – Burning syndrome
Jwara – fever caused by the simultaneous vitiations of an the 3 Doshas,
Trusna – morbid thirst
Poisoning and
Halimaka – A serious type of Jaundice [53-54]

Chitrakadi Ghrutam:

सचित्रकं धान्ययवान्यजाजी सौवर्चलं त्र्यूषणवेतसाम्लम्|
बिल्वात् फलं दाडिम यावशूकौ सपिप्पलीमूलमथापि चव्यम्||५५||
पिष्ट्वाऽक्षमात्राणि जलाढकेन पक्त्वा घृतप्रस्थमथ प्रयुञ्ज्यात्|
अर्शांसि गुल्मं श्वयथुं च कृच्छ्रं निहन्ति वह्निं च करोति दीप्तम्||५६||

Chitrakadi Ghrita:
2 Prasthas of ghee is cooked by adding the paste of
Chitraka – Plumbago zeylanica
Dhanya – Coriander
Yavani – Carum copticum
Ajaji – cumin
Sauvarcala – Sochal salt
Tryusana (Trikatu – Pepper, long pepper and ginger)
Vetasamla
Fruit of
Bilva – Aegle marmelos
Dadima – Punica granatum

Yavakshara
Pippali mula – Piper nigrum and
Chavya – Piper chaba 1 Aksha (12 gram) each
And 2 Adhakas of water
It cures
Arsha – Piles,
Gulma – Tumor
Shotha – Oedema and
Mutra krchrra – Dysuria
It stimulates the power of digestion. [55-56]

Chitrakadi Ghrita:

पिबेद्घृतं वाऽष्टगुणाम्बुसिद्धं स चित्रक क्षारमुदारवीर्यम्‌|
कल्याणकं वाऽपि स पञ्चगव्यं तिक्तं महद्वाऽप्यथ तिक्तकं वा||५७||

Ghee boiled with 8 times of water and the Alkali preparation of Chitraka – Plumbago zeylanica [as paste] can also be given to the patient suffering from oedema.

Alternatively, he is given "Kalyanaka Ghrta' (Chikitsa 9: 33-42) or Pancha Gavya (144-150) or 'Tiktaka Ghrta' (Cikitsa 7: 140- 143) [57]

Chitraka Ghrutam:

क्षीरं घटे चित्रक कल्क लिप्ते दध्यागतं साधु विमथ्य तेन|
तज्जं घृतं चित्रक मूल गर्भ तक्रेण सिद्धं श्वयथुघ्नमग्र्यम्‌||५८||
अर्शोऽतिसारानिल गुल्म मेहांश्चैतन्निहन्त्यग्निबलप्रदं च|
तक्रेण चाद्यात् सघृतेन तेन भोज्यानि सिद्धामथवा यवागूम्‌||५९||
इति चित्रकघृतम्‌|

An earthen jar is smeared with the paste of Chitraka—Plumbago zeylanica
In this Jar, milk is kept and made to curd.
This curd is churned and ghee is prepared out of the butter which comes out.
This ghee is cooked with the paste of Chitraka mula and butter milk (which is already prepared during the process of curing).
This medicated Ghee is an excellent recipe for curing
Svayathu – oedema
Arshas – piles
Atisara – diarrhea
Gulma – tumor caused by Vayu and
Prameha – obstinate urinary disorders including diabetes
It promotes the power of digestion.
Food ingredients are taken along with butter milk and the above mentioned ghee.
Yavagu (thick Gruel) prepared by adding this medicated ghee is administered to the patient suffering from oedema. [58-59]

Yavagu (Thick Gruel):

जीवन्त्यजाजी शटि पुष्कराह्वैः स कारवी चित्रक बिल्व मध्यैः|
सयावशूकैर्बदर प्रमाणैर्वृक्षाम्लयुक्ता घृत तैलभृष्टा||६०||
अर्शोऽतिसारानिलगुल्मशोफहृद्रोगमन्दाग्निहिता यवागूः|
या पञ्चकोलैर्विधिनैव तेन सिद्धा भवेत् सा च समा तयैव||६१||

Yavagu (thick Gruel) is prepared by adding 1 Kola each of

Jivanti – Leptadenia reticulata

Ajaji

Shati – Hedychium spicatum

Puskara mula – Inula racemosa

Karavi – Black cumin

Chitraka – Plumbago zeylanica

Rind of Bilva – Aegle marmelos and

Yava Ksara.

To this, a small quantity of Vrksamla is added and it is sizzled with ghee and oil.

This medicated gruel cures

Arsha – piles,

Atisara – diarrhea,

Gulma – tumor caused by Vayu,

Shyavathu – Oedema,

Hrud roga – heart diseases and

Manda agni -suppression of the power of digestion

Yavagu prepared by adding Pancha Kola (Pippali – Piper longum, Pippalimula, Chavya – Piper retrofractum, Chitraka – Plumbago zeylanica and Nagara – Zingiber officinale), in the above mentioned manner has also the above mentioned properties. [60-61]

Yusha:

कुलत्थ यूषश्च सपिप्पलीको मौद्गश्च सत्र्यूषण यावशूकः।

रसस्तथा विष्किर जाङ्गलानां सकूर्म गोधा शिखि शल्लकानाम्।।६२।।

The soup of Kulattha – Horse gram along with Pippali –Piper longum or the soup of Mudga along with Trikatu (Sunthi—Zingiber officinale, Pippali – Piper longum and Marica – Piper nigrum) and Yava is useful for the patient suffering from oedema.

Similarly, the meat soup of Vishkiras (group of Gallinacious birds) and Jangala group of animals dwelling in dry land forests) and other animals, like Kurma (Tortoise), Godha (Iguana) Sikhi(Peacock) and Sallaka of Sallaki (Pangoline) in wholesome for the patient suffering from oedema. [62]

Vegetables and Cereals:

सुवर्चला गृञ्जनकं पटोलं सवायसीमूलक वेत्र निम्बम्।

शाकार्थिनां शाकमिति प्रशस्तं भोज्ये पुराणश्च यवः सशालिः।।६३।।

For those who are desirous of taking vegetables, Suvarcala or Suvarcika (Suryavarta) Grnjanaka (a type of vegetable similar to garlic) or Sobhanjana, Patola – Trichosanthes dioica, Vayasi (Kakamachi – Solanum xantocarpum), Mulaka – Raphanus sativus, Vetra and Nimba – Azadirachta indica are useful.

Rice prepared from old Sali (a Variety of Paddy which is prepared after harvesting for more than 1 year) or barley is very useful for such patients. [63]

External Therapies for Vatika Oedema:

आभ्यन्तरं भेषज मुक्तमेतद्बर्हिर्हितं यच्छृणु तद्यथावत्।

स्नेहान् प्रदेहान् परिषेचनानि स्वेदांश्च वात प्रबलस्य कुर्यात्।।६४।।

शैलेय कुष्ठागुरुदारु कौन्तीत्वक्पद्मकैलाम्बु पलाश मुस्तैः।

प्रियङ्गु थौणेयक हेम मांसी तालीशपत्र प्लव पत्र धान्यैः।।६५।।

श्रीवेष्टकध्यामक पिप्पलीभिः स्पृक्कानखैश्चैव यथोपलाभम्।

वातान्विते$भ्यङ्गमुशन्ति तैलं सिद्धं सुपिष्टैरपि च प्रदेहम्।।६६।।

जलैश्च वासार्क करञ्ज शिग्रु काश्मर्य पत्रार्जकजैश्च सिद्धैः।

स्विन्नो मृदूष्णै रवितप्ततोयैः स्नातश्च गन्धैरनुलेपनीयः||६७||

In the above mentioned verses, recipes for internal use are prescribed. Now recipes for external use will be appropriately discussed.

If oedema is caused by the aggravation of Vayu, then the patient is given

Oleation

Pradeha – application of thick ointments

Parisechana – sprinkling of mentioned liquids and

Fermentation therapies

Oil is cooked with

Shaileya

Mustha – Cyperus rotundus

Aguru – Aquilaria agallocha

Devadaru—Cedrus deodara

Kaunti

Tvak – Cinnamon

Padmaka

Ela – Elettaria cardamomum

Ambu

Palasa—Butea monosperma

Priyangu – Callicarpa macrophylla

Thauneyaka

Hema

Mamsi – Jatamansi

Talisapatra – Taxus baccata

Plava

Patra – Cinnamon leaf

Dhanya – Coriander

Srivestaka

Dhyanaka

Pippali – Piper longum

Sprukka and

Nakha, whichever is readily available.

This medicated oil is used for oedema caused by Vayu.

The fine paste of the above mentioned drugs can also be used as ointment (Pradeha) externally.

The patient should take fermentations therapy in a bathtub filled with water boiled by adding Vasa – Adhatoda vasica, aksa, Karanja – Pongamia pinnata, Shigru – Moringa oleifera, Kasmarya, Patra, and Arjaka. Thereafter, he should take a bath with water which is made warm by exposing to the rays of the sun.

At the end, he is smeared with the ointment of aromatic drugs. [64-67]

External Therapies for Paittika Oedema

सवेतसाः क्षीरवतां द्रुमाणां त्वचः समञ्जिष्ठलतामृणालाः|

सचन्दनाः पद्मककवालकौ च पैत्ते प्रदेहस्तु सतैलपाकः||६८||

आक्तस्य तेनाम्बु रविप्रतप्तं सचन्दनं साभयपद्मकं च|

स्नाने हितं क्षीरवतां कषायः क्षीरोदकं चन्दनलेपनं च||६९||

Vetasa – Amla vetasa

Bark of Ksiri vrukshas (Nyagrodha—Ficus bengalensis, Udumbara –Ficus racemosa, Asvattha – Ficus religiosa, Parusaka, and Plaksa)

Manjistha – Rubia cordifolia

Mrunala – lotus stalk

Chandana – Santalum album

Padmaka and

Balaka- Hrivera .

These drugs are made to a paste and applied over the body of the patient suffering from Paittika type of oedema.

Oil is cooked with the paste and the decoction of the above mentioned drugs and used for massage.

Having applied the above mentioned medicated oil, the patient should take bath with water which is boiled by adding Chandana – Santalum album; abhaya, Usira – Vetiveria zizanioides and Padmaka and which is further heated through its exposure to the rays of the sun.

The decoction of Ksirivrksas (Nyagrodha – Ficus bengalensis, Udumbara – Ficus racemosa, Asvattha – Ficus religiosa, Parisa – and Plaksa) and milk added with water are useful for the bath of the patient suffering from Paittika type of oedema. After bath he should apply sandal- wood paste over his body. [68-69]

External Therapies for Kaphaja Shotha:

कफे तु कृष्णा सिकता पुराण पिण्याक शिग्रुत्वग्वुमा प्रलेपः|

कुलत्थ शुण्ठी जल मूत्रसेकश्चण्डागुरुभ्यामनुलेपनं च||७०||

Paste of these ingredients is applied to relive oedema caused by Kapha:

Pippali – Piper longum

Sand – Sikata

Pinyaka – old oil cake,

Bark of Sigru – Moringa oliefera and

Atasi – Linum usitaissimum

For this purpose, the body of the patient is sprinkled with the decoction of Kulattha and Sunthi as well as cow's urine. After taking bath, the patient is anointed with the paste of chandana – Santalum album and Aguru – Aquilaria agallocha [70]

External Therapies for All Types of Oedema in General:

बिभीतकानां फल मध्यलेपः सर्वेषु दाहार्तिहरः प्रदिष्टः|

यष्ट्याह्वमुस्तैः स कपित्थ पत्रैः स चन्दनैस्तत्पिडकासु लेपः||७१||

रास्ना वृषार्क त्रिफला विडङ्गं शिग्रु त्वचो मूषिक पर्णिका च|

निम्बार्जकौ व्याघ्रनखः सदूर्वा सुवर्चला तिक्तक रोहिणी च||७२||

स काकमाची बृहती सकुष्ठा पुनर्नवा चित्रक नागरे च|

उन्मर्दनं शोफिषु मूत्रपिष्टं शस्तस्तथा मूलक तोय सेकः||७३||

The pulp of Bibhitaka – Terminalia bellerica is made to a paste and applied externally. This cures burning sensation and pain in all types of oedema.

If this patient of oedema is suffering from pimples associated with burning sensation, etc, then the paste of Madhuyasti – Glycyyrrhiza glabra, Musta – Cyperus rotundus, leaves of Kapittha and Chandana – Santalum album is applied.

Rasna – Pluchea lanceolata

Vasa – Adhatoda vasica

Arka – Calotropis procera

Triphala (Haritaki – Terminalia chebula, Bibhitaki – Terminalia bellerica and Amalaki – Phyllanthus emblica),

Arjaka

Vyaghranakha (Nakhi)

Durva – Cynodon dactylon

Suvarchala – Black salt

Tiktaka rohini

Kakamachi

Brihati – Solanum indicum

Kushta – Saussurea lappa

Punarnava – Boerhavia diffusa

Chitraka – Plumbago zeylanica and

Nagara – Zingiber officinale - the powder of these drugs is made to a paste by triturating with cow's urine and used for unction (Unmardana), which cures [all types of] oedema.

In this condition, sprinkling with the juice or decoction of Mulaka – Raphanus sativus is useful. [71-73]

Localized Oedema:

शोफास्तु गात्रावयवाश्रिता ये ते स्थान दूष्याकृति नाम भेदात्‌‌।

अनेक सङ्ख्याः कतिचिच्च तेषां निदर्शनार्थं गदतो निबोध||७४||

Sometimes oedema is localized in a particular part or organ of the body. Depending upon their locations, tissue elements involved, shape and nomenclatures, these are of innumerable types. By way of example, some of these are being described here. [74]

Sirah Shotha (cellulitis / swelling of the head):

दोषास्त्रयः स्वैः कुपिता निदानैः कुर्वन्ति शोफं शिरसः सुघोरम्‌|७५|

All the 3 Doshas get aggravated by their respective causative factors and caused oedema in the head which is of very serious nature. [75]

Kantha Saluka (Quinsy):

अन्तर्गले घुर्घुरिकान्वितं च शालूक मुच्छ्वास निरोधकारि||७५||

Sometimes oedema occurs inside the throat.

In shape, it is like 'saluka' (rhizome of lotus) because of this the patient gets strenuous breathing. It obstructs inspiration. [75/ ½]

Bidalika (Ludwig's Angina)

गलस्य सन्धौ चिबुके गले च सदाहरागः श्वसनासु चोग्रः।

शोफो भृशार्तिस्तु बिडालिका स्याद्धन्याद्गले चेद्वलयीकृता सा||७६||

Bidalika is characterized by oedema in the joint between the neck and the face, chin and throat.

The swelling is associated with Daha-burning sensation and Raga-redness.

It causes serious impairment of respiration and excruciating pain.

If it surrounds the neck, then the patient succumbs to this disease. [76]

Talu Vidradhi (Palatal Abscess):

स्यातालु विद्रध्यपि दाह राग पाकान्वितस्तालुनि सा त्रिदोषात्‌||७७||

Talu Vidradhi is characterized by an abscess associated with Daha-burning sensation, Raga- redness and Talu pakva – suppuration in the throat.

It is caused by the aggravation of the 3 Doshas. [77½]

Upajihvika and Adhijihvika:

जिह्वोपरिष्टादुप जिह्विका स्यात् कफादधस्तादधि जिह्विका च||७७||

Upajihvika – acute superficial glossitis is located in the exterior of the tongue and Adhijihvika (sub- linglual abscess) which is caused by Kapha afflicts the lower part of the tongue. [77 ½]

Upakusha (Gingivitis):

यो दन्त मांसेषु तु रक्त पित्तात् पाको भवेत् सोपकुशः प्रदिष्टः|

Because of the aggravation of Rakta and Pitta, there is inflammation in gum muscles which is called Upakusa (Gingivitis) [78 1/2]

Danta vidradhi (Dental Abscess)

स्याद्दन्तविद्रध्यपि दन्त मांसे शोफः कफाच्छोणित सञ्चयोत्थः||७८||

Inflammation in the muscles surrounding the teeth is called Danta Vidradhi (dental abscess)

It is caused by the accumulation of aggravated Kapha and blood in that locality. [78 ½]

Galaganda (Goitre) and Gandamala (Cervical adenitis):

गलस्य पार्श्वे गलगण्ड एकः स्याद्गण्डमाला बहुभिस्तु गण्डैः|

साध्याः स्मृताः पीनस पार्श्व शूल कास ज्वरच्छर्दियुतास्त्वसाध्याः||७९||

तेषां सिरा काय शिरो विरेका धूमः पुराणस्य घृतस्य पानम्|

स्याल्लङ्घनं वक्त्रभवेषु चापि प्रघर्षणं स्यात् कवलग्रहश्च||८०||

If there is a single swelling in the side of the throat. It is called Galaganda (Goitre) and if there is a chain of swellings, then it is called Gandamala (cervical adenitis).

These two conditions are curable. But if these conditions are associated with complications in the form of pinasa – rhinitis, Parsva Sula (pain in the rides of the chest), kasa – cough, bronchiectasis, jwara - fever and chardi - vomiting then they are incurable.

For their treatment Sira Vyadha (Venesection), Kaya Vireka (Elimination of the Doshas from the head), Dhuma (therapeutic smoking), intake of old ghee and fasting therapy is administered.

If the swelling occurs inside the mouth, then Pragharsana (rubbing) and Kavalagraha (keeping the paste of drugs in the mouth for a specific period) is administered. [79- 80]

Granthi (Hard Tumour)

अङ्गैकदेशेष्वनिलादिभिः स्यात् स्वरूपधारी स्फुरणः सिराभिः|

ग्रन्थिर्महान्मांसभवस्त्वनर्तिर्मेदोभवः स्निग्धतमश्चलश्च||८१||

संशोधिते स्वेदितमश्म काष्ठैः साङ्गुष्ठदण्डैर्विलयेदपक्वम्|

विपाट्य चोद्धृत्य भिषक् सकोशं शस्त्रेण दग्ध्वा व्रणवच्चिकित्सेत्||८२||

अदग्ध ईषत् परिशेषितश्च प्रयाति भूयोऽपि शनैर्विवृद्धिम्|

तस्मादशेषः कुशलैः समन्ताच्छेद्यो भवेद्वीक्ष्य शरीरदेशान्||८३||

शेषे कृते पाकवशेन शीर्यातः क्षतोत्थः प्रसरेद्विसर्पः|

उपद्रवं तं प्रविचार्य तज्ज्ञस्तैर्भेषजैः पूर्वतरैर्यथोक्तैः||८४||

निवारयेदादित एव यत्नादिविधानवित् स्वस्वविधिं विधाय|

ततः क्रमेणास्य यथाविधानं व्रणं व्रणज्ञस्त्वरया चिकित्सेत्||८५||

विवर्जयेत् कुक्ष्युदराश्रितं च तथा गले मर्मणि संश्रितं च|

स्थूलः खरश्चापि भवेद्विवर्ज्यो यश्चापि बालस्थविराबलानाम्||८६||

Granthi (hard Tumour) occurs in a particular part of the body because of vitiated Vayu, etc. It is associated with the signs and symptoms of the concerned aggravated Dosha.

It is surrounded by vessels, it pulsates.

Granthi in muscles tissue is large in size.

If it is of Medas (fat tissue), then it is free from pain and it is unctuous as well as mobile

First of all, the body of the patient is purified [by the administration of elimination therapies].

Tumour is then fomented with the help of a stone, wood, thumb or a rod.

The physician should dissolve (Vilayana) the tumour if it is not suppurated.

After suppuration, it is excised and removed along with the help of a stone, wood, thumb or a rod.

The physician should dissolve (Vilayana) the tumour if it is not suppurated.

After suppuration, it is excised and removed along with its covering capsule with the help of a sharp instrument.

Thereafter, the stump of the tumour is cauterized. Then the resultant ulcer is treated on the lines suggested for the treatment of urinary Vrana (Ulcer).

If it is not cauterized, and if even a little amount of the tumour tissue remains there, it would likely grow again gradually, even to large size.

Therefore, an expert surgeon should, keeping in view the anatomy of the locality, excise it from all sides without any residual tissue left.

If any residual tissue is left, then it is likely to cause suppuration, which may spread from this ulcer to the nearby tissues. If such a complication arises, the physician, with proper consideration, should apply medicines described earlier and prevent such a spread of suppuration right in the beginning by careful administration of the appropriate therapies.

Thereafter, by the application of appropriate therapies, the skilful physician should make efforts to heal the ulcer quickly.

If the tumour is located in Pelvic region, abdomen, throat or in any vital organ it is incurable. Even if they are not manifested in the mentioned regions, i.e. if they are manifested in the regions of the body other than these places, but are large (thick) in size and rough on touch, they will be considered as incurable. The same tumors / cysts occurring in children, persons of old age and in persons with weak physique then also they will be incurable in nature. [81-86]

Granthi – tumour, fibroid, Arbuda:

ग्रन्थ्यर्बुदानां च यतोऽविशेषः प्रदेश हेत्वाकृति दोष दूष्यैः|
ततश्चिकित्सेद्भिषगर्बुदानि विधान विद्ग्रन्थि चिकित्सितेन||८७||

Since in Granthi (hard tumours) and Arbuda (ordinary tumour), the site of manifestation, shape, causes of manifestation, symptoms, Doshas and dusyas (vitiation of tissue elements) are similar. Therefore, the skilful physician should treat cases of Arbuda (Ordinary tumour) according to the line of treatment suggested for Granthi (hard tumour). [87]

Alaji:

ताम्रा सशूला पिडका भवेद्या सा चालजी नाम परिसुताग्रा|

Copper coloured and painful eruptions associated with discharge from their mouth are called Alaji. [88 ½]

Charma nakhantara Sotha (Whitlow)

शोफोऽक्षत श्चर्म नखान्तरे स्यान्मांसास्रदूषी भृश शीघ्र पाकः||८८||

The oedema appearing to the joint of the skin and the nail without any ulcer is caused by the vitiation of Mamsa (Muscle tissue) and blood.

It gets serious and becomes quickly suppurated. [88 ½]

Vidarika (Inguinal and Axillary Lymphadenitis)

ज्वरान्विता वङ्क्षण कक्षजा या वर्तिर्निरर्तिः कठिनायता च|
विदारिका सा कफमारुताभ्यां

The elongated swelling in the inguinal and axillary regions which is associated with fever, which is painless [some scholars interpret "Nirarti" as having pain], which is hard to touch and which is expansive, is called Vidarika. This condition is caused by the vitiation of both Kapha and Vayu. [89 ¾]

Treatment:

तेषां यथा दोषमुपक्रमः स्यात्||८९||

विस्रावणं पिण्डिकयोपनाहः पक्वेषु चैव व्रणवच्चिकित्सा|९०|

For the treatment of above mentioned ailment (Alaji etc) therapies according to the Doshas involved, is administered. The patient is given blood- letting therapy by venesection, etc. Upanaha type of fomentation is given with the help of drugs, tied to a bolus (Pindika).

After suppuration, these ailments are treated like an ordinary Vrana (Ulcer). [89 ½ – 90½]

Visphotaka – Boils

विस्फोटकाः सर्व शरीरगास्तु स्फोटाः सराग ज्वर तर्ष युक्ताः||९०||

In postural eruptions (Sphota) eruptions appear all over the body.

These eruptions are red in colour and the patient suffers from fever and morbid thirst. [90 ½]

Kaksha (herpes Zoster):

यज्ञोपवीत प्रतिमाः प्रभूताः पित्तानिलाभ्यां जनितास्तु कक्षाः |

याश्चापराः स्युः पिडकाः प्रकीर्णाः स्थूलाणुमध्या अपि पित्तजास्ताः||९१||

In Kaksa, large number of eruptions appear on the line where the Yajnopavita (Sacred thread of Hindus) is worn [i.e. the line connecting the lateral part of the left shoulder with the bottom of the right side chest and then round the back up to the top of the shoulder).

These eruptions are caused by Pitta and Vayu.

Some other miscellaneous varieties of eruptions of big, small and medium size also appear on the body. These are all caused by Pitta. [91]

Romantika:

क्षुद्र प्रमाणाः पिडकाः शरीरे सर्वाङ्गगाः सज्वर दाह तृष्णाः|

कण्डूयुताः सारुचिस प्रसेका रोमान्तिकाः पित्तकफात् प्रदिष्टाः||९२||

Romantika is caused by aggravated Pitta and Kapha, but is characterized by the Pidaka – appearance of small eruptions all over the body and association with

Jwara-fever

Daha – burning sensation

Aruchi – anorexia and

Praseka – excessive salivation [92]

Masurika:

याः सर्व गात्रेषु मसूर मात्रा मसूरिकाः पित्त कफात् प्रदिष्टाः|

वीसर्प शान्त्यै विहिता क्रिया या तां तेषु कुष्ठे च हितां विदध्यात्||९३||

Masurika is caused by aggravated Pitta and Kapha. Here many eruptions which resemble and appear like masura in size and color are formed over the entire body due to aggravation of pitta and kapha. The treatments and medicines explained in the context of treatment of Visarpa and also those prescribed for the treatment of Kustha (skin diseases including leprosy) are also useful for the treatment of the above mentioned diseases, namely Visphota, Kaksha, Romantika , Masurika. [93]

Bradhna (Hernia and Scrotal Tumour):

ब्रध्नोऽनिलाद्यैवृषणे स्व लिङ्गैरन्त्रं निरेति प्रविशेन्मुहुश्च|

मूत्रेण पूर्ण मृदु मेदसा चेत् स्निग्धं च विद्यात् कठिनं च शोथम्||९४||

विरेचनाभ्यङ्ग निरूह लेपाः पक्वेषु चैव व्रणव चिकित्सा|

स्यान्मूत्रसेकः कफजं विपाट्य विशोध्य सीव्येद्व्रणवच्च पक्वम्||९५||

Bradhna is a swelling in the inguinal and scrotal regions caused by aggravated Vayu, Pitta and Kapha.

These are characterized by the signs and symptoms of aggravated Doshas.

Antravrdhi is characterized by frequent entry of the intestines from abdomen into the scrotum and their exit [through the inguinal canal].

Mutra Vrddhi – This is a condition when urine accumulates in excess in the scrotum. Here the scrotum becomes smooth on touch.

Medoja Vrddhi: is characterized by the swelling caused by fat, and then it is unctuous and hard to touch

For their treatment, purgation therapy, massage, Niruha (a type of medicated enema) and Lepa (external application of drugs in a paste form) should be administered. If the swelling gets suppurated, then it should be treated like any other ulcer.

Mutra Vrddhi, Medoja Vrddhi and Kaphaja Vrddhi should be first cleansed (of morbid material) by cutting them with a surgical instrument and later they should be sutured. If these are suppurated or they get suppurated after suturing them then treatment inclusive of shodhana – cleansing and ropana – healing shall be done on the lines of ordinary ulcers. [94-95]

Bhagandara (Fistula in ano):

क्रिम्यस्थि सूक्ष्म क्षणन व्यवाय प्रवाहणान्युत्कटकाश्व पृष्ठैः |

गुदस्य पार्श्वे पिडका भृशार्तिः पक्व प्रभिन्ना तु भगन्दरः स्यात्||९६||

विरेचनं चैषण पाटनं च विशुद्ध मार्गस्य च तैलदाहः|

स्यात् क्षार सूत्रेण सुपाचितेन छिन्नस्य चास्य व्रणवच्चिकित्सा||९७||

Causes: Because of injury caused by parasites or small pieces of bone, Vyavaya-excessive sexual intercourse, Pravhana-excessive straining for passing stool, Utkata ashva -use of hard seat and riding on horseback, abscess appears in the sides of the anal orifice which is exceedingly painful. When abscess gets suppurated and bursts, the condition is known as Bhagandara (fistula- in –ano)

For its treatment, purgation therapy is administered and probing as well as incision is performed.

When the tract is cleansed, it is cauterized with the help of hot oil.

Thereafter with alkaline preparations), the tract is cut open. Then, this is treated like an ordinary ulcer. [96-97]

Shleepada [Elephantiasis]:

जङ्घासु पिण्डीप्रपदोपरिष्टात् स्याच्छलीपदं मांस कफास्र दोषात्|

सिरा कफघ्नश्च विधिः समग्रस्तत्रेष्यते सर्षपलेपनं च||९८||

Slipada (elephantiasis) is caused because of the vitiation of muscle tissue by Kapha and Rakta (blood).

It causes swelling in calf, groin, Pindi (lower part of the leg) and the swelling begins from Prapada (front portion of the leg). Siravedha – venesection and all kapha destroying (mitigating) treatment measures shall be adopted in the treatment of this ailment.

Application of mustard paste over the swelling part it very useful [98]

Jalakagardabha:

मन्दास्तु पित्त प्रबलाः प्रदुष्टा दोषाः सुतीव्रं तनु रक्त पाकम्|

कुर्वन्ति शोथं ज्वर तर्ष युक्तं विसर्पणं जालकगर्दभाख्यम्||९९||

विलङ्घनं रक्त विमोक्षणं च विरूक्षणं काय विशोधनं च|

धात्री प्रयोगात् शिशिरान् प्रदेहान् कुर्यात् सदा जालकगर्दभस्य||१००||

Nidana: Mildly aggravated Doshas with the predominance of Pitta causes serious type of swelling with mild suppuration of blood. This condition is associated with fever and morbid thirst. It spreads from one place to the other. This condition is called 'Jalakagardabha".

Treatment: Langhanam – fasting, Raktamokshana -blood-letting, application of unctuous ointment, elimination of the Doshas from the body (by emesis, purgation, etc) is performed.

Amalaki in different forms is administered to such a patient and cooling ointment should be invariably applied for the treatment of 'Jalakagardabha'. [99-100]

Management of Miscellaneous types of swelling:
एवंविधांश्चाप्यपरान् परीक्ष्य शोथ प्रकारान्निलादि लिङ्गैः|
शान्तिं नयेद्दोषहरैर्यथास्वमालेपनच्छेदनभेददाहैः||१०१||

Similar other varieties of swelling are examined with reference to their signs and symptoms of the concerned aggravated Doshas and appropriate therapies including Alepana (external application of ointment), Chedana (excision), Bhedana (Puncturing) and Daha (Cauterisation) is administered to cure them. [101]

Agantuja Shotha – Exogenous Swelling:
प्रायोऽभिघातादनिलः सरक्तः शोथं सरागं प्रकरोति तत्र|
वीसर्पनुन्मारुत रक्तनुच्च कार्य विषघ्नं विषजे च कर्म||१०२||

Generally (external) when the injury occurs, the vayu aggravated at the site of injury combines along with the blood and causes localized swelling with red colour.

Therapies indicated for the treatment of Visarpa – herpes (vide Cikitsa 21) and those helpful in the alleviation of aggravated Vayu and Vitiated blood are administered.

If the swelling is caused by the contact with [poisonous substances, then appropriate anti- toxic therapies are administered. [102]

Summary:
तत्र श्लोकः-
त्रिविधस्य दोषभेदात् सर्वार्धाव यव गात्रभेदाच्च|
श्वयथोर्द्विविधस्य तथा लिङ्गानि चिकित्सितं चोक्तम्||१०३||

In this chapter the following topics are discussed:
1. These 3 varieties of oedema, depending upon the aggravation of 3 Doshas
2. The varieties of oedema extending all over the body, half of the body or specific parts of the body
3. The two varieties of oedema, viz endogenous and exogenous
4. The signs and symptoms of oedema and
5. The treatment of different varieties of oedema [103]

इत्यग्निवेशकृते तन्त्रेऽप्राप्ते दृढबल सम्पूरिते चिकित्सा स्थाने श्वयथु चिकित्सितं नाम द्वादशोऽध्यायः||१२||
Thus, ends the 12th Chapter dealing with the treatment of oedema (Svayathu), in the section on therapeutics of Agnivesha's work as redacted by Charaka, restored by Drudhabala.

19

Chikitsasthana Chapter 13 Udara Chikitsitam

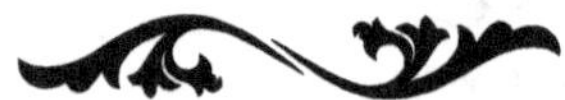

The 13th Chapter of Charaka Samhita Chikitsa Sthana deals with treatment of Udara. The disease Udara encompasses many diseases including ascites, intestinal obstruction, gaseous distension of abdomen etc.

अथात उदर चिकित्सितं व्याख्यास्यामः||१||
इति ह स्माह भगवानात्रेयः||२||
We shall now expound the chapter on the treatment of Udara.

Agnivesha's query to Atreya Punarvasu:
सिद्ध विद्याधराकीर्ण कैलासे नन्दनोपमे|
तप्यमानं तपस्तीव्रं साक्षाद्धर्ममिव स्थितम्||३||
आयुर्वेद विदां श्रेष्ठं भिषग्विद्या प्रवर्तकम्|
पुनर्वसुं जितात्मानमग्निवेशोऽब्रवीद्वचः||४||
भगवन्नुदरैर्दुःखैर्दृश्यन्ते ह्यर्दिता नराः|
शुष्क वक्त्राः कृशैर्गात्रैराध्मातोदरकुक्षयः||५||
प्रनष्टाग्नि बलाहाराः सर्वचेष्टा स्वनीश्वराः|
दीनाः प्रतिक्रिया भावाज्जहतोऽसूननाथवत्||६||
तेषामायतनं सङ्ख्यां प्रागूपाकृति भेषजम्|
यथावच्छ्रोतुमिच्छामि गुरुणा सम्यगीरितम्||७||
सर्वभूत हितायर्षिः शिष्येणैवं प्रचोदितः|
सर्वभूतहितं वाक्यं व्याहर्तुमुपचक्रमे||८||
Thus, said Lord Atreya [1-2]

Once upon a time, Lord Punarvasu was dwelling on mount Kailasa which was the abode of the Siddhas and Vidyadhars and which was charming like Nandana (celestial garden). Punarvasu was dazzling with the practice of severe penance and looked like an incarnate. He was the original profounder of the science of medicine, and he was the first and foremost of the physicians proficient in the science of life, having full control over his senses.

Agnivesha inquired with Atreya as below:

'O Lord! People are seen suffering with maladies of Udara (abdomen) having

Shushka vaktra – dryness of mouth,

Krusha Gatra – emaciation of the body, weight loss

Adhmana Udara Kukshayaha – distension of the abdomen and pelvis

Pranashta Agni, Bala, Ahara – Loss of digestion fire, appetite and strength

Incapability of doing any work;

They are helpless for want of effective remedy and they are breathing their last breath like an orphan. For the welfare of all living beings, I want to hear about the causative factor, types, premonitory signs and symptoms, manifested signs and symptoms and effective therapies of this malady as appropriately instructed by my preceptor like you". Being thus asked by the disciple, the sage initiated his discourse as follows for the welfare of living beings. [3-8]

Udara Samprapti:

अग्निदोषान्मनुष्याणां रोगसङ्घाः पृथग्विधाः|
मलवृद्ध्या प्रवर्तन्ते विशेषेणोदराणि तु||९||
मन्देऽग्नौ मलिनैर्भुक्तैरपाकाद्दोषसञ्चयः|
प्राणाग्न्यपानान् सन्दूष्य मार्गानुद्ध्वाऽधरोत्तरान्||१०||
त्वङ्मांसान्तरमागम्य कुक्षिमाध्मापयन् भृशम्|
जनयत्युदरं तस्य हेतुं शृणु सलक्षणम्||११||

Pathogenesis: of Udara:

Agnidosha – defective digestion strength and

Mala Vruddhi – increase in waste products / morbid matter – These two are the reasons for diseases like Udara (abdominal diseases including ascites).

If there is suppression of Agni (power of digestion and metabolism), and if the person takes Polluted food, this leads to indigestion as a result of which Doshas get accumulated.

This causes vitiation of Prana (a variety of Vata Dosha), Agni (digestive enzymes) and Apana (another variety of Vata, related to expulsion of faeces, flatus, urine etc) and obstruction to the upward and downward channels of circulation.

Thereafter, the vitiated Doshas get lodged between the skin and the muscle tissue and cause extensive distension of the lower part of abdomen.

This gives rise to Udara (obstinate abdominal diseases including Ascites). Now, hear the causative factors, signs and symptoms of this ailment [9-11]

Udara Nidana – Causes:

अत्युष्ण लवण क्षार विदाह्यम्लगराशनात्|
मिथ्या संसर्जनाद्रूक्ष विरुद्धा शुचि भोजनात्||१२||
प्लीहार्शे ग्रहणी दोष कर्शनात् कर्मविभ्रमात्|
क्लिष्टानाम प्रतीकाराद्रौक्ष्याद्वेगविधारणात्||१३||
स्रोतसां दूषणादामात् सङ्क्षोभादतिपूरणात्|
अर्शोबालशकृद्रोधादन्त्रस्फुटनभेदनात्||१४||
अतिसञ्चितदोषाणां पापं कर्म च कुर्वताम्|
उदराण्युपजायन्ते मन्दाग्नीनां विशेषतः||१५||

Etiology:

1. Intake of excessively hot, saline, Alkaline, Vidahi (which causes burning sensation), sour and poisonous food and drinks (Gara visha)
2. Mithya Samsarjana – Improper Samsarjana karma (diet, drinks and other regimens given to the patient after the administration of Pancha karma therapy)
3. Rooksha, Viruddha, Ashuchi Bhojana – Intake of dry, mutually contradictory and unclean food
4. Pleeha Arsha Grahani Dosha Karshana – Emaciation as a consequence of diseases, like Pliha - Splenic disorders), Arsas (piles) and Grahani Dosha (sprue syndrome)
5. Karma Vibhramaat - Improper administration of PanchaKarma therapy, namely emesis, purgation etc.
6. Negligence of treatment of diseases, like Pliha Roga (splenic disorder) and the consequential unctuousness in the body
7. Vega dharanat – Suppression of the manifested natural urges
8. Vitiation of the channels of circulation

9. Continued presence of Ama (product of improper digestion and metabolism) in the body

10. Intake of irritating food and drinks

11. Over nourishment

12. Obstruction by piles, hair and hard stool masses

13. Ulceration and perforation of intestines

14. Excessive accumulation of vitiated Doshas and

15. Indulgence in serious sinful acts

Because of the above-mentioned factors, different varieties of Udara are manifested, especially in those having Mandagni (low digestion strength) [12-15]

Udara Poorvaroopa: Premonitory Signs and Symptoms

क्षुन्नाशः स्वाद्वतिस्निग्धगुर्वन्नं पच्यते चिरात्|

भुक्तं विदह्यते सर्वं जीर्णाजीर्णं न वेत्ति च||१६||

सहते नाति सौहित्यमीषच्छोफश्च पादयोः|

शश्वद्बलक्षयोऽल्पेऽपि व्यायामे श्वासमृच्छति||१७||

वृद्धिः पुरीष निचयो रूक्षोदावर्तहेतुका|

बस्ति सन्धौ रुगाध्मानं वर्धते पाट्यतेऽपि च||१८||

आतन्यते च जठरमपि लघ्वल्प भोजनात्|

राजी जन्म वलीनाश इति लिङ्गं भविष्यताम्||१९||

Premonitory Signs and Symptoms

1. Khsut Nasha – Low digestion strength

2. Late digestion of food - which is sweet, excessively unctuous and heavy

3. Vidaha (burning, indigestion) of all the food and drinks taken by the patient

4. Inability to determine between the digestion and indigestion of the food

5. Inability to tolerate a little excess of food

6. Slight swelling in the legs

7. Constant loss of strength

8. Shortness of breath even with slight exercise

9. Excessive accumulation of stool because of unctuousness and Udavarta (bloating, upward movement of the wind in the abdomen)

10. Pain and Adhmana (distension) in the Basti- Sandhi (lower part of abdomen)

11. Even if a patient takes a small quantity of food, the size of his abdomen considerably increases. The patient experiences bursting pain and the abdomen becomes considerably distended.

12. Raji Janma – Appearance of network of veins and

13. Vali nasha – Disappearance of folds in the abdomen and creases due to swelling [16-19]

Udara Samprapti: Pathogenensis

रुद्ध्वा स्वेदाम्बु वाहीनि दोषाः स्रोतांसि सञ्चिताः|

प्राणाग्न्यपानान् सन्दूष्य जनयन्त्युदरं नृणाम्||२०||

Accumulated Doshas obstruct the channels of water and sweat (Ambuvaha srotas and Swedavaha Srotas) and vitiate Prana Vata, Agni (power of digestion and metabolism) and Apana Vayu, as a result of which Udara (obstinate abdominal diseases including ascites) is manifested in human beings [20]

Udara Samana Lakshana – General Symptoms:

कुक्षेराध्मानमाटोपः शोफः पादकरस्य च|

मन्दोऽग्निः श्लक्ष्णगण्डत्वं कार्श्यं चोदरलक्षणम्||२१||

Kukshe adhmana – Distension in the sides of the abdomen,

Aatopa – gurgling noise

Pada shopha – oedema in the legs and hands,

Suppression of the power of digestion,

Slakshna gandatva – smoothness of the chin and

Karshya – emaciation [21]

Udara Bheda – Types:

पृथग्दोषैः समस्तैश्च प्लीह बद्ध क्षतोदकैः|
सम्भवन्त्युदराण्यष्टौ तेषां लिङ्गं पृथक् शृणु||२२||

8 types –

Vatodara

Pittodara

Kaphodara

Sannipatikodara

Plihodara

Baddhodara

Kshatodara and

Udakodara (Jalodara).

Signs and symptoms of each of these varieties will thereafter be described. [22]

Vatodara – Nidana, Samprapti

रूक्षाल्प भोजनायास वेगोदावर्त कर्शनैः|
वायुः प्रकुपितः कुक्षि हृद्बस्ति गुद मार्गगः||२३||
हत्वाऽग्निं कफमुद्धूय तेन रूद्धगतिस्ततः|
आचिनोत्युदरं जन्तोस्त्वङ्मांसान्तरमाश्रितः||२४||

Vataja Udara causes and pathogenesis:

Vata gets aggravated because of the intake of dry food, less quantity of food,

Ayasa – exertion,

Vega – suppression of natural urges,

Udavarta (upward movement of the wind in the abdomen) and emaciation (fasting , etc which are responsible for emaciation).

This aggravated Vayu, while passing through Kukshi (sides of the abdomen), cardiac region, urinary bladder and anus, suppresses digestion strength and stimulates Kapha.

The Kapha arrests the movement of Vata Dosha, as a result of which the latter gets located between the skin and muscle tissue of the abdomen and causes swelling of the abdomen. [23-24]

Vatodara Lakshana:

तस्य रूपाणि- कुक्षि पाणि पाद वृषण श्वयथुः, उदरविपाटनम्, अनियतौ च वृद्धिह्रासौ, कुक्षि पार्श्व शूलोदावर्ताङ्गमर्द पर्वभेद शुष्ककास कार्श्य दौर्बल्यारोचकाविपाकाः, अधोगुरुत्वं, वातवर्चोमूत्रसङ्गः, श्यावारुणत्वं च नख नयन वदनत्वङ्मूत्र वर्चसाम्, अपि चोदरं तन्वसितराजी सिरा सन्ततम्, आहतमाध्मातर्तिशब्दवद्भवति, वायुश्चोर्ध्वमधस्तिर्यक् च सशूलशब्दश्चरति, एतद्वातोदरमिति विद्यात्||२५||

Signs and symptoms of Vatodara:

The following are the signs and symptoms of Vatika type of Udara

1. Kukshi, Pani, pada vrshana svayathu – Swelling in sides of the abdomen, hands, legs and scrotum

2. Udara vipatanam – Appearance of cracks in the abdomen

3. Increase and decrease of the swelling in the abdomen without any appreciable cause

4. Kukshi parshva shoola -Colic pain in the sides of the abdomen and in the sides of the chest

5. Udavarta (upward movement of wind in the abdomen)

6. Anga marda, Parva bheda, Sushka kasa, Karshya, Daurbalya, Arochaka, Avipaka – Malaise, cracking pain in the phalanges, dry cough, emaciation, weakness, anorexia and indigestion

7. Adho gurutvam – Heaviness in the lower part of the abdomen

8. Vata varcho mutra sanga – non-elimination (blockage) of flatus, stool and urine

9. Shyava aruna cha nakha nayana vadana tvak mutra varchas – Greyish discoloration and reddishness of nails, eyes, face, skin, urine, and stool

10. Appearance of thin and black network of veins over the abdominal wall

11. When percussed by fingers on the abdomen the sounds resembling the sounds coming from an inflated leather bag (when air filled leather bag is percussed or tapped with fingers) can be experienced

12. Movement of Vayu upwards, downwards and sideward along with colic pain and sound [25]

Pittodara Nidana, Samprapti:

कट्वम्ल लवणात्युष्ण तीक्ष्णाग्न्यातप सेवनैः।
विदाह्यध्यशनाजीर्णैश्चाशु पित्तं समाचितम्॥२६॥
प्राप्यानिलकफौ रुद्ध्वा मार्गमुन्मार्गमास्थितम्।
निहन्त्यामाशये वह्निं जनयत्युदरं ततः॥२७॥

Aetiology and Pathogenesis of pittodara:

Pitta gets immediately & excessively accumulated because of intake of

Katu-pungent, Amla – sour, Lavana -saline, Ati ushna and Tiksna ahara -excessively hot and sharp food,

Atapa sevana – exposure to the heat of the fire and sun,

Intake of Vidahi (which causes burning sensation) type of food and intake of food before the previous meal is digested.

Pitta having reached the locations of Vata and Kapha and getting mixed with them, will cause obstruction of their channels and gets displaced (moves) in the upward direction and gets lodged therein. Later these doshas would destroy the Agni (power of digestion and metabolism) in the stomach and causes pittaja type of udara. [26-27]

Pittodara Lakshana:

तस्य रूपाणि- दाह ज्वर तृष्णा मूर्च्छातीसार भ्रमाः, कटुकास्यत्वं, हरित हारिद्रत्वं च नख नयन वदन त्वङ्मूत्र वर्चसाम्, अपि चोदरं नील पीत हारिद्र हरित ताम्रराजी सिरावनद्धं, दह्यते, दूयते, धूप्यते, ऊष्मायते, स्विद्यते, क्लिद्यते, मृदुस्पर्श क्षिप्रपाकं च भवति; एतत् पित्तोदरमिति विद्यात्॥२८॥

Signs and symptoms of Pittodara:

The following are the signs and symptoms of Paittika type of Udara:

1. Daha – Burning sensation, jwara -fever, Trushna – thirst, Murcha -fainting, Atisara -diarrhoea and Bhrama – giddiness

2. Katukasyatvam – Pungent taste in the mouth

3. Harita haridratvam cha nayana, vadana, tvak mutra varchasam – Green and yellowish discoloration of nails, eyes, face, skin, urine and stool

4. Nila pita harita tamra raji sira on Udara – Appearance of the net- work of veins with blue, yellow, Haridra (yellowish like the colour of turmeric), green and coppery colour

5. Daha – Burning sensation, Duyate -sensation of pain as if smoke is coming out, Dhupyate -heating sensation, Usmayate – perspiration, Svidyate – stickiness / sweating and Klidyate-softness to touch and

6. The condition gets converted to Jalodara (Ascites) because of swiftness (Kshiprapaka). [28]

Kaphodara Nidana and Samprapti:

अव्यायाम दिवास्वप्न स्वाद्वति स्निग्ध पिच्छिलैः।
दधि दुग्धौदकानूपमांसैश्चाप्यति सेवितैः॥२९॥
क्रुद्धेन श्लेष्मणा स्रोतःस्वावृतेष्वावृतोऽनिलः।

तमेव पीडयन् कुर्यादुदरं बहिरन्त्रगः ||३०||

Etiology and Pathogenesis of kaphodara:

Kapha gets excessively aggravated due to

Avyayama – owing to lack of exercise

Diva swapna – sleep during day time

Svadati snigdha picchila – intake of sweet, unctuous and slimy food

Dadhi, dugdha Anupa mamsa sevana – curd, milk, and aquatic meat of animals inhabiting marshy land in excess

This aggravated Kapha obstructs the channels of circulation as a result of which Vayu located in the exterior of the intestines gets obstructed. This Vata on its part exercises pressure on Kapha as a result of which [kaphaja type of] Udara is manifested. [29-30]

Kaphodara Lakshana:

तस्य रूपाणि- गौरवारोचका विपाकाङ्गमर्दाः, सुप्तिः, पाणिपादमुष्कोरुशोफः, उत्क्लेश निद्रा कास श्वासाः, शुक्लत्वं च नख नयन वदन त्वङ्मूत्र वर्चसाम्; अपि चोदरं शुक्लराजी सिरा सन्ततं, गुरु, स्तिमितं, स्थिरं, कठिनं च भवति; एतच्छ्लेष्मोदरमिति विद्यात्||३१||

The following are the signs and symptoms of Kaphaja type of Udara:

1. Gaurava – Heaviness, aruchi- anorexia, Avipaka -indigestion and Anga marda -Malaise

2. Supti – Numbness

3. Pani pada mushka sopha – Appearance of swelling in hands, legs, scrotum

4. Utklesha -Nausea, Ati nidra -excessive sleep, Kasa – cough and Svasa -dyspnoea

5. Suklatvam of nakha, nayana, vadana, tvak and mutra varchas - Whiteness of nails, eyes, face, skin, urine and stool

6. Udaram sukla raji sira santatam – Appearance of the network of veins white in colour and

7. Guru – The abdomen becomes heavy, Stimita (timid or fixed), Sthira -immobile and Kathinam -hard. [31]

Sannipatodara Nidana and Samprapti:

दुर्बलाग्नेरपथ्यामविरोधि गुरु भोजनैः|

स्त्रीदतैश्च रजो रोम विण्मूत्रास्थि नखादिभिः||३२||

विषैश्च मन्दैर्वाताद्याः कुपिताः सञ्चयं त्रयः|

शनैः कोष्ठे प्रकुर्वन्तो जनयन्त्युदरं नृणाम्||३३||

Etiology and Pathogenesis of Sannipatikodara:

All the 3 Doshas, namely Vata, Pitta and Kapha get simultaneously aggravated because of the following

1. When a person with a weak power of digestion indulges in unwholesome, uncooked, mutually contradictory and heavy food

2. When unwholesome ingredients, like menstrual blood, hair, stool, urine, bone, nails etc. are administered by women etc and

3. Slow poisoning

These 3 Doshas get accumulated gradually in the Kostha (viscera of the alimentary tract) as a result of which [Sannipatika type of] Udara (obstinate abdominal disease) is caused. [32-33]

Signs and symptoms of Sannipatodara:

तस्य रूपाणि- सर्वेषामेव दोषाणां समस्तानि लिङ्गान्युपलभ्यन्ते, वर्णाश्च सर्वे नखादिषु, उदरमपि नाना वर्ण राजी सिरा सन्ततं भवति; एतत् सन्निपातोदरमिति विद्यात्||३४||

The following are the signs and symptoms of Sannipatika type of Udara:

1. Appearance of signs and symptoms of all the 3 Doshas

2. Affliction of nails etc, with all the types of colours described in respect of the Udaras caused by all 3 Doshas (individual doshas above) and

3. Appearance of network of veins over the abdomen having varieties of colours (described in respect of Vatodara, Pittodara and Kaphodara) [34]

Pleehodara Nidana and Samprapti:

अशितस्यातिसङ्क्षोभाद्यानयानातिचेष्टितैः|

अतिव्यवाय भाराध्व वमन व्याधि कर्शनैः||३५||

वाम पार्श्वाश्रितः प्लीहा च्युतः स्थानात् प्रवर्धते|

शोणितं वा रसादिभ्यो विवृद्धं तं विवर्धयेत्||३६||

तस्य प्लीहा कठिनोऽष्ठीलेवादौ वर्धमानः कच्छपसंस्थान उपलभ्यते; स चोपेक्षितः क्रमेण कुक्षिं जठरमग्न्यधिष्ठानं च परिक्षिपन्नुदरमभिनिर्वर्तयति||३७||

Etiology and Pathogenesis of Plihodara:

Spleen which is located in the left side [of the abdomen] gets displaced and enlarged because of intake of excessively irritating food, travelling in excess, riding a vehicle,

strenuous exercise, over indulgence in sex, lifting heavy weight, walking a long distance and emaciation caused by excessive administration of emetic therapy or by suffering from chronic diseases.

Spleen also gets enlarged because of increase in the quantity of blood as a result of increase in the quantity of Rasa (chyle) etc.

The spleen becomes stony-hard in the beginning of the process of enlargement and [on palpation] feels like a tortoise.

If the treatment of this condition is neglected, it gradually puts pressure and expands over the Kukshi (sides and lower abdomen) and Agni Adhisthana (pancreas) as a result of which Pihodara is manifested. [35-37]

Signs and symptoms of Plihodara

तस्य रूपाणि- दौर्बल्यारोचका विपाक वर्चोमूत्रग्रह तमःप्रवेश पिपासाङ्गमर्द च्छर्दि मूर्च्छाङ्गसाद- कास श्वास मृदुज्वरानाहाग्निनाश काश्यर्स्य वैरस्य पर्वभेद कोष्ठवात शूलानि, अपि चोदरमरुणवर्णं विवर्णं वा नील हरित हारिद्रराजिमद्भवति; एवमेव यकृदपि दक्षिण पार्श्वस्थं कुर्यात्, तुल्य हेतुलिङ्गौषधत्वात्तस्य प्लीह जठर एवावरोध इति; एतत् प्लीहोदरमिति विद्यात्||३८||

Signs and symptoms of Plihodara (splenic enlargement) and Yakrutodara (liver enlargement):

1. Daurbalya -Weakness, Aruchi -anorexia,

avipaka-indigestion, Varcha mutra graha – retention of stool and urine,

Tamah pravesha – entering into darkness,

Pipasa -excessive thirst, Anga marda -malaise,

Chardi -vomiting, Murchha -fainting,

Angasada- prostration, Kasa -cough,

Shwasa-dyspnoea, Mrudu jwara -mild fever,

Anaha (immobility of wind in the abdomen),

Agni nasha -loss of the power of digestion,

Karshya – emaciation, Aasya vairasya – distaste in the mouth,

Parva bheda -pain in finger joints, Kostha vata shula -distension of alimentary tract by wind and colic pain.

2. Shyava aruna udara -Reddishness or discolouration of the abdomen and

3. Appearance of network of veins having blue, green or yellow colour

Similarly signs and symptoms are manifested by the enlargement of the liver (Yakrddalyudara) which is located in the right side of the abdomen. Since its aetiology, signs and symptoms and treatment are similar to those of Plihodara (splenic enlargement), it is included in the description of the latter.

Thus, the ailment Pleehodara (splenic enlargement) is described [38]

Baddhagudodara – Nidana and Samprapti:

पक्ष्मबालैः सहान्नेन भुक्तैर्बद्धायने गुदे|

उदावर्तैस्तथाऽशॉर्भिरन्त्रसम्मूर्च्छनेन वा||३९||

अपानो मार्ग संरोधाद्धत्वाऽग्निं कुपितोऽनिलः|

वर्चःपित्तकफान् रुद्ध्वा जनयत्युदरं ततः॥४०॥

Etiology and Pathogenesis of Baddhagudodara – intestinal obstruction

Vata gets aggravated as a result of obstruction in the passage of the rectum because of:

1. Intake of small hair, like eye – lashes along with food

2. Udavarta – upward movement of the wind in the abdomen

3. Arshas – Piles

4. Antra sammurcchana (Intussusception) or intrusion of the intestine into its lumen and

5. Obstruction to the passage of Apana vayu (flatus)

This aggravated Vayu suppresses Agni (activities of enzymes responsible for digestion and metabolism and obstructs the movement of faeces, Pitta and Kapha as a result of which Baddhagudodara (abdominal swelling caused by obstruction in the intestines) is manifested. [39-40]

Signs and symptoms of Baddhagudodara

तस्य रूपाणि- तृष्णा दाह ज्वर मुख तालु शोषोरुसाद कास श्वास दौर्बल्यारोचका विपाक- वर्चो मूत्र सङ्गाध्मान च्छर्दि क्षवथु शिरोहृन्नाभिगुदशूलानि, अपि चोदरं मूढवातं स्थिरमरुणं नील राजि सिरावनद्धराजिकं वा प्रायो नाभ्युपरि गोपुच्छ वदभिनिर्वर्तत इति; एतद्बद्धगुदोदरमिति विद्यात्॥४१॥

Signs and symptoms of Baddhagudodara (intestinal obstruction)

1. Trushna – Morbid thirst, Daha -burning sensation, Jwara -fever,

Mukha talu sosha – dryness of mouth and Palate,

Uru sada -prostration in the thighs,

Kasa – cough, Shvasa – dysponea,

Daurbalya -weakness, Aruchi -anorexia, Vipaka – indigestion,

Varcho mutra sanga – stoppage of excretion of stool and urine,

Adhmana (abdominal distension), Chardi – vomiting, Ksavathu -sneezing

Shiro shola -headache and Hrut Guda shoola – colic pain in the regions of the heart, umbilicus and anus

2. Mudha vata in udara – Absence of peristaltic movement in the abdomen.

3. Appearance of stable and blue network of veins and

4. Appearance of an elongated swelling of the size and shape of the tail of the cow over the umbilical region.

This is called Baddhagudodara (abdominal swelling caused by obstruction in the intestines) [41]

Etiology and Pathogenesis of Chidrodara: Intestinal perforation

शर्करा तृण काष्ठास्थि कण्टकैरन्नसंयुतैः।

भिद्येतान्त्रं यदा भुक्तैर्जृम्भयाऽत्यशनेन वा॥४२॥

पाकं गच्छेद्रसस्तेभ्यश्छिद्रेभ्यः प्रस्रवद्बहिः।

पूरयन् गुदमन्त्रं च जनयत्युदरं ततः॥४३॥

The intestine gets perforated because of the following

1. Piercing of the intestine by the intake of sand, grass, pieces of wood, bone or nails along with food.

2. Yawning (deeply) and

3. Intake of food in large quantity

The wound in the intestine, thus caused, gets suppurated, and from the wounds the juice (thin paste of food) comes to the exterior of the intestine. The rectum and the intestines get filled up with this juice as a result of which Chidrodara (acute abdominal swelling caused by intestinal perforation) is manifested. [42-43]

Signs and symptoms of Chidrodara:

तस्य रूपाणि- तदधो नाभ्याः प्रायोऽभिवर्धमानमुदकोदरं भवति, यथाबलं च दोषाणां रूपाणि दर्शयति, अपि चातुरः सलोहित नील पीत पिच्छिल कुणपगन्ध्यामवर्च उपवेशते, हिक्का श्वास कास तृष्णा प्रमेहारोचका विपाक दौर्बल्य परीतश्च भवति; एतच्छिद्रोदरमिति विद्यात्॥४४॥

The following are the signs and symptoms of Chidrodara (acute abdominal swelling caused by intestinal perforation):

1. The abdomen gets swollen generally below the Umbilical region; it subsequently grows to cause Udakodara (Ascites)

2. Manifestation of the signs and symptoms of Doshas according to the nature of their affliction

3. Passing of unformed stool which is red, blue, yellow slimy or having the odour of a dead body and

4. Manifestation of hiccup, dyspnoea, cough, excess thirst, Prameha (obstinate urinary disorders), anorexia, indigestion and weakness

This condition is called Chidrodara (acute abdominal swelling caused by intestinal perforation). [44]

Etiology and Pathogenesis of Udakodara (Ascites):

स्नेहपीतस्य मन्दाग्नेः क्षीणस्यातिकृशस्य वा|

अत्यम्बुपानान्नष्टेऽग्नौ मारुतः क्लोम्नि संस्थितः||४५||

स्रोतःसु रुद्धमार्गेषु कफश्चोदकमूच्छितः|

वर्धयेतां तदेवाम्बु स्वस्थानादुदराय तौ||४६||

Agni (digestion strength) loses its power because of excessive intake of water after administration of Snehana treatment (oleation) or by a person suffering from Mandagni (suppressed power of digestion) or by an individual who is suffering from Rajayakshma or excessively emaciated.

As a result of this, Vayu located in Kloman (viscera located adjacent to the heart, i.e right lung) gets interrupted with Kapha and Udaka Dhatu (a liquid element of the body) and increases the quantity of that water in the obstructed channels of circulations. The vitiated Kapha and Vayu from their own locations assist in increasing this water as a result of which Udakodara (ascites) is caused. [45-46]

Signs and Symptoms of Udakodara (Ascites):

तस्य रूपाणि- अनन्नकाङ्क्षा पिपासा गुदस्राव शूल श्वास कास दौर्बल्यानि, अपि चोदरं नाना वर्णराजि सिरा सन्ततमुदकपूर्ण दृति क्षोभ संस्पर्शं भवति, एतदुदकोदरमिति विद्यात्||४७||

The following are the signs and symptoms of Udakodara (Ascites):

1. Loss of appetite, morbid thirst, discharge from the anus, colic pain, Dyspnoea, cough and general debility

2. Appearance of network of veins having different colours over abdomen and

3. In percussion and Palpation, the physician feels as if the abdomen is a leather bag filled with water.

This is called Udakodara (Ascites). [47]

Prognosis:

तत्र अचिरोत्पन्नमनुपद्रवमनुदकम प्राप्तमुदरं त्वरमाणश्चिकित्सेत्; उपेक्षितानां ह्येषां दोषाः स्वस्थानादपवृत्ता परिपाकाद्द्रवीभूताः सन्धीन् स्रोतांसि चोपक्लेदयन्ति, स्वेदश्च बाह्येषु स्रोतःसु प्रतिहत गतिस्तिर्यगवतिष्ठमानस्तदेवोदकमाप्याययति; तत्र पिच्छोत्पत्तौ मण्डलमुदरं गुरु स्तिमितमाकोठितमशब्दं मृदुस्पर्शमपगतराजीकमाक्रान्तं नाभ्यामेवोपसर्पति|

ततोऽनन्तरमुदकप्रादुर्भावः|

तस्य रूपाणि- कुक्षेरतिमात्रवृद्धिः, सिरान्तर्धानगमनम, उदकपूर्णदृतिसङ्क्षोभसंस्पर्शत्वं च||४८||

The physician should immediately treat this condition before the appearance of complications and before water accumulates in the abdomen.

If the treatment is neglected, then the vitiated Doshas get displaced and become liquefied as a result of Paripaka (maturation), causing stiffness in the joints and channels of circulation and diverting sweat from the external channels. The water element moves sideways (Tiryak). It collects in the abdominal cavity. This zigzag- moving sweat adds to the quantity of water already accumulated in the abdomen.

The appearance of this sticky liquid makes the abdomen dull on percussion and soft to touch. The abdomen becomes dull in percussion and soft to touch. Thereafter, the network of veins disappears.

During this period, the umbilical region is primarily afflicted, and from there the disease spreads in the remaining parts of the abdomen, thereafter, states accumulating in the abdomen.

The signs and symptoms of this condition are as follows:

1. Excessive enlargement of the sides of the abdomen

2. Disappearance of the network of the veins and

3. In palpation and percussion, the physician feels as if the abdomen is a leather sack filled with water. [48]

Upadrava – Complications

तदाऽऽतुरमुपद्रवाः स्पृशन्ति- छर्द्यतीसार तमक तृष्णा श्वास कास हिक्का दौर्बल्य पार्श्वशूलारुचि स्वरभेद मूत्रसङ्गादयः; तथा विधमचिकित्स्यं विद्यादिति||४९||

Thereafter, the patient gets afflicted with complications, like

Chardi -vomiting, Atisara – diarrhoea,

Tamaka type of Asthma, |Trushna – Morbid thirst, Svasa – dyspnoea, Kasa – cough, Hikka- hiccup, Daurbalya- debility, Parshva shoola – pain in the sides of the chest, Aruchi -anorexia, Svara bheda -hoarseness of voice and Mutra sanga—anuria (suppression of urine). A patient with these complications is incurable. [49]

भवन्ति चात्र-

वातात्पितात्कफात् प्लीह्नः सन्निपातात्तथोदकात्|

परं परं कृच्छ्रतरमुदरं भिषगादिशेत्||५०||

पक्षाद्बद्धगुदं तूर्ध्वं सर्वं जातोदकं तथा|

प्रायो भवत्यभावाय च्छिद्रान्त्रं चोदरं नृणाम्||५१||

Thus, it is said: of the 6 types of Udara, Viz

Vatodara

Pitodara

Kaphodara

Plihodara

Sannipatodara and

Udakodara,

The subsequent ones are more and more difficult for treatment than the previous ones.

After a fortnight, Baddhagudodara (abdominal swelling caused by the obstruction in the intestine) becomes incurable.

Udakodara (ascites) in its Jata Udaka stage (when water accumulates in the abdomen) and Chidrodara (acute abdominal swelling caused by intestinal perforation) are generally incurable right from the beginning [50-51]

Bad Prognosis

शूनाक्षं कुटिलोपस्थमुपक्लिन्न तनु त्वचम्|

बल शोणित मांसाग्नि परिक्षीणं च वर्जयेत्||५२||

श्वयथुः सर्वमर्मोत्थः श्वासो हिक्काऽरुचिः सतृट्|

मूच्छीं च्छर्दिरतीसारो निहन्त्युदरिणं नरम्||५३||

जन्मनैवोदरं सर्वं प्रायः कृच्छ्रतमं मतम्|

बलिनस्तदजाताम्बु यत्नसाध्यं नवोत्थितम्||५४||

Shoonakshi – Swollen eyes,

Kutila Upastha – curved penis (genital) / pudendum, sticky and thin skin and diminished strength, blood, muscle tissue as well as Agni (Power of digestion and metabolism) – appearance of these signs and symptoms indicates incurability of the condition [even if the patient is otherwise curable].

Occurrence of complications, like swelling in all the vital organs, dyspnoea, hiccup, anorexia, morbid thirst, fainting, vomiting and diarrhoea leads to the death of the patient suffering from Udara (obstinate abdominal disease).

All varieties of Udara, right from the time of their manifestation, are generally considered difficult to cure; however, it can be cured with adequate care soon after its appearance. If the patient is otherwise strong and if water has not started accumulating in the abdomen [52-54]

Signs and symptoms of Ajatodaka Stage of Udara – Ascites

अजात शोथमरुणं सशब्दं नातिभारिकम्|
सदा गुडगुडायच्च सिरा जाल गवाक्षितम्||५५||
नाभिं विष्टभ्य पायौ तु वेगं कृत्वा प्रणश्यति|
हृन्नाभि वङ्क्षण कटी गुद प्रत्येक शूलिनः||५६||
कर्कशं सृजतो वातं नातिमन्दे च पावके|
लोलस्या विरसे चास्ये मूत्रेऽल्पे संहते विषि||५७||
अजातोदकमित्येतैर्लिङ्गैर्विज्ञाय तत्त्वतः|
उपाक्रमेदिभषग्दोषबलकालविशेषवित्||५८||

Ajata means not yet appeared, Udaka means water

Signs and symptoms indicate Ajatodaka (non-appearance of water) stage of Udara Roga

1. There will be either no swelling or less of Swelling in the abdomen and legs

2. The colour of the abdomen will be reddish

3. There will be tympanic sound on percussion

4. The abdomen is not very heavy

5. Always having gurgling sounds in the abdomen

6. The abdomen will be covered with the network of veins

7. There will be movement of wind from rectum to the umbilicus and distension of the umbilical region; the urge will be suppressed after the elimination of stool and flatus

8. There will be colic pain in each of the heart region, umbilicus, inguinal region, lumbar region and anus

9. Flatus will be eliminated with force

10. The power of the digestion of the patient will not be very weak;

11. Because of excessive salivation, there will be imperceptibility of taste in the mouth and

12. There will be scanty urine and hard stool

The above-mentioned signs and symptoms indicate Ajatodaka (non-appearance of water in the abdomen) stage of Udara Roga.

Having ascertained it with care, the physician, well acquainted with dosha, strength and the time of the treatment, should initiate remedial measures for the patient. [55-58]

Vatodara Chikitsa:

वातोदरं बलमतः पूर्वं स्नेहैरुपाचरेत्|
स्निग्धाय स्वेदिताङ्गाय दद्यात् स्नेह विरेचनम्||५९||
हृते दोषे परिम्लानं वेष्टयेद्वाससोदरम्|
तथाऽस्यानवकाशत्वाद्वायुर्नाध्मापयेत् पुनः||६०||
दोषातिमात्रोपचयात् स्रोतोमार्गनिरोधनात्|
सम्भवत्युदरं तस्मान्नित्यमेव विरेचयेत्||६१||
शुद्धं संसृज्य च क्षीरं बलार्थं पाययेतु तम्|
प्रागुत्क्लेशान्निवर्त्यं च बले लब्धे क्रमात् पयः||६२||
यूषै रसैर्वा मन्दाम्ल लवणैरेधितानलम्|
सोदावर्तं पुनः स्निग्धं स्विन्नमास्थापयेन्नरम्||६३||
स्फुरणाक्षेप सन्ध्यस्थि पार्श्व पृष्ठ त्रिकार्तिषु|
दीप्ताग्निं बद्धविड्वातं रूक्षमप्यनुवासयेत्||६४||
तीक्ष्णाधोभागयुक्तोऽस्य निरूहो दाशमूलिकः|
वातघ्नाम्लशृतैरण्ड तिलतैलानुवासनम्||६५||

अविरेच्यं तु यं विद्याद्दुर्बलं स्थविरं शिशुम्|
सुकुमारं प्रकृत्याऽल्पदोषं वाऽथोल्बणानिलम्||६६||
तं भिषक् शमनैः सर्पि यूष मांस रसौदनैः|
बस्त्यभ्यङ्गानुवासैश्च क्षीरैश्चोपाचरेद्बुधः||६७||

Treatment of Vatodara :

If the patient is suffering from Udara Roga caused by the aggravation of Vayu, and if he is strong, then in the beginning, he is given

Snehana – oleation therapy followed by

Swedana – sweating treatment and

Snigdha virechana – Purgation by oils such as castor oil.

After the Doshas (morbid matter) are removed by Virechana treatment, the abdomen of the patient becomes flaccid. Then the abdomen is tightly wrapped with the help of a cloth, so that the Vayu (wind), in view of the empty space in the abdomen, may not cause distension again.

Udara Roga is caused because of excessive accumulation of Doshas (morbid matter) in the gastro- intestinal tract and also because of the obstruction to the opening of channels of circulation (Srotas).

Therefore, the patient is given purgation therapy every day.

After the body is cleansed, the patient is given Samsarjana Krama (administration of a heavier diet gradually). Thereafter, he is made to drink milk for the promotion of strength.

If milk is given continuously for a long time, then the patient is likely to get nausea. Therefore, after he has regained strength and prior to the occurrence of nausea, milk is withdrawn.

The patient is then given vegetable soup or meat soup added with small quantities of sour and salt foods to promote his appetite. If he gets flatulence, then again oleation and fomentation (swedana) therapies are administered. This is followed by Asthapana (decoction enema)

If the patient has itching sensation, cramps, pain in joints, bones, sides of the chest, back and lumbar region, if he has strong power of digestion; and if there is retention of stool and flatus, then even without oleation therapy, the patient is given Anuvasana type of enema (fat enema)

For the purpose of Niruha and Asthapana Basti, the decoction of Dashamoola and such other drugs having Teekshna (sharp) qualities are used.

For the purpose of Anuvasana Basti, castor oil or Sesame oil boiled with sour drugs which help in the alleviation of Vata is used.

If the patient is not suitable for Virechana, if he is weak, old, too young or of tender nature; if there is slight aggravation of Doshas, and if Vayu is aggravated much in excess, then the wise physician should treat him with alleviation therapies. Such a patient is given medicated ghee, vegetable soup and meat soup along with rice, and he should be given massage therapy, anuvasana type of enema and milk (boiled with Vata balancing herbs) [59-67]

Treatment of Pittodara

पित्तोदरे तु बलिनं पूर्वमेव विरेचयेत्|
दुर्बलं त्वनुवास्यादौ शोधयेत् क्षीरबस्तिना||६८||
सञ्जातबलकायाग्निं पुनः स्निग्धं विरेचयेत्|
पयसा सत्रिवृत्कल्केनोरुबूकशृतेन वा||६९||
सातलात्रायमाणाभ्यां शृतेनारग्वधेन वा|
सकफे वा समूत्रेण सवाते तिक्तसर्पिषा||७०||
पुनः क्षीरप्रयोगं च बस्तिकर्म विरेचनम्|
क्रमेण ध्रुवमातिष्ठन् युक्तः पित्तोदरं जयेत्||७१||

If the patient is suffering from Paittika type of Udara Roga and if he is strong, then in the beginning, he is given Virechana – purgation therapy.

If he is weak, then he is given elimination therapies, like Anuvasana Basti or medicated enema prepared by boiling drugs with milk (Ksheera Basti).

After the patient regains his strength, and after the promotion of his digestion strength, he is again given Snehana followed by Virechana therapy for which the following recipes are used:

1. Milk boiled with the paste of Trivrit and castor seed
2. Milk boiled with Satala and Trayamana
3. Milk boiled with fruit- pulp of Aragvadha (Cassia fistula)
4. If Udara Roga is caused by Kapha and Pitta, then for the purpose of purgation, milk is used with cow's urine and
5. If Udara Roga is caused by Pitta and Vata Dosha, then for the purpose of purgation, Tiktaka Ghrta (vide Cikista 7: 140- 150) added with Trivrit etc. is administered.
6. The patient is given milk, medicated enema and purgation therapy repeatedly. The Paittika type of Udara Roga can be certainly cured by Virechana treatment. [68-71]

Treatment of Kaphodara

स्निग्धं स्विन्नं विशुद्धं तु कफोदरिणमातुरम्।
संसर्जयेत् कटु क्षार युक्तैरन्नैः कफापहैः||७२||
गोमूत्रारिष्टपानैश्च चूर्णायस्कृतिभिस्तथा।
सक्षारैस्तैलपानैश्च शमयेत् कफोदरम्||७३||

The patient with Kaphaja type of Udara Roga is given Snehana, Swedana, Vamana treatment. Thereafter, Samsarjana Krama (administration of lighter to heavier food gradually) is given by adding pungent drugs and alkalies to cereals. He is then given other Kapha mitigating herbs, Ayaskriti (special preparations of iron) and medicated oils added with Alkalies. These therapies alleviated Udara Roga caused by Kapha. [72-73]

Treatment of Sannipatodara

सन्निपातोदरे सर्वा यथोक्ताः कारयेत् क्रियाः।
सोपद्रवं तु निर्वृत्तं प्रत्याख्येयं विजानता|७४|

If the patient is suffering from Sannipatika Udara (caused by vitiation of all 3 Doshas) then all the therapies prescribed above for the treatment of Vatodara, Pittodara and Kaphodara are to be suitably employed. If this condition is associated with complications, then the patient is treated keeping in view the incurability of the condition. [74]

Treatment of Pleehodara and Yakruddalyudara:

उदावर्त रुजानाहै र्दाह मोह तृषा ज्वरैः।
गौरवारुचि काठिन्यैश्चानिलादीन् यथाक्रमम्||७५||
लिङ्गैः प्लीहन्यधिकान् दृष्ट्वा रक्तं चापि स्वलक्षणैः।
चिकित्सां सम्प्रकुर्वीत यथादोषं यथाबलम्||७६||
स्नेहं स्वेदं विरेकं च निरूहमनुवासनम्।
समीक्ष्य कारयेद्बाहौ वामे वा व्यधयेत् सिराम्||७७||
षट्पलं पाययेत् सर्पिः पिप्पलीर्वा प्रयोजयेत्।
सगुडामभयां वाऽपि क्षारारिष्टगणांस्तथा||७८||
एष क्रियाक्रमः प्रोक्तो योगान् संशमनाञ्छृणु।
पिप्पली नागरं दन्ती चित्रकं द्विगुणाभयम्||७९||
विडङ्गांशयुतं चूर्णमेतदुष्णाम्बुना पिबेत्।
विडङ्गं चित्रकं शुण्ठीं सघृतां सैन्धवं वचाम्||८०||
दग्ध्वा कपाले पयसा गुल्मप्लीहापहं पिबेत्।
रोहीतकलतानां तु काण्डकानभयाजले||८१||
मूत्रे वा सुनुयातच्च सप्तरात्रस्थितं पिबेत्।

कामलागुल्ममेहार्शःप्लीहसर्वोदरक्रिमीन्||८२||
स हन्याज्जाङ्गलरसैर्जीर्णे स्याच्चात्र भोजनम्|
रोहीतकत्वचः कृत्वा पलानां पञ्चविंशतिम्||८३||
कोलद्विप्रस्थसंयुक्तं कषायमुपकल्पयेत्|
पलिकैः पञ्चकोलैस्तु तैः सर्वैश्चापि तुल्यया||७४||
रोहीतकत्वचा पिष्टैर्घृतप्रस्थं विपाचयेत्|
प्लीहाभिवृद्धिं शमयत्येतदाशु प्रयोजितम्||८५||
तथा गुल्मोदरश्वासक्रिमिपाण्डुत्वकामलाः|
अग्निकर्म च कुर्वीत भिषग्वातकफोल्बणे||८६||
पैतिके जीवनीयानि सर्पींषि क्षीरबस्तयः|
रक्तावसेकः संशुद्धिः क्षीरपानं च शस्यते||८७||
यूषैर्मांसरसैश्चापि दीपनीयसमायुतैः|
यकृति प्लीहवत् सर्वं तुल्यत्वादभेषजं मतम्||८८||
लघून्यन्नानि संसृज्य दद्यात् प्लीहोदरे भिषक्|८९|

Plihodara splenomegaly with Vata Dosha dominance exhibits Udavarta (bloating, upward movement of wind in the abdomen), pain and Anaha (abdominal distension).

Pleehodar with Pitta dominance exhibits – burning sensation, unconsciousness, thirst and fever

With Kapha dominance, heaviness, anorexia as well as hardness.

Based on the dominance of Dosha and with keeping blood vitiation in mind, suitable treatment is adopted.

The patient is given oleation, fomentation, purgation, Niruha Basti, and Anuvasana Basti, as suitable.

The patient can also be given Siravyadha treatment (bloodletting) on the left arm.

The patient is given the following recipes:

1. Shatpala Ghrta (vide Cikitsa 5: 147 – 148)

2. Pippali Rasayana

3. Abhaya (Terminalia chebula) mixed with Jaggery and

4. Recipes of Kshara and Aristas (Alcoholic Preparations) which are described later below, and in chapter 14 and 15.

The following herbal blends are useful in Pleehodar:

1. 1 part each of long pepper, Ginger, Danti, Chitraka, 2 parts of Haritaki and 1 part of Vidanga is given to the patient with hot water.

2. Vidanga – Embelia ribes, Chitraka – Plumbago zeylanica, Sunthi – Ginger, Ghee, Rock-salt and Vacha (Acorus calamus Linn.)- All these herbs are taken in equal quantities, kept over an earthen plate, covered with another earthen plate and the joints are sealed. This is placed over fire to reduce the ingredients into ashes. Intake of this with milk cure Gulma (tumour) and Plihodara (splenic enlargement).

3. Stems of Rohitaka are cut into small pieces. To this, the crushed pulp of Haritaki is added. These ingredients are soaked in adequate quantities of either water or cow's urine and allowed to ferment for 7 nights. Intake of this liquid cures Kamala (Jaundice), Gulma (tumour), Meha (urinary diseases including diabetes), Arsha (piles), Plihodar (splenic enlargement), all the remaining type of Udara rogas and Krimi Roga (parasitic infestation). After this potion is digested, the patient is given the soup of meat of animals inhabiting arid zones, (Jangala mamsarasa).

4. 25 Palas of bark of Rohitaka and 2 Prasthas Kala is boiled with [8 times of] water [and reduced to 1/4th]. To this, 1 pala paste of pippali, 1 Pala Pippali Mula, 1 Pala Ginger, 5 Palas of the bark of Rohitaka and 1 Prastha (768 g) ghee is added and cooked. This medicated ghee instantaneously cures Pleeha (splenic enlargement), Gulma (Phantom tumour), Udara (obstinate abdominal disorder), Asthma, Krmi (Parasitic infestation), Pandu (anaemia) and Kamala (jaundice).

If there is predominance of aggravated Vayu and Kapha in the patient suffering from splenic enlargement then Agni Karma (cauterisation therapy) is administered. If Pitta is aggravated, then Jeevaneeya Ghrta, Ksheera, bloodletting, elimination therapies, light purgation therapy and intake of milk are useful.

Such a patient is given food mixed with vegetable soup and meat soup prepared by boiling with digestive stimulants.

In Yakrdodara (enlargement of liver), all the therapies prescribed for plihodara (enlargement of spleen) are administered because of the similarity between these 2 conditions.

After the administrations of therapies, the patient is given Samsarjana Krama (administration of lighter to heavier food gradually) with the help of food ingredients which are easily digestible [75- 89 ½]

Treatment of Baddhodara: Intestinal obstruction

स्विन्नाय बद्धोदरिणे मूत्र तीक्ष्णौष धान्वितम्||८९||

स तैल लवणं दद्यान्निरूहं सानुवासनम्|

परिसंसीनि चान्नानि तीक्ष्णं चैव विरेचनम्||९०||

उदावर्तहरं कर्म कार्यं वातघ्नमेव च|

To the patient suffering from Baddhodara (intestinal obstruction), fomentation therapy is given thereafter, Niruha (type of medicated enema) and Anuvasana (another type of medicated enema) is given adding cows urine to drugs having Tiksna (sharp) attributes, oil and Salt.

The patient is given such food as would help in the downward movement of Vayu in the abdomen. He is given strong purgative therapies indicated for the treatment of udavarta (upward movement of wind in the abdomen) and such other therapies which are responsible for alleviation of Vayu are administered. [89 ½ – 91½]

Treatment of Chidrodara:

छिद्रोदरमृते स्वेदाच्छ्लेष्मोदरवदाचरेत्||९१||

जातं जातं जलं स्राव्यमेवं तद्यापयेदिभषक्|

तृष्णा कास ज्वरार्तं तु क्षीण मांसाग्नि भोजनम्||९२||

वर्जयेच्छ्वासिनं तद्वच्छूलिनं दुर्बलेन्द्रियम्|९३|

Chidrodara (abdominal swelling caused by the perforation of intestine) is treated on the lines suggested for Kaphodara (vide verses 72- 73) above. However, Swedana is not administered to the patient.

In the patient of Chidrodara suffers from morbid thirst, cough and fever; if there is depletion of his muscle tissue; if his power of digestion and the quantity of food intake are diminished; if he suffers from dyspnoea and colic pain; and if his sense organs become weak, then such a patient is not to be treated [91 ½ – 93 ½]

Treatment of Udakodara:

अपां दोषहराण्यादौ प्रदद्यादुदकोदरे||९३||

मूत्र युक्तानि तीक्ष्णानि विविधक्षारवन्ति च|

दीपनीयैः कफघ्नैश्च तमाहारैरुपाचरेत्||९४||

द्रवेभ्यश्चोदकादिभ्यो नियच्छेदनु पूर्वशः|९५|

In Udakodara (Ascites), the patient is given therapies to correct the defects of the liquid elements (Apam Doshaharani) in the beginning.

The patient is given therapies containing cow's urine, drugs having Tiksna (sharp) attributes and different types of Alkalies. He is given food which is a digestive stimulant and which alleviates Kapha. Gradually, the patient is prohibited to take water and other liquids [93 ½ – 95½]

Involvement of all the 3 Doshas

सर्वमेवोदरं प्रायो दोषसङ्घातजं मतम्||९५||

तस्मात्रिदोषशमनीं क्रियां सर्वत्र कारयेत्|

All the varieties of Udara are generally caused by the involvement of all the three Doshas. Therefore, therapies which cause alleviation of all the 3 Doshas are administered for the treatment of all the varieties of Udara. [95 ½ – 96½]

Diet and regimen

दोषैः कुक्षौ हि सम्पूर्णे वह्निर्मन्दत्वमृच्छति||९६||

तस्माद्भोज्यानि भोज्यानि दीपनानि लघूनि च|
रक्तशालीन् यवान्मुद्गाञ्जाङ्गलांश्च मृगद्विजान्||९७||
पयो मूत्रासवारिष्टान्मधुसीधुं तथा सुराम्|
यवागूमोदनं वाऽपि यूषैरद्याद्रसैरपि||९८||
मन्दाम्ल स्नेह कटुभिः पञ्चमूलोप साधितैः|
औदकानूपजं मांसं शाकं पिष्टकृतं तिलान्||९९||
व्यायामाध्व दिवा स्वप्नं यानयानं च वर्जयेत्|
तथोष्ण लवणाम्लानि विदाहिनि गुरूणि च||१००||
नाद्यादन्नानि जठरी तोयपानं च वर्जयेत्|१०१|

Since the abdomen is filled with vitiated Doshas, the power of digestion gets diminished. Therefore, the patient should take such food which is light to digest. (Laghu ahara)

He should take Raktashali – red rice, Barley, moong dal – green gram, meat of animals and birds inhabiting arid zone (Jangala mamsa), milk, cow's urine, Asava (alcoholic preparation in which drugs are generally added without boiling), Arista (alcoholic preparation), honey, Seedhu (a type of alcohol) and Sura (another type of alcohol).

He may also take Yavagu (thick gruel) and boiled rice prepared by boiling with the decoction of Panchamula (roots of Bilva, Syonaka, Gambhari, Patali and Ganikarika) and added with slightly sour ingredients, unctuous substances, like ghee and oil, and pungent drugs along with vegetable soup or meat soup.

He should avoid aquatic meat and animals inhabiting marshy land; leafy vegetables; pastries, preparations of sesame seeds, exercise, walking long distances, and sleep during day time and travelling by fast moving vehicles.

He should also avoid hot, saline and sour things, ingredients which cause burning sensation (Vidahi) and heavy food. This type of patient should strictly avoid taking water. [96 ½ – 101½]

Use of buttermilk

नाति सान्द्रं हितं पाने स्वादु तक्रमपेलवम्||१०१||
त्र्यूषण क्षार लवणैर्युक्तं तु निचयोदरी|
वातोदरी पिबेत्तक्रं पिप्पली लवणान्वितम्||१०२||
शर्करा मधुकोपेतं स्वादु पित्तोदरी पिबेत्|
यवानी सैन्धवाजाजी व्योष युक्तं कफोदरी||१०३||
पिबेन्मधुयुतं तक्रं कवोष्णं नातिपेलवम्|
मधु तैल वचा शुण्ठी शताह्वा कुष्ठ सैन्धवैः||१०४||
युक्तं प्लीहोदरी जातं सव्योषं तूदकोदरी|
बद्धोदरी तु हपुषा यवान्यजाजि सैन्धवैः||१०५||
पिबेच्छिद्रोदरी तक्रं पिप्पलीक्षौद्रसंयुतम्|
गौरवारोचकार्तानां समन्दाग्न्यतिसारिणाम्||१०६||
तक्रं वात कफार्तानाममृतत्वाय कल्पते|१०७|

Buttermilk for Udara roga:

Buttermilk, which is not very thick, which is sweet (not sour) and which is free from fat, is useful for the patient suffering from Udara Roga.

If the patient is suffering from Sannipatika Udara Roga, then he should take butter milk along with Tryusana (ginger, pepper, long pepper) Alkalies and Rock salt

The patient of Vatika type of Udara Roga should take

• Buttermilk along with Pippali – Piper longum and Rock- salt.

In Paittika type of Udara Roga, the patient should take

• Buttermilk which is freshly churned and sweet and added with sugar and the powder of Madhuka (licorice).

For the patient suffering from Kaphaja type of Udara Roga, buttermilk is added with Yavani, Rock salt, cumin seeds and Trikatu (ginger, pepper and long pepper) and it should not contain much fat.

The patient of Plihodara (abdominal swelling caused by the enlargement of spleen) should take butter milk along with honey, oil and the powder of Vata, Sunthi, Shatahva (dill), Kustha and rock salt.

The patient suffering from Udakodara (Ascites) should take buttermilk prepared with well formed curd along with the powder of Trikatu (ginger, pepper and long pepper).

For the patient suffering from Baddhodara (enlargement of abdomen because of intestinal strangulation), buttermilk added with Hapusha, Yavani, cumin seeds and rock salt is useful.

The patient suffering from Chidrodara (abdominal swelling caused by intestinal perforation) should take buttermilk along with Pippali and honey

Butter milk is like nectar for people suffering from heaviness, anorexia, suppression of the power of digestion, diarrhoea and diseases caused by aggravated Vata and Kapha. [101 ½ – 107½]

Use of milk

शोफानाहार्तितृष्णमूर्च्छा पीडिते कारभं पयः||१०७||

शुद्धानां क्षामदेहानां गव्यं छागं समाहिषम्|

If the patient of Udara is suffering from oedema, Anaha (bloating, abdominal distension because of wind), pain, and thirst and fainting, then camel milk is useful. After administration of Panchakarma treatment, when it has become emaciated, cow milk, goat milk and buffalo milk are useful [107 ½ – 108½]

Recipes for External Use:

देवदारु पलाशार्क हस्तिपिप्पलि शिग्रुकैः||१०८||

साश्वगन्धैः सगोमूत्रैः प्रदिह्यादुदरं समैः|

वृश्चिकालीं वचां कुष्ठं पञ्चमूलीं पुनर्नवाम्||१०९||

भूतीकं नागरं धान्यं जले पक्त्वाऽवसेचयेत्|

पलाशं कत्तृणं रास्नां तद्वत् पक्त्वाऽवसेचयेत्||११०||

The paste of Devadaru – Cedrus deodara, Palasa – Butea monosperma, Arka – Calotropis procera, Gaja Pippali, Shigru—Moringa oliefera and Ashvagandha- Withania somnifera taken in equal quantities, prepared by triturating with cow's urine is applied over the abdomen of the patient suffering from Udara Roga.

Vrushchikali, Vacha – Acorus calamus, Kustha – Saussurea lappa, Panchamula (Bilva – Aegle marmelos, Syonaka – Oroxylum indicum, Gambhari – Gmelina arborea, Patali, and Ganikarika), Punarnava – Boerhavia diffusa, Bhutika, Nagara – Zingiber officinale and Dhanyaka is boiled in water and this decoction is used for sprinkling over the abdomen of the patient suffering from Udara Roga.

Similarly the decoction of Palasa – Butea monosperma, Kattrna and Rasna is used for sprinkling [108 ½ -110]

Use of Urine

मूत्राण्यष्टावुदरिणां सेके पाने च योजयेत्|१११|

8 type of urine [described in Sutra 1/92-104] are used for sprinkling (over the abdomen) and drinking by the patient suffering from Udara Roga. [111½]

Use of Medicated Ghee

रूक्षाणां बहु वातानां तथा संशोधनार्थिनाम्||१११||

दीपनीयानि सर्पींषि जठरघ्नानि चक्ष्महे|११२|

If the patient of Udara Roga has Ruksha-dryness and Bahu vata- excess of Vayu in his body, and if he needs elimination therapy, then medicated ghee which is stimulant of digestion and which cures Udara Roga is administered. These recipes will be described hereafter. [111 ½ – 112½]

Panchakola Ghirta:

पिप्पली पिप्पलीमूल चव्य चित्रक नागरैः||११२||

सक्षारैरर्धपलिकैर्द्विप्रस्थं सर्पिषः पचेत्।
कल्कैर् द्विपञ्चमूलस्य तुलार्ध स्वरसेन च॥११३॥
दधि मण्डाढकोपेतं तत् सर्पि जठरापहम्।
श्वयथुं वात विष्टम्भं गुल्मार्शांसि च नाशयेत्॥११४॥

2 Prasthas of ghee is cooked by adding the following:

1. Paste of ½ Pala each of Pippali – Piper longum, Pippali Mula, Chavya – Piper retrofractum, Chitraka – Plumbago zeylanica, Nagara – Zingiber officinale and Yavaksara

2. ½ Tula of the decoction of Dashamula (Bilva – Aegle marmelos, Syonaka – Oroxylum indicum, Gambhari – Gmelina arborea, Patali, Agnimantha – Clerodendrum phlomidis, prsniparni, Shalaparni, Brhati, Kantakari – Solanum xantocarpum and Goksura – Tribulus terrestris) and

3. 1 Adhaka of Dadhimanda (liquid portion of the curd)

This medicated ghee cures Udara Rogas, oedema, Vatavistambha (immobility of wind in the abdomen), Gulma (Phantom tumour) and piles. [112 ½ – 114]

Nagara Ghrta

नागर त्रिफला प्रस्थं घृत तैलात्तथाऽऽढकम्।
मस्तुनः साधयित्वैतत् पिबेत् सर्वोदरापहम्॥११५॥
कफ मारुत सम्भूते गुल्मे चैतत् प्रशस्यते॥११६।

1 Prastha Ghee and 1 Prastha til oil is cooked by adding [the paste of] Nagara and Triphala (Haritaki – Terminalia bellerica, Bibhitaka – Terminalia chebula and Amalaki – Phyllanthus emblica) [2 palas each] and 2 Adhakas of Mastu (thin butter- milk).

This medicated ghee cures all types of Udara rogas. It is also useful in the treatment of Gulma caused by the vitiation of kapha and vayu. [115 ½ – 116½]

Chitraka Ghrita

चतुर्गुणे जले मूत्रे द्विगुणे चित्रकात् पले॥११६॥
कल्के सिद्धं घृतप्रस्थं सक्षारं जठरी पिबेत्।

2 Prasthas Ghee, 8 Prasthas water, 4 prasthas cow's urine, 1 Pala paste of Citraka and 1 Pala Yavakshara is cooked together.

This medicated ghee is used by the patient suffering from Udara Roga. [116 ½- 117½]

Yavadi Ghrita

यव कोल कुलत्थानां पञ्चमूल रसेन च॥११७॥
सुरा सौवीरकाभ्यां च सिद्धं वाऽपि पिबेद्घृतम्॥११८।

Ghee cooked with the decoction of Yava, Kola, Kulattha and Panchamula (Bilva – Aegle marmelos, Syonaka – Oroxylum indicum, Gambhari – Gmelina arborea, Patali and Agnimantha – Clerodendrum phlomidis) and Sura (a type of alcohol) as well as Savira (a type of vinegar) is useful for a patient suffering from udara Roga (obstinate abdominal disorders) 117 ½- 118½]

Virechana – Purgation Therapy

एभिः स्निग्धाय सञ्जाते बले शान्ते च मारुते॥११८॥
स्रस्ते दोषाशये दद्यात् कल्पदिष्टं विरेचनम्॥११९।

By the administration of the above-mentioned recipes of medicated ghee, the patient becomes oleated; he regains strength; aggravated Vayu in his body gets alleviated and the adhesiveness of the Doshas in various Asayas (visceras) is diminished. Thereafter, the patient of Udara Roga is given purgation therapy described in Kalpa section. [118 ½ – 119½]

Patoladi Churna

पटोल मूलं रजनीं विडङ्गं त्रिफला त्वचम्||११९||

कम्पिल्लकं नीलिनीं च त्रिवृतां चेति चूर्णयेत्|

षडाद्यान् कार्षिकानन्त्यांस्त्रींश्च द्विवित्रिचतुर्गुणान्||१२०||

कृत्वा चूर्णमतो मुष्टिं गवां मूत्रेण ना पिबेत्|

विरिक्तो मृदु भुञ्जीत भोजनं जाङ्गलै रसैः||१२१||

मण्डं पेयां च पीत्वा ना सव्योषं षडहं पयः|

शृतं पिबेत्ततश्चूर्णं पिबेदेवं पुनः पुनः||१२२||

हन्ति सर्वोदराण्येतच्चूर्णं जातोदकान्यपि|

कामलां पाण्डुरोगं च श्वयथुं चापकर्षति||१२३||

पटोलाद्यमिदं चूर्णमुदरेषु प्रपूजितम्|१२४|

1 Karsa Root of Patola, 1 Karsa Rajani, 1 Karsa Vidanga – Embelia ribes, 1 Karsa fruit Pulp of Haritaki, 1 Karsa fruit Pulp of Amalaki, 2 Karsas Kampillaka, 3 Karsa Nilini and 4 Karsas Trivrt all these drugs is made to powders and given to the patient along with 1 Musti (Pala) of cow's urine.

This causes purgation.

Thereafter, the patient is given a light diet along with meat soup of animals inhabiting arid zones.

For 6 days, thereafter, depending upon the power of digestion, the patient is given Manda (exceedingly thin gruel) or Peya (thin gruel) along with milk boiled by adding Trikatu (Sunthi, Pippli and Marica).

The above-mentioned powder is given again and again.

It cures all types of Udara Rogas even in their Jatodaka Stage (when water starts accumulating in the abdomen). It is also useful in the treatment of Jaundice, anaemia and oedema.

This is called Patoladya churna, and it is very effective in the treatment of all types of udara Rogas. [119 ½ – 124½]

गवाक्षीं शङ्खिनीं दन्तीं तिल्वकस्य त्वचं वचाम्||१२४||

पिबेद्द्राक्षाम्बु गोमूत्रकोल कर्कन्धु सीधुभिः|

The patient of Udara Roga should take the powder of Gavaksi, Sankhini (Sveta Bhallataki), Danti, Bark of Tilvaka and Vacha – Acorus calamus along with Cow's urine, decoction of Draksa – Vtis vinfera, juice of Kola, Juice of Karkandhu or Sidhu (a type of alcoholic preparation). [124 ½ – 125½]

Narayana Churna

यवानी हपुषा धान्यं त्रिफला चोपकुञ्चिका||१२५||

कारवी पिप्पलीमूलमजगन्धा शटी वचा|

शताह्वा जीरकं व्योषं स्वर्णक्षीरी सचित्रका||१२६||

द्वौ क्षारौ पौष्करं मूलं कुष्ठं लवण पञ्चकम्|

विडङ्गं च समांशानि दन्त्या भागत्रयं तथा||१२७||

त्रिवृद्द्विशाले द्विगुणे सातला स्याच्चतुर्गुणा|

एतन्नारायणं नाम चूर्णं रोगगणापहम्||१२८||

नैनत् प्राप्यातिवर्तन्ते रोगा विष्णुमिवासुराः|

तक्रेणोदरिभिः पेयं गुल्मिभिर्बदराम्बुना||१२९||

आनद्धवाते सुरया वातरोगे प्रसन्नया|

दधिमण्डेन विट्सङ्गे दाडिमाम्बुभिरर्शसैः||१३०||

परिकर्ते सवृक्षाम्लमुष्णाम्बुभिरजीर्णके|

भगन्दरे पाण्डुरोगे श्वासे कासे गलग्रहे||१३१||

हृद्रोगे ग्रहणीदोषे कुष्ठे मन्देऽनले ज्वरे|

दंष्ट्राविषे मूलविषे सगरे कृत्रिमे विषे||१३२||

यथार्हं स्निग्धकोष्ठेन पेयमेतद्विरेचनम्|
इति नारायणचूर्णम्|

Yavani, Hapusa, Dhanya, Triphala, (Haritaki –Terminalia chebula, Bibhitaka – Terminalia belerica and Amalaki – Phyllanthus emblica), Upakuncika (Krsna Jiraka), Karvi (small variety of Jiraka), Pippali Mula, Ajagandha [see commentary], Shati – Hedychium spicatum, Vacha – Acorus calamus, satahva, Jiraka (large variety of Jiraka), Trikatu (Sunthi – Zingiber officinale, Pippali- Piper longum and Marica – Piper nigrum), Svarnaksiri, Chitraka – Plumbago zeylanica, Yavaksara, Svarajiksara,Puskaramula, Kustha – Sauussera lappa, Lavana Panchaka (Sauvarcala, Saindhava, Vida,Audmula, Kustha, Lavana Pancaka (Sauvarcala, Saindhava, Vida, audbhida and Samudra) and Vidanga – all taken one part each, Dani (three parts), Trivrt – Operculina turpethum(2 parts), Visala (2 Parts) and Satala (4 parts) is made into powder. This is called Narayana Churna. Just like the group of demons would get destroyed just by the glimpse of Lord Narayana, the group of diseases too will get destroyed by the consumption of this powder. It shall be taken along with the following Anupanas depending on the nature of the diseases concerned:

1. In Udara Roga – with ButterMilk
2. In Gulma (Phantom Tumour) – with Juice of Badara
3. In Anaddhavata (Immobility of wind in the abdomen) – with Sura (alcoholic drink)
4. In Diseases caused by Vayu – with Prasanna (another type of alcoholic drink)
5. In Vidsanga (fecal obstruction) – with Dadhimanda (water which is squeezed out of the curd)
6. In Piles – with Juice of Dadima
7. In Parikartika (sawing pain in the abdomen) – with Vrksamla
8. In indigestion – with Hot water

In Bhagandara (fistula- in- ano) Pandu Roga (anemia), Asthma, bronchitis, Galagraha(obstruction in the throat), heart diseases, spue syndrome, Kustha (obstinate skin diseases including leprosy), suppression of the powder of digestion, fever, Damstra visa(biting by an animal having poisonous teeth), Mula Visa (root poisons) Garavisa (a type of Poison artificially prepared by combining different ingredients), and Krtrima Visa (artificial Poison), the patient should first of all be given oleation therapy followed by this recipes for the purpose of purgation [124 ½ – 133½]

Hapushadya Churna

हपुषां काञ्चन क्षीरीं त्रिफलां कटुरोहिणीम्||१३३||
नीलिनीं त्रायमाणां च सातलां त्रिवृतां वचाम्|
सैन्धवं काललवणं पिप्पलीं चेति चूर्णयेत्||१३४||
दाडिम त्रिफला मांसरस मूत्र सुखोदकैः|
पेयोऽयं सर्वगुल्मेषु प्लीहनि सर्वोदरेषु च||१३५||
श्वित्रे कुष्ठे सरुजके सवाते विषमाग्निषु|
शोथार्शःपाण्डुरोगेषु कामलायां हलीमके||१३६||
वातं पित्तं कफं चाशु विरेकात् सम्प्रसाधयेत्|
इति हपुषाद्यं चूर्णम्|

Hapusa, Kancanaksiri, Triphala (Haritaki – Terminalia chebula, Bibhitaki – Terminalia bellerica, and Amalaki – Phyllanthus emblica), Katurohini, Nilini, Trayamana, Satala, Trivrt – Operculina turpethum, Saindhava, Kala lavana (Bida Lavana) and Pippali – Piper longum is made to powder.

This powder is taken along with juice of Dadima – Punica granatum, Decoction of Triphala, meat soup, cow's urine or hot water.

It is useful in the treatment of all types of Gulma (phantom tumour), Plihodara (splenic enlargement), all other forms of Udara roga, Svitra (leucoderma), Kustha (obstinate skin diseases including leprosy), Visamagni (irregular power of digestion) associated with pain and flatulence, Shotha – oedema, Arsha -piles, Pandu – anemia, Kamala – Jaundice and Halimaka (A serious type of Jandice) by causing purgation. This recipe instantaneously corrects aggravated Vayu, Pitta and kapha. [133 ½ – 137½]

Nilinyadya Curna:

नीलिनीं निचुलं व्योषं द्वौ क्षारौ लवणानि च||१३७||

चित्रकं च पिबेच्चूर्णं सर्पिषोदरगुल्मनुत्|

इति नीलिन्याद्यं चूर्णम्|

Nilini, Nicula, Trikatu (Sunthi – Zingiber officinale, Pippali –Piper longum and Maricha – Piper nigrum), Yava, Ksara, Svarjiksara, Pancha Lavana (Sauvarcala, Saindhava, Vida, Audbhida and Samudra) and Chitraka – Plumbago zeylanica is made to a powder.

Intake of this potion along with ghee cures Udara (obstinate abdominal disorders including ascetics) and Gulma (Phantom tumour) [137 ½ – 138½]

Recipes of Snuhi ksheera Ghrta

क्षीर द्रोणं सुधा क्षीर प्रस्थार्धसहितं दधि||१३८||

जातं विमथ्य तद्युक्त्या त्रिवृत्सिद्धं पिबेद्घृतम्|

तथा सिद्धं घृतप्रस्थं पयस्यष्टगुणे पिबेत्||१३९||

स्नुक्क्षीर पल कल्केन त्रिवृता षट्पलेन च|

गुल्मानां गर दोषाणामुदराणां च शान्तये||१४०||

इति स्नुही क्षीरघृतम्|

दधिमण्डाढके सिद्धात् स्नुक्क्षीरपल कल्कितात्|

घृतप्रस्थात् पिबेन्मात्रां तद्वज्जठरशान्तये||१४१||

एषां चानु पिबेत् पेयां पयो वा स्वादु वा रसम्|

घृते जीर्णे विरिक्तस्तु कोष्णं नागरकैः शृतम्||१४२||

पिबेदम्बु ततः पेयां यूषं कौलत्थकं ततः|

पिबेद्रूक्षस्त्र्यहं त्वेवं भूयो वा प्रतिभोजितः||१४३||

पुनः पुनः पिबेत् सर्पिरानुपूर्व्या तयैव च|

घृतान्येतानि सिद्धानि विदध्यात् कुशलो भिषक्||१४४||

गुल्मानां गरदोषाणामुदराणां च शान्तये|

2 Dronas of Cow's milk and 1 Prastha milky latex of Sunhi is mixed together and converted into curd.

It is churned and the ghee that comes out of it is appropriately cooked by adding Trivrt – Operculina turpethum

2 Prasthas of Cow's ghee and 16 Prasthas cow's milk is cooked by adding the paste prepared of 1 Pala of the milky latex of Snuhi and 6 Palas of Trivrt.

The above mentioned 2 recipes are useful in the treatment of Gulma (Phantom tumour), poisoning by artificially poisons and Udara Rogas (obstinate abdominal disorders including ascites).

2 Prasthas of Ghee is cooked along with 2 Adhakas of Dadhimanda (water squeezed out of curd) and 1 pala paste of the milky latex of Snuhi. This is taken by the patient in appropriate dose for the cure of Udara Roga (obstinate abdominal disorders including ascites).

After the intake of these recipes, either

Peya (thin gruel) or

Milk or

Juice of sweet fruits (Kapha, Pitta and Vayu respectively) is taken as a post – prandial drink.

When the ghee is digested and the purgation is over, the patient is given luke- warm water boiled with ginger (prepared according to the procedure laid down for Sadanga Paniya (vide Cikitsa 1: 3: 145).

Thereafter, the patient is given Peya or thin gruel (on the second day) and soup of Kulattha (on the third day). If necessary, these food ingredients can be given for a longer period and the Patient will, thus, become Ruksa (unctuous and dry). The course of medicated ghee along with the food preparations prescribed above is administered to him repeatedly by an expert physician.

These cures:

Gulma (Phantom Tumour),

Poisoning by artificial poisons and

Udara Rogas (obstinate abdominal disorders including ascites) (138 ½ – 145½)

Other recipes of Medicated Ghee

पीलु कल्कोपसिद्धं वा घृतमानाह भेदनम्||१४५||
गुल्मघ्नं नीलिनी सर्पि: स्नेहं वा मिश्रकं पिबेत्|१४६|

Ghee cooked with the paste of Pilu cures anaha (abdominal distension).

Nilini Ghrta (Nilinyadya Ghrta- vide Cikitsa 5: 105- 109) cures Gulma (Phantom Tumour). The patient of Udara (obstinate abdominal disorders including ascites) may also take Misraka Sneha- vide Cikitsa 5: 149: 151. [145 ½ – 146 ½]

Other medicines:

क्रमान्निर्हृतदोषाणां जाङ्गल प्रति भोजिनाम् ||१४६||
दोष शेष निवृत्यर्थं योगान् वक्ष्याम्यतः परम्|
चित्रकामर दारुभ्यां कल्कं क्षीरेण ना पिबेत्||१४७||
मासं युक्तस्तथा हस्ति पिप्पली विश्वभेषजम्|
विडङ्गं चित्रकं दन्ती चव्यं व्योषं च तैः पयः||१४८||
कल्कैः कोलसमैः पीत्वा प्रवृद्धमुदरं जयेत्|
पिबेत् कषायं त्रिफला दन्ती रोहितकैः शृतम्||१४९||
व्योष क्षारयुतं जीर्णे रसैरद्यातु जाङ्गलैः|
मांसं वा भोजनं भोज्यं सुधा क्षीर घृतान्वितम्||१५०||
क्षीरानुपानां गोमूत्रेणाभयां वा प्रयोजयेत्|
सप्ताहं माहिष मूत्रं क्षीरं चानन्नभुक् पिबेत्||१५१||
मासमौष्ट्रं पयश्छागं त्रीन्मासान् व्योषसंयुतम्|
हरीतकी सहस्रं वा क्षीराशी वा शिलाजतु||१५२||
शिलाजतु विधानेन गुग्गुलुं वा प्रयोजयेत्|
शृङ्गवेरार्द्रकरसः पाने क्षीरसमो हितः||१५३||
तैलं रसेन तेनैव सिद्धं दशगुणेन वा|
दन्ती द्रवन्ती फलजं तैलं दूष्योदरे हितम्||१५४||
शूलानाह विबन्धेषु मस्तु यूष रसादिभिः|
सरला मधु शिग्रूणां बीजेभ्यो मूलकस्य च||१५५||
तैलान्यभ्यङ्गपानार्थं शूलघ्नान्यनिलोदरे|
स्तैमित्यारुचिहृल्लासे मन्देऽग्नौ मद्यपाय च||१५६||
अरिष्टान् दापयेत् क्षारान् कफस्त्यानस्थिरोदरे|
श्लेष्मणो विलयार्थं तु दोषं वीक्ष्य भिषग्वरः||१५७||
पिप्पलीं तिल्वकं हिङ्गु नागरं हस्तिपिप्पलीम्|
भल्लातकं शिग्रुफलं त्रिफलां कटुरोहिणीम्||१५८||
देवदारु हरिद्रे द्वे सरलातिविषे वचाम् |
कुष्ठं मुस्तं तथा पञ्च लवणानि प्रकल्प्य च||१५९||
दधि सर्पि र्वसा मज्ज तैल युक्तानि दाहयेत्|
अन्नादूर्ध्वमतः क्षारादिबिडालकपदं पिबेत्||१६०||
मदिरा दधि मण्डोष्णजलारिष्ट सुरासवैः|
हृद्रोगं श्वयथुं गुल्मं प्लीहार्शो जठराणि च||१६१||

विसूचिकामुदावर्तं वाताष्ठीलां च नाशयेत्।
क्षारं चाजकरीषाणां सुतं मूत्रैर्विपाचयेत्॥१६२॥
कार्षिकं पिप्पलीमूलं पञ्चैव लवणानि च।
पिप्पलीं चित्रकं शुण्ठीं त्रिफलां त्रिवृतां वचाम्॥१६३॥
द्वौ क्षारौ सातलां दन्तीं स्वर्णक्षीरीं विषाणिकाम्।
कोलप्रमाणां वटिकां पिबेत् सौवीरसंयुताम्॥१६४॥
श्वयथाविपाके च प्रवृद्धे च दकोदरे।
भावितानां गवां मूत्रे षष्टिकानां तु तण्डुलैः॥१६५॥
यवागूं पयसा सिद्धां प्रकामं भोजयेन्नरम्।
पिबेदिक्षुरसं चानु जठराणां निवृत्तये॥१६६॥
स्वं स्वं स्थानं व्रजन्त्येवं तथा पितकफानिलाः।
शङ्खिनीस्नुक्त्रिवृद्दन्तीचिरबिल्वादिपल्लवैः॥१६७॥
शाकं गाढपुरीषाय प्राग्भक्तं दापयेद्भिषक्।
ततोऽस्मै शिथिली भूत वर्चोदोषाय शास्त्रवित्॥१६८॥
दद्यान्मूत्रयुतं क्षीरं दोष शेषहरं शिवम्।
पार्श्वशूलमुपस्तम्भं हृद्ग्रहं चापि मारुतः॥१६९॥
जनयेद्यस्य तं तैलं बिल्वक्षारेण पाययेत्।
तथाऽग्निमन्थस्योनाक पलाश तिलनालजैः॥१७०॥
बलाकदल्यपामार्गक्षारैः प्रत्येकशः सुतैः।
तैलं पक्त्वा भिषग्दद्यादुदराणां प्रशान्तये॥१७१॥
निवर्तते चोदरिणां हृद्ग्रहश्चानिलोद्भवः।
कफे वातेन पितेन ताभ्यां वाऽप्यावृतेऽनिले॥१७२॥
बलिनः स्वौषधयुतं तैलमेरण्डजं हितम्।
सुविरिक्तो नरो यस्तु पुनराध्मापितो भवेत्॥१७३॥
सुस्निग्धैरम्ललवणैर्निरूहैस्तमुपाचरेत्।
सोपस्तम्भोऽपि वा वायुराध्मापयति यं नरम्॥१७४॥
तीक्ष्णैः सक्षारगोमूत्रैर्बस्तिभिस्तमुपाचरेत्॥१७५॥

After the vitiated Doshas are gradually eliminated, the patient is given the meat of animals inhabiting arid zones for the elimination of the residual Doshas, following recipes is administered to the patient:

1. The paste of Devadaru – Cedrus deodara along with milk is taken for 1 month

2. The powder of Gajapippali and Sunthi along with milk

3. Milk boiled with 1 Kola each of Vidanga – Embelia ribes, Chitraka – Plumbago zeylanica, Danti, Chavya – Piper chaba and Trikatu (Sunthi – Zingiber officinale, Pippali – Piper longum and Marica – Piper nigrum). Intake of this medicated milk cures acute form of Udara (obstinate abdominal disorders including Ascites). For the preparation of this recipe, the powder of above-mentioned drugs is boiled by adding 8 Palas of milk and 32 Palas of water)

4. Decoction of Triphala (Haritaki – Terminalia chebula, Bibhitaka – Terminalia bellerica and Amalaki—Phyllanthus emblica), Danti and Rohitaka along with Trikatu (Sunthi – Zingiber offcinale, Pippali – Piper longum, and Marica -Piper nigrum) and Yavakshara should be consumed. When the medicine gets digested, he should take food along with the soup of meat of animals inhabiting arid zone

5. Meat along with the recipes of Sudhaksira Ghrta or Snuhiksira Ghrta- vde verses 138- 145 above;

6. Harithaki along with cow's urine followed by milk as post prandial drink; the patient should not take any cereal while taking this recipe.

7. Buffalo – urine; this should be taken for one week; during this period the patient should not take any cereal. The patient should take only a milk predominant diet.

9. Camel- milk along with the powder of Trikatu (Sunthi – Zingiber officinale, Pippali – Piper longum and Marica –

Piper nigrum) to be taken for 1 month.

10. Goat- milk along with the powder of trikatu (sunthi, Pippali and Marica) to be taken for 3 months.

11. 1000 fruits of haritaki (to be taken according to the procedure prescribed for Pippali Vardhamana Rasayana- (vide Cikitsa 1: 3: 36-40).

12. Shilajit along with milk

13. Guggulu according to the procedure prescribed above for Silajatu, i.e along with milk

14. Juice of green ginger along with milk

15. Til oil cooked with ten times of ginger- juice

16. Oil of the fruits of Danti and Dravanti; this is useful in Dusodara (sannipatika Udara); if there is Colic Pain, abdominal distension and constipation, then this oil should be taken along with Mastu (thin butter- milk) vegetable soup, meat soup etc

17. Oils collected from the seeds of Sarala, Madhusigru and Mulaka; these are useful for massage as well as for taking internally; these oils cure colic pain in the patient suffering from Vatodara;

18. Aristas (alcoholic preparations) these recipes are useful if there is Staimitya (a feeling as if a person is covered with a wet cloth or leather), anorexia and nausea; if there is suppression of the power of digestion, and if the patient is accustomed to alcoholic drinks

19. Ksharas (Alkaline preparations); these recipes are useful if kapha has become thick and sticky in the patient suffering from Udara Roga it liquefies the Kapha;

20. [Pippalyadi Ksara] Pippali – Piper longum, Tilvaka, Hingu, Sunthi – Zingiber officinale, Gajapippali, Bhallataka – Randia dumetorum, fruit of Sigru – Moringa oliefera, Triphala (Haritaki – Terminalia chebula , Bibhitaki – Terminalia bellerica and Amalaki – Phyllanthus emblica), katurohini, Devadaru – Cedrus deodara, Haridra, Daruharidra — Berberis aristata, Sarala, Ativisa, Dhava, Vida, Audbhida and samudra) – all these drugs are mixed with curd, ghee, muscle fat, bone marrow and oil and burnt over the fire [the quantity of curd, etc. should be sufficient enough to make the powders of drugs to take the shape of bolus; this bolus is kept in an earthen vessel and covered with an earthen plate; the joint between the earthen vessel and earthen plate is sealed with the help of mud seared cloth; this is placed over fire for reducing the ingredients into ashes. 1 Karsa of this powder is taken after food along with Madira (alcoholic drink), Dadhimanda (water squeezed out of curd), hot water, Arista (a type of alcoholic preparation), Sura (alcohol) and Asava (another type of alcoholic preparation). It cures heart disease, oedema, Gulma, (Phantom tumour), enlargement of spleen, piles, various types of Udara Rogas, Visucika (choleric diarrhoea / cholera), Udavarta (upward movement of wind) and Vatasthila (stone like growth in the abdomen caused by vayu).

21. Ksara Vatika- Stool of the goat is burnt, reduced to ashes, diluted with 6 times cow's urine and strained through a cloth twenty -one times to prepare Ksara (Alkaline preparation). This Alkaline preparation is cooked till it becomes thick in consistency. To this, Pippalimula, panca lavana (Sauvarcala, Saindhava, Vida, Audbhida and Samudra), Pippali, Chitraka –Plumbago zeylanica, Sunthi, Triphala (Haritaki, Bibhitaka and Amalaki), Trivrt, Vacha, Yavaksara, Svarjiksara, Satala, Danti, Svarnaksiri and Visanika – 1 Karsa each is added and cooked (the quantity of liquid Ksara should be eight times of the powder). From out of this paste, pills of 1 Kola each are prepared. Intake of this pill along with Sauvira (a type of vinegar) cures oedema, indigestion and acute form of jalodara oedema, indigestion and acute form of Jalodara (Ascites)

22. Shastika type of rice is impregnated with cow's urine. This rice is cooked with milk and given to the patient as much as he could take. Thereafter, he is given sugarcane juice which cures Udara Rogas. By the administration of this recipe, the aggravated Vayu, Kapha and Pitta get restored to their own locations

23. To the patient having costive bowels, vegetable preparation of the leaves of Sankhini, Snuhi, Trivrt, Danti Cirabilva etc. is given before food. By the administration of this recipe, the stool becomes soft and the physician well versed in medical texts should administer milk along with cow's urine for the elimination of the residual Doshas

24. If the patient suffers from Sula (pain in the sides of the chest) Hrdgraha (stiffness and pain in the cardiac region) because of aggravate Vayu, then he is given oil cooked with Bilva Ksara (fruits of Bilva should be burnt for the preparation of ksara or Alkali preparation and the oil is cooked with this Kshara preparation)

25. Similarly, oil cooked with the Ksara (Alkali preparation) of either agnimantha, Syonaka, Palasa, Stems of Tila,

Bala, Kadali or Apamarga should be given to the patient for the cure of Udara Rogas (obstinate abdominal disorders). By the administration of this medicated oil, Hrdgaha (stiffness and pain in the cardiac region) caused by vayu in the patient suffering from Udara Roga gets subsided

26. If Kapha gets occluded (Avrtta) either by Vayu or by Pitta and if Vayu gets afflicted (Avrttta) by Kapha and Pitta, then castor oil added with Drugs appropriate for the alleviation of the respective Doshas is administered.

27. If the patient gets flatulence even after proper purgation, then he is given Niruha basti (a type of enema prepared of Unctuous, sour and saline drugs) and

28. If the patient suffers from flatulence and there is occlusion of Vayu, then he is given medicated enema therapy prepared of Tiksna (having sharp attributes) drugs, alkalies and cow's urine. [145 ½- 175 ½]

Administration of Snake- venom

क्रियातिवृत्ते जठरे त्रिदोषे चा प्रशाम्यति||१७५||
ज्ञातीन् ससुहृदो दारान् ब्राह्मणान्नृपतीन् गुरून्|
अनुज्ञाप्य भिषक् कर्म विदध्यात् संशयं ब्रुवन्||१७६||
अक्रियायां ध्रुवो मृत्युः क्रियायां संशयो भवेत्|
एवमाख्याय तस्येदमनुज्ञातः सुहृद्गणैः||१७७||
पान भोजन संयुक्तं विषमस्मै प्रयोजयेत्|
यस्मिन् वा कुपितः सर्पो विसृजेदिद्धि फले विषम्||१७८||
भोजयेत्तदुदरिणं प्रविचार्य भिषग्वरः|
तेनास्य दोषसङ्घातः स्थिरो लीनो विमार्गगः||१७९||
विषेणाशुप्रमाथित्वादाशु भिन्नः प्रवर्तते|
विषेण हृतदोषं तं शीताम्बुपरिषेचितम्||१८०||
पाययेत भिषग्दुग्धं यवागूं वा यथाबलम्|
त्रिवृन्मण्डूकपर्ण्योश्च शाकं सयववास्तुकम्||१८१||
भक्षयेत् कालशाकं वा स्वरसोदकसाधितम्|
निरम्ललवणस्नेहं स्विन्नास्विन्नमनन्नभुक्||१८२||
मासमेकं ततश्चैव तृषितः स्वरसं पिबेत्|
एवं विनिर्हृते दोषे शाकैर्मासात् परं ततः||१८३||
दुर्बलाय प्रयुञ्जीत प्राणभृत् कारभं पयः|१८४|

If the Udara Roga caused by the simultaneous vitiation of all the 3 Doshas does not yield to the above-mentioned treatment, then the physician should call for patient's relatives, friends, wife Brahmanas, the kin (authorities of the state) and preceptors, and inform them of his doubts about the curability of the disease. In normal course they should also be informed that the patient will certainly die if the risk of toxic therapy is not permitted. After this statement, if the friends, etc, of the patient permits, then he is given snake-venom mixed with his food and drinks.

A (Cobra) snake should be enraged and made to bite a fruit to ejaculate its venom. The physician, after due consideration, should ask the patient to eat that fruit.

The snake-venom is Pramathi (the drug which by its own potency drains out the accumulated Doshas from the channels of circulation is called Pramathi). Because of this, the compact Doshas which are stabilised and completely submerged in the tissues and which have gone astray to channels other than their own, get instantaneously separated from tissues and come out.

When the aggravated Doshas are eliminated, then the patient is sprinkled with cold water and the physician should give him either milk or Yavagu (thick gruel) in adequate quantity depending upon his strength.

Then for 1 month, the patient should not take any cereal and depend upon the leaves of Trivrit – Operculina turpethum, Mandukaparni, Barley, Vastuka and Kalasaka. These leafy vegetables can be either boiled or taken in unboiled form.

No sour drug, salt or fat is added to these vegetables. These are to be prepared along with their own juice or by adding water.

If during this 1 month, the patient feels thirsty, then he is given the juice of above-mentioned plants, specially or Kalasaka to drink.

Intake of these leafy vegetables will eliminate the accumulated Doshas, and after 1 month, the patient who has already become weak is given camel- milk to restore his vitality. [175 ½ – 184 ½]

Surgical Measures

इदं तु शल्यहर्तॄणां कर्म स्यादृष्टकर्मणाम्||१८४||
वामं कुक्षिं मापयित्वा नाभ्यधश्चतुरङ्गुलम्|
मात्रा युक्तेन शस्त्रेण पाटयेन्मतिमान् भिषक्||१८५||
विपाट्यान्त्रं ततः पश्चाद्वीक्ष्य बद्ध क्षतान्त्रयोः|
सर्पिषाऽभ्यज्य केशादीनवमृज्य विमोक्षयेत्||१८६||
मूर्च्छनाद्यच्च सम्मूढमन्त्रं तच्च विमोक्षयेत्|
छिद्राण्यन्त्रस्य तु स्थूलैर्दर्शयित्वा पिपीलिकैः||१८७||
बहुशः सङ्गृहीतानि ज्ञात्वा च्छित्वा पिपीलिकान्|
प्रतियोगैः प्रवेश्यान्त्रं प्रेयैः सीव्येद्व्रणं ततः||१८८||

The following surgical measures are performed by the physician having practical experience for the removal / correction of Shalya (foreign bodies including perforation etc).

An expert surgeon should do an incision in the left pelvic region below the umbilicus leaving 4 fingers breadth of space (from the level of the umbilicus) with the help of an appropriate surgical instrument.

After opening the abdomen, the physician should carefully examine the intestines for strangulation and perforation. The afflicted part is anointed with ghee and foreign bodies, like hair etc, is removed from the intestine. Thereafter, the afflicted part is put in its appropriate place.

If there is perforation in the intestine, it is made to be bitten by big- black- ants (Pipilikas). If the perforation is bigger, it should be made to be bitten by 4-10 big ants. Having ascertained that the ants have properly bitten the edges, their bodies are cut off and separated. Then the intestine is placed back into their appropriate place and the incised abdominal skin is sutured with the help of a needle. [184 ½- 188]

Abdominal Tapping

तथा जातोदकं सर्वमुदरं व्यधयेद्भिषक्|
वाम पार्श्वे त्वधो नाभेर्नाडीं दत्वा च गालयेत्||१८९||
विस्राव्य च विमृद्यैतद्वेष्टयेद्वाससोदरम्|
तथा बस्ति विरेकाद्यैर्म्लानं सर्वं च वेष्टयेत्||१९०||

If liquid is already accumulated in the abdomen (Jatodaka stage) in all types of Udara (Ascites) Rogas, the physician should tap in the left side of the abdomen below the umbilicus (with the help of torchar and canula). Later, with the help of the canula all the fluid is removed by applying pressure. The abdomen is tied tightly with the help of a cloth- bandage, the retraced abdomen is required to be similarly tied with the help of a cloth- bandaged after the administration of enema or purgation therapy and after similar other measures. [189- 190]

Diet

निःसुते लङ्घितः पेयामस्नेहलवणां पिबेत्|
अतः परं तु षण्मासान् क्षीरवृत्तिर्भवेन्नरः||१९१||
त्रीन् मासान् पयसा पेयां पिबेत्त्रींश्चापि भोजयेत्|
श्यामाकं कोरदूषं वा क्षीरेणा लवणं लघु||१९२||
नरः संवत्सरेणैवं जयेत् प्राप्तं जलोदरम्|

After the fluid from the abdomen is drained out, the patient is made to fast and thereafter, he is given (thin gruel) which is prepared without adding fat and salt. Thereafter, for 6 months, the patient should live only on milk. Thereafter, for 3 months, the patient should take Peya (thin Gruel) prepared with milk. For 3 months, thereafter, he is given cereals like Syamaka or Koradusa along with milk. These are light for digestion and no salt is given to the patient during this period.

Thus, the patient having reached the Jatodaka stage of ascites should overcome the ailment in 1 year. [191- 193½]

Utility of Milk

प्रयोगाणां च सर्वेषामनु क्षीरं प्रयोजयेत्||१९३||
दोषानु बन्धरक्षार्थं बलस्थैर्यार्थमेव च|
प्रयोगापचिताङ्गानां हितं ह्युदरिणां पयः|
सर्वधातुक्षयार्तानां देवानाममृतं यथा||१९४||

After the administration of all therapies, the patient should invariably be given milk to take for maintaining the harmony of Doshas and for promoting strength as well as stability in the body.

By the administration of different therapies, the body of the patient becomes emaciated and all the tissue elements in his body get diminished.

For such patients, milk is very useful. It is as good as the ambrosia for the gods. [193 ½- 194]

Thus, it is said: -

तत्र श्लोकौ-

हेतुं प्रागूपमष्टानां लिङ्गं व्याससमासतः|
उपद्रवान् गरीयस्त्वं साध्यासाध्यत्वमेव च||१९५||
जाता जाताम्बु लिङ्गानि चिकित्सां चोक्तवानृषिः|
समासव्यास निर्देशैरुदराणां चिकित्सिते||१९६||

In this chapter dealing with the treatment of Udara Rogas the Sage Atreya has described in brief as well as in detail the following topics.

1. Causative factors
2. Premonitory signs and symptoms
3. Signs and symptoms of eight varieties of Udara Roga (obstinate abdominal diseases including ascites) in detail as well as in brief;
4. Complications and their seriousness
5. Curability and incurability
6. Signs and symptoms of Jatodaka (where fluid has started accumulating in the abdomen) and Ajatodaka abdomen stages of this disease and
7. Treatment [195- 196]

इत्यग्निवेशकृते तन्त्रेऽप्राप्ते दृढबल पूरिते चिकित्सा स्थान उदर चिकित्सितं नाम त्रयोदशोऽध्यायः||१३||

Thus, ends the 13th chapter dealing with the treatment of Udara Roga (obstinate abdominal disorders including ascites) in the section on therapeutics of Agnivesha's work as redacted by Charaka, restored by Drudhabala.

20

Chikitsasthana Chapter 14 Arsha Chikitsitam

The 14th chapter of Charaka Samhita Chikitsa Sthana is Arsha Chikitsa, explains in detail about causes, types, signs and symptoms and treatment of haemorrhoids.

अथातोऽर्शश्चिकित्सितं व्याख्यास्यामः||१||
इति ह स्माह भगवानात्रेयः||२||

We shall now expound the chapter on the treatment of Arsas (piles). Thus said Lord Atreya [1-2]

आसीनं मुनिमव्यग्रं कृतजाप्यं कृतक्षणम्|
पृष्ट्वानर्शसां युक्तमग्निवेशः पुनर्वसुम्||३||

To Punarvasu, who was seated without any anxiety after completing his religious and secular duties, Agnivesha inquired about various aspects of Arshas (haemorrhoids) [3]

Topics covered in this chapter:
प्रकोप हेतुं संस्थानं स्थानं लिङ्गं चिकित्सितम्|
साध्यासाध्य विभागं च तस्मै तन्मुनिरब्रवीत्||४||

Lord Punarvasu explained to Agnivesha, the following topics relating to Arsa:

1. Causative and aggravating factors
2. Different forms (Samsthana)
3. The places of manifestation
4. Signs and symptoms
5. Treatment and
6. Classification of the disease depending upon its curability and incurability [4]

Classification
इह खल्वग्निवेश! द्विविधान्यर्शांसि- कानिचित् सहजानि, कानिचिज्जातस्योत्तरकालजानि|
तत्र बीजं गुदवलि बीजोप तप्तमायतनमर्शसां सहजानाम्|
तत्र द्विविधो बीजोपतप्तौ हेतुः- मातापित्रोरपचारः, पूर्वकृतं च कर्म; तथाऽन्येषामपि सहजानां विकाराणाम्|
तत्र सहजानि सह जातानि शरीरेण, अर्शांसीत्यधिमांसविकाराः||५||

Types of hemorrhoids as per Ayurveda:

O Agnivesha! Piles are of 2 types;

Sahaja Arsas – congenital or hereditary

Jatasya Uttara Kalaja Arsas – acquired which are manifested after birth.

Sahaja Arsha – Congenital Piles:

Caused by vitiation of seeds (sperm and ovum), specially the part of the seed responsible for the formation of the anal sphincters,

The cause for Sahaja Arshas are –

(i) wrong diet and regimen of father and mother, and

(ii) Sinful acts of past life.

These two categories of causative factors are applicable to all the other hereditary diseases also.

Sahaja means which is manifested (Jata) along with (Saha) the appearance of body (birth)

Arshas is a disease characterized by Adhimamsa Vikara – morbid growth in the muscle tissue [5]

Locations of Piles – Utpatti Kshetra:

सर्वेषां चार्शसां क्षेत्रं- गुदस्यार्ध पञ्चमाङ्गुलावकाशे त्रिभागान्तरास्तिस्रो गुदवलयः क्षेत्रमिति; केचित्तु भूयांसमेव देशमुपदिशन्त्यर्शसां-शिश्नमपत्यपथं गल तालु मुख नासिका कर्णाक्षि वर्त्मानि त्वक् चेति।

तदस्त्यधि मांस देशतया, गुदवलिजानां त्वर्शांसीति सञ्ज्ञा तन्त्रेऽस्मिन्।

Locations of Piles

All types of piles are located in the space of 4 ½ Angulas (8-10 cm. approx) in the lower part of the colon. This area has 3 sphincters dividing the space into 3 parts- Guda valaya.

According to some other physicians, Arshas has several other locations in the body, like pudendum, female genital tract, throat, palate, mouth, nose, ears, eyelids and skins because in the above mentioned locations, excessive and unnatural growth of the muscle tissue also take place. However, in the present text, those occurring in the anal region are specifically considered as Arshas.

Arsha Adhishtana: Tissues involved:

सर्वेषां चार्शसामधिष्ठानं- मेदो मांसं त्वक् च||६||

Adhishtana – tissues involved in Arsham are –

Medas – fat tissue

Mamsa – muscle tissue and

Tvak – skin including mucous membrane [6]

Forms and structures of Congenital Piles

तत्र सहजान्यर्शांसि कानिचिदणूनि, कानिचिन्महान्ति, कानिचिद्दीर्घाणि, कानिचिद्ध्रस्वानि, कानिचिद्वृतानि, कानिचिद्विषमविसृतानि, कानिचिदन्तःकुटिलानि, कानिचिद्बहिःकुटिलानि, कानिचिज्जटिलानि, कानिचिदन्तर्मुखानि, यथास्वं दोषानुबन्धवर्णानि||७||

Among the congenital piles, some are small, some are large, some are long, some are short, some are round, some are irregularly spread, some are curved internally, some are curved externally, some are matted together, and some are introverted. Their characteristic colours are based on Dosha aggravation. [7]

Signs and symptoms of Congenital Piles

तैरुपहतो जन्म प्रभृति भवत्यतिकृशो विवर्णः क्षामो दीनः प्रचुर विबद्ध वात मूत्र पुरीषः शर्कराश्मरीमान्, तथाऽनियतविबद्धमुक्तपक्वामशुष्कभिन्नवर्चा अन्तरान्तरा श्वेत पाण्डु हरित पीत रक्तारुण तनु सान्द्र पिच्छिल कुणपगन्ध्याम पुरीषोपवेशी, नाभि बस्ति वङ्क्षणोद्देश प्रचुर परिकर्तिकान्वितः, सगुदशूल प्रवाहिका परिहर्ष प्रमेह प्रसक्त विष्टम्भान्त्रकूजोदावर्त हृदयेन्द्रियोपलेपः प्रचुर विबद्ध तिक्ताम्लोद्गारः, सुदुर्बलः, सुदुर्बलाग्निः, अल्पशुक्रः, क्रोधनो, दुःखोपचारशीलः, कास श्वास तमक तृष्णा हल्लास च्छर्द्यरोचका विपाक पीनस क्षवथु परीतः, तैमिरिकः, शिरःशूली, क्षामभिन्नसन्नसक्तजर्जरस्वरः, कर्णरोगी, शून पाणिपाद वदनाक्षिकूटः, सज्वरः, साङ्गमर्दः, सर्व पर्वास्थि शूली च, अन्तरान्तरा पार्श्व कुक्षि बस्ति हृदय पृष्ठ त्रिकग्रहोपतप्तः, प्रध्यानपरः, परमालसश्चेति; जन्म प्रभृत्यस्य गुदैरावृतो मार्गोपरोधाद्वायुरपानः प्रत्यारोहन् समानव्यानप्राणोदानान् पित्तश्लेष्माणौ च प्रकोपयति, एते सर्व एव प्रकुपिताः पञ्च वायवः पित्तश्लेष्माणौ चार्शसमभिद्रवन्त एतान् विकारानुपजनयन्ति; इत्युक्तानि सहजान्यर्शांसि||८||

Person afflicted with congenital piles has the following signs and symptoms

1. Right from birth, he is lean and thin, discoloured, emaciated, weak, having flatus, urine and stool in excessive quantities and sometimes having their obstruction, and having urinary gravels and stone in the urinary tract.

2. His stool is irregular- sometimes it is constipated and sometimes it is normal; sometimes it is Pakva (free from Ama) and sometimes it is associated with Ama (Mucus or products of improper digestion) and sometimes it is dry and sometimes it is loose;

3. His stool, at times, is white, pale yellow, green, yellow, red, reddish, thin, dense, slimy, having the smell of dead body and associated with Ama (Mucus or products of improper digestion)

4. He suffers severe type of sawing pain in umbilicus, urinary bladder region and pelvis

5. He suffers from pain in anus, dysentery, horripilation, Prameha (urinary disorders including diabetes), continuous constipation, gurgling sound in the intestine, abdominal distension and a feeling as if the heart and the sense organs are covered with sticky material. (Hrudaya Indriya Upalepa)

6. He gets excessive eructation, which are often obstructed and associated with bitter and sour taste

7. He is extremely weak and has very weak digestion strength, he has very little semen; he is irritable and he is difficult to treat.

8. He frequently gets cough, dyspnoea, asthma, morbid thirst, nausea, vomiting, anorexia, indigestion, chronic rhinitis and sneezing

9. He gets fits, fainting and headache

10. His voice is weak, broken, of low pitch, impeded and hoarse

11. He suffers from fever, Malaise and pain in all the joints and bones

12. Occasional chest stiffness, stiffness in the sides of the abdomen, region of urinary bladder, cardiac region, back and lumbar region

13. Dizziness and extremely lazy

14. Right from birth, his Apana Vayu gets obstructed by the piles- mass. Because of this obstruction to the passage, the Apana Vayu moves upwards and causes aggravation of Samana Vayu, Prana Vayu, Vyana Vayu, Pitta and Kapha. When all these 5 varieties of Vayu, pitta and Kapha get aggravated the individual succumbs to the above mentioned symptoms.

Thus ends the description of the congenital type of piles. [8]

Etiology and Pathogenesis of Acquired Piles:

अत ऊर्ध्वं जातस्योतरकालजानि व्याख्यास्यामः- गुरु मधुर शीताभिष्यन्दि विदाहि विरुद्धाजीर्ण प्रमिताशना सात्म्य भोजनाद्गव्य मात्स्य वाराह माहिष जाविक पिशित भक्षणात् कृश शुष्क पूतिमांस पैष्टिक परमान्न क्षीर दधि मण्ड तिलगुड विकृति सेवनान्माषयूषेक्षुरस पिण्याक पिण्डालुक शुष्क शाक- शुक्तल शुन किलाट तक्र पिण्डक बिस मृणाल शालूक क्रौञ्चादन कशेरुक शृङ्गाटकतरूट विरूढ नव शूक शमी- धान्याममूलकोपयोगाद्गुरु फल शाक राग हरितक मर्दक वसा शिरस्पद पर्युषित पूति शीत सङ्कीर्णान्नाभ्यवहारान्मन्द- कातिक्रान्त मद्यपानाद्व्यापन्न गुरु सलिलपानादति स्नेहपानादसंशोधनाद्बस्तिकर्म विभ्रमाद् व्यायामाद व्यवायादिदिवास्वप्नात् सुख शयनासन स्थान सेवनाच्चोपहताग्नेर्मलोपचयो भवत्यतिमात्रं, तथोत्कटक विषम कठिनासनसेवनादुद्भ्रान्तयानोष्ट्रयानादति व्यवायाद्बस्तिनेत्रा सम्यक्प्रणिधानाद्गुदक्षणनाद भीक्ष्णं शीताम्बु संस्पर्शाच्चेललोष्ट तृणादि घर्षणात् प्रततति निर्वाहणाद्वातमूत्रपुरीषवेगोदीरणात् समुदीर्ण वेग विनिग्रहात् स्त्रीणां चामगर्भभ्रंशाद्गर्भोत्पीडनादिविषमप्रसूतिभिश्च प्रकुपितो वायुरपानस्तं मलमुपचितमधोगमासाद्य गुदवलिष्वाधत्ते, ततस्तास्वर्शांसि प्रादुर्भवन्ति||९||

Hemorrhoids which occur after birth (acquired):

In a person whose power of digestion is afflicted, Mala (waste products) get accumulated in excess because of the following:

1. Intake of heavy, sweet, cold, Abhisyandi (which causes obstruction in the channels), Vidahi (causes burning sensation) and Viruddha (mutually contradictory) food; intake of food before the previous meal is digested; intake of small quantity of food and intake of unwholesome food.

2. Excess intake of flesh of cattle, fish, pig, buffalo, goat and sheep

3. Intake of the meat of emaciated animals, dried meat and spoilt milk; Excess intake of pastries, Paramanna or Payasa (a preparation of milk, rice and sugar), milk, Dadhimanda (whey) preparations of sesame seed and jaggery- products

4. Excess intake of Masha (black gram), sugarcane juice, oil cake, Pindaluka, dry vegetables, vinegar, garlic, Kilata (cream of milk), buttermilk, Pindaka (cream of curd), Bisa (thick lotus stalk), Mrinala (thin lotus Stalk), Shaluka,

Kraunchadana, Kasheruka (Scripus grossus), Sringataka, Taruta, germinated corns and pulses, freshly harvested corns and cereals and tender radish;

5. Intake of heavy fruits, vegetables, pickles, haritaka (vegetables used uncooked), Mardaka, Vasa (muscle fat), meat of head and legs of animals, stale, putrid and sankeerna anna (food prepared by the mixture of different items, like rice and meat)

6. Intake of Mandaka (immature, thick curds) and wrongly fermented alcohol preparations;

7. Drinking of polluted and heavy water

8. Excess intake of Sneha (oleation therapy)

9. Non-use of elimination of Basti Karma (enema therapy)

10. Wrong application of Basti Karma (enema therapy)

11. Lack of exercise

12. Avyavaya or Ativyavaya (lack of sexual act or excess of it)

13. Sleep during day time and

14. Habitually resorting to pleasant beds, seats and location

Following factors are responsible for the aggravation of Apana Vayu:

1. Use of rough, irregular and hard seats

2. Use of vehicles carried by improperly trained animals or vehicles carried by camels

3. Excessive indulgence in sex

4. Improper insertion of enema nozzle and frequent injury in the anal region

5. Frequent application of cold water

6. Use of rags, colds of grass etc, for rubbing [the anus]

7. Continuous and excessive straining during defecation

8. Forcible attempt for passing flatus, urine and stool

9. Suppression of manifested strain / urges

10. Miscarriage, pressure of the pregnant uterus and abnormal delivery in case of women

The Apana Vayu aggravated by the above-mentioned factors, brings down the accumulated waste products [reasons for their accumulations are already described above] and so afflict the anal sphincters. Because of this, piles are manifested in the sphincters. [9]

Different Shapes of the Piles

सर्षप मसूर माष मुद्गमकुष्ठ कयव कलाय पिण्डिटिण्टिकेर केबुक तिन्दुक कर्कन्धु काकणन्तिका बिम्बी बदर करीरोदुम्बर- खर्जूर जाम्बव गोस्तनाङ्गुष्ठ कशेरु शृङ्गाटक शृङ्गीदक्ष शिखि शुक्तुण्ड जिह्वा पद्ममुकुलकर्णिका संस्थानानि सामान्याद्वात पित्त कफ प्रबलानि॥१०॥

Piles have different shapes in as much as they look like mustard, Masura, Masha (black gram), Makustha – Phaseolus aconitifolius, Yava – Barley, Kalaya – green pea, Pindi, Tintikera (fruit of Karira), Kebuka, Tinduka, Karkandhu Kakanantika, Bimbi –Coccinia indica, Badara – (ber fruit), Kareera, Udumbara – Ficus racemosa, Kharjura- Phoenix sylvestris, Jambu (Jamun fruit), Gostana (cow's udder), Thumb, Kaseruka – Scripus grossus, Sringataka, Srungi, beaks or tongues of cock, peacock or parrot, and buds of lotus or Karnika(ra).

These are, in general the characteristic shapes of piles caused by excessive aggravation of vayu, Pitta and Kapha. [10]

Vataja Arshas – Signs and symptoms:

तेषामयं विशेषः- शुष्कम्लान कठिन परुष रूक्ष श्यावानि, तीक्ष्णाग्राणि, वक्राणि, स्फुटित मुखानि, विषम विसृतानि, शूलाक्षेपतोदस्फुरण चिमिचिमासंहर्ष परीतानि, स्निग्धोष्णोपशयानि, प्रवाहिका ध्मान शिशन वृषण बस्ति वङ्क्षण हृद्ग्रहाङ्गमर्द हृदय द्रव प्रबलानि, प्रतत विबद्ध वात मूत्र वर्चांसि, ऊरु कटी पृष्ठ त्रिक पार्श्व कुक्षि बस्ति शूल शिरोऽभिताप क्षवथूद्गार प्रतिश्याय कासोदावर्तायाम शोष शोथ- मूर्च्छारोचक मुखवैरस्य तैमिर्य कण्डू नासा कर्ण शङ्ख शूल स्वरोपघातकराणि, श्यावारुण परुष नख नयन वदन त्वङ्मूत्र पुरीषस्य वातोल्बणान्यर्शांसीति विद्यात्॥११॥

Piles caused by the predominance of aggravated Vata Dosha:

1. The mass of piles is dry, wrinkled, hard, rough and greyish in colour; these masses have sharp tips; curved, have

cracks, and spread irregularly.
2. The pile is associated with pain, cramps, Toda (Piercing pain), itching, numbness and tingling sensation in excess.
3. Oily and hot things give relief to the patient
4. The patient suffers from dysentery, abdominal distension and stiffness of genitals, testicles, the region of urinary bladder, pelvis and cardiac region; he also suffers from malaise and palpitation in excess.
5. His flatus, urine and stool are constantly obstructed – constipation and dysuria
6. He suffers from pain in thighs, lumbar region, back, Trika (Sacral region), Parshva (sides of the chest), Kukshi (sides of abdomen) and in the region of urinary bladder.
7. He has burning sensation in the heart; suffers from sneezing, coryza, cough, Udavarta, (upward movement of wind in the abdomen), Ayama, Ayasa, odema, fainting, anorexia, distaste in mouth Timira (impairment of vision) itching pain in the nose, ears and temporal region, and impairment of the voice and
8. Greyish colour, reddishness and roughness of nails, eyes, face, skin, urine and stool. [11]
Vataja Arsha Causes:

भवतश्चात्र-
कषाय कटु तिक्तानि रूक्ष शीत लघूनि च|
प्रमितल्पाशनं तीक्ष्ण मद्य मैथुन सेवनम्||१२||
लङ्घनं देशकालौ च शीतौ व्यायामकर्म च|
शोको वातातपस्पर्शो हेतुर्वातार्शसां मतः||१३||
Etiology of Vatik type of Piles:
1. Intake of astringent, pungent, bitter, un-unctuous, cold and light food
2. Habitual intake of food in extremely small quantities (Pramitashana) intake of less quantities of food, intake of alcoholic drinks having sharp quality and indulgence in sexual acts
3. Fasting, residing in cold climate, excess physical exercise and
4. Grief and exposure to sun and wind [12-13]

Pittaja Arsha Lakshana:
मृदु शिथिल सुकुमाराण्य स्पर्शसहानि, रक्त पीत नील कृष्णानि, स्वेदोपक्लेद बहुलानि, विस्र गन्धि तनु पीत रक्त स्राविणि, रुधिरवहानि, दाह कण्डू शूल निस्तोद पाकवन्ति, शीतोपशयानि, सम्भिन्नपीत हरित वर्चांसि, पीत विस्रगन्धि प्रचुर विण्मूत्राणि, पिपासा ज्वर तमक सम्मोह भोजन द्वेषकराणि पीत नख नयन त्वङ्मूत्र पुरीषस्य पित्तोल्बणान्यर्शांसीति विद्यात्||१४||
Signs and symptoms of Pittaja Arsh:
1. Pile mass is Mrudu – soft, Shithila – flabby, fragile, Sukumara -delicate and tender touch
2. Pile mass is Rakta – red, Pita – yellow, Neela – blue or Krishna – black in colour
3. The mass of piles is associated with Sveda upakleda – excessive sweating and sticky discharge
4. The discharges from the piles mass is Visra (smelling like raw- meat), thin, yellow or red
5. Blood discharge
6. Associated with burning sensation, itching colic pain, pricking pain and suppuration
7. There will be relief by resorting to cold things
8. The stool of the patient is loose yellow or green
9. Increased volume of urine and stool and these are yellow in colour and smell like raw meat
10. The individual suffers from excess thirst, fever Asthma, fainting and disliking for food
11. The Nails, eyes, skin urine and stool of the patient are yellow in colour [14]

Pittaja Arsha Nidana:
भवतश्चात्र-
कटूष्ण लवण क्षार व्यायामाग्न्यातप प्रभाः |
देश कालावशिशिरौ क्रोधो मद्यमसूयनम्||१५||

विदाहि तीक्ष्णमुष्णं च सर्वं पानान्नभेषजम्|
पित्तोल्बणानां विज्ञेयः प्रकोपे हेतुरर्शसाम्||१६||

Paittik piles is caused by the following:

1. Intake of pungent, hot, saline and alkaline food

2. Excercise in a place and season which are not cold

3. Intake of alcohol and envy, jealousy and

4. Intake of all types of drinks, food and drugs which are Vidahi (causing burning sensation), sharp and hot [15-16]

Kaphaja Arsha Lakshana:

तत्र यानि प्रमाणवन्ति, उपचितानि, श्लक्ष्णानि, स्पर्शसहानि, स्निग्ध श्वेत पाण्डु पिच्छिलानि, स्तब्धानि, गुरूणि, स्तिमितानि, सुप्त सुप्तानि, स्थिर श्वयथूनि, कण्डू बहुलानि, बहुप्रतत पिञ्जर श्वेतरक्त पिच्छा स्रावीणि, गुरु पिच्छिल श्वेत मूत्र पुरीषाणि, रूक्षोष्णोपशयानि, प्रवाहिकातिमात्रोत्थानवङ्क्षणानाहवन्ति, परिकर्तिका हृल्लास निष्ठीविका कासारोचक प्रतिश्याय गौरव च्छर्दि मूत्रकृच्छ्र शोष शोथ- पाण्डु रोग शीतज्वराश्मरी शर्करा हृदयेन्द्रियोपलेपास्य माधुर्य प्रमेहकराणि, दीर्घकालानुबन्धीनि, अतिमात्रमग्निमार्दव क्लैब्यकराणि, आम विकार प्रबलानि, शुक्ल नख नयन वदन त्वङ्मूत्रपुरीषस्य श्लेष्मोल्बणान्यर्शांसीति विद्यात्||१७||

Signs and symptoms of Kaphaja types of piles:

1. The mass of piles is large in size, swollen, smooth, painless to touch, unctuous, white, slimy, having stiffness, heavy, rigid, benumbed, having constant oedema with severe itching

2. Large and continuous discharge from the piles mass, reddish, white or red colour, slimy

3. Urine and stool of the patient are heavy, slimy and white

4. The disease gets alleviated by dry and hot therapies

5. The patient has excessive desire to pass stool with gurgling sound

6. There is distension in the lower pelvic region

7. The patient suffers from sawing pain, nausea, excessive spitting, cough, anorexia, cold, heaviness, vomiting, dysuria, consumption, oedema, anaemia, fever associated with cold, stone and gravels in genitourinary tract, feeling as if the heart and sense organs are covered with sticky material, sweet taste in the mouth and Prameha (urinary disorders including diabetes)

8. Symptoms are chronic

9. Low digestion strength, impotence

10. Associated with acute disease caused by Ama (product of improper digestion and metabolism)

11. The nails eyes, skin, urine and stool are white in colour. [17]

Kaphaja Arsha Nidana:

भवतश्चात्र-
मधुर स्निग्ध शीतानि लवणाम्ल गुरूणि च|
अव्यायामो दिवास्वप्नः शय्यासनसुखे रतिः||१८||
प्राग्वातसेवा शीतौ च देशकालावचिन्तनम्|
श्लैष्मिकाणां समुद्दिष्टमेतत् कारणमर्शसाम्||१९||

Causes for Kaphaja type of Arsha:

1. Intake of Madhura – Sweet, Snigdha – unctuous, Shita – cold, Lavana – saline, Amla – sour and Guru – heavy food, Avyayama – lack of exercise, Diva swapna – sleeping during day time and Shayyana sukha – indulgence in the pleasure of beds and seats

2. Prag vata sevana – Exposure to easterly wind

3. Shitau desha kala – Residing in cold place and cold season and

4. Achintanam – Mental inactivity [18-19]

Dwandwaja and Sannipataja Arsha – Piles caused by aggravations of 2 Doshas and all the 3 Doshas:

हेतु लक्षण संसर्गादिवद्याद्द्वन्द्वोल्बणानि च|

सर्वो हेतुस्त्रिदोषाणां सहजैर्लक्षणैः समम्||२०||

Dvandvolbana types of Arshas (in which 2 doshas are predominantly aggravated) are caused by the combination of 2 types of etiological factors. Here, a combination of symptoms of the two Doshas are exhibited.

In Sannipataja Arshas, all the three Doshas are aggravated. The symptoms resemble Sahaja Arsha symptoms that have been explained above. [20]

Arsha Poorvaroopa – Premonitory symptoms:

विष्टम्भोऽन्नस्य दौर्बल्यं कुक्षेराटोप एव च|
कार्श्यमुद्गारबाहुल्यं सक्थिसादोऽल्पविट्कता||२१||
ग्रहणीदोषपाण्डुवर्तेराशङ्का चोदरस्य च|
पूर्वरूपाणि निर्दिष्टान्यर्शसामभिवृद्धये||२२||

Premonitory symptoms:

Vistambha – constipation,

Daurbalya – weakness

Kukshi aatopa – gurgling sound in the lower abdomen

Karshya – emaciation

Bahula udgara – frequent eructation,

Sakti sada – weakness in the thighs,

Alpa vit kata – voiding less of stool,

Grahani – sprue syndrome, IBS

Pandu – anaemia,

Udara shanka – apprehension of the manifestation of Udara Roga (abdominal disorders including ascites) [21-22]

Involvement of 3 Doshas:

अर्शांसि खलु जायन्ते नासन्निपतितैस्त्रिभिः|
दोषैर्दोषविशेषात्तु विशेषः कल्प्यतेऽर्शसाम्||२३||

Piles never occur without the aggravation of all the 3 Doshas. It is because of the predominance of one or all the Doshas that different types of piles are determined. [23]

Reason for bad Prognosis:

पञ्चात्मा मारुतः पित्तं कफो गुदवलित्रयम्|
सर्व एव प्रकुप्यन्ति गुदजानां समुद्भवे||२४||
तस्मादर्शांसि दुःखानि बहुव्याधिकराणि च|
सर्वदेहोपतापीनि प्रायः कृच्छ्रतमानि च||२५||

5 kinds of Vayu (Prana, Apana, Vyana, Udana and Samana)

Pitta and Kapha- all these morbid factors in their aggravated form afflict the 3 anal sphincters, as a result of which piles are manifested. Therefore these piles are painful and are associated with several complications. They afflict the entire body, and generally, these are difficult to cure. [24-25]

Prognosis: Arsha Upashaya

हस्ते पादे मुखे नाभ्यां गुदे वृषणयोस्तथा|
शोथो हृत्पार्श्वशूलं च यस्यासाध्योऽर्शसो हि सः||२६||
हृत्पार्श्वशूलं सम्मोहश्छर्दिरङ्गस्य रुग् ज्वरः|
तृष्णा गुदस्य पाकश्च निहन्यर्गुदजातुरम्||२७||
सहजानि त्रिदोषाणि यानि चाभ्यन्तरां वलिम्|
जायन्तेऽर्शांसि संश्रित्य तान्यसाध्यानि निर्दिशेत्||२८||

शोषत्वादायुषस्तानि चतुष्पादसमन्विते|
याप्यन्ते दीप्तकायाग्नेः प्रत्याख्येयान्यतोऽन्यथा||२९||
द्वन्द्वजानि द्विताीयायां वलौ यान्याश्रितानि च|
कृच्छ्रसाध्यानि तान्याहुः परिसंवत्सराणि च||३०||
बाह्यायां तु वलौ जातान्येकदोषोल्बणानि च|
अर्शांसि सुखसाध्यानि न चिरोत्पाततानि च||३१||
तेषां प्रशमने यत्नमाशु कुर्यादिवचक्षणः|
तान्याशु हि गुदं बद्ध्वा कुर्युर्बद्धगुदोदरम्||३२||

Prognosis of Arshas:

If the patient suffering from piles develops oedema in hands, legs, face, umbilicus, anus and testicles, and if he suffers from pain in cardiac region and in the sides of the chest, then he is incurable.

Pain in the cardiac region and sides of the chest, fainting, vomiting, pain in the limbs, fever, excess thirst and inflammation of the anus- these complications lead to the death of the patient suffering from piles.

Hereditary piles caused by the simultaneous aggravation of all the three Doshas and piles located in the internal sphincter of the anus is incurable.

Considering residual life span, the piles may become palliative (Yapya) if all the four constituents of treatment (physician, drugs, attendants and patient) are in the state of their excellence and if the patient has strong Kayagni (powder of digestion and metabolism). Otherwise, such patient should not be entertained because they are incurable.

Kashta Sadhya: If piles are caused by the simultaneous vitiation of 2 Doshas (Dwandwaja), if they are located in second anal- sphincter and if these are one year old, then such patients are difficult of cure – Kashta Sadhya

Sukha Sadhya: If piles are located in the external anal sphincter, if they are caused by the dominance of one aggravated Dosha, and if they are not very chronic, then such a patient is easily curable. A wise physician should immediately take necessary steps for the cure of such patients. Otherwise, the piles mass will cause obstruction in the passage of the rectum. [25- 32]

Indication of Shastra, Kshara and Agnikarma:

तत्राहुरेके शस्त्रेण कर्तनं हितमर्शसाम्|
दाहं क्षारेण चाप्येके, दाहमेके तथाऽग्निना||३३||
अस्त्येतद्भूरितन्त्रेण धीमता दृष्टकर्मणा|
क्रियते त्रिविधं कर्म भ्रंशस्तत्र सुदारुणः||३४||
पुंस्त्वोपघातः श्वयथुर्गुदे वेगविनिग्रहः|
आध्मानं दारुणं शूलं व्यथा रक्तातिवर्तनम्||३५||
पुनर्विरोहो रूढानां क्लेदो भ्रंशो गुदस्य च|
मरणं वा भवेच्छीघ्रं शस्त्रक्षाराग्निविभ्रमात्||३६||
यत्तु कर्म सुखोपायमल्पभ्रंशमदारुणम्|
तदर्शसां प्रवक्ष्यामि समूलानां विवृत्तये||३७||

Indication of Shastra, Kshara and Agnikarma:

Some physicians advocate surgical excision of pile mass as a useful therapy. Some others recommended cauterization (Agnikarma) and some – application of alkalies (Kshara);

These 3 types of therapies are administered only by a physician who is wise and who has previous experience of performing such surgical operations. If there is any mistake in these operative processes, then the consequences can be serious.

Complications of Shastra, Kshara and AgniKarma:

Pumsatvahara – Impotency,

Shvayathu – swelling in the anus,

Vega vinigraha – lack of urge for defecation,

Adhamanam – abdominal distension

Shoolam – excruciating pain,

Vyatha – feeling of discomfort

Rakta ati vartanam – excessive bleeding,

Punar viho vruddhanam – recurrence of the piles mass after these are healed, sticky discharge,

Guda bhramsha – prolapse of the rectum or

Maranam – even instant death.

Hence, alternative methods are explained below[33-37]

Classification of Piles

वातश्लेष्मोल्बणान्याहुः शुष्काण्यशांसि तद्विदः।
प्रस्रावीणि तथाऽऽर्द्राणि रक्तपित्तोल्बणानि च॥३८॥

Piles are broadly classified into 2 groups, namely

(i) dry piles, which are caused by predominance of aggravated Vayu and Kapha, and

(ii) Exudation or wet piles, which are caused by predominance of aggravated Rakta (blood) and Pitta. [38]

Treatment of Dry Piles:

तत्र शुष्कार्शसां पूर्वं प्रवक्ष्यामि चिकित्सितम्।

Swedana Yogas:

स्तब्धानि स्वेदयेत् पूर्वं शोफशूलान्वितानि च॥३९॥
चित्रक क्षार बिल्वानां तैलेनाभ्यज्य बुद्धिमान्।
यव माष कुलत्थानां पुलाकानां च पोट्टलैः॥४०॥
गोखराश्वशकृत्पिण्डैस्तिलकल्कैस्तुषैस्तथा।
वचाशताह्वापिण्डैर्वा सुखोष्णैः स्नेहसंयुतैः॥४१॥
शक्तूनां पिण्डिकाभिर्वा स्निग्धानां तैलसर्पिषा।
शुष्कमूलकपिण्डैर्वा पिण्डैर्वा कार्ष्णगन्धिकैः॥४२॥
रास्नापिण्डैः सुखोष्णैर्वा सस्नेहैर्हाषुषैरपि।
इष्टकस्य खराह्वायाः शाकैर्गृञ्जनकस्य वा॥४३॥
अभ्यज्य कुष्ठतैलेन स्वेदयेत् पोट्टलीकृतैः।

Swedana for Arsha:

If there is numbness, oedema and pain in the piles, then first of all, the mass is smeared with oil prepared by boiling with Chitraka – Leadword – Plumbago zeylanica, Kshara and Bilva – Aegle marmelos.

Thereafter, Swedana (sweating) therapy is administered with below methods.

1. Pottali (medicines tied in a piece of clothing in the form of a bolus) containing Yava – Barley, Black gram, Horse gram and Pulaka (Tuccha dhanya).

2. Pinda (lump) containing the dung of cow, donkey or horse:

3. Pinda (Lump) prepared of the cake of the sesame seed

4. Pinda (Lump) of Vacha (Acorus calamus Linn.) and Shatahva

5. Pinda (Lump) containing husk of Paddy

The above-mentioned recipes of Pottali and Pindas are tolerably warm and should are added with fat.

6. Pinda (Lump) containing the pulp of dry radish

7. Pinda (Lump) containing Saktu (Roasted corn flour) added with unctuous substances, like oil and ghee

8. Pinda (Lump) containing Krsnagandha (sobhanjana)

9. Pinda (Lump) containing Rasna (Vanda roxburghi / Pluchea lanceolata)

10. Pinda (Lump) containing Hapusha

The above mentioned recipes (nos. 6 – 10) should be luke-warm and is added with fat.

11. The piles mass should be smeared with oil prepared by boiling with Kushta – Saussurea lappa. Thereafter, it is

fomented. With the help of a Pottali (medicines tied in a piece of cloth in the form of a bolus) containing brick powder, Kharahva (Ajamoda – Ajowan (fruit) – Trachyspermum roxburghianum) and the pulp of Grunjanaka. [39 ½ – 44½]

Recipe for Sprinkling – Sechana

वृषार्कैरण्डबिल्वानां पत्रोत्क्वाथैश्च सेचयेत्||४४||

The piles mass is sprinkled with decoction of the leaves of Vrusha, Arka – Calotropis gigantea, Castor and Bilva. [44 ½]

Recipes for Bath:

मूलक त्रिफलार्काणां वेणूनां वरुणस्य च|
अग्निमन्थस्य शिग्रोश्च पत्राण्यश्मन्तकस्य च||४५||
जलेनोत्क्वाथ्य शूलार्तं स्वभ्यक्तमवगाहयेत्|
कोलोत्क्वाथेऽथवा कोष्णे सौवीरक तुषोदके||४६||
बिल्वक्वाथेऽथवा तक्रे दधिमण्डाम्लकाञ्जिके|
गोमूत्रे वा सुखोष्णे तं स्वभ्यक्तमवगाहयेत्||४७||

If there is pain in piles mass, then it is well smeared with medicated oil and the patient is given sitz- bath with the help of decoction prepared by boiling with leaves of Radish, triphala (Haritaki, Bibhitaki, and Amalki), Arka – Calotropis gigantea, Venu, Varuna (Crataeva nurvala), Agnimantha – Clerodendrum phlomidis, Shigru – Moringa oliefera and Ashmantaka

The patient can also be given a sitz bath with the decoction of Kola (ber) or Sauviraka or Tushodaka or decoction of Bilva or butter milk or Dadhimanda (Whey) or Sour kanjika or cow's urine. Before giving a sitz bath, the piles mass is well smeared with medicated oil, and the decoction should be tolerably warm. [45-47]

Abhyanga and Dhoopana – Smearing and Fumigation:

कृष्ण सर्प वराहोष्ट्र जतुकावृषदंशजाम्|
वसामभ्यञ्जने दद्याद्धूपनं चार्शसां हितम्||४८||
नृकेशाः सर्पनिर्मोको वृषदंशस्य चर्म च|
अर्कमूलं शमीपत्रमर्शोभ्यो धूपनं हितम्||४९||
तुम्बुरूणि विडङ्गानि देवदार्वक्षता घृतम्|
बृहती चाश्वगन्धा च पिप्पल्यः सुरसा घृतम्||५०||
वराहवृषविट् चैव धूपनं सक्तवो घृतम्|
कुञ्जरस्य पुरीषं तु घृतं सर्जरसस्तथा||५१||

Abhyanga and Dhoopana – Smearing and Fumigation:

The fat of Krisna Sarpa (black snake), pig, camel, Jatuki (Carma Catika) and cat is smeared over piles mass. These fats are used for fumigation of piles also.

Fumigation with human hair, serpent's slough, cat's skin, root of Arka – Calotropis gigantea and leaf of Shami is useful for piles.

Fumigation is given with Tumburu—Zanthoxylum alatum, Vidanga – Embelia ribes, Devadaru – Cedrus deodara and Aksata (Barley) mixed with ghee.

Brihati – Solanum indicum, Ashwagandha – Withania somnifera, Pippali – Long pepper fruit and Surasa (Tulsi) mixed with ghee is used for fumigation.

Dung of pig or goat, Saktu (roasted corn- flour) and ghee is used for fumigation.

Fumigation with the dung of elephant mixed with ghee and Sarjarasa is also useful for piles. [48-51]

Recipes for Ointment:

हरिद्रा चूर्ण संयुक्तं सुधा क्षीरं प्रलेपनम्|
गोपित्त पिष्टाः पिप्पल्यः सहरिद्राः प्रलेपनम्||५२||
शिरीष बीजं कुष्ठं च पिप्पल्यः सैन्धवं गुडः|
अर्क क्षीरं सुधा क्षीरं त्रिफला च प्रलेपनम्||५३||
पिप्पल्यश्चित्रकः श्यामा किण्वं मदन तण्डुलाः|
प्रलेपः कुक्कुट शकृद्धरिद्रा गुडसंयुतः||५४||
दन्ती श्यामाऽमृतासङ्गः पारावतशकृद्गुडः|
प्रलेपः स्याद्गजास्थीनि निम्बो भल्लातकानि च||५५||
प्रलेपः स्यादलं कोष्णं वासन्तकवसायुतम्|
शूलश्वयथुहृद्युक्तं चुलूकीवसयाऽथवा||५६||
आर्क पयः सुधाकाण्डं कटुकालाबुपल्लवाः|
करञ्जो बस्तमूत्रं च लेपनं श्रेष्ठमर्शसाम्||५७||

Ointment recipes:

The following recipes are used as ointments in the treatment of piles:

1. Latex of Snuhi – Euphorbia nerifolia mixed with the powder of turmeric

2. Fruits of long pepper and turmeric made to a paste by adding cow's bile

3. Paste prepared of the seeds of Sirisha, Kushta – Saussurea lappa, Pippali – Long pepper fruit – Piper longum, Saindhava, Jaggery, latex of Arka – Calotropis gigantea and Snuhi – Euphorbia neriifolia and Triphala (Haritaki – Terminalia chebula, Bibhitaka – Terminalia bellerica and Amalaka – Embelica officinalis)

4. Paste prepared of Pippali – Long pepper fruit – Piper longum, Chitraka – Leadword – Plumbago zeylanica, Syamaka, Kinva (yeast), fruit Pulp of Madana – Randia dumetorum, droppings of cock, turmeric and jaggery

5. Paste of Danti – Baliospermum montanum, Shyama (Trivrit), Mrutasanga (Mayuratuttha – Copper sulphate) droppings of pigeon and jaggery

6. Paste prepared of elephant bone, Nimba – Neem (Azadirachta indica) and Bhallataka – Semecarpus anacardium.

7. Paste prepared of Ala (Haritala) mixed with the fat of camel or the fat of Culuki is applied lukewarm. It cures pain and oedema in the piles mass and

8. Paste of the latex of Arka, stem of Snuhi – Euphorbia neriifolia , leaf of bitter variety of Alabu, and urine of goat is excellent for curing piles. [52-57]

अभ्यङ्गाद्याः प्रदेहान्ता य एते परिकीर्तिताः|
स्तम्भ श्वयथु कण्डुवर्ति शमनास्तेऽर्शसां मताः||५८||

All the recipes enumerated above beginning with Abhyanga (recipes for smearing) and ending with Pradeha (recipes for preparing ointment) are useful for curing piles associated with stiffness, odema, itching and pain. [58]

प्रदेहान्तैरुपक्रान्तान्यर्शांसि प्रस्रवन्ति हि|
सञ्चितं दुष्टरुधिरं ततः सम्पद्यते सुखी||५९||

By the application of the above recipes the vitiated blood which is accumulated in the pile mass oozes out which gives relief to the patient [59]

Raktamokshana – Bloodletting:

शीतोष्णा स्निग्ध रूक्षैर्हि न व्याधि रुपशाम्यति|
रक्ते दुष्टे भिषक् तस्माद्रक्तमेवावसेचयेत्||६०||
जलौकोभिस्तथा शस्त्रैः सूचीभिर्वा पुनः पुनः|
अवर्तमानं रुधिरं रक्तार्शोभ्यः प्रवाहयेत्||६१||

If the disease doesn't subside by the application of cold, hot and oily recipes, then it is determined to be caused by vitiated blood. To such patients, Raktamokshana therapy is administered.

In the case of Raktaja type of piles, if blood doesn't come out on its own, then it is taken out by the repeated leech therapy or sharp edged instruments or needles. [60-61]

Trayushanadi Curna:

गुद श्वयथु शूलार्तं मन्दाग्निं पाययेत्तु तम्।
त्र्यूषणं पिप्पलीमूलं पाठां हिङ्गु सचित्रकम्॥६२॥
सौवर्चलं पुष्कराख्यमजाजीं बिल्वपेषिकाम्।
बिडं यवानीं हपुषां विडङ्गं सैन्धवं वचाम्॥६३॥
तिन्तिडीकं च मण्डेन मद्येनोष्णोदकेन वा।
तथाऽर्शोग्रहणीदोषशूलानाहादिमुच्यते॥६४॥
पाचनं पाययेद्वा तद्यदुक्तं ह्यातिसारिके।

If the patient suffers from oedema and pain in the anus, and if there is suppression of the power of the digestion, then he is given Trayushanadi Churna –

powder of Tryusana (Ginger, pepper and long pepper fruit), Pippali Mula, Patha – Cyclea peltata, Hingu – Asafoetida, Chitraka – Leadword – Plumbago zeylanica, Sauvarcala, Puskara – Inula racemosa, Ajaji – Nigella sativa, Pulp of Bilva – Aegle marmelos, Bida, Yavani – Carum copticum, Hapusa, Vidanga – Embelia ribes, Saindhava, Vacha (Acorus calamus Linn.) and Tintidika along with heavy, alcoholic drinks or hot water.

This recipe also cures piles, Grahani (Sprue syndrome), colic pain and Anaha (constipation).

The above mentioned patient can also be given recipes for Pachana (which help in the digestion of undigested food), which are described for the treatment of Atisara (Diarrhoea) in Chikitsa 19th chapter [62- 65½]

Recipes:

सगुडामभयां वाऽपि प्राशयेत् पौर्वभक्तिकीम्॥६५॥
पाययेद्वा त्रिवृच्चूर्णं त्रिफलारससंयुतम्।
हृते गुदाश्रये दोषे गच्छन्त्यर्शांसि सङ्क्षयम्॥६६॥
गोमूत्राध्युषितां दद्यात् सगुडां वा हरीतकीम्।
हरीतकीं तक्रयुतां त्रिफलां वा प्रयोजयेत्॥६७॥
सनागरं चित्रकं वा सीधुयुक्तं प्रयोजयेत्।
दापयेच्चव्ययुक्तं वा सीधुं साजाजिचित्रकम्॥६८॥
सुरां सहपुषापाठां दद्यात् सौवर्चलान्विताम्।
दधित्थ बिल्व संयुक्तं युक्तं वा चव्यचित्रकैः॥६९॥
भल्लातक युतं वाऽपि प्रदद्यात्क्रतर्पणम्।
बिल्व नागर युक्तं वा यवान्या चित्रकेण च॥७०॥
चित्रकं हपुषां हिङ्गुं दद्याद्वा तक्रसंयुतम्।
पञ्चकोल युतं वाऽपि तक्रमस्मै प्रदापयेत्॥७१॥

The patient of piles is given following recipes

1. Abhaya along with Jaggery is given before taking food

2. Powder of Trivrt along with decoction of Triphala (Haritaki, Bibhitaki and Amalaka)

With the above mentioned two recipes, the accumulated Doshas [in the anal region get eliminated as a result of which piles subside]

3. Haritaki – Terminalia chebula soaked overnight. It is given along with Jaggery

4. Haritaki along with buttermilk

5. Triphala (Haritaki, Vibhitaki and Amalaki) along with buttermilk

6. Chitraka – Plumbago zeylanica and Nagara – Zingiber officinale along with Sidhu (a type of alcoholic drink)

7. Ajaji – Nigella sativa, Chitraka – Leadword – Plumbago zeylanica and Chavya – Piper retrofractum along with Sidhu (a type of alcoholic drink)

8. Sura (a type of alcoholic drink) added with Hapusa – Juniperus communis and Patha –Cyclea peltata mixed with Sauvarcala salt.

9. Taphana (refreshing drink prepared of roasted corn- flour) mixed with butter-milk and added with either Kapitha and Bilva – Aegle marmelos or Chavya – Piper retrofractum and Chitraka – Leadword – Plumbago zeylanica or Bhallataka (Semecarpus anacardium Linn.) or Bilva – Aegle marmelos and Nagara or Chitraka – Leadword – Plumbago zeylanica

10. Chitraka – Plumbago zeylanica , Hapusa – Juniperus communis and Hingu mixed Butter- milk and

11. Butter added with Panchakola (Sunthi – Zingiber officinale, Pippali – Long pepper fruit – Piper longum, Pippali – Long pepper fruit – Piper longum Mula, Chavya – Piper retrofractum and Chitraka – Plumbago zeylanica. [65 ½ – 71]

Takrarista:

हपुषां कुञ्चिकां धान्यमजाजीं कारवीं शटीम्।
पिप्पलीं पिप्पलीमूलं चित्रकं हस्तिपिप्पलीम्॥७२॥
यवानीं चाजमोदां च चूर्णितं तक्रसंयुतम्।
मन्दाम्लकटुकं विद्वान् स्थापयेद्धृतभाजने॥७३॥
व्यक्ताम्लकटुकं जातं तक्रारिष्टं मुखप्रियम्।
प्रपिबेन्मात्रया कालेष्वन्नस्य तृषितस्त्रिषु॥७४॥
दीपनं रोचनं वर्ण्यं कफवातानुलोमनम्।
गुद श्वयथु कण्डुवर्तिनाशनं बलवर्धनम्॥७५॥
इति तक्रारिष्टः।

In a jar, the inside wall of which is smeared with ghee, butter- milk is kept. To this, the powder of Hapusa –Juniperus communis, Kuncika, Dhanya, Ajaji – Nigella sativa, Karavi, Shati – Hedychium spicatum, Pippali – Long pepper fruit – Piper longum, mula Chitraka – Leadword – Plumbago zeylanica, Gajapippali, Yavani and Ajamoda – Ajowan (fruit) – Trachyspermum roxburghianum is added.

The paste of the ingredients to keep in jar will be slightly sour and pungent. When it is well fermented, the sour and pungent tastes become well manifested. This is called Takararista, which is very delicious. This drink is taken in appropriate doses during the beginning, middle and end of meals, to overcome thirst.

It stimulates digestion, improves appetite for food, promotes complexion, helps in downward movement of Kapha and Vayu, cures swelling, itching and pain in anus and promotes strength. [72-75]

Buttermilk for haemorrhoids:

त्वचं चित्रक मूलस्य पिष्ट्वा कुम्भं प्रलेपयेत्।
तक्रं वा दधि वा तत्र जातमर्शोहरं पिबेत्॥७६॥
वातश्लेष्मार्शसां तक्रात् परं नास्तीह भेषजम्।
तत् प्रयोज्यं यथादोषं सस्नेहं रूक्षमेव वा॥७७॥
सप्ताहं वा दशाहं वा पक्षं मासमथापि वा।
बलकालविशेषज्ञो भिषक् तक्र प्रयोजयेत्॥७८॥
अत्यर्थमृदुकायाग्नेस्तक्रमेवावचारयेत्।
सायं वा लाजशक्तूनां दद्यात्तक्रावलेहिकाम्॥७९॥
जीर्णे तक्रे प्रदद्याद्वा तक्रपेयां ससैन्धवाम्।
तक्रानुपानं सस्नेहं तक्रौदनमतः परम्॥८०॥
यूषैर्मांसरसैर्वाऽपि भोजयेत्तक्रसंयुतैः।
यूषै रसेन वाऽप्यूर्ध्वं तक्रसिद्धेन भोजयेत्॥८१॥
कालक्रमज्ञः सहसा न च तक्रं निवर्तयेत्।
तक्रप्रयोगो मासान्तः क्रमेणोपरमो हितः॥८२॥

अपकर्षो यथोत्कर्षो न त्वन्नादपकृष्यते|
शक्त्यागमनरक्षार्थं दाढ्यर्थमनलस्य च||८३||
बलोपचयवर्णार्थमेष निर्दिश्यते क्रमः|
रूक्षमर्धोद्धृतस्नेहं यतश्चानुद्धृतं घृतम्||८४||
तक्रं दोषाग्निबलवित्त्रिविधं तत् प्रयोजयेत्|
हतानि न विरोहन्ति तक्रेण गुदजानि तु||८५||
भूमावपि निषिक्तं तद्दहेतक्रं तृणोलुपम्|
किं पुनर्दीप्तकायाग्नेः शुष्काण्यर्शांसि देहिनः||८६||
स्रोतःसु तक्रशुद्धेषु रसः सम्यगुपैति यः|
तेन पुष्टिर्बलं वर्णः प्रहर्षश्चोपजायते||८७||
वातश्लेष्मविकाराणां शतं चापि निवर्तते|
नास्ति तक्रात् परं किञ्चिदौषधं कफवातजे||८८||

The inside wall of an earthen jar is smeared with the paste of the root bark of Chitraka – Plumbago zeylanica, and in this Jar, curd is prepared. Intake of this curd or the butter milk prepared out of it cures piles.

There is no medicine better than butter-milk for the cure of piles caused by the predominance of aggravated Vayu and kapha depending upon the Dosha involved, it is taken along with fat (for Vayu) or in an unctuous form (for Kapha).

The physician, acquainted with the specifications of the strength of the patient as well as the nature of the season is given butter-milk for either one week or for 10 days or for 15 days or for a month.

If the Kayagni (power of digestion and metabolism) of the patient is very weak, then he is given only butter- milk [both morning and evening], other- wise Takravalehika (linctus prepared by adding butter- milk to the flour of fried paddy) is given in the evening. After the butter- milk (taken in the morning) is digested, [in the evening] the patient is given Takrapeya (thin gruel prepared by adding butter-milk) along with rock- salt, thereafter, Takraudana (rice mixed with butter-milk) added with fat is given and butter-milk is given to such a patient as post-prandial drink. As food, he may be given vegetable soup or meat soup along with butter-milk. Alternatively, vegetable soup and meat soup prepared by boiling with butter-milk can be given to him.

The physician acquainted with the time (Kala) and procedure of administration (Krama) of buttermilk should take care that consumption of buttermilk should not be discontinued all of a sudden.

Butter milk is administered for up to 1 month, and thereafter, it is gradually withdrawn. It is withdrawn gradually in the same quantity in which it was increased [in the beginning].

While reducing butter- milk, the patient's total food intake is reduced. Adoption of this procedure will promote and maintain his energy, maintain the strength of his digestive power and promote his strength, plumpness as well as completion.

Butter-milk is of 3 types. Viz

1) From which fat is completely removed

2) From which half of the fat is removed and

3) From which fat is not at all removed.

The physician acquainted with the nature of the Doshas involved in the causation of the disease, Agni (power of digestion and metabolism) of the patient and his strength should administer any of the above mentioned 3 types of butter – milk appropriately.

Piles in the anus, once cured by the administration of butter- milk, do not recur. When sprinkled over the ground, butter- milk burns all grass thereon let alone the dry type of piles in a patient whose Agni (power of digestion and metabolism) has been kindled through this therapy.

Butter- milk cleans the channels of circulation as a result of which Rasa (end product of the food after digestion) reaches [the tissue elements] appropriately. This produces proper nourishment, strength, completion and exhilaration, and cures 100 diseases including those caused by Vayu (80 in number) and Kapha (20 in number).

There is no medicine better than butter- milk, for the treatment of piles caused by Vayu and Kapha. [76- 88]

Recipes:

पिप्पलीं पिप्पलीमूलं चित्रकं हस्तिपिप्पलीम्|
शृङ्गवेरमजाजीं च कारवीं धान्यतुम्बुरु||८९||
बिल्वं कर्कटकं पाठां पिष्ट्वा पेयां विपाचयेत्|
फलाम्लां यमकैर्भृष्टां तां दद्याद्गुदजापहाम्||९०||
एतैश्चैव खडान् कुर्यादेतैश्च विपचेज्जलम्|
एतैश्चैव घृतं साध्यमर्शसां विनिवृत्तये||९१||

Peya (thin gruel) is prepared by cooking with Pippali – Long pepper fruit – Piper longum, Pippali Moola, Chitraka – Plumbago zeylanica, Gaja Pippali, Srngavera, Ajaji – Nigella sativa, Karavi, Dhanya, Tumburu – Zanthoxylum alatum, Bilva (unripe fruit), Karkataka and Patha – Cyclea peltata.

It is made sour by adding [the juice of] sour fruits and sizzled with ghee and oil. Intake of this Peya (thin gruel) cures piles.

With the above mentioned ingredients, Khada (a type of sour drink) is prepared and given to the patient. Water boiled with the above mentioned ingredients is useful for the patient suffering from piles. Ghee boiled with the above ingredients is also useful in curing piles [89-91]

Yavagu (thick Gruel):

शटी पलाश सिद्धां वा पिप्पल्या नागरेण वा|
दद्याद्यवागूं तक्राम्लां मरिचैरवचूर्णिताम्||९२||

Yavagu (thick gruel) is prepared by boiling with either Shati – Hedychium spicatum or Palasha – Butea monosperma or Pippali – Piper longum and Nagara – Zingiber officinale, made sour by adding buttermilk and sprinkled with the powder of Maricha – Piper nigrum is useful for the patient suffering from piles. [92]

Yusha (Vegetable soup):

शुष्क मूलक यूषं वा यूषं कौलत्थमेव वा|
दधित्थ बिल्व यूषं वा सकुलत्थमकुष्ठकम्||९३||
छागलं वा रसं दद्याद्यूषैरेभिर्विमिश्रितम्|
लावादीनां फलाम्लं वा सतक्रं ग्राहिभिर्युतम्||९४||
रक्तशालिर्महाशालिः कलमो लाङ्गलः सितः|
शारदः षष्टिकश्चैव स्यादन्नविधिरर्शसाम्||९५||
इत्युक्तो भिन्नशकृतामर्शसां च क्रियाक्रमः||९६|

Vegetable soup prepared of dried radish or horse gram or Kapittha, Bilva – Aegle marmelos, horse gram and Makustha is useful for piles. This soup can be added with goat-meat soup. The soup of the meat of lava etc. added with the juice of sour fruit, butter milk or astringent drugs is given to such a patient.

Rakta Sali, Maha Sali, Kalama, Langala, Sita, Sarada and Sustika types of rice can be given as food to the patient suffering from piles.

Thus, the therapeutic measures for the patients of piles having loose motions are described. [93-96 1/2]

Treatment of piles with bulky Bowels:

येऽत्यर्थं गाढशकृतस्तेषां वक्ष्यामि भेषजम्||९६||
सस्नेहैः शक्तुभिर्युक्तां प्रसन्नां लवणी कृताम्|
दद्यान्मत्स्यण्डिकां पूर्वं भक्षयित्वा सनागराम्||९७||
गुडं सनागरं पाठां फलाम्लं पाययेच्च तम्|
गुडं घृत यव क्षार युक्तं वाऽपि प्रयोजयेत्||९८||
यवानी नागरं पाठां दाडिमस्य रसं गुडम्|

सतक्र लवणं दद्याद्वातवर्चोऽनुलोमनम्||९९||
दुःस्पर्शकेन बिल्वेन यवान्या नागरेण वा|
एकैकेनापि संयुक्ता पाठा हन्त्यर्शसां रुजम्||१००||
प्राग्भक्तं यमके भृष्टान् सक्तुभिश्चावचूर्णितान्|
करञ्ज पल्लवान् दद्याद्वातवर्चोऽनुलोमनान्||१०१||
मदिरां वा सलवणां सीधुं सौवीरकं तथा|
गुड नागरसंयुक्तं पिबेद्वा पौर्वभक्तिकम्||१०२||

Now, recipes for the treatment of patients suffering from piles and having excessively costive bowels will be described, these are as follows:

i) Prasanna (a type of alcoholic drink) mixed with Saktu (Roasted corn- flour) and salt before administering this potion, the patient is given matsyandika (a preparation of sugar-cane juice) along with Nagara (dry ginger)

ii) Jaggery along with Nagara (dry Ginger), Patha – Cyclea peltata and Juice of sour fruit. this is given as a drink

iii) jaggery mixed with the ghee and Yava Ksara (Alkali preparation of Barley)

iv) Yavani – Carum copticum, Ginger, Patha – Cyclea peltata, Pomegranate juice and jaggery along with butter milk and salt (in adequate quantity to make it saline in taste). this potion helps in the downward movement of flatus and stool

v) Patha – Cyclea peltata along with either Duhsparsa or Bilva Yavani or Nagara, This cures pain in the piles.

vi) Tender leaves of Karanja – Pongamia pinnata fried with ghee and oil, and sprinkled with the powder of Saktu (Roasted corn flour). This is given before food. It helps in the downward movement of flatus and stool

vii) Madira (a type of alcohol) or Sauvira (a type of Vinegar) along with Jaggery and Nagara (dry ginger). This is administered before food. [96 ½ – 102]

Pippalyadi Ghrita:

पिप्पली नागर क्षार कारवी धान्य जीरकैः|
फाणितेन च संयोज्य फलाम्लं दापयेद्घृतम्||१०३||

Ghee added with Pippali—Piper longum, Nagara – Zingiber officinale, Ksara (alkali preparation), Karavi, Dhanya, Jiraka – Cuminum cyminum and Phanita (penidium) and juice of sour fruits is given [to the patient suffering from piles. [103]

Pippalyadya Ghruta:

पिप्पली पिप्पलीमूलं चित्रको हस्तिपिप्पली|
शृङ्गवेरयवक्षारौ तैः सिद्धं वा पिबेद्घृतम्||१०४||

Ghee cooked with Pippali – Piper longum, Pippali Mula, Chitraka – Plumbago zeylanica, Gaja Pippali, Srngavera and Yavaksara (Alkali preparation of Barley) is taken by the patient suffering from piles [104]

Recipes of Medicated Ghee:

चव्य चित्रक सिद्धं वा गुड क्षार समन्वितम्|
पिप्पलीमूल सिद्धं वा सगुडक्षार नागरम् ||१०५||

Ghee cooked with the paste of Chavya – Piper retrofractum and Chitraka – Plumbago zeylanica and added (at the final stage of cooking) with jaggery, Ksara (Alkali preparation) and Nagara (Dry ginger powder) is given to the patient suffering from piles

Ghee cooked with the paste of Pippali Mula and added (at the final stage of cooking) with jaggery, Ksara (Alkali preparation) and Nagara (dry ginger powder) is given to the patient suffering from piles [105]

Pippalyadya Ghritham

पिप्पली पिप्पलीमूल दधि दाडिम धान्यकैः |
सिद्धं सर्पि विधातव्यं वात वर्चो विबन्धनुत्||१०६||

Ghee cooked with the paste of Pippali – Piper longum, Pippali Mula, Dadima –Punica granatum and Dhanyaka – Coriander and curd (which is to be used as liquid) is given to the patient suffering from piles. It helps in the movement of flatus and stool. [106]

Chavyadya Ghrita:

चव्यं त्रिकटुकं पाठां क्षारं कुस्तुम्बुरूणि च|
यवानीं पिप्पलीमूलमुभे च विडसैन्धवे||१०७||
चित्रकं बिल्वमभयां पिष्ट्वा सर्पिर्विपाचयेत्|
शकृद्वातानुलोम्यार्थं जाते दध्नि चतुर्गुणे||१०८||
प्रवाहिकां गुदभ्रंशं मूत्रकृच्छ्रं परिस्रवम्|
गुदवङ्क्षणशूलं च घृतमेतद्व्यपोहति||१०९||

Ghee is cooked with the paste of Chavya – Piper chaba, Trikatuka (Sunthi – Zingiber officinale, Pippali – Long pepper fruit – Piper longum and Maricha – Black pepper fruit – Piper nigrum), Patha – Cyclea peltata, Ksara (Alkali preparation), Dhanyaka, Yavani, Pippali Mula – Long pepper fruit – Piper longum, Vida, Saindhava (Rock- Salt) Chitraka – Leadword – Plumbago zeylanica, Bilva and Abhaya – Terminalia chebula. To this, well fermented curd (4 times the quantity of ghee) is added while cooking.
It helps in
Pravahika – downward movement of stool with tensmus,
Guda bhramsha – prolapse of rectum,
Mutra krchrra – dysuria,
Parisravam – incontinence of urine and
Guda vankshana shoolam – pain in the anus as well pelvic region / groins [107-109]

Nagaradya Ghruta:

नागरं पिप्पलीमूलं चित्रको हस्तिपिप्पली|
श्वदंष्ट्रा पिप्पली धान्यं बिल्वं पाठा यवानिका||११०||
चाङ्गेरीस्वरसे सर्पिः कल्कैरेतैर्विपाचयेत्|
चतुर्गुणेन दध्ना च तद्घृतं कफवातनुत्||१११||
अर्शांसि ग्रहणीदोषं मूत्रकृच्छ्रं प्रवाहिकाम्|
गुदभ्रंशार्तिमानाहं घृतमेतद्व्यपोहति||११२||

Ghee is cooked with the paste of Nagara – Zingiber officinale, Pippali – Long pepper fruit – Piper longum Mula, Chitraka – Leadword – Plumbago zeylanica, Gaja Pippali – Long pepper fruit – Piper longum, Svadamstra, Pippali – Long pepper fruit – Piper longum, Dhanya, Bilva – Aegle marmelos, Patha – Cyclea peltata and Yavani – Carum copticum, juice of Changeri (4 times the quantity of ghee)
This medicated ghee alleviates Kapha and Vayu and cures piles, Grahani Dosa (sprue syndrome), Dysuria, Pravahika (Passage of stool with Tenesmus), prolapsed of rectum, pain in the anal region and constipation. [110-112]

Pippalyadya Ghrita:

पिप्पलीं नागरं पाठां श्वदंष्ट्रां च पृथक् पृथक्|
भागांस्त्रिपलिकान् कृत्वा कषायमुपकल्पयेत्||११३||
गण्डीरं पिप्पलीमूलं व्योषं चव्यं च चित्रकम्|
पिष्ट्वा कषाये विनयेत् पूते द्विपलिकं भिषक्||११४||
पलानि सर्पिषस्तस्मिंश्चत्वारिंशत् प्रदापयेत्|
चाङ्गेरीस्वरसं तुल्यं सर्पिषा दधि षड्गुणम्||११५||
मृद्वग्निना ततः साध्यं सिद्धं सर्पिर्निधापयेत्|
तदाहारे विधातव्यं पाने प्रायोगिके विधौ||११६||

ग्रहण्यर्शोविकारघ्नं गुल्महृद्रोगनाशनम्।
शोथप्लीहोदरानाहमूत्रकृच्छ्रज्वरापहम्॥११७॥
कासहिक्कारुचिश्वाससूदनं पार्श्वशूलनुत्।
बलपुष्टिकरं वर्ण्यमग्निसन्दीपनं परम्॥११८॥

Decoction is prepared of Pippali – Long pepper fruit – Piper longum, Nagara – Zingiber officinale, Patha – Cyclea peltata and Svadamstra, taken 3 Palas of each (for the preparation of decoction, these drugs is boiled by adding 160 palas of water and reduced to 1/4th , i.e 40 Palas). In this decoction, the paste of Gandira, Pippali – Long pepper fruit – Piper longum Mula, Vyosa (Sunthi Pippali – Long pepper fruit – Piper longum and Maricha – Black pepper fruit – piper nigrum), Chavya – Piper retrofractum and Chitraka – Leadword – Plumbago zeylanica, taken 2 Palas of each, is added, to this, 40 Palas of ghee, 40 Palas of juice of Changeri and 240 Palas of curd is kept in kept in a clean jar and used in food and as a drink regularly.

It cures

Grahani (Sprue syndrome)

Arshas – piles

Gulma (Phantom tumor),

Hrd roga – heart diseases,

Shotha – Oedema,

Plihodara – splenic disorders,

constipation,

Mutra krchra – dysuria,

Jwara – fever,

Kasa – cough,

Hikka – hiccup,

Aruchi – anorexia,

Shvasa – asthma and

Parshva shoola – pain in the sides of the chest

It is an excellent promoter of strength, plumpness of the body, complexions and the power of digestion as well as metabolism [113- 118]

Administration of Haritaki:

सगुडां पिप्पली युक्तां घृतभृष्टां हरीतकीम्।
त्रिवृद्दन्तीयुतां वाऽपि भक्षयेदानुलोमिकीम्॥११९॥
विड्वात कफ पित्तानामानुलोम्येऽथ निर्वृते।
गुदेऽर्शांसि प्रशाम्यन्ति पावकश्चाभिवर्धते॥१२०॥

For the downward movement of Vayu, the patient is given Haritaki fried in ghee along with either Jaggery and Pippali – Long pepper fruit – Piper longum, or Trivrt – Operculina turpethum and Danti. By the downward movement of stool, flatus, Kapha and Pitta and by their elimination, piles of the anal region are cured and the power of digestion is increased. [119-120]

Meat Soup:

बर्हि तित्तिरि लावानां रसानम्लान् सुसंस्कृतान्।
दक्षाणां वर्तकानां च दद्यादिवड्वातसङ्ग्रहे॥१२१॥

If there is obstruction to the movement of stool and flatus, then the patient is given the meat- soup of peacock, partridge, grey quail, cock and bustard quail. This meat soup is made sour and well sizzled. [121]

Leafy Vegetables:

त्रिवृद्दन्तीपलाशानां चाङ्गेर्याश्चित्रकस्य च।

यमके भर्जितं दद्याच्छाकं दधि समन्वितम्||१२२||

उपोदिकां तण्डुलीयं वीरां वास्तुक पल्लवान्|

सुवर्चलां सलोणीकां यव शाकमवल्गुजम्||१२३||

काकमाचीं रुहापत्रं महापत्रं तथाऽम्लिकाम्|

जीवन्तीं शटिशाकं च शाकं गृञ्जनकस्य च||१२४||

दधि दाडिम सिद्धानि यमके भर्जितानि च|

धान्य नागर युक्तानि शाकान्येतानि दापयेत्||१२५||

[Leaves of] Trivrt – Operculina turpethum, Danti – Baliospermum montanum, Palasa – Butea monosperma, Changeri – Oxalis corniculata and Chitraka – Leadword – Plumbago zeylanica is fried with ghee and oil. This is given along with curd [to the patient suffering from piles].

[Leaves of] Upodika, Tanduliya, Vira, Vastuka, Suvarcala, Lonika, Yava – Barley (Hordeum vulgare), Avalguja, Kakamaci, Ruha Patra – Cinnamomum tamala Nees and Eberum. (Udagra Saka) Maha Patra – Cinnamomum tamala Nees and Eberum. (Syonaka), Amlika, Jivanti – Leptadenia reticulata, Sati and Grnjanaka is cooked with curd and fried with ghee as well as oil. This is given [to the patient suffering from piles] mixed with Dhanya and Nagara. [122-125]

Other food ingredients

गोधालोपाक मार्जार श्वाविदुष्ट्रगवामपि|

कूर्म शल्लकयोश्चैव साधयेच्छाकवद्रसान्||१२६||

रक्त शाल्योदनं दद्याद्रसैस्तैर्वात शान्तये|१२७|

This meat soup of Godha, Lopaka, Marjara, Svavit, Ustro, cow Kurma and Sallaka is prepared on the line suggested above for leafy vegetables.

Along with this meat soup, red variety of Sali rice is given [to the patient suffering from piles] for the alieviation of Vayu. [126- 127 ½]

Anupana after drink

ज्ञात्वा वातोल्बणं रूक्षं मन्दाग्निं गुदजातुरम्||१२७||

मदिरां शार्करं जातं सीधुं तक्रं तुषोदकम्|

अरिष्टं दधिमण्डं वा शृतं वा शिशिरं जलम्||१२८||

कण्टकार्या शृतं वाऽपि शृतं नागरधान्यकैः|

अनुपानं भिषग्दद्याद्वातवर्चोऽनुलोमनम्||१२९||

The patient having piles caused by the predominance of aggravated vayu, having unctuousness and having less power of digestion is given Madira (a type of alcoholic drink), butter- milk, Tusodaka (a type of Vinegar prepared of barley), Arista (recipes to be described in verses 138- 1680, whey, boiled, and cooled water, decoction of Kantakari – Solanum xanthocarpum or decoction of Nagara – Zingiber officinale and Dhanyaka as Anupana (post prandial drink) for the downward movement of flatus and stool. [127 ½ – 129]

Anuvasana type of Enema

उदावर्त परीता ये ये चात्यर्थं विरूक्षिताः|

विलोमवाताः शूलार्तास्तेष्विष्टमनुवासनम्||१३०||

It is desirable to administer Anuvasana type of enema to the patient suffering from Udavarta (upward movement of wind in the abdomen), who is extremely devoid of unctuousness whose wind in the stomach moves in the opposite direction and who is suffering from colic pain. [130]

Pippalyadya Taila

पिप्पलीं मदनं बिल्वं शताह्वां मधुकं वचाम्|

कुष्ठं शटी पुष्कराख्यं चित्रकं देवदारु च||१३१||
पिष्ट्वा तैलं विपक्तव्यं पयसा द्विगुणेन च|
अर्शसां मूढवातानां तच्छ्रेष्ठमनुवासनम्||१३२||
गुदनिःसरणं शूलं मूत्रकृच्छ्रं प्रवाहिकाम्|
कट्यूरुपृष्ठदौर्बल्यमानाहं वङ्क्षणाश्रयम्||१३३||
पिच्छास्रावं गुदे शोफं वातवर्चोविनिग्रहम्|
उत्थानं बहुशो यच्च जयेत्तच्चानुवासनात्||१३४||

Oil is cooked with the paste of pippali – Piper longum, Madana – Randia dumetorum, Bilva – Aegle marmelos, Satahva, Madhuka – Terminalia madhuca, Vaca—Acorus calamus, Kustha – Saussurea lappa, Sati – Hedychium spicatum, Pushkaramula, Citraka – Plumbago zeylanica and Devadaru – Cedrus deodara by adding milk (taken in double the quantity of oil).

This is an excellent recipe for the administration of Anuvasana type of medicated enema for piles and Mudha Vata (immobility of wind in abdomen).

This cure:

Guda nissarana – prolapse of rectum,

Shoola – colic pain,

Mutrakruchra – dysuria,

Kati, uru, Prushta Daurbalya – weakness in the pelvic region, thighs and back,

Vankshana anaha – distension in groin

Pichcha sravam -slimy discharge from the anus,

Gude shopham – edema in the anus,

Vata varcho vinigraha – frequent desire for passing fart and stool [131-134]

Paste for External Application

आनुवासनिकैः पिष्टैः सुखोष्णैः स्नेहसंयुतैः|
दार्वन्तैः स्तब्ध शूलानि गुदजानि प्रलेपयेत्||१३५||
दिग्धास्तैः प्रस्रवन्त्याशु श्लेष्म पिच्छां सशोणिताम्|
कण्डूः स्तम्भः सरुक् शोफः सूतानां विनिवर्तते||१३६||

The above mentioned drugs ending with Devadaru – Cedrus deodara (vide verse 131) is made to a paste.

This paste is mixed with fat, made luke-warm and applied over piles having numbness and pain. By its application, slimy Kapha along with blood will ooze out, and because of this pile will be free from itching, stiffness, pain and oedema [135-136]

Niruha Type of Enema:

निरूहं वा प्रयुञ्जीत सक्षीरं दाशमूलिकम्|
समूत्र स्नेह लवणं कल्कैर्युक्तं फलादिभिः||१३७||

Enema should contain milk, decoction of Dashamula (Bilva – Aegle marmelos, syonaka, Gambhari – Gmelina arborea, Patali, Ganikarika, Shalaparni, Prsniparni, Brhati – Solanum indicum, Kantakari – Solanum surattense and Goksura – Tribulus terrestris), cow's urine, fat, salt and the paste of Madana Phala – Randia dumetrom, etc(vide Sutra 4:13). [137]

Abhayarista:

हरीतकीनां प्रस्थार्धं प्रस्थमामलकस्य च|
स्यात् कपित्थाद्दशपलं ततोऽर्धा चेन्द्रवारुणी||१३८||
विडङ्गं पिप्पली लोधं मरिचं सैलवालुकम्|
द्विपलांशं जलस्यैतच्चतुर्द्रोणे विपाचयेत्||१३९||

द्रोणशेषे रसे तस्मिन् पूते शीते समावपेत्।
गुडस्य द्विशतं तिष्ठेतत् पक्षं घृतभाजने॥१४०॥
पक्षादूर्ध्वं भवेत् पेया ततो मात्रा यथाबलम्।
अस्याभ्यासादरिष्टस्य गुदजा यान्ति सङ्क्षयम्॥१४१॥
ग्रहणी पाण्डु हृद्रोग प्लीह गुल्मोदरापहः।
कुष्ठ शोफारुचिहरो बलवर्णाग्निवर्धनः॥१४२॥
सिद्धोऽयमभयारिष्टः कामलाश्वित्रनाशनः।
कृमिग्रन्थ्यर्बुद व्यङ्ग राजयक्ष्म ज्वरान्तकृत्॥१४३॥
इत्यभयारिष्टः।

½ Prastha Haritaki—Terminalia chebula, 1 Prastha Amalaki – Phyllanthus emblica, 10 Palas Kapittha – Feronia limonia ,5 Pala Indra Varuni – Citrullus colocynthis, 2 Palas Vidanga – Embelia ribes, 2 Palas Pippali – Piper longum, 2 Palas Lodhra – Symplocos racemosa, 2 Palas Maricha – Piper nigrum and 2 Palas Elavaluka is added with 8 Dronas of water and boiled till 2 Dronas remain.

The decoction is filtered and allowed to cool. To this, 200 Palas of Jaggery is given in an appropriate dose depending upon the strength of the patient.

By the regular intake of this Arista, Piles get cured. This effective recipe is called Abhayarista.

It cures

Grahani dosha (sprue syndrome)

Pandu – anemia,

Hrudi roga – heart diseases,

Pliha – splenic disorders,

Gulma – Tumors of the abdomen (Phantom tumour),

Udara – ascites, enlargement of the abdomen (obstinate abdominal diseases including Ascites),

Kustha (obstinate skin diseases including leprosy),

Shotha – oedema,

Anorexia,

Kamala – Jaundice

Leucoderma,

Krmi – infestation with intestinal parasites,

Granthi (adenitis) Tumour

Vyanga – discoloured patch on face (Freckles),

Raja yakshma – Tuberculosis and

Jwara – fever.

It promotes strength, complexion and the power of digestion [138-143]

Dantyarista

दन्ती चित्रक मूलानामुभयोः पञ्चमूलयोः।
भागान् पलांशानापोथ्य जलद्रोणे विपाचयेत्॥१४४॥
त्रिपलं त्रिफलायाश्च दलानां तत्र दापयेत्।
रसे चतुर्थ शेषे तु पूते शीते समावपेत्॥१४५॥
तुलां गुडस्य तत्तिष्ठेन्मासार्ध घृतभाजने।
तन्मात्रया पिबन्नित्यमर्शोभ्यो विप्रमुच्यते॥१४६॥
ग्रहणी पाण्डु रोगघ्नं वातवर्चोऽनुलोमनम्।
दीपनं चारुचिघ्नं च दन्त्यरिष्टमिमं विदुः॥१४७॥
इति दन्त्यरिष्टः।

Roots of Danti – Baliospermum montanum, Chitraka – Plumbago zeylanica and Dashamula (Bilva – Aegle marmelos,

Syonaka, Gambhari—Gmelina arborea, Patali, Ganikarika, Sala parni, Prsni Parni, Brhati – Solanum indicum, Kantakari and Goksura – Tribulus terrestris), taken 1 pala each is boiled by adding 2 eDronas of water.

To this, fruits pulp of Triphala (3 Palas in total) is added.

It is boiled till 1/4th remains. The decoction is strained through a cloth and cooled.

To this, 1 Tula (100 pala - 4.8 kg) of Jaggery is added and kept in a ghee smeared jar for 15 days. Regular intake of this in appropriate doses makes a person free from piles. This is called Dantyarista and it cures Grahani (sprue syndrome) and Pandu – Anemia, initial stages of liver disorders.

It helps in the downward movement of flatus and stool.

It stimulates the power of digestion and cures anorexia [144-147]

Phalarista:

हरीतकी फलप्रस्थं प्रस्थमामलकस्य च|

विशालाया दधित्थस्य पाठाचित्रकमूलयो:||१४८||

द्वे द्वे पले समापोथ्य द्विद्रोणे साधयेदपाम्|

पादावशेषे पूते च रसे तस्मिन् प्रदापयेत्||१४९||

गुडस्यैकां तुलां वैद्यस्तत् स्थाप्यं घृतभाजने|

पक्षस्थितं पिबेदेनं ग्रहण्यर्शोविकारवान्||१५०||

हृत्पाण्डुरोगं प्लीहानं कामलां विषमज्वरम्|

वर्चोमूत्रानिलकृतान् विबन्धानग्निमार्दवम्||१५१||

कासं गुल्ममुदावर्तं फलारिष्टो व्यपोहति|

अग्निसन्दीपनो ह्येष कृष्णात्रेयेण भाषित:||१५२||

इति फलारिष्ट:|

Fruits pulp of 1 Prastha Haritaki – Terminalia chebula, 1 Prastha Amalaki – Phyllanthus emblica; 2 Palas Visala, 2 Palas Kapittha, 2 Palas Patha – Cissampelos parriera and 2 Palas Root of Chitraka – Plumbago zeylanica is added with 4 Dronas of water and boiled till 1/4th remains.

The decoction is then stained out through a cloth. To this, 1 Tula (100 pala - 4.8 kg) of jaggery is added and kept in ghee.

It cures

Grahani (sprue syndrome),

Arshas – piles,

Hrt roga – heart diseases,

Pliha roga – splenic this obstruction to the passage of stool, urine and flatus, low power of digestion,

Kasa – cough,

Gulma – Phantom Tumor and

Udavarta – bloating (upward movement of wind in the abdomen),.

It stimulates the power of digestion.

It called Phalarista, and is propounded by the sage Krsna Atreya. [148- 152]

Phalarista (second Recipe)

दुरालभायाः प्रस्थः स्याच्चित्रकस्य वृषस्य च|

पथ्यामलकयोश्चैव पाठाया नागरस्य च||१५३||

दन्त्याश्च द्विपलान् भागाञ्जलद्रोणे विपाचयेत्|

पादावशेषे पूते च सुशीते शर्कराशतम्||१५४||

प्रक्षिप्य स्थापयेत् कुम्भे मासार्धं घृतभाविते|

प्रलिप्ते पिप्पली चव्य प्रियङ्गु क्षौद्र सर्पिषा||१५५||

तस्य मात्रां पिबेत् काले शर्करस्य यथाबलम्|

अर्शांसि ग्रहणीदोषमुदावर्तमरोचकम्||१५६||
शकृन्मूत्रानिलोद्गारविबन्धानग्निमार्दवम्|
हृद्रोगं पाण्डुरोगं च सर्वमेतेन साधयेत्||१५७||
इति द्वितीयफलारिष्टः |

1 Prastha of Duralabha – Fagonia cretica and 2 Palas of each of Chitraka – Plumbago zeylanica, Ursa, Haritaki – Terminalia chebula, Amalaki – Phyllanthus emblica, Patha – Cissampelos pariera, Nagara – Zingiber officinale and Danti – Baliospermum montanum is added with 2 Dronas of water and boiled till 1/4th remains.

The decoction is strained out through a cloth and cooled. To this, 100 Palas of Sugar is added. It is kept in a jar for15 days. The inside wall of the jar is smeared with the paste containing Pippali – Piper nigrum, Chavya, Priyangu, honey and ghee.

This preparation of sugar (Sarkara) is taken in appropriate doses depending upon the strength of the patient.

It cures

Arshas – Piles,

Grahani – Malabsorption syndrome, Irritable Bowel Syndrome (sprue Syndrome), Udavarta – bloating upward movement of wind in the stomach,

Arochaka – anorexia,

Sakrt anila mutra udgara – obstruction to the movement of stool, urine, flatus and eructation,

Agni mandya – low power of digestion,

Hrud roga – heart diseases and

Pandu – Anemia, initial stages of liver disorders (anemia) [153-157]

Kanakarista

नवस्यामलकस्यैकां कुर्याज्जर्जरितां तुलाम्|
कुडवांशाश्च पिप्पल्यो विडङ्गं मरिचं तथा||१५८||
पाठां च पिप्पली मूलं क्रमुकं चव्य चित्रकौ|
मञ्जिष्ठैल्वालुकं लोध्रं पलिकानुपकल्पयेत्||१५९||
कुष्ठं दारुहरिद्रां च सुराह्वं सारिवाद्वयम्|
इन्द्राह्वं भद्रमुस्तं च कुर्यादर्धपलोन्मितम्||१६०||
चत्वारि नागपुष्पस्य पलान्यभिनवस्य च|
द्रोणाभ्याममम्भसो द्वाभ्यां साधयित्वाऽवतारयेत्||१६१||
पादावशेषे पूते च शीते तस्मिन् प्रदापयेत्|
मृद्वीकाद्व्याढकरसं शीतं निर्यूहसम्मितम्||१६२||
शर्करायाश्च भिन्नाया दद्यादि्द्वगुणितां तुलाम्|
कुसुमस्य रसस्यैकमर्धप्रस्थं नवस्य च||१६३||
त्वगेलाप्लवपत्राम्बुसेव्यक्रमुककेशरान्|
चूर्णयित्वा तु मतिमान् कार्षिकानत्र दापयेत्||१६४||
तत् सर्वं स्थापयेत् पक्षं सुचौक्षे घृतभाजने|
प्रलिप्ते सर्पिषा किञ्चिच्छर्करागुरुधूपिते||१६५||
पक्षादूर्ध्वमरिष्टोऽयं कनको नाम विश्रुतः|
पेयः स्वादुरसो हृद्यः प्रयोगाद्भक्तरोचनः||१६६||
अर्शांसि ग्रहणीदोषमानाहमुदरं ज्वरम्|
हृद्रोगं पाण्डुतां शोथं गुल्मं वर्चोविनिग्रहम्||१६७||
कासं श्लेष्मामयांश्चोग्रान् सर्वानेवापकर्षति|
वलीपलितखालित्यं दोषजं च व्यपोहति||१६८||
इति कनकारिष्टः|

1 Tula (100 pala - 4.8 kg) of freshly collected Amalaki – Phyllanthus emblica is coarsely pounded. To this, 4 Palas of each Pippali – Piper nigrum, Vidanga – Embelia ribes and Maricha – Piper nigrum, 1 Pala of each of Patha – Cissampelos parieira, Pippali Mula, Kramuka (Puga or Pattika Lodhra) Chavya – Piper retrofractum, Chitraka – Plumbago zeylanica, Manjistha –Rubia cordifolia, Elavauka and Lodhra –Symplocos racemosa ,

½ Pala of each of Kustha—Saussurea lappa, Daruharidra – Berberis aristata, Surahva (Goraksa Karkatika), Sariva – Hemidesmus indicus, Krsna sariva, indrahva and bhadramusta, and 4 Palas of freshly collected Naga Puspa is added. To this, two Dronas of water are added and boiled till 1/4th remains.

The decoction is strained out through a cloth and collected. Honey and the powder of Tvak, Ela, Plava patra, Ambu, Sevya, Karmuka and Kesara, taken in the quantity of 1 Karsa each, is added. This is kept in a clean and vessel-smeared with ghee and fumigated with sugar and Aguru. After 15 days, the recipe is filtered out.

This is called Kanakarista. This drink is sweet in taste and cardiac tonic.

It produces relish in the food and cures

Arshas – piles,

Grahani – Malabsorption syndrome, Irritable Bowel Syndrome Dosa (Sprue syndrome),

Anaha (flatulence),

Udara – Ascites (obstinate abdominal diseases including ascites),

Jwara – fever,

Hrud roga – heart diseases,

Pandu – Anemia, initial stages of liver disorders,

Shotha – Oedema,

Gulma – abdominal tumor, distension (Phantom tumour), Obstruction to the Passage of Stool,

Kasa – cough and other diseases caused by Kapha.

Vali (Appearance of wrinkles in the body),

Palita (appearance of Premature grey hair) and

Khalitya caused by the vitiation of Doshas. [158-168]

Water for Washing

पत्रभङ्गोदकैः शौचं कुर्यादुष्णेन वाऽम्भसा।

इति शुष्कार्शसां सिद्धमुक्तमेतच्चिकित्सितम्||१६९||

For cleansing the anus, the patient of piles should use the decoction of leaves (which are curative of piles) or warm water. Thus, the effective treatment for dry type of piles is described [169]

Treatment of Bleeding Piles:

चिकित्सितमिदं सिद्धं सा विणां शृण्वतः परम् |

तत्रानुबन्धो द्विविधः श्लेष्मणो मारुतस्य च||१७०||

Hereafter, the effective treatment of bleeding piles will be described. In this type of piles, kapha or Vayu remain aggravated secondarily [170]

Signs of Bleeding Piles Associated with Vayu

विट् श्यावं कठिनं रूक्षं चाधो वायुर्न वर्तते।

तनु चारुणवर्णं च फेनिलं चासृगर्शसाम्||१७१||

कट्यूरुगुदशूलं च दौर्बल्यं यदि चाधिकम्।

तत्रानुबन्धो वातस्य हेतुर्यदि च रूक्षणम्||१७२||

One should determine the bleeding associated with the secondarily aggravated Vayu if un-uncutuous / dry food and regimens are its causative factors and if the following signs and symptoms are manifested:

(i) Grayish colour, hardness and un-unctuousness of tract,

(ii) non-elimination of the flatus through the downward tract,

(iii) the blood which exudes from the piles is thin, reddish in colour and foamy,

(iv) pain in the lumbar region, thighs and anus and

(v) Excessive weakness. [171- 172]

Signs of bleeding Piles associated with Kapha

शिथिलं श्वेतपीतं च विट् स्निग्धं गुरु शीतलम्|

यद्यर्शसां घनं चासृक् तन्तुमत् पाण्डु पिच्छिलम्||१७३||

गुदं सपिच्छं स्तिमितं गुरु स्निग्धं च कारणम्|

श्लेष्मानुबन्धो विज्ञेयस्तत्र रक्तार्शसां बुधैः||१७४||

स्निग्धशीतं हितं वाते रूक्षशीतं कफानुगे|

One should determine the bleeding piles as secondarily associated with Kapha if food and regimens which are heavy and unctuous are the causative factors and if the following signs and symptoms are manifested:

(i) stool is loose, white, yellow, unctuous, heavy and cold,

(ii) the blood which exudes from the piles is dense, therapy, pale yellow and slimy and

(iii) The anus is smeared with slimy material and there is numbness in that region. [173-174]

Line of Treatment

स्निग्धशीतं हितं वाते रूक्षशीतं कफानुगे|

चिकित्सितमिदं तस्मात् सम्प्रधार्य प्रयोजयेत्||१७५||

पित्तश्लेष्माधिकं मत्वा शोधनेनोपपादयेत्|

स्रवणं चाप्युपेक्षेत लङ्घनैर्वा समाचरेत्||१७६||

If Vayu is secondarily vitiated in this type of (bleeding) piles then unctuous and cold things and medicinesare useful. If however, Kapha is secondarily vitiated, then un-unctuous and cold things are useful. Therefore, therapies are administered keeping these points in view.

If there is predominance of Pitta and kapha, the patient is administered elimination therapies: However, bleeding is not stopped immedietly and one should wait for appropriate time. The patient can be given "fasting "therapy.[175-176]

Complications of Immediate Hemostasis

प्रवृत्तमादावशोंभ्यो यो निगृह्णात्यबुद्धिमान्|

शोणितं दोषमनिलं तद्रोगाञ्जनयेद्बहून्||१७७||

रक्तपित्तं ज्वरं तृष्णामग्निसादमरोचकम्|

कामलां श्वयथुं शूलं गुद वङ्क्षण संश्रयम्||१७८||

कण्डवरुःकोठपिडकाः कुष्ठं पाण्डवाहवयं गदम्|

वात मूत्र पुरीषाणां विबन्धं शिरसो रुजम्||१७९||

स्तैमित्यं गुरुगात्रत्वं तथाऽन्यान् रक्तजान् गदान्|

तस्मात् सुते दुष्टरक्ते रक्तसङ्ग्रहणं हितम्||१८०||

हेतु लक्षण कालज्ञो बल शोणित वर्णवित्|

कालं तावदुपेक्षेत यावन्नात्ययमाप्नुयात्||१८१||

If the bleeding containing material polluted by Doshas, which comes out from the piles is arrested in the beginning by an unwise physician, then it gives rise to several other diseases, viz, Rakta Pitta (a diseases characterised by bleeding from various part of the body), Jwara – fever, Trushna – morbid thirst, Suppression of the power of digestion, Aruchi -Anorexia, Kamala – Jaundice, Shotha – Odema, colic pain in the Anus and pelvic region, urticaria and pimples in the lumer region and things, kustha(obstinate skin diseases including leprosy), Pandu – Anemia, initial stages of liver disorders(anemia, (arrest of the flatus, urine and stool, headache, Staimitya(a feeling as if the body is covered with a wet cloth), heaviness of the body and other diseases caused by vitiated blood. Therefore, only after the polluted blood is eliminated, haemostatic measures are useful.

The physician well acquainted with the causative factors, signs and symptoms, nature of the time, strength and colour of the blood should wait for an appropriate time before administering hemostatic therapies unless it is an emergency. [177-181]

Administration of Bitter Drugs

अग्नि सन्दीपनार्थं च रक्त सङ्ग्रहणाय च|
दोषाणां पाचनार्थं च परं तिक्तैरुपाचरेत्||१८२||

The patient is given bitter drugs for stimulation of the power of digestion, hemostasis and Pachana (metabolic transformation) of Doshas. [182]

Use of Sneha

यत्तु प्रक्षीणदोषस्य रक्तं वातोल्बणस्य च|
वर्तते स्नेहसाध्यं तत् पानाभ्यङ्गानुवासनैः||१८३||

If in the Piles having predominance of Vayu, bleeding continues even after the aggravated Doshas are eliminated then the patient is given unctuous therapies in the form of Drinks, massage and Anuvasana type of enema. [183]

Indication for Hemostatic Therapy

यत्तु पित्तोल्बणं रक्तं घर्मकाले प्रवर्तते|
स्तम्भनीयं तदेकान्तान्न चेद्वातकफानुगम्||१८४||

If Vayu and Kapha are not secondarily predominant, if piles are caused by the exclusive predominance of Pitta and if it occurs in summer, then hemostratic therapies are administered immediately to stop bleeding. [184]

Hemostatic Recipes

कुटज त्वङिनर्यूहः सनागरः स्निग्ध रक्त सङ्ग्रहणः|
त्वग्दाडिमस्य तद्वत् सनागरश्चन्दनरसश्च||१८५||
चन्दन किराततिक्तक धन्वयवासाः सनागराः क्वथिताः|
रक्तार्शसां प्रशमना दार्वीत्वगुशीर निम्बाश्च||१८६||
सातिविषा कुटज त्वक् फलं च सरसाञ्जनं मधुयुतानि|
रक्तापहानि दद्यात् पिपासवे तण्डुलजलेन||१८७||

The decoction of the bark of Kutaja mixed with the powder of Nagara – Zingiber officinale stops exudation of unctuous blood. Similarly, the decoction of the bark (of stem or fruit) of Dadima along with the powder of Nagara and the decoction of Candana along with the powder of Nagara are hemostatic.

Decoction of Chandana – Santalum album, Kiratatikta, Dhanvayasa and Nagara – Zingiber officinale, and the decoction of darvi, Tvak, Aguru – Aquilaria agallocha Usira and nimbi alleviate piles caused by the vitiation of blood (bleeding piles).

Bark and fruits of Kutaja – Holarrhena antidysenterica along with Ativisa and Rasanjana is mixed with honey and used as a hemostatic. If the patient is suffering from morbid thirst, then this potion is given along with Tandulodaka (rice- wash). [185- 187]

Kutajadi Rasakriya

कुटज त्वचो विपाच्यं पलशतमार्द्रे महेन्द्रसलिलेन|
यावत्स्याद्गतरसं तद्द्रव्यं पूतो रसस्ततो ग्राह्यः||१८८||
मोचरसः ससमङ्गः फलिनी च समांशिकैस्त्रिभिस्तैश्च|
वत्सकबीजं तुल्यं चूर्णितमत्र प्रदातव्यम्||१८९||
पूतोत्क्वथितः सान्द्रः स रसो दर्वीप्रलेपनो ग्राह्यः|

मात्राकालोपहिता रसक्रियैषा जयत्यसृक्स्रावम्||१९०||
छगली पयसा पीता पेयामण्डेन वा यथाग्निबलम्|
जीर्णौषधश्च शालीन् पयसा छागेन भुञ्जीत||१९१||
रक्तार्शास्यतिसारं रक्तं सासृग्रुजो निहन्त्याशु|
बलवच्च रक्तपित्तं रसक्रियैषा जयत्युभयभागम्||१९२||
इति कुटजादिरसक्रिया|

100 Palas of the freshly collected bark of Kutaja – Holarrhena antidysenterica is boiled with 1 Drona rain water till the entire essence of the bark comes to water (i.e till 1/8th remains).

This decoction is then strained out through a cloth. To this, the powders of 1 Pala Mocarasa, 1 Pala Samanga1 Pala Phalini and 3 Palas seeds of Kutaja is added and boiled again till it becomes semi- soild extract, administered in appropriate dose and time, stops bleeding, depending upon the strength of the patient, this recipe is administered along with goat- milk to eat.

It instantaneously cures rakta arsha – bleeding piles, Atisara -diarrhoea with bleeding, blood- diseases and serious types of Urdhvaga Rakthapitta (disease characterised by bleeding from upward tracts of the body) as well as Adhoga Rakta Pitta (a disease characterised by bleeding from downward tract of the body). [188-192]

Recipes for Piles

नीलोत्पलं समङ्गा मोचरसश्चन्दनं तिला लोध्रम्|
पीत्वा च्छगलीपयसा भोज्यं पयसैव शाल्यन्नम्||१९३||

Powder of Nilotpala, Samanga, Mocarasa, Chandana – Santalum album, Tila and Lodhra is taken along with goat- milk. Thereafter, the patient should eat Sali type of rice along with goat milk [193]

छागलि पयः प्रयुक्तं निहन्ति रक्तं सवास्तुकरसं च|
धन्व विहङ्ग मृगाणां रसो निरम्लः कदम्लो वा||१९४||

Intake of the juice of Vastuka along with goat- milk stops bleeding. The soup of the meat of birds and animals inhabiting arid zone is taken without any sour ingredient or with small quantity of sour drugs, which is useful for bleeding piles.1[94]

पाठा वत्सकबीजं रसाञ्जनं नागरं यवान्यश्च|
बिल्वमिति चार्शसैश्चूर्णितानि पेयानि शूलेषु||१९५||

The powder of Patha—Cissampelos pariera, seed of Kuthaja – Holarrhena antidysenterica, Rasanjana, Nagara – Zingiber officinale, Yavani and Bilva – Aegle marmelos is taken in the form of a drink if there is pain in piles.[195]

दार्वी किराततिक्तं मुस्तं दुःस्पर्शकश्च रुधिरघ्नम्|

The powder of Darvi, Kiratatikta, Musta and Duhsparsa stops bleeding [1961/2]

रक्तेऽतिवर्तमाने शूले च घृतं विधातव्यम्||१९६||
कुटजफल वल्क केशर नीलोत्पल लोध्र धातकी कल्कैः|
सिद्धं घृतं विधेयं शूले रक्तार्शसां भिषजा||१९७||
सर्पिः सदाडिमरसं सयावशूकं शृतं जयत्याशु
रक्तं सशूलमथवा निदिग्धिकादुग्धिकासिद्धम्||१९८||

If there is excessive bleeding and pain in the piles, then medicated ghee is administered.

If bleeding – piles are associated with pain, then ghee cooked with the paste of the fruits and barks of Kutaja –Holarrhena antidysenterica , Kesara, Nilotpala, Lodhra and Dhataki – Woodfordia floribunda is administered by the physician.

Ghee cooked with the juice of Dadima – Punica granatum and Yava Ksara (Alkali prepared of barley) instantaneously cures bleeding and piles.

Ghee cooked with Nidigdhika and Dugdhika, similarly, cures bleeding and pain in the piles instantaneously. [196 ½-198]

Recipes of Peya (Thin Gruel)

लाजापेया पीता सचुक्रिका केशरोत्पलैः सिद्धा|
हन्त्याश्वस्रस्रावं तथा बला पृश्निपर्णीभ्याम्||१९९||
ह्रीवेर बिल्व नागर निर्यूहे साधितां सनवनीताम्|
वृक्षाम्ल दाडिमाम्लामम्लीकाम्लां सकोलाम्लाम्||२००||
गृञ्जनकसुरासिद्धां दद्याद्यमकेन भर्जितां पेयाम्|
रक्तातिसार शूल प्रवाहिका शोथ निग्रहणीम्||२०१||

Peya (thin gruel) of Laja (fried paddy) prepared by adding Cukrika, Kesara and Nilotpala, or Bala and Prsniparni instantaneously cures bleeding in piles.

Peya (thin gruel) prepared by adding the decotion of Haridra, Bilva – Aegle marmelos and Nagara – Zingiber officinale, added with butter and made sour by adding Vrksamula, Amulika and Kola cures raktatisara (diarrhoea with bleeding), colic pain, Pravahika (dysentery) and oedema.

Similarly, Peya (thin Gruel) prepared by adding Grnjanaka and Sura (a type of alcohol), and sizzled with ghee and oil is taken for the cure of Raktatisara (Diarrhoea with bleeding), colic pain, Pravahika (dysentery) and oedema. [199-201]

Recipes of Curds

काश्मर्यामलकानां सकर्बुदारान् फलाम्लांश्च|
गृञ्जनक शाल्मलीनां क्षीरिण्याश्चुक्रिकायाश्च||२०२||
न्यग्रोध शुङ्गकानां खण्डांस्तथा कोविदार पुष्पाणाम्|
दध्नः सरेण सिद्धान् दद्याद्रक्ते प्रवृत्तेऽति||२०३||

The khadayusha prepared with the decoction or juice of the below mentioned recipes should be processed with cream of curds and administered if there is excessive bleeding –

i) Kasmari, Amalaka, Karbudara and sour fruits
ii) Grnjanaka and Shalmali – Salmalia malabarica
iii) Kstrini and Cukrika
iv) adventitious roots of Nyagrodha and
v) Flowers of Kovidara[202-203]

Diet

सिद्धं पलाण्डुशाकं तक्रेणोपोदिकां सबदराम्लाम्|
रुधिरस्रवे प्रदद्यान्मसूरसूपं च तक्राम्लम्||२०४||

To stop bleeding, the patient is given onion cooked with butter-milk, Upodika along with Badaramla) sour vinegar prepared of Badara) or the soup of Masura made sour by adding butter- milk. [204]

पयसा शृतेन यूषै र्मसूर मुद्गाढकीमकुष्ठानाम् |
भोजनमद्यादम्लैः शालि श्यामाक कोद्रवजम्||२०५||

The patient of bleeding piles should take the food containing Sali rice, Syamaka and Kodrava along with the boiled milk or the soup of Masura, Mudga, Adhaki and Makustha, and added with sour ingredients. [205]

शश हरिण लाव मांसैः कपिञ्जलैणेयकैः सुसिद्धैश्च|
भोजनमद्यादम्लैर्मधुरैरीषत् समरिचैर्वा||२०६||

The patient suffering from bleeding piles should take food along with the meat of Sasa, Harina, Lava, Kapinjala and

Ena.

He can add sour or slightly sweet ingredients to his food or sprinkle powder of Marica on his food [206]

दक्ष शिखि तितिरि रसैर्दिर्वककुदलो पाकजैश्च मधुराम्लैः|
अद्याद्रसैरतिवहेष्वर्शःस्वनिलोल्बणशरीरः||२०७||

If there is excessive bleeding from the piles and if there is excessive aggravation of Vayu in the body of the patient, then he should take food along with the soup of cock, peacock, Tittiri bird, camel and Jackal. This meat soup should be suitably mixed with sweet and sour ingredients. [207]

Yusha of Onion

रस खड यूष यवागू संयोगतः केवलोऽथवा जयति|
रक्तमतिवर्तमानं वातं च पलाण्डु रुपयुक्तः||२०८||

Onion taken alone or along with Rasa (meat soup), Khada (a sour and pungent drink), Yusa (vegetable soup) and Yavagu (thick gruel) cures excessive bleeding and aggravated Vayu. [208]

छागान्तराधि तरुणं सरुधिरमुपसाधितं बहु पलाण्डु|
व्यत्यासान्मधुराम्लं विट्शोणितसङ्क्षये देयम्||२०९||

The trunk of a young goat along with its blood is well cooked by adding a large quantity of Onion. It is given by adding alternatively, sweet and sour ingredients if there is diminution of stool and blood. [209]

नवनीत तिलाभ्यासात् केशर नवनीत शर्कराभ्यासात्|
दधि सर मथिताभ्यासादर्शास्यपयान्ति रक्तानि||२१०||

Bleeding piles gets cured by the habitual intake of the following recipes:
I) Navanita (Butter) and Tila (sesame seed)
II) Kesara , Navanita (Butter) and Sharkara (sugar) and
III) The cream of curd after churning [210]

नवनीतघृतं छागं मांसं च सषष्टिकः शालिः|
तरुणश्च सुरा मण्डस्तरुणी च सुरा निहन्त्यसम्||२११||

Bleeding stops if the patient takes freshly collected ghee from butter, goat meat, Sastika or Sali types of rice, the scum of freshly fermented Sura (a type of alcoholic drink) or freshly fermented Sura [211]

Predominance of Vayu

प्रायेण वात बहुलान्यशांसि भवन्त्यतिसुते रक्ते|
दुष्टेऽपि च कफ पित्ते तस्मादनिलोऽधिको ज्ञेयः||२१२||

Generally all kinds of piles are predominant in vayu. This is because due to excessive bleeding and due to excessive aggravation of kapha and pitta the vata will eventually get aggravated. Therefore the vayu is essentially aggravated in all kinds of piles. [212]

Cooling therapy

दृष्ट्वा तु रक्तपित्तं प्रबलं कफ वात लिङ्गमल्पं च|
शीता क्रिया प्रयोज्या यथेरिता वक्ष्यते चान्या ||२१३||

If there is predominance of Rakta and Pitta, and there is less of the signs and symptoms of aggravated Kapha as well as Vayu, then the patient should be given cooling remedies which are already described and some of which are to be described later. [213]

Sprinkling

मधुकं सपञ्चवल्कं बदरीत्वगुदुम्बरं धवपटोलम्‌|
परिषेचने विदध्याद्वृषककुम यवास निम्बांश्च||२१४||

To stop bleeding in piles, these are sprinkled with the decoctions of Madhuka , Pancavalka (barks of Nyagrodha – Ficus bengalensis, Udumbara –Ficus racemosa, Asvattha, Parisha and Plaksa), Bark of Badari, Udumbara – Ficus racemosa, Dhava and Patola or Vasa – Adhathoda vasica, Kakubha, yavasaka (Duralabha) and Nimba.[214]

Bath

रक्तेऽतिवर्तमाने दाहे क्लेदेऽवगाहयेच्चापि|
मधुक मृणाल पद्मक चन्दन कुश काश निष्क्वाथे||२१५||
इक्षुरस मधुक वेतस निर्यूहे शीतले पयसि वा तम्‌|
अवगाहयेत् प्रदिग्धं पूर्वं शिशिरेण तैलेन||२१६||

If there is Rakta ativartamaane – excessive bleeding, Daha – burning sensation and Kleda – stickiness, then the patient is given bath with the decoction of madhuka, Mrnala, padmaka, Chandana – Santalum album, Kusa and Kasa. If there is excessive bleeding the anus of the patient is first of all anointed with cold oil and then he is given sitz bath with sugar- cane juice and the decoctions of Madhuka and Vetasa or with cold water. [215- 216]

Hemostatic Douche

दत्वा घृतं सशर्करमुपस्थदेशे गुदे त्रिकदेशे च|
शिशिर जल स्पर्श सुखा धारा प्रस्तम्भनी योज्या||२१७||

External application of Leaves

To stop bleeding, the piles mass is frequently covered with the tender leaves of banana, and leaves of Puskara sprinkled with cooled water. Similarly, covering these masses with the leaves of Padma and Utapala is useful. [217]

कदलीदलैरभिनवैः पुष्करपत्रैश्च शीतजलसिक्तैः|
प्रच्छादनं मुहुर्मुहुरिष्टं पद्मोत्पलदलैश्च||२१८||
दुर्वाघृतप्रदेहः शतधौतसहस्रधौतमपि सर्पिः|
व्यजनपवनः सुशीतो रक्तस्रावं जयत्याशु||२१९||

Banana leaves, and puskara sprinkled with cold water and Hemorrhoid mass should be covered with this. Leaves of padma and utpala is usefulfor covering pile mass. Durvaghrita, shatadhauta ghrita and sahasradhauta ghrita, and fanning of cold air helps to stops bleeding. [219]

Rubbing

समङ्गा मधुकाभ्यां तिल मधुकाभ्यां रसाञ्जनवृताभ्याम्‌|
सर्जरस घृताभ्यां वा निम्बघृताभ्यां मधुघृताभ्यां वा||२२०||
दार्वीत्वक्सर्पिभ्र्यां सचन्दनाभ्यामथोत्पलघृताभ्याम्‌|
दाहे क्लेदे च गुदभ्रंशे गुदजाः प्रतिसारणीयाः स्युः||२२१||

If there is prolapse of rectum, burning sensation or stickiness in the anus, then the following recipes are gently rubbed over the anus:

i) Samanga and Madhuka
ii) Tila and Madhuka
iii) Rasanjana and Ghee
iv) Sarjarasa and Ghee
v) Nimba and ghee
vi) Honey and Ghee
vii) Bark of Darvi and Ghee
viii) Chandana – Santalum album and Rakta- Chandana and

ix) Utpala and Ghee [220- 221]

Management of Continuous Bleeding

आभिः क्रियाभिरथवा शीताभिर्यस्य तिष्ठति न रक्तम्।
तं काले स्निग्धोष्णैर्मांसरसैस्तर्पयेन्मतिमान्||२२२||
अवपीडक सर्पिर्भिः कोष्णे घृत तैलिकैस्तथाऽभ्यङ्गैः।
क्षीर घृत तैल सेकैः कोष्णैस्तमुपाचरेदाशु||२२३||

If bleeding continues in spite of the above mentioned remedies and cooling therapies, then a wise physician should administer at the appropriate time, meat- soup which is unctuous and hot.

Such a patient is given Avapidaka Sarpis (medicated ghee which is administered prior to taking food or which is administered in large quantities). His anus is massaged with luke-warm milk, ghee or oil. These remedies are administered instantaneously. [222-223]

Piccha Basti

कोष्णेन वातप्रबले घृतमण्डेनानुवासयेच्छीघ्रम्।
पिच्छाबस्तिं दद्यात् काले तस्याथवा सिद्धम्||२२४||
यवास कुश काशानं मूलं पुष्पं च शाल्मलम्।
न्यग्रोधोदुम्बराश्वत्थ शुङ्गाश्च द्विपलोन्मिताः||२२५||
त्रिप्रस्थं सलिलस्यैतत् क्षीरप्रस्थं च साधयेत्।
क्षीरशेषं कषायं च पूतं कल्कैर्विमिश्रयेत्||२२६||
कल्काः शाल्मलि निर्यास समङ्गा चन्दनोत्पलम्।
वत्सकस्य च बीजानि प्रियङ्गुः पद्मकेशरम्||२२७||
पिच्छाबस्तिरयं सिद्धः सघृतक्षौद्रशर्करः।
प्रवाहिका गुदभ्रंश रक्तस्राव ज्वरापहः||२२८||
प्रपौण्डरीकं मधुकं पिच्छाबस्तौ यथेरितान्।
पिष्ट्वाऽनुवासनं स्नेहं क्षीरद्विगुणितं पचेत्||२२९||
इति पिच्छाबस्तिः।

If bleeding doesn't stop and there is aggravation of Vayu, then the patient is given instantaneously Anuvasana type of enema with the help of Luke-warm Ghrtamanda (Upper portion of the ghee). He is given the effective piccha basti (recipe of which is described below) at the appropriate hour.

In 6 prasthas of water, 2 Prasthas of milk and 2 Palas each of Duralabha, kusa, Kasa, roots and flowers of Salmali – Salmalia malabarica and adventitious roots of Nyagrodha, udumbara and Asvattha is added and boiled till 2 prasthas remain. This is strained through a cloth, and to this, the paste of the resin from Salmali, Samanga, Chandana, utpala, seeds of kutaja – Holarrhena antidysenterica, Priyangu and padmakesara is added. This effective recipe is called piccha basti and it is administered along with ghee, honey and sugar. It cures dysentery, prolapse of rectum, bleeding and fever.

Prapaundarika and madhuka along with the drugs described in piccha basti (in verse no 227) is made into a paste. The paste is added to oil and doubled the quantity of milk, and cooked. This medicated oil is used for anuvasana type of medicated enema for the patients suffering from piles. [224- 229]

Hriveradi Ghrta

ह्रीवेरमुत्पलं लोध्रं समङ्गा चव्य चन्दनम्।
पाठा सातिविषा बिल्वं धातकी देवदारु च||२३०||
दार्वी त्वङ् नागरं मांसी मुस्तं क्षारो यवाग्रजः।
चित्रकश्चेति पेष्याणि चाङ्गेरीस्वरसे घृतम्||२३१||
ऐकध्यं साधयेत् सर्वं तत् सर्पिः परमौषधम्।

अर्शोतिसार ग्रहणी पाण्डुरोगे ज्वरेऽरुचौ||२३२||
मूत्रकृच्छ्रे गुदभ्रंशे बस्त्यानाहे प्रवाहणे|
पिच्छास्रावेऽर्शसां शूले योज्यमेतत्त्रिदोषनुत्||२३३||
इति ह्रीवेरादिघृतम्|

Ghee is cooked by adding the paste of Hrivera,Utpala, lodhra, Samanga, Chavya, Chandana – Santalum album, Patha – Cissampelos pareira , Ativisa – Aconitum heterophyllum, Bilva – Aegle marmelos, Dhataki – Woodfordia floribunda, Devadaru – Cedrus deodara, bark of Daru Haridra – Curcuma longa, Nagara – Zingiber officinale, jatamamsi, Musta – Cyperus rotundus, Yavaksara and Chitraka – Plumbago zeylanica and the juice of Changeri.

It is an excellent remedy for Arshas – piles, Atisaar – diarrhoea, Grahani (sprue syndrome),Pandu (anemia) Jwara-fever, Aruchi – anorexia, Mutrakrchhra- dysuria, Guda bhramsha – Prolapse of rectum, Basti anaha – distension in the region of urinary bladder, tenesmus, voiding of slimy material and pain in the piles. It alleviates all the three aggravated Doshas [230-233]

SuniSannaka-cangeri- ghrta

अवाक्पुष्पी बला दार्वी पृश्निपर्णी त्रिकण्टकः|
न्यग्रोधोदुम्बराश्वत्थशुङ्गाश्च द्विपलोन्मिताः||२३४||
कषाय एषां पेष्यास्तु जीवन्ती कटुरोहिणी|
पिप्पली पिप्पलीमूलं नागरं सुरदारु च||२३५||
कलिङ्गाः शाल्मलं पुष्पं वीरा चन्दनमुत्पलम्|
कट्फलं चित्रको मुस्तं प्रियङ्ग्वतिविषास्थिराः||२३६||
पद्मोत्पलानां किञ्जल्कः समङ्गा सनिदिग्धिका|
बिल्वं मोचरसः पाठा भागाः कर्षसमन्विताः||२३७||
चतुष्प्रस्थे शृतं प्रस्थं कषायमवतारयेत्|
त्रिंशत्पलानि प्रस्थोऽत्र विज्ञेयो द्विपलाधिकः||२३८||
सुनिषण्णकचाङ्गेर्योः प्रस्थौ द्वौ स्वरसस्य च|
सर्वैरेतैर्यथोदिदष्टैर्घृतप्रस्थं विपाचयेत्||२३९||
एतदर्शःस्वतीसारे रक्तस्रावे त्रिदोषजे|
प्रवाहणे गुदभ्रंशे पिच्छासु विविधासु च||२४०||
उत्थाने चातिबहुशः शोथशूले गुदाश्रये|
मूत्रग्रहे मूढवाते मन्देऽग्नावरुचावपि||२४१||
प्रयोज्यं विधिवत् सर्पिर्बलवर्णाग्निवर्धनम्|
विविधेष्वन्नपानेषु केवलं वा निरत्ययम्||२४२||
इति सुनिषण्णकचाङ्गेरीघृतम्|

Avakpuspi (Adhah Puspi), Bala, Darvi, Prsniparni, Goksura and adventitious roots of Nyagrvodha, udumbara and Asvattha these drugs are added and boiled till 1 Prastha of water remains. This decoction is strained through a cloth. In the context of preparation of the decotion, 32 palas constitute 1 prastha.

Jivanti, Katurohini, pippali – Piper longum, pippali mula, Nagara – Zingiber officinale , devadaru, Kalinga, flower of Salmali, Vira, Chandana, Utpala, Katphala, Chitraka – Plumbago zeylanica, Musta – Cyperus rotundus, priyangu, Ativisa – Aconitum heterophyllum, Sthira, pollens of Padma and utpala, Samanga, kantakari, Bilva – Aegle marmelos, mocarasa and Patha- these drugs are taken in the quantity of karsa each and made to a paste.

The above mentioned decoction and paste is added with the juice of Sunisannaka and Changeri, 2 Prasthas of each and 1 Prastha of ghee and cooked. This medicated ghee cures Arshas-piles, Atisara – diarrhoea, bleeding by the simultaneous aggravation of all the 3 Doshas, tenesmus, prolapse of rectum, voiding of different types of slimy material, excessive and frequent urge for motion, odema and pain in the anus, anuria, immobility of wind in the abdomen, suppression of the power of digestion and anorexia.

Appropriate administration of this medicated ghee helps in the

Promotion of strength,

Complexion and

Agni – The power of digestion

This medicated ghee is harmless, and it can be administered alone or along with different type of food and drinks. [234-242]

भवन्ति चात्र-

व्यत्यासान्मधुराम्लानि शीतोष्णानि च योजयेत्|

नित्यमग्निबलापेक्षी जयत्यर्शःकृतान् गदान्||२४३||

Thus it is said

Depending upon the power of digestion and the strength, the patient is given alternatively sweet as well as sour, and cold as well as hot therapies. This cures the ailments caused by piles. [243]

Inter dependency of Diseases

त्रयो विकाराः प्रायेण ये परस्परहेतवः|

अर्शांसि चातिसारश्च ग्रहणीदोष एव च||२४४||

एषामग्निबले हीने वृद्धिर्वृद्धे परिक्षयः|

तस्मादग्निबलं रक्ष्यमेषु त्रिषु विशेषतः||२४५||

Arshas – Piles, Atisara – diarrohea and Grahani – Malabsorption syndrome, Irritable Bowel Syndrome (sprue syndrome) – these 3 diseases are interdependent in as much as one of them can cause the other. They get aggravated if there is reduction in the power of digestion and when the power of digestion is increased, they get cured. Therefore, Agni (Enzymes responsible for digestion) is protected specifically for (keeping) these 3 ailments under control [244-245]

Treatment in General

भृष्टैः शाकै यवागूभिर्यूषैर्मांसरसैः खडैः|

क्षीर तक्र प्रयोगैश्च विविधैर्गुदजाञ्जयेत्||२४६||

The physician should overcome piles by the use of different

Bhrsta shaka – types of fried vegetables

Yavagu – thick gruel

Yusha – vegetable soup,

Mamsa rasa – meat soup,

Khada – as sour preparation

Kshira – milk and

Takra – butter- milk. [246]

Treatment in Brief

यद्वायोरानुलोम्याय यदग्निबलवृद्धये|

अन्नपानौषधद्रव्यं तत् सेव्यं नित्यमर्शसैः||२४७||

यदतो विपरीतं स्यान्निदाने यच्च दर्शितम्|

गुदजाभिपरीतेन तत् सेव्यं न कदाचन||२४८||

Food ingredients and drugs which cause downward movements of Vayu and which are the promoters of the power of digestion are all invariably useful for piles. Those having opposite properties and those described in the etiology of piles should never be used by the patient suffering from this disease. [247- 248]

तत्र श्लोकाः-

अर्शसां द्विविधं जन्म पृथगायतनानि च|

स्थान संस्थानलिङ्गानि साध्यासाध्यविनिश्चयः||२४९||
अभ्यङ्गाः स्वेदनं धूमाः सावगाहाः प्रलेपनाः|
शोणितस्यावसेकश्च योगा दीपनपाचनाः||२५०||
पानान्न विधिरङ्ग्यश्च वातवर्चोऽनुलोमनः|
योगाः संशमनीयाश्च सर्पींषि विविधानि च||२५१||
बस्तयस्तक्रयोगाश्च वरारिष्टाः सशर्कराः|
शुष्काणामर्शसां शस्ताः स्राविणां लक्षणानि च||२५२||
द्विविधं सानुबन्धानां तेषां चेष्टं यदौषधम्|
रक्त सङ्ग्रहणाः क्वाथाः पेष्याश्च विविधात्मकाः||२५३||
स्नेहाहार विधिश्चाब्यो योगाश्च प्रतिसारणाः|
प्रक्षालनावगाहाश्च प्रदेहाः सेचनानि च||२५४||
अतिवृत्तस्य रक्तस्य विधातव्यं यदौषधम्|
तत्सर्वमिह निर्दिष्टं गुदजानां चिकित्सिते||२५५||

Summary:

In this chapter on "The treatment of piles" all the following points pertaining to piles are discussed:

i) 2 different ways in which this diseases are produced

ii) Location, appearance and signs as well as symptoms

iii) Determination of curability and incurability

iv) Recipes for massage, fomentation, fumigation, bath, external application, blood-letting and digestive stimulation and of carminatives.

v) Most useful modes of taking drinks and food

vi) Recipes for the downward movement of flatus and stools

vii) Alleviating recipes

viii) Different types of medicated ghee

ix) Recipes for medicated Enemas and butter- milk

x) Excellent Aristas including Sarkararista

xi) Wholesome regimes for dry piles

xii) Signs and symptoms of bleeding piles

xiii) 2 different types of Anubandhas (secondary aggravations of Doshas) and their appropriate remedies

xiv) Hemostatic decoctions

xv) Pastes of different types

xvi) Excellent modes of giving oleation therapy and food

xvii) Recipes for rubbing over the piles mass

xviii) Recipes for washing, bath, ointment and sprinkling over piles and

xix) Remedies for excessive bleeding in piles. [249- 255]

इत्यग्निवेशकृते तन्त्रे चरकप्रतिसंस्कृते चिकित्सास्थानेऽर्शश्चिकित्सितं नाम चतुर्दशोऽध्यायः||१४||

Thus, ends the 14th chapter dealing with the treatment of Arshas in Chikitsa Sthana of Agnivesha's work as redacted by Charaka.

21

Chikitsasthana Chapter 15
Grahanidosha Chikitsitam

The 15th chapter of Charaka Samhita Chikitsa Sthana is Grahani Dosha Chikisa. Grahani disease is correlated with irritable bowel syndrome, sprue, malabsorption syndrome. This chapter also explains in detail about the food digestion process as per Ayurveda.

अथातो ग्रहणीदोष चिकित्सितं व्याख्यास्यामः||१||

इति ह स्माह भगवानात्रेयः||२||

Let us now explore the chapter on the treatment of Grahani dosha

Thus, said lord Atreya. [1-2]

In the previous chapter (chikitsa 14), treatment of arshas (piles) is presented. Grahani dosha (sprue-syndrome) is [often] caused by arshas (piles). Therefore, the chapter on the treatment of grahani dosha follows that of arshas.

Functions of Agni – Digestive fire:

आयुर्वर्णो बलं स्वास्थ्यमुत्साहोपचयौ प्रभा|

ओजस्तेजोऽग्नयः प्राणाश्चोक्ता देहाग्निहेतुकाः||३||

शान्तेऽग्नौ म्रियते, युक्ते चिरं जीवत्यनामयः|

रोगी स्यादिवकृते, मूलमग्निस्तस्मान्निरुच्यते||४||

Functions of Agni – Digestive fire:

Dehagni or Jatharagni (power of digestion and metabolism) is the reason for

Ayu – life,

Varna – colour, complexion

Bala – strength and immunity

Swasthya – good health

Utsaha – energy, enthusiasm

Upachaya – bulk, shape, plumpness of body

Ojas – immunity, disease resisting power (read more about Ojas)

Tejas – aura, complexion, radiance

Maintenance of other varieties of Agni and

Prana elan vitae, Vital breath.

Extinction of Agni leads to death. Its proper maintenance helps a person to live longer and its impairment gives rise to diseases. Therefore, Jataragni is considered to be the root or the most important sustaining factor (mula) of living beings. [3-4]

Importance of Agni

यदन्नं देह धात्वोजो बल वर्णादि पोषकम्|
तत्राग्निर्हेतुराहारान्न ह्यपक्वाद्रसादयः||५||

Food provides nourishment to the body and tissues and it is the reason for Ojas (vital essence, immunity), strength and complexion. But in effect, it is the agni (digestive strength) that plays a vital role in this connection because tissue elements like, rasa, etc., cannot even originate from undigested food particles, if Agni is not present.[5]

Process of digestion

अन्नमादान कर्मा तु प्राणः कोष्ठं प्रकर्षति|
तद्द्रवैर्भिन्नसङ्घातं स्नेहेन मृदुतां गतम्||६||
समानेनावधूतोऽग्निरुदर्यः पवनोद्वहः|
काले भुक्तं समं सम्यक् पचत्यायुर्विवृद्धये||७||
एवं रस मलायान्नमाशयस्थमधः स्थितः|
पचत्यग्निर्यथा स्थाल्यामोदनायाम्बु तण्डुलम्||८||

Process of digestion:

Prana Vata, draws the ingested food into the koshta – alimentary tract. In the stomach, the food gets softened by the unctuous (oily) substance after which it gets split into small particles by the liquid.

The Agni (enzymes) located in the udara (stomach), gets stimulated by Samana vata. This Agni, stimulated by vata, digests the food that is taken in the required quantity and at the right time for the promotion of longevity.

Consider a cooking pot containing rice and water, placed on fire. As the fire, placed below the cooking pot helps in the cooking of food, similarly, Agni (enzyme) helps in the digestion of food located in the Amashaya – stomach. This leads to the production of Rasa – chyle – nutrition rich resultant of digestion and Mala (waste products). [6-8]

Avastha-paka – three stages of digestion process
1. Madhura Avastha Paka

अन्नस्य भुक्तमात्रस्य षड्रसस्य प्रपाकतः|
मधुराद्यात् कफो भावात् फेनभूत उदीर्यते||९||

As soon as the food consisting of 6 rasa (tastes) is taken, it goes to the stomach and sweetness (madhura-bhava) is manifested during the 1st stage of digestion. It results in the stimulation of kapha which is thin and frothy in nature.[9]

2. Amla Avastha Paka

परं तु पच्यमानस्य विदग्धस्याम्लभावतः|
आशयाच्च्यवमानस्य पित्तमच्छमुदीर्यते||१०||

During the second stage of digestion, the food remains in semi digested form (vidagdha) which results in sourness. While moving downwards from the amashaya (stomach), this (semi digested and sour stuff) stimulates the production of a transparent liquid called pitta (bile). Pitta itself has a sour taste. [10]

3. Katu Avastha Paka

पक्वाशयं तु प्राप्तस्य शोष्यमाणस्य वह्निना|
परिपिण्डितपक्वस्य वायुः स्यात् कटुभावतः||११||

When this food product reaches pakvashaya (large intestine), it gets further digested (cooked) and dehydrated by the agni (enzymes), and it takes a bolus-form resulting in pungent taste. This stimulates Vata Dosha. [11]

Satiation of sense organs by food:

अन्नमिष्टं ह्युपहितमिष्टैर्गन्धादिभिः पृथक्|
देहे प्रीणाति गन्धादीन् घ्राणादीनीन्द्रियाणि च||१२||

Intake of delicious and wholesome food that has pleasant appearance, smell, colour, touch and sound nourishes and satiates the sense organs – nose, eyes, skin, tongue and ears. [12]

Bhutagni paka – digestion by elemental fires

भौमाप्याग्नेय वायव्याः पञ्चोष्माणः सनाभसाः|
पञ्चाहारगुणान्स्वान्स्वान्पार्थिवादीन्पचन्ति हि||१३||
यथास्वं स्वं च पुष्णन्ति देहे द्रव्यगुणाः पृथक्|
पार्थिवाः पार्थिवानेव शेषाः शेषांश्च कृत्स्नशः||१४||

There are five types of Agni (digestive factors) based on 5 basic elements.
Parthivagni – responsible for digestion of solid food matters
Apyagni – responsible for digestion of liquid foods
Tejasagni - responsible for digestion of foods with fire element
Vayuvagni – responsible for digestion of air element and
Akashagni – responsible for digestion of food with ether element
They digest the respective elements and nourish the respective elements in the body. For example, Parthivagni digests solid foods and nourishes the solid body elements. [13-14]

Dhatvagni- paka – absorption of digested foods at tissue level:

सप्तभिर्देहधातारो धातवो द्विविधं पुनः|
यथास्वमग्निभिः पाकं यान्ति किट्टप्रसादवत् ||१५||

Thereafter, the digested food is subjected to Dhatu Paka. Dhatu means 7 types of tissues (Rasa, Rakta, Mamsa, Meda, Asthi, Majja and Shukra). Each of these Dhatu has their own Agni – digestion power. With this again, the digested food gets divided into
Sara bhaga – essence part. This nourishes the respective Dhatu.
Kitta bhaga – waste product – this forms the waste product (Mala) of the respective Dhatu. [15]

Process of metabolic transformation

रसाद्रक्तं ततो मांसं मांसान्मेदस्ततोऽस्थि च|
अस्थ्नो मज्जा ततः शुक्रं शुक्राद्गर्भः प्रसादजः||१६||

The nutrient fraction of Rasa dhatu provides nourishment to Rakta (blood).
The nutrient part of Rakta (blood) nourishes mamsa (muscle tissue),
that of mamsa to medas (fat),
that of medas to asthi (bone),
that of asthi to majja (bone marrow), and
The nutrient fraction of majja nourishes Shukra (semen). The foetus (garbha) is the product of nutrients of sukra or semen (sperm). [16]

Nourishment of upadhatus (subsidiary / secondary tissue elements)

रसात् स्तन्यं ततो रक्तमसृजः कण्डराः सिराः|
मांसादवसा त्वचः षट् च मेदसः स्नायुसम्भवः ||१७||

Breast milk (Stanya) and menstrual blood (Arthava) are formed out of Rasa
Kandara (tendons) and vessels (Sira) are formed out of Rakta,
Vasa (muscle fat) and 6 layers of skin are formed out of Mamsa and
Snayus (sinews) are formed out of medo-dhatu. [17]

Malas (waste-products)

किट्टमन्नस्य विण्मूत्रं, रसस्य तु कफोऽसृजः|
पित्तं, मांसस्य खमला, मलः स्वेदस्तु मेदसः||१८||

स्यात्किट्टं केश लोमास्थ्नो, मज्जः स्नेहोऽक्षि विट्त्वचाम्|
प्रसाद किट्टे धातूनां पाकादेवंविधच्छेतः ||१९||
परस्परोपसंस्तब्धा धातु स्नेह परम्परा |२०|

The following are the malas (waste products) of anna (food) and dhatus (tissue elements):

1. Anna (food) yields stool and urine as waste products

2. Rasa yields Kapha (phlegm) as waste product

3. Rakta (blood) gives out pitta

4. Mamsa (muscle tissue) produces kha-mala (waste products excreted from the cavities like eras, eyes, nose, mouth and genital organs)

5. Medas (fat tissue) – produces sweat

6. Asthi (bone) makes kesa (big hair) and loma (small hair)

7. Majja (bone-marrow) produces the unctuous substance present in the eyes, stool and skin

Thus, Prasada (nutrient fraction) and Kitta (waste product) these 2 categories of products arise out of the paka (metabolic transformation) of the dhatus (tissue elements). Therefore, the process of successive transformation of the dhatus is mutually inter- woven. [18 - 201/2]

Prabhava –

Usually, for the nourishment of Shukra Dhatu (semen and female reproductive components) first, Rasa dhatu should be nourished, then Rakta etc. and at the end, the nourishment reaches Shukra.

But some herbs when administered bypass nourishing all the other Dhatus and directly nourish Shukra dhatu. They act as aphrodisiac herbs – Vrushya. This action is caused by special efficacy of that herb – called Prabhava. [20 ½]

Time taken for metabolic transformation

षड्भिः केचिदहोरात्रैरिच्छन्ति परिवर्तनम्|
सन्तत्या भोज्यधातूनां परिवृत्तिस्तु चक्रवत्||२१||

According to some scholars, the transformation of dhatus from rasa to Shukra is affected in 6 days and nights. This process of transformation of the tissue elements requiring nourishment is a continuous one, like a moving wheel. [21]

Answer to query about metabolic transformation

इत्युक्तवन्तमाचार्यं शिष्यस्त्विदमचोदयत्|
रसाद्रक्तं विसद्दशात् कथं देहेऽभिजायते||२२||
रसस्य च न रागोऽस्ति स कथं याति रक्तताम्|
द्रवाद्रक्ता तिस्थिरं मांसं कथं तज्जायते नृणाम्||२३||
द्रवधातोः स्थिरान्मांसान्मेदसः सम्भवः कथम्|
श्लक्ष्णाभ्यां मांस मेदोभ्यां खरत्वं कथमस्थिषु||२४||
खरेष्वस्थिषु मज्जा च केन स्निग्धो मृदुस्तथा|
मज्जश्च परिणामेन यदि शुक्रं प्रवर्तते||२५||
सर्वं देहगतं शुक्रं प्रवदन्ति मनीषिणः|
तथाऽस्थि मध्य मज्जश्च शुक्रं भवति देहिनाम्||२६||
छिद्रं न दृश्यतेऽस्थनां च तन्निःसरति वा कथम्|
एवमुक्तस्तु शिष्येण गुरुः प्राहेदमुत्तरम्||२७||
तेजो रसानां सर्वेषां मनुजानां यदुच्यते|
पित्तोष्मणः स रागेण रसो रक्तत्वमृच्छति||२८||
वाय्वम्बु तेजसा रक्तमूष्मणा चाभिसंयुतम्|
स्थिरतां प्राप्य मांस स्यात् स्वोष्मणा पक्वमेव तत्||२९||
स्वतेजोऽम्बुगुणस्निग्धोद्रिक्तं मेदोऽभिजायते|

पृथिव्यग्न्यनिलादीनां सङ्घातः स्वोष्मणा कृतः||३०||
खरत्वं प्रकरोत्यस्य जायतेऽस्थि ततो नृणाम्|
करोति तत्र सौषिर्यमस्थ्नां मध्ये समीरणः||३१||
मेदसस्तानि पूर्यन्ते स्नेहो मज्जा ततः स्मृतः|
तस्मान्मज्जस्तु यः स्नेहः शुक्रं सञ्जायते ततः||३२||
वाय्वाकाशादिभिर्भावैः सौषिर्यं जायतेऽस्थिषु|
तेन स्रवति तच्छुक्रं नवात् कुम्भादिवोदकम्||३३||
स्रोतोभिः स्यन्दते देहात् समन्ताच्छुक्रवाहिभिः |
हर्षणोदीरितं वेगात् सङ्कल्पाच्च मनोभवात्||३४||
विलीनं घृतवद्व्यायामोष्मणा स्थानविच्युतम्|
बस्तौ सम्भृत्य निर्याति स्थलान्निम्नादिवोदकम्)||३५||

On hearing the discussion or discourse from Lord Punarvasu, Agnivesha enquired: "How is rakta (blood) produced out of dissimilar rasa (plasma) in the body?

Rasa is free from any colour. How does it acquire colour (redness)? Raktha is liquid by nature and how does the compactness and stability of Mamsa (muscle tissue) come out of raktha?

How is medas (fat tissue), which is semisolid, produced out of compact Mamsa? How do the bones attain kharatva (roughness and hardness) when they are produced out of mamsa and medas, that are smooth and soft?

On the other hand, the bones being so hard, how does majja (bone-marrow) which is so smooth and soft come out of them? How does majja (bone marrow) get transformed into Shukra (semen)? According to the wise, sukra pervades the entire body and majja from out of which it is produced is located inside the bone. No holes are visible in the bones. So, how does Shukra (semen) ooze out through the bones?

Lord Punarvasu replied as follows:

"Rasa dhatu (chyle, blood plasma) represents the essence (tejas) of all the rasas (ingredients of food and drinks having six tastes). That essence of rasa gets transformed into rakta (blood) by virtue of the colour (raga) imparted by the heat of Pitta.

This rakta again, accompanied by Vayu (air), Jala (water), tejas (fire) and heat (ushma) attains compactness and gets transformed into Mamsa (muscle tissue).

That mamsa cooked by its own heat (ushma = enzymes), gets transformed into medas (fat tissue) with the influence of liquidity (Ambu Guna) and Snigdha (unctuousness).

The Asthi dhatu (bone tissue) is produced by the transformation of medas (fat tissue) into a compact form. This compactness is brought about by the action of the Ushma (enzymes) of Medas. It is influenced by Pruthvi (earth), jala, and vayu elements. This enzymatic action gives rise to kharatva (hardness and roughness), with the result that asthi (bone) is manifested.

Vayu causes porosity in the interior of bones, and this porous space gets filled up with medas (fat). This unctuous substance is, thereafter, called majjja (bone marrow)

The unctuous substance (essence) of that majja (bone marrow), thereafter, gives rise to Shukra (male and female reproductive system). Porosity of bones is caused by vayu, akasha etc., and through these porous holes, exudation of Shukra takes place. This can be compared to exudation of water through the porous walls of a new earthen pot. The entire body is pervaded by fine channels carrying semen.

When a person gets excited because of the sexual urge, determination and amorous mental attitude, then semen comes out from the entire body through pores to the testicle. The displacement (ejaculation) of semen takes place because of the heat that is produced during the physical exercise involved at the time of sexual intercourse. This heat causes melting of semen. This happens on the analogy of the melting of ghee by the application of physical heat. From the testicles, semen gets ejaculated as water flows from a higher altitude to a place of lower altitude. [22-35]

Circulation of Rasa

व्यानेन रस धातुर्हि विक्षेपो चित कर्मणा|

युगपत् सर्वतोऽजसं देहे विक्षिप्यते सदा||३६||
क्षिप्यमाणः खवैगुण्याद्रसः सज्जति यत्र सः|
करोति विकृतिं तत्र खे वर्षमिव तोयदः||३७||
दोषाणामपि चैवं स्यादेक देश प्रकोपणम् |३८|

Circulation of Rasa

Vyana-vata (a type of Vata Dosha), which by nature stimulates the process of circulation, causes circulation of Rasa-dhatu all over the body simultaneously and continuously.

Rasa- dhatu during the process of circulation, gets stuck up due to the vitiation of the channels of circulation (Kha Vaigunya). It is at this very site of morbidity, that the disease is manifested. As the rains are caused by the (obstructed) cloud in the sky, similarly, the Doshas get vitiated in that particular spot to cause morbidity in a part of the body. [36- 381/2]

Importance of Jatharagni – digestive fire

इति भौतिक धात्वन्न पक्तृणां कर्म भाषितम्||३८||
अन्नस्य पक्ता सर्वेषां पक्तृणामधिपो मतः|
तन्मूलास्ते हि तद्वृद्धि क्षय वृद्धि क्षयात्मकाः||३९||
तस्मातं विधि वद्युक्तैरन्नपानेन्धनैर्हितैः|
पालयेत् प्रयतस्तस्य स्थितौ ह्ययुर्बलस्थितिः||४०||
यो हि भुङ्क्ते विधिं त्याक्त्वा ग्रहणी दोषजान् गदान्|
स लौल्याल्लभते शीघ्रं, वक्ष्यन्तेऽतः परं तु ते||४१||

Importance of Jataragni – digestive fire

Thus, 5 Bhautikagni (elemental digestive fire), 7 Dhatvagnis (tissue level digestive fire) and 1 Jatharagni (digestive enzymes in stomach and intestines) are responsible for food digestion and assimilation.

In all these 13 types of Agnis, Jatharagni (digestive fire in the stomach and intestines) is the chief. Bhutagni and Dhatvagni s are dependent upon it.

Aggravation or diminution of Jathatagni results in the aggravation or diminution of Bhutagni and Dhatvagni. Therefore, with appropriate types of fuel in the form of wholesome foods and drinks, the Jataragni should be carefully maintained. The strength of a person depends upon the strength of the Jataragni.

If a person takes food without following appropriate procedure, then he quickly succumbs to disease caused by the vitiation of Grahani (duodenum and the upper part of the small intestine) because of these uncontrolled habits. These ailments will be described hereafter. [38 ½- 41]

Ajeerna Nidana and Samprapti:

अभोजनादजीर्णाति भोजनादिवषमाशनात्|
असात्म्य गुरु शीताति रूक्ष सन्दुष्ट भोजनात्||४२||
विरेक वमन स्नेह विभ्रमाद्व्याधिकर्षणात्|
देशकालर्तुवैषम्याद्वेगानां च विधारणात्||४३||
दुष्यत्यग्निः, स दुष्टोऽन्नं न तत् पचति लघ्वपि|
अपच्यमानं शुक्तत्वं यात्यन्नं विषरूपताम् ||४४||

Ajeerna – Low digestion, causes and pathogenesis:

Agni (enzymes responsible for digestion and metabolism) gets vitiated of the following:

Abhojanat – Excessive fasting

Ajeernati Bhojanaat – Eating when digestion strength is low

Vishamashana – irregular eating

Asatmya – Intake of unwholesome,

Guru, Sheeta, Atirooksha Sandushta Bhojana – intake of heavy, cold excessively unctuous and polluted food

Improper administration of Vamana, Virechana, and Snehana therapies
Vyadhi Karshanat – Emaciation as a result of affliction by diseases
Residing in improper country and in inappropriate time
Seasonal perversions (raining during summer, high temperature during winter etc) and
Vega Vidharana – Suppression of manifested natural urges.
The above activities cause vitiation of Agni. The agni becomes so weak that it cannot digest even light foods. The undigested food becomes sour and it works like poison. This leads to the manifestation of Ajeerna. [42-44]

Ajirna Lakshana:
तस्य लिङ्गमजीर्णस्य विष्टम्भः सदनं तथा|
शिरसो रुक् च मूर्च्छा च भ्रमः पृष्ठकटिग्रहः||४५||
जृम्भाङ्गमर्दस्तृष्णा च ज्वरश्छर्दिः प्रवाहणम्|
अरोचको ऽविपाकश्च, घोरमन्नविषं च तत्||४६||
General signs and symptoms of Ajeerna
Vistambha – abdominal distension
Sadana – felling of prostration,
Shira ruk – headache,
Murcchha – fainting,
Bhrama – giddiness,
Prshta kati graha -stiffness of the back and lumber region,
Jrumbha – yawning,
Anga marda – malaise,
Trshna – morbid thirst,
Jwara – fever,
Chardi – vomiting,
Pravahanam – tenesmus
Aruchi – anorexia and
Avipaka – indigestion of food
This is a serious condition called Anna – visha – food turning into poison. [45-46]

Ajeerna Bheda Lakshana:
संसृज्यमानं पित्तेन दाहं तृष्णां मुखामयान्|
जनयत्यम्लपित्तं च पित्तजांश्चापरान् गदान्||४७||
यक्ष्म पीनस मेहादीन् कफजान् कफसङ्गतम्|
करोति वात संसृष्टं वातजांश्च गदान् बहून्||४८||
मूत्र रोगांश्च मूत्रस्थं कुक्षि रोगान् शकृद्गतम्|
रसादिभिश्च संसृष्टं कुर्याद्रोगान् रसादिजान्||४९||
Signs and symptoms of different types of Ajeerna:
Ajeerna when associated with Pitta, causes below symptoms –
Daha -burning sensation,
Trushna – morbid thirst and
Mukha roga – mouth ulcer
Amla pitta – hyper acidity and such other Paittik diseases.
When associated with kapha it gives rise to
Yakshma – tuberculosis,
Peenasa – chronic rhinitis, coryza
Meha – urinary diseases, diabetes and such other morbidities.

When associated with Vata Dosha, it gives rise to several vatika diseases.

When located in the urine, it causes urinary diseases and when located in the stools, it gives rise to diseases of the pelvic region. When associated with tissue elements, like rasa etc. it causes diseases of the concerned tissues, viz Rasa. etc [47-49]

Vishamagni and Teekshnagni:

विषमो धातुवैषम्यं करोति विषमं पचन्।

तीक्ष्णो मन्देन्धनो धातून् विशोषयति पावकः||५०||

Vishamagni – irregular type of Agni causes irregularity in the digestion of food, leading to discordance of tissue elements.

Teekshnagni – when digestive fire is intense, but the food quantity is low, it causes emaciation of tissue elements. [50]

Samagni – Normal state of Agni

युक्तं भुक्तवतो युक्तो धातुसाम्यं समं पचन्||५१|

If Agni is in normal state and if the individual takes an appropriate quantity of food, then there will be proper digestion of food, which leads to the maintenance of the equilibrium of all tissue elements. [1/2 51]

Signs of Mandagni and Grahani Gada

दुर्बलो विदहत्यन्नं तद्यात्यूर्ध्वमधोऽपि वा||५१||

अधस्तु पक्वमामं वा प्रवृत्तं ग्रहणीगदः|

उच्यते सर्वमेवान्नं प्रायो ह्यस्य विदह्यते||५२||

अतिसृष्टं विबद्धं वा द्रवं तदुपदिश्यते|

तृष्णारोचकवैरस्यप्रसेकतमकान्वितः||५३||

शूनपादकरः सास्थिपर्वरुक् छर्दनं ज्वरः|

लोहामगन्धिस्तिक्ताम्ल उद्गारश्चास्य जायते||५४||

Mandagni (weak digestion strength) brings about vidaha (semi-digested food) of food. Such a food is called vidagdha (partly digested) ahara. The disease in which such type of food moves downwards and gets excreted in the form of unformed (undigested) or formed (digested) stools is called Grahani. Here, the food remains in the state of vidagdha (partly undigested) avastha whether it is digested or not digested.

This leads to below symptoms:

Constipation or diarrhea.

Trushna – excess thirst

Arochaka – anorexia

Vairasya – distaste in mouth,

Praseka – excessive salivation and

Tamaka shvasa (asthma),

Parvaruk – pain in small joints,

Chardi – vomiting,

Jwara – fever and

Udgara – belching, eructation having metabolic smell, smell of ama (undigested food) and bitter and sour tastes. [51 ½- 54]

Grahani Poorvaroopa:

पूर्वरूपं तु तस्येदं तृष्णाssलस्यं बलक्षयः|

विदाहोऽन्नस्य पाकश्च चिरात् कायस्य गौरवम्||५५||

Premonitory signs and symptoms

Trushna – excess thirst

Alasya – laziness

Bala kshaya – diminution of strength

Vidaho annasya –partial digestion of food

Chirat anna paka – delay in the digestion of food and

Kaya Gauravam – heaviness of the body [55]

Definition of Grahani:

अग्न्यधिष्ठानमन्नस्य ग्रहणाद्ग्रहणी मता|

नाभेरुपर्यह्यग्निबलेनोपष्टब्धोप बृंहिता ||७६||

अपक्वं धारत्यन्नं पक्वं सृजति पार्श्वतः|

दुर्बलाग्निबला दुष्टा त्वाममेव विमुञ्चति||७७||

Definition of Grahani:

Grahani (duodenum, first part of intestine), which is the site of Agni (digestive enzymes), is called so, because of its power to restrain (Grahanat) the downward movement of food. It is located above the umbilical region, and is supported and nourished by the strength of Agni.

Normally, it restrains the downward movement of undigested food and after the digestion it releases the food through its Lumen. In the abnormal condition, when it gets vitiated because of weakness of Agni (power of digestion), it releases the food in undigested form only. [56-57]

Grahani Roga Bheda

वातात् पित्तात् कफाच्च स्यात्द्रोगस्त्रिभ्य एव च|

हेतुं लिङ्गं रूपभेदात् शृणु तस्य पृथक् पृथक्||७८||

Grahaniroga is of 4 types, viz,

Vatika – caused by the aggravation of vata

Paittika – caused by the aggravation of pitta

Kaphaja – caused by the aggravation of kapha and

Sannipatika – caused by the simultaneous aggravation of all the 3 Doshas

Their etiology, signs and symptoms (linga and rupa) are explained below. [58]

Vataja Grahani Nidana, Samprapti, lakshana –

कटु तिक्त कषायातिरूक्ष शीतल भोजनैः|

प्रमितानशनात्यध्व वेग निग्रह मैथुनैः||७९||

करोति कुपितो मन्दमग्निं सञ्छाद्य मारुतः |

तस्यान्नं पच्यते दुःखं शुक्त पाकं खराङ्गता||६०||

कण्ठास्य शोषः क्षुतृष्णा तिमिरं कर्णयोः स्वनः|

पार्श्वोरुवङ्क्षण ग्रीवारुजोऽभीक्ष्णं विसूचिका||६१||

हृत्पीडा कार्श्यं दौर्बल्यं वैरस्यं परिकर्तिका|

गृद्धिः सर्व रसानां च मनसः सदनं तथा||६२||

जीर्णे जीर्यति चाध्मानं भुक्ते स्वास्थ्यमुपैति च|

स वातगुल्म हृद्रोग प्लीहा शङ्की च मानवः||६३||

चिरादुःखं द्रवं शुष्कं तन्वामं शब्दफेनवत्|

पुनः पुनः सृजेद्वर्चः कास श्वासार्दितोऽनिलात्||६४||

Etiology, signs and symptoms of vatika grahani

Causes:

Intake of

Katu – pungent,

Tikta – bitter,

Kashaya – astringent,

Rooksha Sheetala bhojana – dry, cold foods

Pramitashana – intake of less of food, fasting,

Atyadhva – walking long distance,

Vega nigraha – suppression of natural urges and

Ati maithuna – excessive sexual intercourse.

Because of the above-mentioned factors, Vata Dosha gets aggravated and covers (Sanchadya) the suppressed Agni (power of digestion). As a result of this, the food taken by the patient does not get easily digested.

Symptoms:

This leads to acidity and roughness in the body,

Kanta Asya Shosha – dryness of throat and mouth,

Kshut, Trushna – excessive hunger & thirst,

Timira – appearance of darkness in the eyes,

Karnayo Swana – abnormal sound in the ears, tinnitus

Parshwa ruk – frequent pain in the sides of the chest, thighs, pelvic region and neck, pain in the cardiac region and neck,

Visucika – severe diarrhoea,

pain in the cardiac region, emaciation, weakness, distaste in the mouth, sawing pain in the abdomen, craving for (ingredients of food having) all tastes, mental frustration, flatulence after and burning the process of digestion, and temporary feeling of relief immediately after the intake of food.

The patient suspects as if he is suffering from Vatika Gulma (tumors), Hrdroga – heart diseases and splenic disorders. He passes stools with difficulty. Stool is liquid mixed, hard stool, thin and associated with ama (mucous), produces gurgling sounds and froth. He voids stools frequently and gets afflicted with cough and dyspnoea. All these signs and symptoms are manifested because of the aggravated Vata Dosha. [59-64]

Pittaja Grahani Nidana, Lakshana:

कट्वजीर्ण विदाह्यम्लक्षाराद्यैः पित्तमुल्बणम्।

अग्निमाप्लावयद्दधन्ति जलं तप्तमिवानलम्||६५||

सोऽजीर्ण नीलपीताभं पीताभः सार्यते द्रवम्।

पूत्यम्लोद्गार हृत्कण्ठदाहारुचि तृड्दितः||६६||

Causes, signs and symptoms of paittika grahani

Pitta gets aggravated by the intake of food ingredients which are

Katu – pungent,

Ajirna – Indigestion

vidahi – which cause burning sensation

Amla – sour

Kshara – alkaline etc.

The aggravated pitta suppresses and extinguishes agni (digestive enzymes), as hot water causes extinction of physical fire. The patient voids loose stool containing undigested material, which is bluish-yellow or yellow in colour.

He also suffers from eructation, foul smell and sour taste.

Hrut Kanta Daha – Burning sensation in the cardiac region and throat,

Aruchi – anorexia as well as

Trushna – excess thirst [65-66]

Kaphaja Grahani – Nidana, Lakshana

गुर्वति स्निग्ध शीतादि भोजनादतिभोजनात्‌|
भुक्तमात्रस्य च स्वप्नाद्धन्त्यग्निं कुपितः कफः||६७||
तस्यान्नं पच्यते दुःखं हृल्लास च्छर्द्यरोचकाः|
आस्योप देह माधुर्य कास ष्ठीवन पीनसाः||६८||
हृदयं मन्यते स्त्यानमुदरं स्तिमितं गुरु|
दुष्टो मधुर उद्गारः सदनं स्त्रीष्वहर्षणम्||६९||
भिन्नामश्लेष्म संसृष्ट गुरु वर्चःप्रवर्तनम्|
अकृशस्यापि दौर्बल्यमालस्यं च कफात्मके||७०||

Causes, signs and symptoms of Kaphaj Grahani:
Kapha gets aggravated by the intake of food, which is
Guru – heavy,
Snigdha – excessively unctuous,
Sheeta – cold etc.
By the intake of food in excess quantity and by sleeping immediately after food, in such circumstances, food does not get easily digested and the patient suffers from
Hrullasa – nausea,
Chardi – vomiting
Aruchi – anorexia
Stickiness and
Madhura aasya – sweet taste in the mouth,
Kasa – cough
Sthivana – spitting (excessive salivation) and
Pinasa – chronic rhinitis
A feeling of sluggishness in the cardiac region,
Stimita – Numbness and
Udara gurutvam – heaviness in the abdomen
Eructation with foul smell and sweet taste
Low libido.
He voids stool which is split into pieces, mixed with mucous and phlegm, and heavy. Even if not emaciated, the patient feels weak and indolent. [67-70]

यश्चाग्निः पूर्वमुद्दिष्टो रोगानीके चतुर्विधः|
तं चापि ग्रहणी दोषं समवर्जं प्रचक्ष्महे||७१||

In roganika chapter (Vimana sthana 6:12), 4 types of Agni, viz,
Tiksnagni – sharp
Mandagni – mild
Vishamagni —irregular and
Samagni – regular digestive fire are explained.
The first 3 types of disorders of agni also constitute Grahani dosha. [71]

Signs and symptoms of sannipatika grahani –
पृथग्वातादि निर्दिष्ट हेतु लिङ्ग समागमे|
त्रिदोष निर्दिशेतेषां भेषजं शृण्वतः परम्||७२||

The sannipatika (where all the 3 doshas are simultaneously vitiated) type of grahani gada is to be determined on the basis of simultaneous manifestation of all signs and symptoms pertaining to the 3 doshas (vide verse nos. 59-70). The treatment of these varieties of agni- dosha is expounded hereafter. [72]

Description of Ama-grahani –

ग्रहणीमाश्रितं दोषं विदग्धाहार मूर्च्छितम्|
सविष्टम्भ प्रसेकार्ति विदाहारुचि गौरवैः||७३||
आमलिङ्गान्वितं दृष्ट्वा सुखोष्णेनाम्बुनोद्धरेत्|
फलानां वा कषायेण पिप्पली सर्षपैस्तथा||७४||
लीनं पक्वाशयस्थं वाऽऽप्यामं स्राव्यं सदीपनैः|
शरीरानुगते सामे रसे लङ्घनपाचनम्||७५||
विशुद्धामाशयायास्मै पञ्चकोलादिभिः शृतम्|
दद्यात् पेयादि लघ्वन्नं पुनर्योगांश्च दीपनान्||७६||

Ama-grahani – when Grahani disease is associated with Ama (product of altered digestion and metabolism)

When Dosha is located in Grahani is afflicted by food, which is not fully digested (vidagdha – partly digested), then the signs of ama (product of improper digestion and metabolism) are manifested –

Vistambha – constipation

Praseka – salivation

Shoola – Pain

Vidaha – burning sensation

Aruchi – anorexia and

Gauravam – heaviness is manifested.

Such a patient is administered emetic therapy with the help of lukewarm water.

Alternatively, the decoction of Madanaphala – Randia dumetorum mixed with Pippali – long pepper- Piper longum and Sarshapa is used for Vamana – emetic therapy.

If the Ama (undigested food mix) moves downwards and remains adhered to the colon, then the patient is given Virechana purgation therapy with such herbs that stimulate digestion strength.

If the dosha in its ama (undigested) stage is converted into Rasa (chyle) and pervades other parts of the body, then the patient is made to fast, and should be given medicines conducive to Pachana (digestion) of the undigested material, e.g., yavagu (thick gruel).

After the amashaya is cleared, by the administration of appropriate Vamana (purgation) and Langhanam (fasting) therapies, the patient is given – Peya (thin gruel) prepared of the decoction of Panchakola (pippali—Piper longum, pippalimula – long pepper root, Chavya – Piper retrofractum, chitraka – Plumbago zeylanica and nagara – Zingiber officinale), etc.

He may also be given light food and such other ingredients as are stimulants of digestion. [73-76]

Treatment for Vataja Grahani

ज्ञात्वा तु परिपक्वामं मारुत ग्रहणी गदम्|
दीपनीय युतं सर्पिः पाययेताल्पशो भिषक्||७७||
किञ्चित्सन्धुक्षिते त्वग्नौ सक्त विण्मूत्र मारुतम्|
द्व्यहं त्र्यहं वा संस्नेह्य स्विन्नाभ्यक्तं निरूहयेत्||७८||
तत एरण्ड तैलेन सर्पिषा तैल्वकेन वा|
स क्षारेणानिले शान्ते स्रस्त दोषं विरेचयेत्||७९||
शुद्धं रूक्षाशयं बद्धवर्चसं चानुवासयेत्|
दीपनीयाम्ल वातघ्न सिद्धा तैलेन मात्रया||८०||
निरूढं च विरिक्तं च सम्यक् चैवानुवासितम्|
लघ्वन्नं प्रति सम्भुक्तं सर्पिरभ्यासयेत् पुनः||८१||

Treatment for Vataja Grahani:

Having ascertained that Vata and Grahani roga has become free from Ama, the physician should administer medicated ghee prepared with Deepaneeya herbs (improving digestion strength) in small quantities.

After the agni (power of digestion) is slightly stimulated, the patient becomes capable of retaining the stool, urine and flatus. To such a patient, Snehaha (oleation) therapy is administered for 2 or 3 days, followed by fomentation and massage therapies. Thereafter, niruha type of medicated enema is administered.

After the Dosha has become loosened (free from adhesion, Srastha Dosha), and the Vata is eliminated or alleviated as a result of the administration of niruha enema, the patient is given purgation therapy with the help of castor-oil or Tilvaka- Ghrita mixed with Kshara.

Even after the colon is cleansed, stool has become well formed; the dryness of the colon might persist. For correcting this dryness, the patient is given anuvasana basti (oil / fat enema) with the help of an appropriate quantity of oil cooked with drugs which stimulates digestion, which are sour in taste and which balance Vata Dosha.

After the appropriate administration of Niruha, Virechana and Anuvasana therapies the patient is given light food, and a course of medicated ghee is administered. [77-81]

Dashamuladya Ghrita

द्वे पञ्चमूले सरलं देवदारु सनागरम्|
पिप्पलीं पिप्पलीमूलं चित्रकं हस्ति पिप्पलीम्||८२||
शणबीजं यवान् कोलन् कुलत्थान् सुषवीं तथा |
पाचयेदारनालेन दध्ना सौवीरकेण वा||८३||
चतुर्भागावशेषेण पचेतेन घृताढकम्|
स्वर्जिकायावशूकाख्यौ क्षारौ दत्त्वा च युक्तितः||८४||
सैन्धवौद्भिद सामुद्र बिडानां रोमकस्य च|
स सौवर्चल पाक्यानां भागान्द्विपलिकान् पृथक्||८५||
विनीय चूर्णितान् तस्मात् पाययेत् प्रसृतं बुधः|
करोत्यग्निं बलं वर्णं वातघ्नं भुक्तपाचनम्||८६||
इति दशमूलाद्यं घृतम्|

Dashamuladi Ghrita

2 varieties of Panchamula, Sarala, Devadaru – Cedrus deodara, Nagara – Zingiber officinale, pippali – long pepper- Piper longum mula, gaja-pippali, seeds of sana, Yava, kola, kulattha and Suravi is boiled in Aranala, Dadhi manda or sauvira and reduced to 1/4th .

To this, 1 adhaka (2 adhakas according to general rule for manufacture) of ghee is mixed and reduced to 1/4th .To this, 1 adhaka (2 adhakas according to general rule for manufacture) palas of each of the powders of Svarjiksara,Yavaksara, Saindhava, Audbhida, Samudra, Vida, Romaka, Sauvarchala and pakya (pakaja) types of salt in appropriate time. After the recipe is cooked, it is administered to the patient in the dose of 1 prastha.

It promotes Agni – power of digestion, Bala – strength and Varnam – complexion.

It alleviates vayu, and helps in the digestion of the undigested food. Thus, ends the description of Dashamuladya-ghrta. [82-86]

Tryusanadi- ghritam

त्र्यूषण त्रिफला कल्के बिल्वमात्रे गुडात् पले|
सर्पिषोऽष्टपलं पक्त्वा मात्रां मन्दानलः पिबेत्||८७||
इति त्र्यूषणाद्यं घृतम्|

8 palas (384 g) of ghee is cooked by adding 1 pala (48 g) of the paste of Trikatu (ginger, pepper and long pepper) and Triphala (Haritaki, Vibhitaki and Amalki) taken together and 1 pala (48 g) of guda – Jaggery. This medicated ghee is taken by a person suffering from mandagni (suppressed power of digestion). [87]

Panhcamuladhya ghrta [taila] and churna

पञ्चमूलाभया व्योष पिप्पलीमूल सैन्धवैः|

रास्ना क्षार द्वयाजाजी विडङ्ग शटिभि घृतम्||८८||
शुक्तेन मातुलुङ्गस्य स्वरसेनार्द्रकस्य च|
शुष्कमूलक कोलाम्बु चुक्रिका दाडिमस्य च||८९||
तक्र मस्तु सुरामण्ड सौवीरक तुषोदकैः|
काञ्जिकेन च तत् पक्वमग्नि दीप्तिकरं परम्||९०||
शूल गुल्मोदर श्वास कासानिल कफापहम्|
स बीजपूरकरसं सिद्धं वा पाययेद्घृतम्||९१||
सिद्धमभ्यञ्जनार्थं च तैलमेतैः प्रयोजयेत्|
एतेषामौषधानां वा पिबेच्चूर्णं सुखाम्बुना||९२||
वाते श्लेष्मावृते सामे कफे वा वायुनोद्धते|
दद्याच्चूर्णं पाचनार्थमग्नि सन्दीपनं परम्||९३||
इति पञ्चमूलाद्यं घृतं चूर्णं च|

Panhcamuladya Ghrita, Taila and Churna

Ghee is cooked by adding the paste of Panchamula (bilva – Aegle marmelos, Shyonaka - Oroxylum indicum, Gambhari – Gmelina arborea, Patali – Stereospermum suaveolens and ganikarika), Haritaki – Terminalia chebula, Trikatu (Sunthi – Zingiber officinale, pippali- Piper longum and Maricha – Piper nigrum) pippali mula , Saindhava, Rasna – Alpinia galanga, Svarji- ksara, Yavaksara, Ajaji – Nigella sativa, Vidanga – Embelia ribes and Sati—Hedychium spicatum and liquids, viz sukta, Matulunga(juice), Ardraka – wet ginger (rhizome)(juice) suska- mulaka (decoction), kolambu, Chukrika, dadima – Punica granatum(juice), takra, mastu, Suramanda, Sauviraka, Tusodaka and kanjika.

It is an excellent promoter of the power of digestion.

It cures

Shoola – colic pain

Gulma – abdominal tumour distension (phantom tumour)

Udara – ascites (obstinate abdominal diseases including ascites),

Shvasa – asthma and

Kasa – cough

It also alleviates Vata and Kapha.

Alternatively, this medicated ghee can be prepared by adding the juice of Bijapuraka – Citrus medica to the above given to the patient.

Oil cooked with the above mentioned ingredients is useful for massage.

The powder of panchamula (Bilva – Aegle marmelos, Shyonaka – Oroxylum indicum, Gambhari – gmelina arborea , Patala – Stereospermum suaveolens and ganikarika), haritaki – Terminalia chebula,Trikatu (Ginger, pepper and long pepper), Pippali mula – long pepper root, Saindhava, Rasna – Alpinia galanga, Svarji ksara, Yava ksara, Ajaji – Nigella sativa, Vidanga – Embelia ribes and Shati – Hedychium spicatum (which are mentioned to be added as paste in the above recipe) can be given to the patient along with luke- warm water.

This powder is useful for alleviating vayu occluded by kapha in its association with ama (product of improper digestion); or kapha stimulated by vayu. This powder recipe is carminative and it is an excellent stimulator of the power of digestion.

Thus, ends the description of Panchamula- ghrta and Panchamuladya churna. [88-93]

Determination of Sama and nirama types of grahani roga:

मज्जत्यामा गुरुत्वादिट् पक्वा तूत्प्लवते जले|
विनाऽति द्रव सङ्घात शैत्य श्लेष्म प्रदूषणात्||९४||
परीक्ष्यैवं पुरा सामं निरामं चामदोषिणम्|
विधिनोपाचरेत् सम्यक् पाचनेनेतरेण वा||९५||

The stool associated with ama sinks in water due to its heaviness. If the stool is voided after proper digestion (pakva, i.e if it is not associated with ama), then it floats over the water.

This rule does not hold good or apply in cases where the consistency of the stool is thin or exceedingly compact, and if the stool is afflicted with excessive cold or Kapha. Therefore, the Nirama (Ama – less) or Sama nature of the stools should be tested well before administering suitable therapies.[94-95]

Chitrakadya gutika

चित्रकं पिप्पलीमूलं द्वौ क्षारौ लवणानि च|

व्योषं हिङ्ग्वजमोदां च चव्यं चैकत्र चूर्णयेत्||९६||

गुटिका मातुलुङ्गस्य दाडिमस्य रसेन वा|

कृता विपाचयत्यामं दीपयत्याशु चालनम्||९७||

इति चित्रकाद्या गुटिका|

Chitrakadi gutika

Chitraka – Plumbago zeylanica, Pippali mula – long pepper- Piper longum, Yavaksara, Svarjiksara (5 types of) salt, Sunthi – Zingiber officinale, pippali , maricha – Piper nigrum, Hingu – Asaefetida, Ajamoda – ajowan seed – Trachyspermum ammi and chavya – Piper chaba—all these drugs taken together, is made to a powder. This is then triturated by adding juice of Matulunga – Citrus medica or dadima – Punica granatum and made to pills. Intake of these pills is efficacious for the metabolic transformation (cooking) of ama (product of improper digestion and metabolism). It also stimulates agni (power of digestion and metabolism).

Thus, ends the description of Chitrakadhya –gutika [96-97]

Nagaradi Kwatha

नागरातिविषा मुस्त क्वाथः स्यादाम पाचनः|

मुस्तान्त कल्कः पथ्या वा नागरं चोष्णवारिणा||९८||

Nagaradi Kashaya, Churna

Intake of the decoction of Nagara – Zingiber officinale, Ativisha – Aconitum heterophyllum and Musta – Cyperus rotundus (root) helps in the metabolic transformation (cooking) of ama (product of improper digestion and metabolism).

Similarly, the paste / powder of the above herb is taken along with hot water for pachana (cooking or metabolic transformation) of ama.

Intake of the powder of Haritaki – Terminalia chebula or Nagara – ginger along with hot water also helps in the Pachana of Ama. [98]

Devadarvadi Churna with varuni:

देवदारु वचा मुस्त नागरातिविषाभयाः|

वारुण्यामासुतास्तोये कोष्णे वाऽलवणाः पिबेत्||९९||

वर्चस्यामे सशूले च पिबेद्वा दाडिमाम्बुना|

Devadaru – Cedrus deodara,

Vacha –Acorus calamus,

Musta –Cyperus rotundus (root),

Nagara – ginger – Zingiber officinale,

Ativisha – Aconitum heterophyllum and

Abhaya – harad –Terminalia chebula is soaked in Varuni (an alcoholic preparation) and taken by the patient by adding a small quantity of salt along with hot water. This recipe is used if there is ama (mucus) in the stool and if the patient is having colic pain.

Alternatively, the above powder is administered along with pomegranate juice. [99 – 100½]

Vida lavanadi churna:

विडेन लवणं पिष्टं बिल्वं चित्रक नागरम्||१००||
सामे वा सकफे वाते कोष्ठशूलकरे पिबेत्|

If the pain in the kostha (abdomen, pelvis) is caused by Vata and is associated with ama (mucus) or kapha, then the patient should take the paste of bilva – bael – Aegle marmelos, Chitraka – Plumbago zeylanica and Nagara – ginger which is made saline by adding Vidalavana (Bida salt). [100½ - 1011/2]

Kalingadi Churna:

कलिङ्ग हिङ्ग्वतिविषा वचा सौवर्चलाभयाः||१०१||
छर्द्यर्शो ग्रन्थि शूलेषु पिबेदुष्णेन वारिणा|
पथ्या सौवर्चलाजाजी चूर्ण मरिचसंयुतम्||१०२||

If there is vomiting, piles and colic pain, then the patient should take the powder of kalinga, Hingu – Asafoetida, ativisha – Aconitum heterophyllum, Vacha – Acorus calamus, Sauvarchala- Black salt and Abhaya – harad – along with hot water.
Alternatively, the patient having vomiting etc., (mentioned above) should take the powder of Pathya, Sauvarcala and Ajaji – Nigella sativa mixed with Maricha – Black pepper. [101 ½- 102]

Abhayadi kashaya / Churna:

अभयां पिप्पलीमूलं वचां कटुक रोहिणीम्|
पाठां वत्सक बीजानि चित्रकं विश्वभेषजम्||१०३||
पिबेन्निष्क्वाथ्य चूर्ण वा कृत्वा कोष्णेन वारिणा|
पित्त श्लेष्माभिभूतायां ग्रहण्यां शूलनुद्दिधतम्||१०४||

Abhayadi kashaya / Churna:
The patient should take the decoction or the powder of
Abhaya – harad – Terminalia chebula,
Pippalimula – Long pepper root,
Vacha – Acorus calamus,
Katuka rohini – Picrorhiza kurroa,
Patha – Cyclea peltata,
seeds of Vatsaka – Kutaja beeja,
Chitraka – Plumbago zeylanica and
Vishvabheshaja – ginger along with lukewarm water, which is useful for curing colic pain in Grahani roga caused by the affliction of Pitta and kapha. [103- 104]

सामे सातिविषं व्योषं लवणक्षार हिङ्गु च|
निःक्वाथ्य पाययेच्चूर्ण कृत्वा वा कोष्णवारिणा||१०५||

If grahani is associated with ama (mucus), then the patient is given the decoction or powder of abhaya – harad – Terminalia chebula, pippali moola – long pepper root Piper longum, Vacha, Katukarohini – Picrorhiza kurroa, patha – Cyclea peltata, seeds of vatsaka, chitraka – Plumbago zeylanica and visvabhesaja) along with ativisha – Aconitum heterophyllum, shunthi – Zingiber officinale, pippali – long pepper- Piper longum, maricha – Piper nigrum, lavana ksara and hingu with luke-warm water. [105]

Pippalyadya- curna

पिप्पली नागरं पाठां सारिवां बृहती द्वयम्|
चित्रकं कौटजं बीजं लवणान्यथ पञ्च च||१०६||
तच्चूर्ण सयवक्षारं दध्युष्णाम्बुसुरादिभिः|
पिबेदग्नि विवृद्ध्यर्थं कोष्ठ वातहरं नरः||१०७||

The powder of

Pippali — Piper longum

Nagara – Zingiber officinale

Patha – Cyclea peltata

Sariva –Hemidesmus indicus

Brhati – Solanum indicum

Kantakari – Solanum xanthocarpum

Chitraka – Plumbago zeylanica

Seed of kutaja – Holarrhena antidysenterica

Saindhava – rock salt

Samudra lavana

Vida lavana

Audbhida

Sauvarcala is given along with

Yavaksara

Yoghurt, hot water and different types of alchoholic drinks for the promotion of agni (power of digestion) and elimination of vayu (flatus) from the kostha (gastro- intestinal tract). [106-107]

Marichadya- curna for Vataja Grahani

मरिचं कुञ्चिकाम्बष्ठा वृक्षाम्लाः कुडवाः पृथक्|

पलानि दश चाम्लस्य वेतसस्य पलार्धिकम्||१०८||

सौवर्चलं बिडं पाक्यं यवक्षारः ससैन्धवः|

शटी पुष्कर मूलानि हिङ्गु शिवाटिका||१०९||

तत् सर्वमेकतः सूक्ष्मं चूर्णं कृत्वा प्रयोजयेत्|

हितं वाताभिभूतायां ग्रहण्यामरुचौ तथा||११०||

इति मरिचाद्यं चूर्णम्|

1 kudava of each of

Maricha – Piper nigrum

Kunchika

Ambastha – Cyclea peltata

Vruksamla – Garcinia ambogia

10 palas of

Amla vetasa – Garcinia pedunculata

½ palas of each of sauvarcala

Vida salt

Pakya (pamsuja-lavana)

Yavaksara saindhava

Sati – Hedychium spicatum

Puskaramula – Inula racemosa

Hingu – Asafoetida

Hingu-sivatika (vamsapatri) is taken together and made to a fine powder.

Administration of this recipe is useful in grahani, caused by the affliction of vayu and in anorexia.

Thus, ends the description of marichadya – churna. [108- 1101/4]

चतुर्णां प्रस्थमम्लानां त्र्यूषणस्य पलत्रयम्|

लवणानां च चत्वारि शर्करायाः पलाष्टकम्|

सञ्चूर्ण्य शाक सूपान्नरागादिष्ववचारयेत्||१११||

कासाजीर्णारुचि श्वासा हृत्पाण्ड्वामय शूलनुत्||११२|
1 prastha (768 g) of 4 sour herbs
1 pala of
Sunthi – Zingiber officinale
Pippali – long pepper- Piper longum
Maricha – Piper nigrum taken together 4 palas of salts
Saindhava
Sauvarcala
Bida
Audbhida
Samudra types of salt taken together and 8 palas of sugar is made into a powder.
This powder is added to vegetable preparations, dals, rice, raga (pickles and similar other preparations), which cures
Kasa – cough
Ajirna – indigestion
Aruchi – anorexia
Shvasa – asthma
Hrud roga – heart diseases
Pandu – anaemia and
Shula – colic pain [111-3/4 - 1121/2]

Yavagu for Vataja Grahani
चव्य त्वक्पिप्पलीमूल धातकी व्योष चित्रकान्||११२||
कपित्थं बिल्वमम्बष्ठां शाल्मलं हस्ति पिप्पलीम्|
शिलोद्भेदं तथाऽजाजीं पिष्ट्वा बदर सम्मितम्||११३||
परिभर्ज्य घृते दध्ना यवागूं साधयेद्भिषक्|
रसैः कपित्थ चुक्रिका वृक्षाम्लैर्दाडिमस्य च||११४||
सर्वातिसार ग्रहणी गुल्मार्शःप्लीहनाशिनी|
1 kola (6 g) of each of chavya – Piper retrofractum
Tvak – Cinnamomum zeylanica
Pippali mula – Piper longum
Dhataki – Woodfordia fruticosa
Sunthi – Zingiber officinale
Pippali – Piper longum
Maricha – Piper nigrum
Chitraka – Plumbago zeylanica
Kapittha -Feronia limonia
Bilva – bael – Aegle marmelos
Ambastha – Cyclea peltata
Gum of shalmali – Salmalia malabarica
Gaja pippali
Silodbheda (sailaja)
Ajaji – Nigella sativa is made into a paste.
This paste with curd is fried by adding ghee. With the help of this paste gruel is prepared by adding the juice of
Kapittha –Feronia limonia
Cukrika (changeri) — Oxalis corniculata
Vrksamla — Garcinia indica
Dadima – Punica granatum

Intake of this medicated gruel cures all types of

Atisara — diarrohea,

Grahani,

Gulma – phantom tumour

Arshas — piles and

Pliha — splenic disorders. [112 ½- 115½]

Diet and drinks for Vataja Grahani

पञ्चकोलक यूषश्च मूलकानां च सोषणः||११५||

स्निग्धो दाडिम तक्राम्लो जाङ्गलः संस्कृतो रसः|

क्रव्याद स्वरसः शस्तो भोजनार्थै सदीपनः||११६||

तक्रारनाल मद्यानि पानायारिष्ट एव च|११७|

Soup of Panchakola

Pippali – long pepper- Piper longum

Pippali mula – long pepper- Piper longum

Chavya – Piper chaba

Chitraka – Plumbago zeylanica

Nagara – Zingiber officinale

Or the soup of mulaka prepared by adding marica and ghee or oil, or the soup of the meat of birds and animals inhabiting arid land prepared by sizzling (with ghee etc) or the soup of the meat of kravyada (meat eating) types of birds and animals prepared by adding drugs, which stimulate the power of digestion is made sour by adding dadima – Punica granatum and buttermilk and administered as food to the patient suffering from grahani. He is given buttermilk, aranala (a sour drink), alcoholic drinks and arista (a type of alcoholic drink) as drinks.[1151/2 - 1171/2]

Butter milk for Vataja Grahani

तक्रं तु ग्रहणीदोषे दीपन ग्राहि लाघवात्||११७||

श्रेष्ठं मधुर पाकित्वान्न च पित्तं प्रकोपयेत्|

कषायोष्ण विकाशित्वाद्रौक्ष्याच्चैव कफे हितम्||११८||

वाते स्वाद्वम्ल सान्द्रत्वात् सद्यस्कम विदाहि तत्|

तस्मात् तक्र प्रयोगा ये जठराणां तथाऽर्शसाम्||११९||

विहिता ग्रहणीदोषे सर्व शस्तान् प्रयोजयेत्|

For a patient suffering from grahani, butter milk is an excellent drink because it stimulates the power of digestion, it is grahi – absorbent, bowel binding, useful in IBS, diarrhoea (constipative) and light for digestion.

It is sweet in vipaka (the taste thet emerges after digestion) and therefore, it does not cause aggravation of pitta.

Because of its astringent taste, hot potency, vikasitva (which relieves the stiffness and causes looseness of joints and ununctuousness, it is useful for counteracting the aggravated kapha.

Because of the sweet and sour tastes and density, it is useful for counter-acting aggravated vayu.

When freshly prepared, it does not cause a burning sensation. Therefore, all the recipes of buttermilk described for the treatment of Udara (ascites) and piles is used for the treatment of Grahani. [117½ - 120½]

Takrarista for Vataja Grahani

यवान्यामलके पथ्या मरिचं त्रिपलंशिकम्||१२०||

लवणानि पलांशानि पञ्च चैकत्र चूर्णयेत्|

तक्रे तदासुतं जातं तक्रारिष्टं पिबेन्नरः|

दीपनं शोथ गुल्मार्शःक्रिमि मेहोदरापहम्||१२१||

इति तक्रारिष्टः|

3 palas each of Yavani

Amalaki (indian gooseberry fruit –Emblica officinalis gaertn)

Pathya

Maricha – Piper nigrum as well as one pala each of saindhava, sauvarcala

Audbhida

Bida

Samudra types of salt are made into a powder.

To this, butter- milk is added and kept till it is fermented and becomes sour. This recipe is called "takrarista".

Intake of this recipe stimulates the power of digestion and cures

Shotha — oedema,

Gulma – abdominal tumor, distension (phantom tumor),

Arshas — piles, parasitic infestation,

Meha – urinary tract disorders, diabetes (obstinate urinary disorders including diabetes) and

Udara – ascites (obstinate abdominal disorders including ascites).

Thus ends the description of takrarista [120 ½ – 121]

This ends the treatment for Vataja Grahani.

Treatment for Pittaja type of Grahani:

Panchakarma therapy in Pittaja Grahani:

स्वस्थानगतमुत्क्लिष्टमग्नि निर्वापकं भिषक्|

पित्तं ज्ञात्वा विरेकेण निर्हरेद्वमनेन वा||१२२||

Having ascertained that the aggravated pitta is located in its natural habitat, the physician should administer Virachana treatment – Purgation or Vamana – emetic therapy for the removal of aggravated Pitta from the body. [122]

Diet for Paittika Grahani

अविदाहिभिरन्नैश्च लघुभिस्तिक्त संयुतैः|

जाङ्गलानां रसै यूषै मुद्गादीनां खडैरपि||१२३||

दाडिमाम्लैः स सर्पिष्कैर्दीपन ग्राहि संयुतैः|

तस्याग्निं दीपयेच्चूर्णैः सर्पिर्भिश्चापि तिक्तकैः||१२४||

The patient suffering from Paittika grahani is given such a diet which does not cause Vidaha (burning sensation), which is light and which is added with the powder of bitter ingredients.

He is given the soup of the meat of animals inhabiting arid zones (Jangala mamsarasa), the soup of vegetable products like mudga (green gram) and khasa (a sour drink).

These food preparations are added with sour dadima – Punica granatum, ghee, herbs which cause stimulation of the digestion and which are constipative, absorbent (grahi).

His power of digestion is stimulated by the administration of the powder of bitter herbs. [123-124]

Chandanadya ghruta for Pittaja Grahani

चन्दनं पद्मकोशीरं पाठां मूर्वा कुटन्नटम्|

षड्ग्रन्था सारिवास्फोता सप्तपर्णाटरूषकान्||१२५||

पटोलोदुम्बराश्वत्थ वट प्लक्ष कपीतनान्|

कटुकां रोहिणीं मुस्तं निम्बं च द्विपलांशिकम्||१२६||

द्रोणेऽपां साधयेत् पादशेषे प्रस्थं घृतात् पचेत्|

किराततिक्तेन्द्र यव वीरामागधिकोत्पलैः||१२७||

कल्के रक्ष समैः पेयं तत् पित्तग्रहणीगदे|

2 palas each of chandana – Santalum album

Padmaka — Prunus cerasoides

Ushira — Vetiveria zizanioides

Patha – Cyclea peltata

Murvakutannata (kaivarta-mustaka)

Shadgrantha (vacha) – Acorus calamus

Sariva – Hemidesmus indicus

Asphota (asphura-mallika)

Saptaparna – Alstonia scholaris

Atarusaka – Vasa – Adhatoda vasica

Patola – Trichosanthes dioica

Udumbara — Ficus racemosa

Asphura

Vata – Ficus bengalensis

Plaksa – Ficus lacor

Kapitana (gandha-munda)

Asvattha – Ficus religiosa

Katuka rohini — Picrorhiza kurroa

Musta – nut grass (root) – Cyperus rotundus

Nimba — Azadirachta indica is boiled in 2 dronas (double the prescribed quantity in view of mana-pribhasa) of water and reduced to 1/4th.

To this decoction, 2 prasthas (double the prescribed quantity in view of mana paribhasa) of ghee and the paste of 1 aksa of each of

Kiratatikta – Swertia chirata

Indrayava – Holarrhena antidysenterica

Vira

Magadhika and

Utpala – water lilies are added and cooked.

This medicated ghee is taken by a patient suffering from paittika type of grahani.

Thus, ends the description of chandanadya ghrta. [125 – 128½]

Tikata grtha for Pittaja Grahani

तिक्तकं यद्घृतं चोक्तं कौष्ठिके तच्च दापयेत्||१२८||

इति चन्दनाद्यं घृतम्|

Tikata ghrita described for the treatment of kustha (skin diseases) may also be administered to the patient suffering from grahani. [128 ½]

Nagaradya Churna for Pittaja Grahani

नागरातिविषे मुस्तं धातकीं च रसाञ्जनम्|

वत्सक त्वक्फलं बिल्वं पाठां कटुकरोहिणीम्||१२९||

पिबेत् समांशं तच्चूर्णं सक्षौद्रं तण्डुलाम्बुना|

पैतिके ग्रहणी दोषे रक्तं यच्चोपवेश्यते||१३०||

अर्शांसि च गुदे शूलं जयेच्चैव प्रवाहिकाम्|

नागराद्यमिदं चूर्णं कृष्णात्रेयेण पूजितम्||१३१||

इति नागराद्यं चूर्णम्|

Nagaradi Churna:

Nagara – Zingiber officinale

Ativisa – Aconitum heterophyllum

Musta – nut grass (root) – Cyperus rotundus

Dhataki – Woodfordia fruticosa

Rasanjana

Bark and fruit of Vatsaka

Bilva – bael – Aegle marmelos

Patha – Cyclea peltata

Katuka-rohini — Picrorhiza kurroa is taken in equal quantities and made into a powder.

This powder is taken along with honey and tandulambu (rice water) by the patient suffering from paittika type of grahani with the symptomatic voiding of blood along with stool, and suffering from piles and pain in anal region. It also cures pravahika (dysentery). This recipe is called nagaradya-curna. This is highly esteemed by lord krsnatreya.

Thus, ends the description of nagaradya- curna. [129-131]

Bhunimbadya churna for Pittaja Grahani

भूनिम्ब कटुका व्योष मुस्तकेन्द्रयवान् समान्‌।

द्वौ चित्रकाद्वत्सकत्वग्भागान् षोडश चूर्णयेत्‌।।१३२।।

गुड शीताम्बुना पीतं ग्रहणीदोष गुल्मनुत्‌।

कामला ज्वर पाण्डुत्वमेहारुच्यतिसारनुत्‌।।१३३।।

इति भूनिम्बाद्यं चूर्णम्‌।

1 part of each of Bhunimba – Andrographis paniculata

Katuka

Sunthi – Zingiber officinale

Pippali- long pepper fruit – Piper longum

Maricha – Piper nigrum

Musta – nut grass (root) – Cyperus rotundus

Indrayava

2 parts of chitraka and 16 parts of the bark of vatsaka is made into a powder.

Intake of this recipe along with cold water mixed with jaggery cures

Grahani,

Gulma – abdominal tumor, distension (phantom tumour)

Kamala — Jaundice

Jwara — Fever,

Pandu — anemia,

Meha — obstinate urinary disorders including diabetes),

Aruch — anorexia and

Atisara – diarrhoea

Thus ends the description of bhunimbadya — churna [132- 133]

Supplement to bhunimbadya- churna

वचामतिविषां पाठां सप्तपर्णं रसाञ्जनम्‌।

स्योनाकोदीच्य कट्वङ्ग वत्सक त्वग्दुरालभाः।।१३४।।

दार्वी पर्पटकं पाठां यवानीं मधु शिग्रुकम्‌।

पटोलपत्रं सिद्धार्थान् यूथिकां जाति पल्लवान्‌।।१३५।।

जम्ब्वाम्र बिल्व मध्यानि निम्ब शाक फलानि च।

तद्रोगशममन्विच्छन् भूनिम्बाद्येन योजयेत्‌।।१३६।।

Vacha – Acorus calamus

Ativisha – Aconitum heterophyllum

Patha – Cyclea peltata

Saptaparna – Alstonia scholaris

Rasanjana

Shyonaka – Oroxylum indicum

Udichya

Katvanga (a type of syonaka having smaller fruits),

Bark of vatsaka

Duralabha – Fagonia arabica

Darvi – Berberis aristata

Parpataka

Yavani – Carum copticum

Madhu

Shigru – Moringa oleifera

Leaf of patola — Trichosanthes dioica

Siddhartha

Yuthika

Leaves of Jati – Jasminum grandiflorum

Seed pulp of jambu — Syzygium cumini

Seed-pulp of amra – Mangifera indica

Pulp of (unripe) bilva – Aegle marmelos

Leaves and fruits of nimba – Azadirachta indica is used in a powder form along with the ingredients of bhunimbadya-churna (described above) [134-136]

Kiratadya Churna for Pittaj Grahni:

किराततिक्तः षड्ग्रन्था त्रायमाणा कटुत्रिकम्|
चन्दनं पद्मकोशीरं दार्वी त्वक् कटुरोहिणी||१३७||
कुटज त्वक्फलं मुस्तं यवानी देवदारु च|
पटोल निम्बपत्रैलासौराष्ट्रयतिविषा त्वचः||१३८||
मधु शिग्रोश्च बीजानि मूर्वा पर्पटकस्तथा|
तच्चूर्णं मधुना लेह्यं पेयं मद्यैर्जलेन वा||१३९||
हृत्पाण्डु ग्रहणीरोग गुल्म शूलारुचि ज्वरान्|
कामलां सन्निपातं च मुखरोगांश्च नाशयेत्||१४०||
इति किराताद्यं चूर्णम्|

Kiratadi Churna:

The powder of kirta-tikta — Swertia chirata

Shadgrantha – Acorus calamus

Trayamana – Gentiana kurroo

Sunthi – Zingiber officinale

Pippali – Piper longum

Maricha – Piper nigrum

Chandana – Santalum album

Padmaka — Prunus cerasoides

Ushira –Vetiveria zizanoides

Bark of daru-haridra – Berberis aristata

Katuka-rohini — Picrorhiza kurroa

Bark and fruits of kutaja – Hollarhena anti dysentrica

Musta – Cyperus rotundus

Yavani – Carum copticum

Devadaru — Cedrus deodara

Patola — Trichosanthes dioica
Nimba – neem (Azadirachta indica)
Patra – Cinnamon leaves
Ela – Cardamom
Saurastri
Ativisha – Aconitum heterophyllum
Tvak – Cinnamomum zeylanica
Seeds of madhu-sigru – Moringa oliefera
Murva — Marsedenia tenacissima
Parpataka is made to linctus by adding honey, and taken by the patient. This recipe may also be taken along with alcohol or water.
It cures
Hrud roga — heart diseases,
Pandu — anemia,
Grahani- roga,
Gulma (phantom tumor),
Shoola — colic pain,
Aruchi — anorexia,
Jwara — fever,
Kamala — jaundice,
Sannipatika type of diarrhea and
Mukha roga — diseases of the mouth
Thus ends the description of kiratadya — curna [137-140]
This ends the treatment for Pittaja Grahani.

Treatment for Kaphaja Grahani:
Elimination therapy for kaphaja grahani
ग्रहण्यां श्लेष्मदुष्टायां वमितस्य यथाविधि|
कट्वम्ल लवण क्षारैस्तिक्तैश्चाग्निं विवर्धयेत्||१४१||
If the Grahani is caused by aggravated kapha, then the patient is given Vamana – emetic therapy according to the prescribed procedure. Thereafter pungent, sour, saline, alkaline and bitter drugs are administered for the promotion of this power of digestion. [141]

Drinks for kaphaja grahani
पलाशं चित्रकं चव्यं मातुलुङ्गं हरीतकीम्|
पिप्पलीं पिप्पलीमूलं पाठां नागर धान्यकम्||१४२||
कार्षिकाण्युदकप्रस्थे पक्त्वा पादावशेषितम्|
पानीयार्थं प्रयुञ्जीत यवागूं तैश्च साधयेत्||१४३||
1 karsa (12 g) of each of
Palasha — Butea monosperma
Chitraka – leadword – Plumbago zeylanica,
Chavya – Piper chaba
Matulunga – lemon variety citrus limon
Haritaki – Terminalia chebula
Pippali mula – long pepper fruit – Piper longum
Patha – Cyclea peltata
Nagara – Zingiber officinale and

Dhanyaka is boiled in 1 prastha (2 prasthas is taken according to mana- paribhasa) of water, and reduced to 1/4th. This decoction is given as a drink to the patient. With the help of this decoction, gruel is prepared and given to the patient (suffering from kaphaja type of grahani) [142-143]

Diet and kaphaja grahani

शुष्क मूलक यूषेण कौलत्थेनाथवा पुनः|

कट्वम्ल क्षारपटुना लघून्यन्नानि भोजयेत्||१४४||

Ingredients of food which are light for digestion, along with the soup of dried radish or kulattha (horse gram) mixed with pungent, sour, alkaline and saline drugs. [144]

Butter milk in kaphaja grahani

अम्लं चानु पिबेतक्रं तक्रारिष्टमथापि वा|

मदिरां मध्वरिष्टं वा निगदं सीधुमेव वा||१४५||

After taking light food, the patient should drink sour butter-milk or takrarista, madira (a type of alcohol), madhvarista and well- fermented sidhu (a type of alcohol). [145]

Madhukasava (first recipe) for Kaphaj Grahni:

द्रोणं मधूक पुष्पाणां विडङ्गानां ततोऽर्धतः|

चित्रकस्य ततोऽर्धं स्यातथा भल्लातकाढकम्||१४६||

मञ्जिष्ठाष्टपलं चैव त्रिद्रोणेऽपां विपाचयेत्|

द्रोणशेषं तु तच्छीतं मध्वर्धाढक संयुतम्||१४७||

एला मृणालागुरुभिश्चन्दनेन च रूषिते|

कुम्भे मासस्थितं जातमासवं तं प्रयोजयेत्||१४८||

ग्रहणीं दीपयत्येव बृंहणः कफपित्तजित्|

शोथं कुष्ठं किलासं च प्रमेहांश्च प्रणाशयेत्||१४९||

इति मधूकासवः|

Madhukasav (first recipe) for Kaphaj Grahni:

1 drona (12.288 g) of the flowers of madhuka– licorice – Glycyrrhiza glabra,

½ drona of vidanga – Embelia ribes

1/4th drona of chitraka – Plumbago zeylanica

1 adhaka of bhallataka – Semecarpus anacardium linn

8 palas of manjistha – rubia cordifolia is boiled with 3 dronas (in actual practice 6 dronas to be used according to mana-paribhasa) of water till 1 drona (2 dronas according to manna-paribhasa) of water remains.

The decoction is cooled. To this, ½ adhaka (1 adhaka according to mana- paribhasa) of honey is added. This is kept in a jar, the interior wall of which is smeared with the paste of

Ela (Elettaria cardamomum maton)

Mrunala – lotus stalk

Aguru – Aquallaria agallocha

Chandana (sandalwood – Santalum album) for 1 month till it is well fermented.

Administration of this asava (medicated alcoholic drink) stimulates the grahani (enzymes in the duodenum and small intestine), promotes nourishment, alleviates kapha and pitta, and cures oedema, kushta (skin diseases), kilasa (a type of leucoderma) and prameha (obstinate urinary diabetes).

Thus, ends the description of madhukasava. [146-149]

Madhukasava (second recipe)

मधूकपुष्प स्वरसं शृत मर्धक्षयीकृतम्|

क्षौद्रपादयुतं शीतं पूर्ववत् सन्निधापयेत्||१५०||

तं पिबन् ग्रहणीदोषाञ्जयेत् सर्वान् हिताशनः।
तद्वद्द्राक्षेक्षु खर्जूर स्वरसानासुतान् पिबेत्॥१५१॥

The juice of the flower of madhuka – Madhuka longifolia is boiled, reduced to ½ and cooled.

To this, 1/4th in quantity of honey is added and kept in a jar as described above. Intake of this potion cures all types of grahani-dosha. While using this recipe, the patient should take wholesome food.

In the above-mentioned manner, the juice of grape, sugar-cane and date-palm is got fermented and taken by the patient [150-151]

Duralabhasava for Kaphaja Grahani

प्रस्थौ दुरालभाया द्वौ पस्थमामलकस्य च।
दन्तीचित्रकमुष्टी द्वे प्रत्यग्रं चाभयाशतम्॥१५२॥
चतुर्द्रोणेऽम्भसः पक्त्वा शीतं द्रोणावशेषितम्।
सगुडद्विशतं पूतं मधुनः कुडवायुतम्॥१५३॥
तद्वत् प्रियङ्गोः पिप्पल्या विडङ्गानां च चूर्णितैः।
कुडवैर्घृतकुम्भस्थं पक्षाज्जातं ततः पिबेत्॥१५४॥
ग्रहणी पाण्डुरोगार्शःकुष्ठ वीसर्प मेहनुत्।
स्वर वर्णकरश्चैष रक्तपित्तकफापहः॥१५५॥
इति दुरालभासवः।

Duralabhasav

2 prasthas of duralabha —

2 prasthas of amalaki – Phyllanthus emblica

1 musti of danti – Baliospermum montanum

1 musti of chitraka – Plumbago zeylanica

200 matured fruits of haritaki – Terminalia chebula is boiled by adding 4 dronas (in actual practice 8 dronas to be taken according to mana-paribhasa) of water and reduced to 1 drona (actual practice, 2 dronas according to mana-paribhasa). The decoction, thus obtained, is cooled. To this, 200 palas of jaggery and 1 kudava of honey are added.

1 kudava each of priyangu — Callicarpa macrophylla

Pippali – long pepper fruit – Piper longum

Vidanga – false black pepper – Embelia ribes in powder from is added in this and kept in a ghee- smeared jar for 15 days, till it becomes well- fermented.

Intake of this potion cures

Grahani, Pandu — anemia,

Arshas – piles,

Kustha (skin diseases), erysipelas and

Meha (obstinate urinary disorders including diabetes)

It promotes Swara – voice and Varna – complexion and cures raktapitta- bleeding disorders like nasal bleeding, ulcerative colitis and menorrhagia (a disease characteris erminalia bellerica is made to a paste and added wited by bleeding from different parts of the body) and diseases caused by aggravated kapha.

Thus ends the description of duralabhasava. [152-155]

Moolasava

हरिद्रा पञ्चमूले द्वे वीरर्षभक जीवकम्।
एषां पञ्च पलान् भागांश्चतुर्द्रोणेऽम्भसः पचेत्॥१५६॥
द्रोणशेषे रसे पूते गुडस्य द्विशतं भिषक्।
चूर्णितान् कुडवार्धांशान् प्रक्षिपेच्च समाक्षिकान्॥१५७॥
प्रियङ्गु मुस्त मञ्जिष्ठा विडङ्ग मधुक प्लवान्।

लोध्रं शाबरकं चैव मासार्धस्थं पिबेतु तम्||१५८||
एष मूलासवः सिद्धो दीपनो रक्तपित्तजित्|
आनाह कफ हृद्रोग पाण्डुरोगाङ्गसादनुत्||१५९||
इति मूलासवः|

Moolasav

5 palas each of haridra – Berberis aristata

Bilva – bael – Aegle marmelos

Shyonaka – Oroxylum indicum

Gambhari – Gmelina arborea

Patala – Stereospermum suaveolens

Ganikarika – Clerodendrum phlomidis

Shalaparni – Desmodium gangeticum

Prsniparni – Uraria picta

Brhati – Solanum indicum

Kantakari – Solanum surratense

Gokshura – Tribulus terrestris

Vira (shatavari) – Asparagus racemosus

Rishabhaka

Jivaka is boiled by adding 4 dronas (in actual practice 8 dronas according to mana-paribhasa) of water till 1 drona (2 dronas according to mana- paribhasa) remains. To this, 200 palas of jaggery and palas (4 palas according to mana-paribhasa) of honey and 2 palas each of priyangu – Callicarpa macrophylla

Musta – Cyperus rotundus

Manjistha – Rubia cordifolia

Vidanga – Embelia ribes

Madhuka – Madhuca longifolia

Plava —

Lodhra — Symplocos racemosa in powder form is added.

This potion is then kept in an earthern jar for 15 days till well fermented. This is called mulasava.

This is an effective recipe for stimulating the power of digestion and cures

Raktapitta (a diseases characterised by bleeding) and

Anaha (abdominal tymphanitis),

Diseases caused by aggravated kapha,

Hrid roga – heart diseases

Pandu — anaemia and

Angasada — prostration of limbs / weakness of body parts

Thus, ends the description of mulasava [156- 159]

Pindasava for Kaphaj Grahani:

प्रास्थिकं पिप्पलीं पिष्ट्वा गुडं मध्यं बिभीतकात्|
उदक प्रस्थ संयुक्तं यवपल्ले निधापयेत्||१६०||
तस्मात् पलं सुजातातु सलिलाञ्जलि संयुतम्|
पिबेत्पिण्डासवो ह्येष रोगानीक विनाशनः||१६१||
स्वस्थोऽप्येनं पिबेन्मासं नरः स्निग्ध रसाशनः |
इच्छंस्तेषामनुत्पत्तिं रोगाणां येऽत्र कीर्तिताः||१६२||
इति पिण्डासवः|

1 prastha each of

Pippali – long pepper fruit – Piper longum,

Jaggery and

Seeds of bibhitaka – Terminalia bellerica are made into a paste and added with 1 prastha (2 prasthas according to mana-pribhasa) of water.

These are placed in a jar the inside of which is smeared with ghee and its opening is closed and sealed with a lid. This jar is now kept in the heap of grains of barley for 15 days (at the end of which it gets well fermented). This is called pindasava.

1 pala of this medicated alcoholic drink is mixed with 1 anjali of water and taken after food.

This recipe cures all the diseases (described earlier). Even a healthy person is advised to take this potion for 1 month in order to prevent the occurrence of these diseases. While taking this medicine, he should take soups added with ghee or oil.

Thus ends the description of pindasava. [160-162]

Madhvarista for Kaphaja Grahni

नवे पिप्पलिमध्वाक्ते कलसेऽगुरुधूपिते|
मध्वाढकं जलसमं चूर्णानीमानि दापयेत्||१६३||
कुडवार्धं विडङ्गानां पिप्पल्याः कुडवं तथा|
चतुर्थिकांशां त्वक्क्षीरीं केशरं मरिचानि च||१६४||
त्वगेलापत्रक शटी क्रमुकातिविषाघनान्|
हरेण्वेल्वालुतेजोह्वा पिप्पलीमूल चित्रकान्||१६५||
कार्षिकांस्तत् स्थितं मासमत ऊर्ध्वं प्रयोजयेत्|
मन्दं सन्दपयत्यग्निं करोति विषमं समम्||१६६||
हृत्पाण्डु ग्रहणी रोग कुष्ठार्शःश्वयथु ज्वरान्|
वातश्लेष्मामयांश्चान्यान्मध्वरिष्टो व्यपोहति||१६७||
इति मध्वरिष्टः|

The interior wall of a new earthen jar is smeared with the paste of pippali – Piper longum and honey, and then the inside of the jar is fumigated with the smoke of aguru – Aquallaria agallocha. In this jar, 1 adhaka (2 adhakas according to mana- paribhasa) each of honey and water is kept.

To this liquid, the powders of

½ kudava of vidanga – Embelia ribes,

1 kuduva of pippali – long pepper fruit – Piper longum

1/4th kuduva of vamsa-lochana

1 karsa each of

Keshara

Maricha – black pepper fruit – Piper nigrum,

Tvak — Cinnamomum zeylanica

Ela – Elettaria cardamomum

Patraka,

Sati – Hedychium spicatum

Karmuka,

Ativisha – Aconitum heterophyllum

Ghana,

Harenu

Elvau,

Tejohva — Zanthoxylum alatum

Pippali mula – long pepper fruit – Piper longum- and

Chitraka – leadwort – Plumbago zeylanica is added and kept for 1 month.

Thereafter, it is administered to the patient.

It stimulates the power of digestion, and makes the irregular agni (powder of digestion) regular.

This recipe called madhvarista cures

Hrid roga — heart diseases

Pandu – anaemia

Grahani

Kushta – skin diseases,

Arshas – piles,

Shotha – oedema,

Jwara – fever and other diseases caused by aggravated vayu and kapha.

Thus, ends the description of madhvarista [163-167]

Pippalyadya churna

समूलां पिप्पलीं क्षारौ द्वौ पञ्च लवणानि च|
मातुलुङ्गाभया रास्ना शटी मरिच नागरम्||१६८||
कृत्वा समांशं तच्चूर्णं पिबेत् प्रातः सुखाम्बुना|
श्लेष्मिके ग्रहणीदोषे बलवर्णाग्निवर्धनम्||१६९||

Pippali – long pepper fruit – Piper longum

Pippali mula – long pepper fruit – Piper longum-

Yavaksara

Svarjiksara

Saindhava

Samudra

Bida

Audbhida

Sauvarcala

Matulunga – Citrus medica

Abhaya – Terminalia chebula

Rasna – Alpinia galangal

Sati – Hedychium spicatum

Marica – Piper nigrum

Nagara – Zingiber officinale taken in equal quantities is made of powder.

This recipe is taken early in the morning with luke-warm water.

It cures Kaphaja type of grahani and promotes strength, complextion and the power of digestion. [168-169]

Recipes

एतैरेवौषधैः सिद्धं सर्पिः पेयं समारुते|
गौल्मिके षट्पलं प्रोक्तं भल्लातक घृतं च यत्||१७०||

If grahani is caused by kapha along with aggravated vayu, then the patient is given medicated ghee prepared by boiling with the above-mentioned herbs. He may also be given satpala ghrta (vide- chikitsa 5: 147- 148) and bhallataka ghrta (vide chikitsa 5: 143-146) described in the chapter dealing with the treatment of gulma – abdominal tumour, distension (phantom tumour) [170]

Kshara ghrita for Kaphaja grahani

बिडं कालोत्थलवणं सर्जिका यव शूकजम्|
सप्तलां कण्टकारीं च चित्रकं चेति दाहयेत्||१७१||
सप्तकृत्वः सुतस्यास्य क्षारस्य द्व्याढकेन तु|
आढकं सर्पिषः पक्त्वा पिबेदग्निविवर्धनम्||१७२||

इति क्षारघृतम्।

Bida lavana

Kalottha-lavana – Sauvarchala

Svarji- ksara

Yava-ksara

Saptala –

Kantakari – yellow berried nightshade (whole plant) – solanum xanthcarpum

Chitraka – Plumbago zeylanica is burnt, mixed with water and filtered for 7 times.

From out of this, ksara (alkaline part of these plants) is collected.

2 adhakas of this ksara is cooked with 1 adhaka (2 adhakas according to mana paribhasa) of ghee.

Intake of this medicated ghee promotes agni (power of digestion). Thus, ends the description of ksara-ghrta. [171-172]

Pippalimooladi Yoga:

समूलां पिप्पली पाठां चव्येन्द्र यव नागरम्।

चित्रकातिविषे हिङ्गु श्वदंष्ट्रां कटुरोहिणीम्||१७३||

वचां च कार्षिकं पञ्च लवणानां पलानि च।

दध्नः प्रस्थद्वये तैल सर्पिषोः कुडव द्वये||१७४||

खण्डीकृतानि निष्क्वाथ्य शनैरन्तर्गते रसे।

अन्तर्धूमं ततो दग्धवा चूर्णं कृत्वा घृताप्लुतम्||१७५||

पिबेत् पाणितलं तस्मिञ्जीर्णं स्यान्मधुराशनः।

वातश्लेष्मामयान्सर्वान्हन्यादिविषगरांश्च सः||१७६||

1 karsa each of pippali – long pepper fruit – Piper longum

Pippali mula – long pepper fruit – Piper longum

Patha — Cyclea peltata

Chavya – Piper retrofractum

Indra-yava

Nagara – Zingiber officinale

Chitraka – Plumbago zeylanica

Ativisha – Aconitum heterophyllum

Hingu — Asafoetida

Svadamstra – Tribulus terrestris

Katuka-rohini — Picrorhiza kurroa

Vacha – Acorus calamus is made into pieces, and 1 pala each of

Saindhava

Sauvarcala

Bida

Audbhida

Samudra types of salt are added with

2 prasthas (4 prasthas according to mana-paribhasa) of curd,

1 kudava (2 kudavas according to mana-paribhasa) of each of oil and ghee

It is then boiled over mild fire till the water portion of the recipe gets evaporated.

The recipe is kept inside a jar and cooked according to antardhuma method.

After cooking, the recipe is then culled from the jar and made into a powder. This is then mixed with appropriate quantity of ghee and taken in the dose of 1 panitala.

After the recipe is digested, the patient should take sweet food.

It cures all the diseases caused by vayu and kapha. It also cures poisoning caused by visha (natural poison) and gara (artificially prepared poison). [173-176]

Bhallatakadya- kshara

भल्लातकं त्रिकटुकं त्रिफलां लवणत्रयम्|
अन्तर्धूमं द्विपलिकं गोपुरीषाग्निना दहेत्||१७७||
स क्षारः सर्पिषा पीतो भोज्ये वाऽप्यवचूर्णितः|
हृत्पाण्डु ग्रहणीदोष गुल्मोदावर्त शूलनुत्||१७८||

2 palas each of bhallataka – Semecarpus anacardium

Sunthi – Zingiber officinale

Pippali – long pepper fruit – Piper longum

Maricha – Piper nigrum

Haritaki – Terminalia chebula

Bibhitaka – Terminalia bellerica

Amalaki – Pjyllanthus emblica

Saindhava

Sauvarcala

Bida should be cooked by antaradhuma method with the help of the fire of cow-dung cakes.

Intake of this alkaline preparation along with ghee or by sprinkling over food-ingredients cures

Hrud roga — heart diseases,

Pandu — anaemia,

Grahani dosha

Gulma – phantom tumour

Udavarta – bloating (upward movement of wind in the abdomen) and colic pain [177-178]

Duralabhadya-kshara

दुरालभां करञ्जौ द्वौ सप्तपर्णं सवत्सकम्|
षड्ग्रन्थां मदनं मूर्वां पाठामारग्वधं तथा||१७९||
गोमूत्रेण समांशानि कृत्वा चूर्णानि दाहयेत्|
दग्ध्वा च तं पिबेत् क्षारं ग्रहणीबलवर्धनम्||१८०||

Duralabha — Fagonia arabica

Karanja – Pongamia pinnata

Lata-karanja

Saptaparna – Alstonia scholaris

Vatsaka

Sadgrantha

Madana – Randia dumetorum

Murva — Marsedenia tenacissima

Patha – Cyclea peltata

Aragvadha – Cassia fistula is made into a powder and triturated by adding equal quantites of cow's urine.

This is cooked.

Intake of this alkaline preparation promotes the strength of grahani (small intestine including duodenumn). [179-180]

Bhunimbadya kshara

भूनिम्बं रोहिणीं तिक्तां पटोलं निम्ब पर्पटम्|
दहेन्माहिषमूत्रेण क्षार एषोऽग्निवर्धनः||१८१||

Bhunimba — Andrographis paniculata

Rohini – Kutki

Tikta – Kiratatikta

Patola — Trichosanthes dioica

Nimba – Azadirachta indica

Parapata is [made to a powder] and triturated with buffalo-urine

Thereafter, the recipe is cooked (by antardhuma method). Intake of this alkali preparation promotes agni (power of digestion). [181]

Haridradya- ksara

द्वे हरिद्रे वचा कुष्ठं चित्रकः कटुरोहिणी|

मुस्तं च बस्तमूत्रेण दहेत् क्षारोऽग्निवर्धनः||१८२||

Haridra – Berberis aristata

Daru-haridra

Vacha – Acorus calamus

Kustha – Sausserea lappa

Chitraka – Plumbago zeylanica

Katuka-rohini – Piccrorhiza kurroa

Musta – nut grass (root) – cyperus rotundus is [made to a powder] and triturated by adding goat's urine

Thereafter, the recipe is cooked by antardhuma method. Intake of this alkali preparation promotes agni (power of digestion). [182]

Kshara gutika

चतुष्पलं सुधा काण्डात्रिपलं लवणत्रयात्|

वार्ताकी कुडवं चार्कादष्टौ द्वे चित्रकात् पले||१८३||

दग्धानि वार्ताकुरसे गुटिका भोजनोतराः|

भुक्तं भुक्तं पचन्त्याशु कास श्वासार्शसां हिताः||१८४||

विसूचिका प्रतिश्याय हृद्रोग शमनाश्च ताः|

इत्येषा क्षारगुटिका कृष्णात्रेयेण कीर्तिता||१८५||

इति क्षारगुडिका|

4 palas of the stems of sudha

1 pala of each

Saindhava

Sauvarcala

Bida

2 palas of chitraka – Plumbago zeylanica is cooked by antardhuma method.

This alkali preparation is then triturated with the juice of vartaki and made into pills.

Intake of his pill after meals helps in quick digestion of food and it is beneficial for patients suffering from Kasa — coughing, Svasa — asthma and Arshas — piles.

It also cures

Visuchika — choleric diarrhoea

Pratisyaya — chronic cold and

Hrud roga — heart diseases

This is called ksara-gutika and it is propunded by Lord Krsnatreya.

Thus, ends the description of ksara- gutika. [183-185]

Fourth recipe of ksara

वत्सकातिविषे पाठां दुःस्पर्शा हिङ्गु चित्रकम्|

चूर्णीकृत्य पलाशाग्रक्षारे मूत्रसुते पचेत्||१८६||
आयसे भाजने सान्द्रात्स्मात् कोलं सुखाम्बुना|
मद्यैर्वा ग्रहणीदोष शोथार्शःपाण्डुमान् पिबेत्||१८७||
इति चतुर्थक्षारः|

Vatsaka – Kutaja – Holarrhena antidysenterica

Ativisa – Aconitum heterophyllum

Patha – Cyclea peltata

Duhsparsha

Hingu and

Chitraka – Plumbago zeylanica is made to a powder

This is mixed with the alkaline liquid of palasha-ksara – Butea monosperma prepared by adding cow's urine and straining and cooked in an iron-pan till it becomes semi- solid.

1 kola of this paste is taken along with luke-warm water or alcohol by a person suffering from grahani -dosha, Shotha — oedema, Arshas — piles and Pandu — anaemia.

Thus, ends the description of the fourth recipes of ksara [186- 187]

Fifth recipe of ksara

त्रिफलां कटभीं चव्यं बिल्व मध्यमयोरजः|
रोहिणीं कटुकां मुस्तं कुष्ठं पाठां च हिङ्गु च||१८८||
मधुकं मुष्कक यवक्षारौ त्रिकटुकं वचाम्|
विडङ्गं पिप्पलीमूलं स्वर्जिकां निम्बचित्रकौ||१८९||
मूर्वाजमोदेन्द्रयवान् गुडूचीं देवदारु च|
कार्षिकं लवणानां च पञ्चानां पलिकान्पृथक्||१९०||
भागान् दध्नि त्रिकुडवे घृततैलेन मूर्च्छितम्|
अन्तर्धूमं शनैर्दग्ध्वा तस्मात् पाणितलं पिबेत्||१९१||
सर्पिषा कफवातार्शी ग्रहणी पाण्डुरोगवान्|
प्लीह मूत्रग्रह श्वास हिक्का कास क्रिमि ज्वरान्||१९२||
शोषातिसारौ श्वयथुं प्रमेहानाहहृद्ग्रहान्|
हन्यात् सर्वविषं चैव क्षारोऽग्निजननो वरः||१९३||
जीर्णे रसैर्वा मधुरैरश्नीयात् पयसाऽपि वा|
इति पञ्चमक्षारः|

One karsha (12 g) of each of

Haritaki – Terminalia chebula

Bibhitaka – Terminalia bellerica

Amalaka – Phyllanthus emblica

Katabhi

Chavya – Piper retrofractum

Pulp of bilva – bael – Aegle marmelos

Powder (bhasma) of iron

Katuka rohini – Picrrorhiza kurroa

Musta – nut grass (root) – Cyperus rotundus

Kustha – Saussurea lappa

Patha – Cyclea peltata

Hingu

Madhuka alkali preparations of

Mushkaka

Yava – Barley

Sunthi – Zingiber officinale

Pippali – long pepper fruit – Piper longum

Maricha – Piper nigrum

Vacha – Acorus calamus

Vidanga – false black pepper – Embelia ribes

Svarjika kshara

Nimba – Azadirachta indica

Chitraka – Plumbago zeylanica

Murva — Marsedenia tenacissima

Ajamoda – ajowan seed – Trachyspermum ammi

Indrayava

Guduchi — Tinospora cordifolia

Devadaru – Cedrus deodara

1 pala of each of the 5 kudavas of curd (yoghurt)

It is mixed with 3 small quantities of ghee and oil.

This is then cooked by air-tight (antardhuma) method over slow fire.

Intake of 1 panitala of this recipe along with ghee is useful for a patient suffering from

Kaphaja and vatika types of Arshas — piles

Grahani and pandu – anemia, initial stages of liver disorders (anaemia).

It cures

Pleeha (splenic disorders)

Mutra graha – anuria

Shvasa – asthma

Hikka – hiccup

Kasa – cough

Krimi – parasitic infection

Jwara – fever

Sosha – consumption,

Atisara – diarrhoea,

Shotha – oedema,

Prameha — obstinate urinary disorders including diabetes

Anaha – constipation

Hrd-graha – cardiac spasm and all types of toxicosis

This alkaline preparation is an excellent stimulant of gastic fire.

After this potion is digested, the patient should take food along with meat-soup, sweet ingredients or milk.

Thus, ends the description of the fifth variety of alkali preparation (ksara). [188 - 194½]

This ends the treatment for Kaphaja Grahani.

Treatment of Tridoshaja grahani

त्रिदोषे विधिविद्वैद्यः पञ्च कर्माणि कारयेत्||१९४||

घृतक्षारासवारिष्टान् दद्याच्चाग्निविवर्धनान्|

क्रिया या चानिलादीनां निर्दिष्टा ग्रहणीं प्रति||१९५||

व्यत्यासातां समस्तां वा कुर्याद्दोषविशेषवित्|१९६|

Tridoshaja Grahani chikitsa:

Grahani caused by the simultaneous vitiation of all the 3 Doshas is treated by the physician with the appropriate administration of Panchakarma.

The patient is given medicated ghee, alkalies, asavas (medicated wine) and aristas (medicated wine of another type)

which stimulate the power of digestion (gastric fire).

For the patient suffering from different types of grahani various therapeutics for the alleviation of vayu, etc are described.

These are administered by the physician either separately or jointly after ascertaining the nature of the doshas involved in the causation of this ailment. [194 ½- 196½]

Summary of therapies

स्नेहनं स्वेदनं शुद्धिर्लङ्घनं दीपनं च यत्||१९६||

चूर्णानि लवण क्षार मध्वरिष्ट सुरासवाः|

विविधास्तक्रयोगाश्च दीपनानां च सर्पिषाम्||१९७||

ग्रहणीरोगिभिः सेव्याः, ...|१९८|

The patient suffering from grahani should, in brief use the following categories of therapies:

1. Snehana or oleation therapy

2. Svedana of fomentation therapy

3. Suddhi or elimination (purificatatory) therapies

4. Langhana or fasting therapy

5. Dipana or the therapy for the stimulation of the power of digestion

6. Churna or recipes in the form of powder

7. Lavana or recipes containing salt

8. Kshara or recipes containing alkalies

9. Madhvarista, i.e an alcoholic preparation containing honey

10. Sura or alcohol

11. Asava or a type of alcoholic preparation or wine

12. Takra-yoga or various recipes containing butter-milk and

13. Deepana- sarpis or recipes of medicated ghee which stimulate the power of digestion. [196 ½- 198½]

Treatment of associated conditions

... क्रियां चावस्थिकीं शृणु|

ष्ठीवनं श्लैष्मिके रूक्षं दीपनं तिक्त संयुतम्||१९८||

सकृद्रूक्षं सकृत्स्निग्धं कृशे बहु कफे हितम्|

परीक्ष्यामं शरीरस्य दीपनं स्नेह संयुतम्||१९९||

दीपनं बहुपित्तस्य तिक्तं मधुर संयुतम्|

बहुवातस्य तु स्नेह लवणाम्लयुतं हितम्||२००||

सन्धुक्षति तथा वह्निरेषां विधिवदिन्धनैः|२०१|

Now the treatment of grahani according to the stages of the disease shall be explained –

In kaphaja type of grahani steevana (spitting therapy), medicines that are dry, digestion stimulants containing bitter herbs are administered.

If kapha is excessively aggravated and the patient is weak, then alternatively dry (rookshana treatment) and unctuous therapies (snehana) is administered.

If the body is pervaded with ama (product of improper digestion and metabolism) then after proper examination, the patient is given digestive stimulants along with sneha (ghee / oil).

If pitta is aggravated in excess, then digestive stimulants which are bitter in taste are administered along with sweet ingredients. If vayu is aggravated in excess, then it is administered along with sweet ingredients.

If Vata is aggravated in excess, then the administration of digestive stimulants mixed with sneha (ghee) and saline as well as sour ingredients is useful.

The above recipes will work as fuel, and when appropriately administered, they will stimulate the gastric fire (power of digestion). [198 ½- 201½]

Use of fats

स्नेहमेव परं विद्याद्दुर्बलानल दीपनम्||२०१||
नालं स्नेह समिद्धस्य शमायान्नं सुगुर्वपि|
मन्दाग्निरविपक्वं तु पुरीषं योऽतिसार्यते||२०२||
दीपनीयौषधैर्युक्तां घृतमात्रां पिबेतु सः|
तया समानः पवनः प्रसन्नो मार्गमास्थितः||२०३||
अग्नेः समीपचारित्वादाशु प्रकुरुते बलम्|
काठिन्याद्यः पुरीषं तु कृच्छ्रान्मुञ्चति मानवः||२०४||
सघृतं लवणैर्युक्तं नरोऽन्नावग्रहं पिबेत्|
रौक्ष्यान्मन्दे पिबेत्सर्पिस्तैलं वा दीपनैर्युतम्||२०५||

Sneha – fat / ghee is excellent for stimulating the Jataragni – digestive fire. If Jataragni is stimulated (kindled) by the fuel in the form of fat (ghee), then it cannot be suppressed even by heavy-to-digest food.

If the patient has weak digestive power and he voids undigested stool in excess, he is given ghee cooked with Deepaniya drugs (ingredients that stimulate the power of digestion) in proper dose.

The Samana Vata is located in the abdomen regulating the functions of digestive fire in the stomach). Since this samana-vayu has its functions near the gastric fire, it instantaneously promotes the strength of digestion.

If the patient finds it difficult to avoid stool because of the latter's hardness, then he should take his food, the middle portion (avagraha) of which is mixed with ghee and salt.

If the gastric fire is suppressed because of the excessive intake of unctuous ingredients, then the patient should drink medicated ghee or medicated oil prepared by cooking with dipaniya drugs (which stimulate the power of digestion) [201 ½ – 205]

Treatment of suppressed Agni

अतिस्नेहात्तु मन्देऽग्नौ चूर्णारिष्टासवा हिताः|
भिन्ने गुदोपलेपात्तु मले तैलसुरासवाः||२०६||
उदावर्तात्तु मन्देऽग्नौ निरूहाः स्नेहबस्तयः|
दोषवृद्ध्या तु मन्देऽग्नौ शुद्धो दोषविधिं चरेत्||२०७||
व्याधि युक्तस्य मन्दे तु सर्पिरेवाग्नि दीपनम्|
उपवासाच्च मन्देऽग्नौ यवागूभिः पिबेद्घृतम्||२०८||
अन्नावपीडितं बल्यं दीपनं बृंहणं च तत्|
दीर्घकाल प्रसङ्गात्तु क्षाम क्षीण कृशान्नरान्||२०९||
प्रसहानां रसैः साम्लैर्भोजयेत् पिशिताशिनाम्|
लघु, तीक्ष्णोष्ण शोधित्वाद्दीपयन्त्याशु तेऽनलम्||२१०||
मांसोपचितमांसत्वात्तथाऽऽशुतरबृंहणाः||२११|

If the gastric fire becomes suppressed because of excessive intake of ghee (Fat), then recipes in the form of powder, asava (medicated wine) and Arista (medicated wine) are useful. If the anus gets adhered with stool because of loose motions [and there is suppression of the gastric fire], then the patient should be given oil, sura (alchohol) and asava (medicated wine, prepared without boiling).

If the digestion strength is suppressed because of urdhva-vata (bloating, upward movement of the vayu), the patient is given niruha and anuvasana types of medicated enema.

If the Agni gets suppressed because of aggravated Doshas, then the patient is given appropriate Panchakarma and thereafter, he should take appropriate medicines for the alleviation of the aggravated Dosha.

If Agni gets suppressed because of Grahani, then the patient is given medicated ghee which stimulates the power of digestion.

If Agni is suppressed because of fasting (upavasa), then the patient should take yavagu (gruels like manda, peya, vilepi) mixed with ghee. The recipe i.e., the ghee mixed with the rice / food promotes strength, stimulates the power of digestion and enhances nourishment.

If the suppression of Agni has become chronic as a result of which the patient has become indolent, weak and emaciated, then he should be given the meat soup of Prasaha type of animals (that eat food by snatching), which are carnivorous and whose meat is light for digestion. Such meat-soups instantaneously stimulates the gastric fire because of their sharp, hot and Shodhana (which purifies the body by elimination of Doshas) properties. The meat of these carnivorous animals is nourished by the meat of other animals; hence it causes nourishment of the body more quickly. [206- 211½]

Food and digestion fire

नाभोजनेन कायाग्निर्दीप्यते नातिभोजनात्||२११||
यथा निरिन्धनो वह्निरल्पो वाऽतीन्धनावृतः|
स्नेहान्न विधिभिश्चित्रैश्चूर्णारिष्ट सुरासवैः ||२१२||
सम्यक्प्रयुक्तैर्भिषजा बलमग्नेः प्रवर्धते|
यथा हि सारदार्वग्निः स्थिरः सन्तिष्ठते चिरम्||२१३||
स्नेहान्न विधिभिस्तद्वदन्तरग्निर्भवेत् स्थिरः|
हितं जीर्ण मितं चाश्नंश्चिरमारोग्यमश्नुते||२१४||
अवैषम्येण धातूनामग्निवृद्धौ यतेत ना|
समैर्दोषैः समो मध्ये देहस्योष्माऽग्निसंस्थितः||२१५||
पचत्यन्नं तदारोग्यपुष्ट्यायुर्बलवृद्धये|
दोषैर्मन्दोऽतिवृद्धो वा विषमैर्जनयेद्गदान्||२१६||
वाच्यं मन्दस्य तत्रोक्तमतिवृद्धस्य वक्ष्यते|२१७|

The Agni is not stimulated by fasting or by over-eating, just as the physical fire is not kindled without fuel or with too much of fuel.

Intake of ghee / fat along with food according to the prescribed procedure, and with appropriate administration of the different recipes of powders, Arishtas, Asava (medicated wines), the strength of digestion is improved. As the physical fire for which hard-wood is used as fuel remains stable for a long time, similarly intake of ghee with food according to the prescribed procedure brings about stability in digestion.

Intake of wholesome food in appropriate quantities after the digestion of the previous meal helps a person to enjoy good health for a long time. A person should strive to promote the gastric fire without provoking the discordance of Dhatus (tissue elements including doshas).

Digestion strength and Tridosha balance:

The digestion fire remains in a balanced state if the Doshas are in balance. This type of agni (gastric fire) helps in proper digestion of food resulting in good health, proper nourishment and promotion of longevity as well as strength. If there is imbalance in Doshas, then the digestion fire becomes either weak or exceeding sharp (ati-vrddha) giving rise to several diseases.

The management of the condition caused by the weak gastric fire is already explained. The same in respect of the gastric fire which is exceedingly sharp is going to be splet out in the succeeding verses. [211 ½- 217 ½]

Etiology and pathogenesis of Atyagni

नरे क्षीणकफे पित्तं कुपितं मारुतानुगम्||२१७||
स्वोष्मणा पावकस्थाने बलमग्नेः प्रयच्छति|
तदा लब्धबलो देहे विरूक्षे सानिलोऽनलः||२१८||
परिभूय पचत्यन्नं तैक्ष्ण्यादाशु मुहुर्मुहुः|
पक्त्वाऽन्नं स ततो धातून्छोणितादीन् पचत्यपि||२१९||
ततो दौर्बल्यमातङ्कान्मृत्युं चोपनयेन्नरम्|

Causes and pathogenesis of Atyagni – excess digestion strength:

In a person with diminished kapha, if Pitta located in the site of Agni (gastric fire) gets aggravated, then along with Vata, it makes the Agni very strong.

Because of the under-nourishment of the body along with Vayu, the strengthened Agni surrounds the food, and by its sharpness (Teekshna), immediately digests the food taken frequently. After digesting the food, it even consumes tissue elements etc. Thereafter, the patient becomes weak and succumbs to death being afflicted by diseases. [217 ½ – 220½]

Signs and symptoms of Atyagni

भुक्तेऽन्ने लभते शान्तिं जीर्णमात्रे प्रताम्यति||२२०||

तृट्श्वास दाह मूर्च्छाद्या व्याधयोऽत्यग्निसम्भवाः|

A person having atyagni (excessively sharp gastric fire) feels pacified after food. But after the food is digested, he gets tremors. Because of this atyagni, he suffers from morbid thirst, dyspnoea, burning sensation in the body, fainting etc. [220 ½- 221½]

Management of atyagni

तमत्यग्निं गुरु स्निग्ध शीतै र्मधुर विज्जलैः||२२१||

अन्नपानैर्नयेच्छान्तिं दीप्तमग्निमिवाम्बुभिः|

मुहुर्मुहुर जीर्णेऽपि भोज्यान्यस्योपहारयेत्||२२२||

निरिन्धनोऽन्तरं लब्ध्वा यथैनं न विपादयेत्|

पायसं कृशरां स्निग्धं पैष्टिकं गुडवैकृतम्||२२३||

अद्यात्तथौदकानूपपिशितानि भृतानि च|

मत्स्यान्विशेषतः श्लक्ष्णान्स्थिरतोयचरांस्तथा||२२४||

आविकं च भृतं मांसमद्यादत्यग्निनाशनम्|

यवागूं स मधूच्छिष्टां घृतं वा क्षुधितः पिबेत्||२२५||

गोधूमचूर्ण मन्थं वा व्यधयित्वा सिरां पिबेत्|

पयो वा शर्करा सर्पि जीवनीयौषधैः शृतम्||२२६||

फलानां तैलयोनीनामुत्क्रुञ्चाश्च सशर्कराः|

मार्दवं जनयन्त्यग्नेः स्निग्धा मांसरसास्तथा||२२७||

पिबेच्छीताम्बुना सर्पि र्मधूच्छिष्टेन संयुतम्|

गोधूमचूर्ण पयसा ससर्पिष्कं पिबेन्नरः||२२८||

आनूप रस सिद्धान् वा त्रीन् स्नेहांस्तैल वर्जितान्|

पयसा सम्मितं चापि घनं त्रिस्नेहसंयुतम्||२२९||

नारि स्तन्येन संयुक्तां पिबेदौदुम्बरीं त्वचम्|

ताभ्यां वा पायसं सिद्धमद्यादत्यग्निशान्तये||२३०||

श्यामात्रिवृद्विपक्वं वा पयो दद्यादि्वरेचनम्|

असकृत् पित्तशान्त्यर्थं पायस प्रतिभोजनम्||२३१||

प्रसमीक्ष्य भिषक् प्राज्ञस्तस्मै दद्यादि्वधानवित्|

यत्किञ्चिन्मधुरं मेद्यं श्लेष्मलं गुरुभोजनम्||२३२||

सर्वं तदत्यग्निहितं भुक्त्वा प्रस्वपनं दिवा|

मेद्यान्यन्नानि योऽत्यग्नावप्रतान्तः समश्नुते||२३३||

न तन्निमित्तं व्यसनं लभते पुष्टिमेव च|

कफे वृद्धे जिते पित्ते मारुते चानलः समः||२३४||

समधातोः पचत्यन्नं पुष्ट्यायुर्बलवृद्धये|२३५|

As a burning fire is extinguished by water, similarly Atyagni (excessively strong digestive fire) is pacified with heavy, unctuous, cold, sweet and slimy food and drinks

Even if the indigestion occurs due to the intake of heavy, unctuous foods, foods should be repeatedly given to the patient. This will prevent the digestive fire from killing the person (causing death) due to the non-availability of the fuel in the form of food.

He is given payasa (milk-pudding), krishara (thick gruel prepared of rice and lentils), pastries added with ghee (fat), preparations of jaggery and minced as well as roasted meat of aquatic and marshy land, inhabiting creatures (Jaleshaya).

He should particularly take fish (without scales, smooth skinned) inhabiting stagnant water and minced as well as roasted sheep which counteract the excessively sharp gastric fire.

The patient, when hungry should take Yavagu (thick gruel) mixed with bee's wax or should take ghee or should take wheat flour mixed with liberal quantity of water (Mantha) after venesection (Raktamokshana). He may also take milk boiled with Jeevaneeya Gana herbs after adding sugar and ghee.

Intake of paste (utkrunca or utkarika) of oil- bearing seeds (fruits) along with sugar, and meat- soup mixed with ghee(fat) reduces the excessive sharpness of the agni (gastric fire) the patient should take ghee with bee's wax along with cold water. He may also take wheat-flour added with milk and mixed with ghee.

For the alleviation of atyagni (excessively sharp gastric fire), the patient may take the following recipes:

1. Excluding oil, three unctuous substances [out of the 4] viz: ghee vasa – (muscle fat) and majja (bone –marrow) boiled with the soup of the meat of the marshy- land inhabiting birds/ animals.

2. Wheat flour mixed with milk

3. Curd mixed with ghee, vasa (muscle fat) and majja (bone- marrow) powder of the bark of Udumbara – Ficus racemosa mixed with woman's milk and

4. Milk pudding (payasa) prepared with the powder of the bark of udumbara – Ficus racemosa and woman's milk.

For the alleviation of pitta, purgation therapy is administered frequently with the milk boiled by adding shyama and trivrt – Operculina turpethum.

The purgation therapy is followed by a diet of milk pudding (payasa). This therapy is administered after proper examination by an expert physician who is proficient in these methods.

Intake of any of such ingredients of food such as sweet, fatty, aggravator of kapha and heavy for digestion and sleep during the day time after meals are useful for the patients suffering from atyagni (excessively sharp gastric fire)

If a patient of atyagni, even if he is hungry, takes different types of fat-producing food he does not succumb to death. On the other hand, this type of food causes robustness of such patients.

When the kapha is aggravated and pitta as well as the vata is subdued. Then the Agni (gastric fire) regains its normal (equilibrium) state. In a patient whose tissue dhatus are in a state of equilibrium, the gastric fire digests food resulting in the promotion of strength and longevity. [221½ –235½]

Different types of meal

भवन्ति चात्र-

पथ्यापथ्यमिहैकत्र भुक्तं समशनं मतम्||२३५||

विषमं बहु वाऽल्पं वाऽप्य प्राप्तातीत कालयोः|

भुक्तं पूर्वान्नशेषे तु पुनरध्यशनं मतम्||२३६||

त्रीण्यप्येतानि मृत्युं वा घोरान् व्याधीन्सृजन्ति वा|

प्रातराशे त्वजीर्णेऽपि सायमाशो न दुष्यति||२३७||

दिवा प्रबुध्यतेऽर्केण हृदयं पुण्डरीकवत्|

तस्मिन्निबुद्धे स्रोतांसि स्फुटत्वं यान्ति सर्वशः||२३८||

व्यायामाच्च विहाराच्च विक्षिप्तत्वाच्च चेतसः|

न क्लेदमुपगच्छन्ति दिवा तेनास्य धातवः||२३९||

अक्लिन्नेष्वन्नमासिक्तमन्यतेषु न दुष्यति|

अविदग्ध इव क्षीरे क्षीरमन्यदिवमिश्रितम्||२४०||

नैव दूष्यति तेनैव समं सम्पद्यते यथा|
रात्रौ तु हृदये म्लाने संवृतेष्वयनेषु च|
यान्ति कोष्ठे परिक्लेदं संवृते देहधातवः||२४१||
क्लिन्नेष्वन्यदपक्वेषु तेष्वासिक्तं प्रदुष्यति|
विदग्धेषु पयःस्वन्यत् पयस्तप्तमिवार्पितम्||२४२||
नैशेष्वाहारजातेषु नाविपक्वेषु बुद्धिमान्|
तस्मादन्यत्समश्नीयात्पालयिष्यन्बलायुषी||२४३||

Definition of Samashana:

When the wholesome and unwholesome ingredients of food are taken together, intake of such mixed food, according to this treatise, is called Samashana (mixed food).

Definition of Vishamashana:

If the food is too much or too little in quantity, and if it is taken too early or too late, then it is called Visamashana (irregular food).

Definition of Adhyashana If food is taken again, even before the previous meal is digested, then it is called adhyasana (predigestion – food).

All the above mentioned three types of meal cause death or give rise to serious diseases.

However, taking food in the evening, even if the morning meal is not digested is not injurious. As the lotus flower blossoms during the daytime because of the sun, similarly the heart of a person becomes awakened (more active) during the day time, and because of this awakened (stimulated) heart, all the channels in the body become more dilated. Because of exercise and physical – mental activities during day time, the Dhatus of a person do not develop stickness (kleda). As a result of this non- stickness, when the food components after digestion of the subsequent meal reach these tissues is on the analogy of the unspoiled milk being added with fresh milk which does not get spoiled (curdled) and gets mixed up uniformly.

In the night, however, the heart becomes sluggish (mlana) or contracted, and thus, the channels of circulation become contracted. Therefore, the food in the kostha (abdominal and thoracic visceras) becomes sticky, and it surrounds (adheres to) the tissues elements. If these sticky undigested materials are further added with other similar material, then this produces injurious effects. This is on the analogy of adding warm milk to curdled milk both of which get spoiled. Therefore, a wise person, with a view to protecting his strength and life, should avoid taking food if the night meal is not digested. [235 ½ – 243]

Summary:

तत्र श्लोकाः:-

अन्तरग्निगुणा देहं यथा धारयते च सः|
यथाऽन्नं पच्यते यांश्च यथाऽऽहारः करोत्यपि||२४४||
येऽग्नयो यांश्च पुष्यन्ति यावन्तो ये पचन्ति यान्|
रसादीनां क्रमोत्पत्तिर्मलानां तेभ्य एव च||२४५||
वृष्याणामाशुकृद्धेतुर्धातुकालोद्भवक्रमः|
रोगैकदेशकृद्धेतुरन्तरग्निर्यथाऽधिकः||२४६||
प्रदुष्यति यथा दुष्टो यान् रोगाञ्जनयत्यपि|
ग्रहणी या यथा यच्च ग्रहणीदोषलक्षणम्||२४७||
पूर्वरूपं पृथक् चैव व्यञ्जनं सचिकित्सितम्|
चतुर्विधस्य निर्दिष्टं तथा चावस्थिकी क्रिया||२४८||
जायते च यथाऽत्यग्निर्यच्च तस्य चिकित्सितम्|
उक्तवानिह तत् सर्वं ग्रहणीदोषके मुनिः||२४९||

In this chapter dealing with the treatment of grahani, the topics described by the sage are as follows:

1. Attributes of antaragni (enzymes inside the body that help in the digestion and metabolism)

2. The manner in which the agni helps in the sustenance of the body

3. The process of food digestion

4. The ultimate functions of the food

5. various types of the agni and their support to different attributes in the body

6. The method of providing nourishment to different attributes in the body

7. different agnis which help in the nourishment of different tissue elements

8. The order of synthesis of tissue elements, etc. Serious

9. The waste products coming out of the tissue elements during the metabolic process

10. The reasons why aphordisiacs produce their effects instantaneously

11. The time taken for the synthesis of tissue- elements

12. The reason for the location of diseases in a particular part of the body

13. The importance of antaragni or jatharagni

14. The manner in which abnormal agni produces diseases

15. The diseases which are caused by the abnormal agni

16. Identification of grahani

17. Signs and symptoms of grhani- dosha in general

18. Premonitory signs and symptoms of grahani-dosha

19. Signs and symptoms of 4 different types of grahani dosha

20. Treatment of different types of grahani dosha

21. Treatment of different states of grahani dosha

22. Causative factors of atyagni

23. Treatment of atyagni[244-249]

इत्यग्निवेशकृते तन्त्रेऽप्राप्ते दृढबल सम्पूरिते चिकित्सास्थाने ग्रहणी चिकित्सितं नाम पञ्चदशोऽध्यायः||१५||

Thus, ends the 15th chapter of Chikitsa Sthana dealing with Granahi, in the work of Agnivesha which was redacted by charaka, and supplemented by Dridhabala.

22

Chikitsasthana Chapter 16 Pandu Chikitsitam

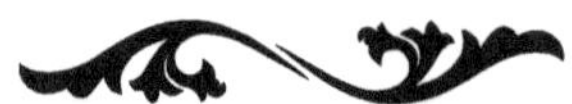

The 16th chapter of Charaka Samhita Chikitsa Sthana is called Pandu Roga Chikitsa. It deals with causes, symptoms and treatment of anemia, jaundice and other liver disorders.

अथातः पाण्डुरोगचिकित्सितं व्याख्यास्यामः||१||

इति ह स्माह भगवानात्रेयः||२||

Let us explore the chapter on the Treatment of Pandurog.

Thus said Lord Atreya [1-2]

Types of Pandu Roga

पाण्डुरोगाः स्मृताः पञ्च वात पित्त कफैस्त्रयः|

चतुर्थः सन्निपातेन पञ्चमो भक्षणान्मृदः||३||

Pandu – Roga is of 5 varieties as follows:

1. Vataja Pandu caused by Vata Dosha

2. Pitta Pandu caused by Pitta

3. Kaphaja Pandu caused by Kapha

4. Sannipatika Pandu Roga caused by the simultaneous aggravation of all the 3 Doshas (Sannipatika) and

5. MrutBhakshaJanya Pandu Roga caused by eating clay or Mrttika (Geographism) [3]

Pandu Samanya Samprapti: General pathology:

दोषाः पित्तप्रधानास्तु यस्य कुप्यन्ति धातुषु|

शैथिल्यं तस्य धातूनां गौरवं चोपजायते||४||

ततो वर्ण बल स्नेहा ये चान्येऽप्योजसो गुणाः|

व्रजन्ति क्षयमत्यर्थं दोष दूष्य प्रदूषणात्||५||

सोऽल्परक्तोऽल्पमेदस्को निःसारः शिथिलेन्द्रियः|

वैवर्ण्य भजते, तस्य हेतुं शृणु सलक्षणम्||६||

Pandu Samanya Samprapti: General pathology:

When the Doshas, with Pitta as the dominant one, are aggravated in the Dhatus, then the Dhatus get afflicted. This results in weakening (Shithila) and heaviness (Gaurava) of Dhathu – body tissues.

Thereafter, the complexion, strength and unctuousness, and the properties of Ojas get reduced on account of the vitiation of the Doshas and Dhatus.

The patient becomes

poor in blood – Alpa Rakta

low in fat tissue – Alpa medaska

Nissara – lack of vitality:

Shithilendriya – His sense organs become weak: and he suffers from discoloration, leading to manifestation of Pandu Roga.

The aetiology and pathogenesis and the signs including symptoms of this disease will be explained hereafter. [4-6]

Panduroga Nidana and Samprapti: Causes and pathology

क्षाराम्ल लवणात्युष्ण विरुद्धा सात्म्य भोजनात्|
निष्पाव माष पिण्याक तिलतैल निषेवणात्||७||
विदग्धेऽन्ने दिवा स्वप्नाद्व्यायामान्मैथुनात्तथा|
प्रतिकर्मर्तुवैषम्याद्वेगानां च विधारणात्||८||
काम चिन्ता भय क्रोध शोकोपहत चेतसः|
समुदीर्ण यदा पित्तं हृदये समव स्थितम्||९||
वायुना बलिना क्षिप्तं सम्प्राप्य धमनीर्दश|
प्रपन्नं केवलं देहं त्वङ्मांसान्तरमाश्रितम्||१०||
प्रदूष्य कफ वातासृक्त्वङ्मांसानि करोति तत्|
पाण्डु हारिद्र हरितान् वर्णान् बहुविधांस्त्वचि||११||
स पाण्डुरोग इत्युक्तः ...|१२|

Causes and pathology of Pandu – Anemia / initial stages of liver disorders:

Pitta gets aggravated by the following:

1. Excessive intake of Kshara, sour, saline, hot and mutually contradictory food, unwholesome food, Nishpava (cow pea) Masha Pinyaka (oil cake) and til oil.

2. Sleeping during day time, and exercise as well as sexual intercourse when the food is not properly digested (Vidagdha Anna)

3. Improper administration of Panchakarma therapies and transgression of prescribed seasonal regimens (rutu-vaishamya) and

4. Suppression of natural urges

In a person with his mind afflicted with worry, fear, anger and grief, aggravation of Pitta located in the cardiac region takes place. Then this Pitta being forcefully propelled by Vata Dosha, enters into the 10 vessels [attached to the heart] and circulates in the entire body.

Being located between the skin and the muscle tissue, this aggravated Pitta vitiates Kapha, Vayu, Asruk (blood), skin and muscles as a result of which different types of coloration, like Pandu (pale yellow), Haridra (yellow) and Harita (green) appear in the skin. This is called Pandu Roga (a type of Anemia) [7- 121/2]

Pandu roga purvaroopa:

... तस्य लिङ्गं भविष्यतः|
हृदय स्पन्दनं रौक्ष्यं स्वेदाभावः श्रमस्तथा||१२||

The premonitory signs and symptoms of Pandu are:

Hrudaya spandana – palpitation

Raukshyam – dryness

Sweda abhava – absence of sweating and

Shrama –fatigue [12 ½]

Pandu Roga Samanya Lakshana – General symptoms:

सम्भूतेऽस्मिन् भवेत् सर्वः कर्ण क्ष्वेडी हतानलः|
दुर्बलः सदनोऽन्नद्विट् श्रम भ्रम निपीडितः||१३||
गात्रशूल ज्वर श्वास गौरवारुचिमान्नरः|

मृदितैरिव गात्रैश्च पीडितोन्मथितैरिव||१४||
शूनाक्षि कूटो हरितः शीर्ण लोमा हतप्रभः|
कोपनः शिशिर द्वेषी निद्रालुः ष्ठीवनोऽल्पवाक्||१५||
पिण्डिकोद्वेष्ट कट्यूरु पादरुक्सदनानि च|
भवन्त्यारोहणायासैर्विशेषश्चास्य वक्ष्यते||१६||

General symptoms:

Any of the varieties of Pandu Roga leads to below listed general symptoms.

Karna Ksveda – tinnitus

Hata anala – suppression of the power of digestion

Durbala – weakness

Sadana – prostration

Anna divshta – repugnance against food

Shrama – fatigue

Bhrama – giddiness

Gatra shoola – pain in the body

Jwara – fever

Shwasa – dyspnoea

Gaurava – heaviness and

Aruchi – anorexia

Mruditagatra – He feels as if all the limbs of his body are being kneaded, squeezed and churned.

Shunakshikoota – He suffers from swelling of the orbital region

Harita– His complexion becomes green.

Sheerna loma hata prabha – The small hair of his body fall out: he loses his bodily lustre:

Kopana – he becomes irritable and angry

Shishira dweshi – hates cold things

Nidralu – tends to sleep at all times

Steevana – keeps spitting

Alpavak – speaks less / avoid speaking to anyone

Pindikodveshtana – he suffers from cramps in the calf region: and while making efforts for climbing,

Kati ura pada ruk sadana – he suffers from pain and weakness in the lumbar region, thighs and feet.

Arohana ayasa – shortness of breath or fatigue while climbing stairs

The signs and symptoms specific to each variety of Pandu will be described hereafter. [13-16]

Vatika Pandu Nidana, lakshana

आहारैरुपचारैश्च वातलैः कुपितोऽनिलः|
जनयेत्कृष्ण पाण्डुत्वं तथा रूक्षारुणाङ्गताम्||१७||
अङ्गमर्दं रुजं तोदं कम्पं पार्श्व शिरो रुजम्|
वर्चःशोषास्य वैरस्य शोफानाह बलक्षयान्||१८||

Aetiology, Signs and Symptoms of Vatika Pandu:

Vata gets vitiated by the Vayu- aggravating diet and regimen which brings about

Krsihnapandu anga – black and pale-yellow complexion,

Ruksha anga – dryness,

Aruna anga – reddishness of the body,

Anga marda – malaise

Ruja – ache

Toda – pricking pain

Kampa – tremor

Parshav ruja – pain in the sides of the chest,

Shiro ruja – headache

Varcha Shosha – dryness of feces

Mukha Vairasya – distaste in the mouth,

Shopha – swelling,

Anaha – flatulence / constipation and

Bala kshaya – Weakness [17-18]

Pittaja pandu Nidana, Lakshana

पितलस्याचितं पित्तं यथोक्तैः स्वैः प्रकोपणैः|

दूषयित्वा तु रक्तादीन् पाण्डुरोगाय कल्पते||१९||

स पीतो हरिताभो वा ज्वर दाह समन्वितः|

तृष्णा मूर्च्छा पिपासार्तः पीतमूत्र शकृन्नरः||२०||

स्वेदनः शीत कामश्च न चान्नमभिनन्दति|

कटुकास्यो न चास्योष्णमुपशेतेऽम्लमेव च||२१||

उद्गारोऽम्लो विदाहश्च विदग्धेऽन्नेऽस्य जायते|

दौर्गन्ध्यं भिन्नवर्चस्त्वं दौर्बल्यं तम एव च||२२||

Aetiology, signs and Symptoms of Paittika Pandu:

If a person of Pitta body type indulges in Pitta increasing diet and regime, then increased Pitta vitiates blood and causes Pittala type of Pandu roga giving rise to below mentioned signs and symptoms:

1. Peeta Harita Varna – complexion becomes yellow or green

2. Jwara Daha Samanvitah – fever and burning sensation

3. Trushna Murccha Pipasa – Faints, because of excessive thirst and suffers from morbid thirst

4. Pita mutra – His urine and stool becomes yellow in colour

5. Svedanah Sheeta kamita – Sweating and develops longing for cold things

6. Na ca Annam Abhinandati – He does not relish food

7. Katuka Aasya – Feeling pungent taste in mouth and

8. Na cha asya Ushnam Upashete Amlameva cha – hot and sour things do not suit him

9. Amla udgara – sour eructation and

10. VidahaVidagdhe Anne – burning sensation due to indigestion of food

11. Mukha Daurgandhya – bad breath and

12. Bhinna varchas, Daurbalyam, tama eva cha – He gets loose motions, weakness and fainting. [19-22]

Kaphaja Pandu Nidana, Lakshana:

विवृद्धः श्लेष्मलैः श्लेष्मा पाण्डुरोगं स पूर्ववत्|

करोति गौरवं तन्द्रा छर्दिं श्वेतावभासताम्||२३||

प्रसेकं लोमहर्षं च सादं मूर्च्छा भ्रमं क्लमम्|

श्वासं कासं तथाऽऽलस्यमरुचिं वाक्स्वरग्रहम्||२४||

शुक्ल मूत्राक्षि वर्चस्त्वं कटु रूक्षोष्ण कामताम्|

श्वयथुं मधुरास्यत्वमिति पाण्डवामयः कफात्||२५||

Aetiology Signs and Symptoms of Kaphaja Pandu:

Kapha vitiated by its aggravating food and drinks gives rise to Kaphaja type of pandu roga as per the pathogenesis described before.

The signs and symptoms of this type of this sub-type of Pandu are as follows:

1. Gauravam – Heaviness,

2. Tandra – Drowsiness,

3. Chardim – Vomiting,

4. Shvetavabhasa – whitish complexion,

5. Prasekam – Salivation,

6. Loma harsha – Horripilation,

7. Murchha- fainting,

8. Bhrama – Giddiness,

9. Klama – mental fatigue,

10. Shvasa – dyspnoea,

11. Kasa – cough,

12. Aalasya – laziness,

13. Aruchi – anorexia,

14. Vaksha savara graham – obstruction in speech and voice,

15. Shukla akshi varchas – whitishness of urine, eyes and faeces

16. Katu ruksha ushna kamata – Longing for pungent, un-unctuous and hot things and

17. Shvathu – Oedema and

18. Madhura aasya – sweet taste in the mouth. [23-25]

Aetiology, Signs and Symptoms of Tridoshaja Pandu Roga:

सर्वान्नसेविनः सर्वे दुष्टा दोषास्त्रिदोषजम्।

त्रिदोषलिङ्गं कुर्वन्ति पाण्डुरोगं सुदुःसहम्॥२६॥

If a person indulges in all types of unwholesome food, then all the 3 Doshas get vitiated to cause Tridoshaja Pandu. This type of Sannipatika Pandu is extremely intolerable (difficult to cure). [26]

Mrud-bhakshanaja Pandu Nidana, Lakshana:

मृत्तिकादन शीलस्य कुप्यत्यन्यतमो मलः।

कषाया मारुतं, पित्तमूषरा, मधुरा कफम्॥२७॥

कोपयेन्मृद्रसादींश्च रौक्ष्यादभुक्तं विरूक्षयेत्।

पूरयत्यविपक्वैव स्रोतांसि निरुणद्धि च॥२८॥

इन्द्रियाणां बलं हत्वा तेजो वीर्याँजसी तथा।

पाण्डुरोगं करोत्याशु बलवर्णाग्निनाशनम्॥२९॥

शून गण्डाक्षिकूट भ्रूःशूनपान्नाभिमेहनः।

क्रिमि कोष्ठोऽतिसार्येत मलं सासृक् कफान्वितम्॥३०॥

MrutBhakshanJanya Pandu – Anaemia due to mud eating:

Habitual indulgence in eating clay (Mrttika) aggravates one of the 3 Doshas.

If the mud is of astringent taste, then it aggravates Vayu: if it is saline with alkaline as a subsidiary taste, then Pitta gets aggravated: and if it is sweet in taste, then Kapha gets aggravated.

Because of its dryness, the clay (Mrut) causes dryness in the Rasa Dhatu (Chyle) and the ingredients of food. Thus, the undigested clay, i.e in its crude from, fills up the channels of circulation and blocks them. It afflicts the sharpness of senses, lustre, energy and Ojas which results in the loss of strength, complexion and Agni (power of digestion and metabolism).

In this type of Pandu, the signs and symptoms manifested are as follows:

1. Shunagandaakshi kuta – Oedema in the cheek, eye sockets and eye bones

2. Oedema in feet, umbilical region and the pudendum

3. Krimi koshta – Appearance of worms in Kostha (intestine) and

4. Atisara – Loose motions, the stool being associated with blood and mucus (Kapha). [27-30]

Prognosis: Pandu Upashaya:

पाण्डुरोगश्चिरोत्पन्नः खरीभूतो न सिध्यति।

काल प्रकर्षाच्छूनो ना यश्च पीतानि पश्यति||३१||
बद्धाल्पविट्कं सकफं हरितं योऽतिसार्यते|
दीनः श्वेतातिदिग्धाङ्गश्छर्दि मूर्च्छा तृषार्दितः||३२||
स नास्त्यसृक्क्षयाद्यश्च पाण्डुः श्वेतत्वमाप्नुयात्|
इति पञ्चविधस्योक्तं पाण्डुरोगस्य लक्षणम्||३३||

Prognosis:

Signs and symptoms indicating incurability of Panduroga are as follows

1. The disease has become chronic

2. Excessive dryness has appeared in the patient

3. When the patient has oedema owing to chronicity of this disease

4. When the patient gets yellow vision

5. When the patient is fully or partially constipated

6. When the patient passes loose stool which is green in colour and which is mixed with mucus

7. When the patient feels exceeding prostrated

8. When the body is exceedingly white as if besmeared (with whiteness)

9. When the patient is exceedingly afflicted with vomiting, fainting and morbid thirst and

10. When the body of the patient becomes pale on account of loss of blood. Such a patient never survives

Thus, the signs and symptoms of all 5 types of Pandu Roga (Vatika, Pittaja, Kaphaja, Sannipatika and Mrd-Bhaksanaja) are discussed. [31-33]

Kamala – Jaundice:

पाण्डुरोगी तु योऽत्यर्थं पित्तलानि निषेवते|
तस्य पित्तमसृग्मांसं दग्ध्वा रोगाय कल्पते||३४||
हारिद्रनेत्रः स भृशं हारिद्रत्वङ्नखाननः|
रक्तपीत शकृन्मूत्रो भेकवर्णो हतेन्द्रियः||३५||
दाहाविपाक दौर्बल्य सदनारुचि कर्षितः|
कामला बहुपित्तैषा कोष्ठ शाखाश्रया मता||३६||

If the patient suffering from Pandu indulges in Pitta aggravating diet and regimen, the Pitta so aggravated burns the Rakta (blood) and Mamsa (Muscle tissue) to cause the disease Kamala [Jaundice].

The signs and symptoms of Kamala are as follows:

Haridra Netra – yellowish discolouration of sclera of eyes

Haridra twak, Nakha, Anana – yellowish discoloration of skin, nails and face

Urine and faeces turns red and yellow

Bheka Varna – He develops complexion like that of a frog

Hatendriya – sense organs are impaired and

Daha – burning sensation

Avipaka, Aruchi – indigestion, anorexia

Daurbalya, Sadana – weakness, bodyache

Kamala disease is caused by an excess of Pitta. It is of two types -

Koshtashrita Kamala – one is located in the gastro- intestinal tract

Shakhashrita Kamala – located in the peripheral tissues (Sakhashraya)[34-36]

Kumbha Kamala

कालान्तरात् खरीभूता कृच्छ्रा स्यात् कुम्भकामला|
कृष्णपीत शकृन्मूत्रो भृशं शूनश्च मानवः||३७||
सरक्ताक्षि मुख च्छर्दि विण्मूत्रो यश्च ताम्यति|
दाहारुचि तृषानाहतन्द्रा मोह समन्वितः||३८||

नष्टाग्निसञ्ज्ञः क्षिप्रं हि कामलावान् विपद्यते।३९।

After some time if not treated properly, the Kamala [Jaundice] becomes deep-seated (Kharibhuta – roughened, hardened) and thus, becomes difficult to cure. This condition is called Kumbha-Kamala (a type of Jaundice).

The signs and symptoms of this Kumbha Kamala are:

1. Krishna pita shakrut mutra – The stool and urine of the patient become black and yellow

2. Bhrusham shunashcha manavah- Excess of oedema in the body

3. Sa Rakta Akshi, Mukha – Blood appears in the eyes and face of the patient (bloody colour in eyes and face)

4. Chardi vin mutro rakta – His vomit, stool and urine are mixed with blood

5. The patient develops tremors

6. Daha, Aruchi, Trushna, Anaha,Tandra, Moha – He is afflicted with burning sensation, anorexia, morbid thirst, constipation, drowsiness and fainting and

7. Nashta Agni – He loses Agni (the power of digestion and metabolism) and consciousness.

A person having this type of Kumbha-Kamala succumbs to death quickly. [37-391/2]

Panduroga Chikitsa Sutra – Line of Treatment:

साध्यानामितरेषां तु प्रवक्ष्यामि चिकित्सितम्||३९||

तत्र पाण्डवामयी स्निग्धस्तीक्ष्णैरूर्ध्वानुलोमिकैः|

संशोध्यो मृदुभिस्तिक्तैः कामली तु विरेचनैः||४०||

ताभ्यां संशुद्ध कोष्ठाभ्यां पथ्यान्यन्नानि दापयेत्|

शालीन् सयव गोधूमान् पुराणान् यूष संहितान्||४१||

मुद्गाढकी मसूरैश्च जाङ्गलैश्च रसैर्हितैः|

यथादोषं विशिष्टं च तयोर्भैषज्यमाचरेत्||४२||

पञ्चगव्यं महातिक्तं कल्याणकमथापि वा|

स्नेहनार्थं घृतं दद्यात् कामला पाण्डु रोगिणे||४३||

Line of Treatment:

Now the treatment for curable patients of Pandu Roga and Kamala (Jaundice) are being described.

The patient suffering from Pandu Roga is given –

Vamana – emetic therapy and

Virechana – Purgation therapies with Snigdha – unctuous and Teekshna – sharp drugs for the cleansing of his body.

The patient suffering from Kamala (jaundice) is given Virechana – purgation therapy with mild and bitter medicines.

After the gastro-intestinal tract is cleansed by the above mentioned elimination therapies, patient is given wholesome food containing old rice, barley and wheat mixed with the Yusha (vegetable soup) of Mudga (green gram), Adhaki (pigeon pea) and Masura (lentil) and the Jangala Mamsarasa (meat soup) of animals inhabiting arid zone.

On the basis of Doshas aggravated to cause these diseases, specific medicines are to be administered to these 2 categories of patients (which will be described later in this chapter)

For the purpose of oleation, the patient suffering from Pandu Roga (Anemia) and Kamala (Jaundice) is given PanchagavyaGrutha, [39 ½ -43]

Dadimadya Ghrta:

दाडिमात् कुडवो धान्यात् कुडवार्ध पलं पलम्|

चित्रकाच्छृङ्गवेराच्च पिप्पल्यष्टमिका तथा||४४||

तैः कल्कैर्विंशतिपलं घृतस्य सलिलाढके|

सिद्धं हृत्पाण्डु गुल्मार्शःप्लीह वात कफार्तिनुत्||४५||

दीपनं श्वास कासघ्नं मूढवाते च शस्यते|

दुःख प्रसविनीनां च वन्ध्यानां चैव गर्भदम्||४६||

इति दाडिमाद्यं घृतम्|

Dadimadi Ghrita: 20 Palas of ghee is cooked by adding 1 Adhaka of water, and the paste of 1 Kudava of Dadima – Punica granatum,

½ Kudava of Dhanya

1 Pala of each of Chitraka – Plumbago zeylanica and Srngavera and

1 Astamika of Pippali- Piper longum

This medicated ghee stimulates the power of digestion.

It is useful for curing

Shvasa – Asthma

Kasa – bronchitis

Mudha-Vata (Claudication of Vayu) and

Duhkha-prasava (difficult labour)

It also helps a sterile woman to beget an offspring.

Thus, ends the description of Dadimadya –Ghrta [44-46]

KatukadyaGhritham

कटुका रोहिणी मुस्तं हरिद्रे वत्सकात् पलम्।

पटोलं चन्दनं मूर्वा त्रायमाणा दुरालभा॥४७॥

कृष्णा पर्पटको निम्बो भूनिम्बो देवदारु च।

तैः कार्षिकै घृत प्रस्थः सिद्धः क्षीर चतुर्गुणः॥४८॥

रक्तपित्तं ज्वरं दाहं श्वयथुं स भगन्दरम्।

अर्शास्यसृग्दरं चैव हन्ति विस्फोटकांस्तथा॥४९॥

इति कटुकाद्यं घृतम्।

Katukadya Ghrita:

1 prastha (768 g) of ghee is cooked by adding 4 Prasthas of milk and

The paste of 1 Pala each of

Katukarohini

Musta – Cyperus rotundus

Haridra – Curcuma longa

Daru- Haridra – Berberis aristata and

Vatsaka and

1 Karsha – 12 g of each of

Patola – Trichosanthes dioica

Chandana – Santalum album

Murva – Marsedenia tenacissima

Trayamana

Duralabha

Krishna – Long pepper

Parpataka – Fumaria indica

Nimba – Azadirachta indica

Bhunimba – Phyllanthus niruri and

Devadaru – Cedrus deodara

This medicated ghee cures

Raktha-Pitta (a disease characterized by bleeding from different parts of the body),

Jwara – fever,

Daha – burning syndrome,

Shotha – oedema,

Bhagandara- fistula-in ano,

Arshas – piles,

Arsgdara – menorrhagia and

Visphotaka (a disease characterized by pustular eruptions in the body).

Thus, ends the description of Katukadya Grtha [47-49]

Pathya Ghruta

पथ्या शतरसे पथ्यावृन्तार्ध शत कल्कवान्‌|

प्रस्थः सिद्धो घृतात् पेयः स पाण्ड्वामय गुल्मनुत्‌||५०||

इति पथ्याघृतम्‌||

1 Prastha of ghee is cooked by adding decoction of 100 fruits of Haritaki – Terminalia bellerica, and the paste of 50 fruits of Haritaki fruit.

This medicated ghee cures Pandu (Anemia) and Gulma (Phantom tumor)

Thus ends the description of Pathya- Ghrta [50]

Danti- Ghrita

दन्त्याश्चतुष्पलरसे पिष्टैर्दन्तीशलाटुभिः|

तद्वत्प्रस्थो घृतात्सिद्धः प्लीहपाण्ड्वर्तिशोफजित्‌||५१||

इति दन्तीघृतम्‌|

Accordingly, 1 Prastha of ghee is cooked by adding 1 Prastha of the decoction of 4 Palas of Danti, and the paste of the cut-pieces of green fruits of danti.

Intake of this medicated ghee cures

Pliha – Splenic disorders

Pandu – Anemia and

Shopha – oedema.

Thus, ends the description of Danti - ghruta [51]

Draksha Ghruta

पुराण सर्पिषः प्रस्थो द्राक्षार्ध प्रस्थ साधितः|

कामला गुल्म पाण्ड्वर्ति ज्वर मेहोदरापहः||५२||

इति द्राक्षाघृतम्‌

1 Prastha of old ghee is added with ½ Prastha of Draksha – Vitis vinfera and cooked.

This medicated ghee cures

Kamala – jaundice

Gulma – Phantom tumor

Pandu – Anaemia,

Jwara – fever,

Meha – obstinate urinary diseases including diabetes and

Udara – obstinate abdominal diseases including ascites

Thus ends the description of Draksha ghrta [52]

HaridradiGhrta

हरिद्रा त्रिफला निम्ब बला मधुक साधितम्‌|

सक्षीरं माहिषं सर्पिः कामलाहरमुत्तमम्‌||५३||

इति हरिद्रादिघृतम्‌|

Ghee collected from buffalo milk is cooked by adding milk and [the paste of] Haridra – Berberis aristata, Triphala, Nimba – Azadirachta indica, Bala and Madhuka – Madhuca longifolia.

This medicated ghee is an excellent recipe for the cure of Jaundice.

Thus, ends the description of Haridradi Ghrta. [53]

Two recipes for medicated Ghee

गोमूत्रे द्विगुणे दार्व्याः कल्काक्षद्वयसाधितः।
दार्व्याः पञ्चपल क्वाथे कल्के कालीयके परः।।५४।।
माहिषात् सर्पिषः प्रस्थः पूर्वः पूर्वे परे परः।५५।

1 Prastha (768 g) of ghee collected from buffalo milk is boiled by adding 2 Prasthas of Cow's urine, and 2 Aksas of the paste of Darvi, this medicated ghee cures Pandu- Roga (Anemia).
1 Prastha of the ghee collected from buffalo milk is boiled by adding the decoction of 5 Palas of Darvi and the paste of Kaliyaka.
This medicated ghee cures Kamala (jaundice) [54 -¼ 55]

Virechana – Purgation therapy

स्नेहैरेभिरुपक्रम्य स्निग्धं मत्वा विरेचयेत्।।५५।।
पयसा मूत्रयुक्तेन बहुशः केवलेन वा।
दन्तीफल रसे कोष्णे काश्मर्याञ्जलिना शृतम्।।५६।।
द्राक्षाञ्जलिं मृदित्वा वा दद्यात् पाण्ड्वामयापहम्।
द्विशर्करं त्रिवृच्चूर्णं पलार्धं पैत्तिकः पिबेत्।।५७।।
कफपाण्डुस्तु गोमूत्र क्लिन्न युक्तां हरीतकीम्।
आरग्वधं रसेनेक्षो विदार्यामलकस्य च।।५८।।
सत्र्यूषणं बिल्वपत्रं पिबेन्ना कामलापहम्।
दन्त्यर्धपल कल्कं वा द्विगुडं शीतवारिणा।।५९।।
कामली त्रिवृतां वाऽपि त्रिफलाया रसैः पिबेत्।

Virechana – Purgation therapy
After the patient is properly oleated by the intake of the above mentioned recipes of medicated ghee, he is given purgation therapy frequently with the following recipes:
1. Milk added with cow's urine
2. Milk alone
3. Luke- warm infusion of Danti sprinkled with the powder of 1 Anjali of Kasmarya (fruit of Gambhari – Gmelina arborea) or mixed with the paste of 1 Anjali of Draksa – Vitis vinfera
The above mentioned recipes cure Pandu- Roga (Anaemia) in general.
4. The patient suffering from the Paittika type of Pandu- Roga should take ½ Pala of the powder of trivrt – Operculina turpethum mixed with 1 Pala of sugar.
5. The patient suffering from Kaphaja type of Pandu- Roga should take haritaki – Terminalia chebula impregnated with cow's urine.
The patient suffering from Kamala (Jaundice) should take Aragvadha – Cassia fistula added with Sunthi – Zingiber officinale, Pippali – Piper longum, Maricha – Piper nigrum and leaves of bilva – Aegle marmelos along with the juice of sugar-cane, vidari – Pueraria tuberosa and Amalaki – Phyllanthus emblica for the cure of the diseases
7. The patient suffering from Kamala (Jaundice) may also take the paste of ½ Pala of Danti mixed with 1 pala jaggery along with cold water and
8. The patient suffering from Kamala (jaundice) may also take Trivrt – Operculina turpethum along with the decoction of Triphala [55 ½- 60 ½]

Vishaladi –Phanta

विशाला त्रिफला मुस्त कुष्ठदारु कलिङ्गकान्।।६०।।
कार्षिकानर्धकर्षांशां कुर्यादतिविषां तथा।

कर्षौ मधुरसाया द्वौ सर्वमेतत् सुखाम्बुना||६१||
मृदितं तं रसं पूतं पीत्वा लिह्याच्च मध्वनु|
कासं श्वासं ज्वरं दाहं पाण्डुरोगमरोचकम्||६२||
गुल्मानाहामवातांश्च रक्तपित्तं च नाशयेत्|

1 Karsha of each of

Vishala

Haritaki – Terminalia chebula,

Bibhitaka – Terminalia bellerica,

Amalaki – Phyllanthus emblica,

Musta – Cyperus rotundus,

Kustha – Sausserea lappa,

Devadaru – Cedrus deodara and

Kalingaka,

½ Karsha – 12 g of

Ativisa – Aconitum heterophyllum,

2 Karsha – 12 gs of Madhurasa (Murva) is made to a paste by triturating with luke-warm water and strained.

After taking this infusion, the patient is given honey.

This phanta cures

Kasa – bronchitis

Shvasa – Asthma

Jwara – fever

Daha – burning sensation

Pandu-Roga – Anemia

Aruchi – anorexia,

Gulma – Phantom tumour

Anaha – constipation

Amavata – rheumatism and

Rakta-Pitta – a diseases characterised by bleeding from different parts of the body [60 ½- 63½]

Medicines:

त्रिफलाया गुडूच्या वा दार्व्या निम्बस्य वा रसम्||६३||
शीतं मधुयुतं प्रातः कामलार्तः पिबेन्नरः|
क्षीरमूत्रं पिबेत् पक्षं गव्यं माहिषमेव वा||६४||
पाण्डुर्गोमूत्रयुक्तं वा सप्ताहं त्रिफलारसम्|
तरुजान् ज्वलितान्मूत्रे निर्वाप्यामृद्य चाङ्कुरान्||६५||
मातुलुङ्गस्य तत् पूतं पाण्डुशोथहरं पिबेत्|
स्वर्णक्षीरी त्रिवृच्छ्यामे भद्रदारु सनागरम्||६६||
गोमूत्राञ्जलिना पिष्टं मूत्रे वा क्वथितं पिबेत्|
क्षीरमेभिः शृतं वाऽपि पिबेद्दोषानुलोमनम्||६७||
हरीतकीं प्रयोगेण गोमूत्रेणाथवा पिबेत्|
जीर्णे क्षीरेण भुञ्जीत रसेन मधुरेण वा||६८||
सप्तरात्रं गवां मूत्रे भावितं वाऽप्ययोरजः|
पाण्डुरोग प्रशान्त्यर्थं पयसा पाययेदिभषक्||६९||

Other recipes which are useful for these ailments are as follows:

1. The patient suffering from Kamala (jaundice) should take in the morning the decoction of Triphala, Guduchi – Tinospora cordifolia, Devadaru – Cedrus deodara or Nimba – Azadirachta indica after cooling and adding honey

2. The patient suffering from Pandu-Roga may take milk or urine of cow or buffalo for 1 fortnight.

3. The patient suffering from Pandu-Roga should take the decoction of Triphala along with cow's urine for 1 week

4. The tender branches of Matulunga – Citrus medica is set on fire, and then immersed in cow's urine. Thereafter, a paste is prepared of these tender branches and strained. The liquid, thus obtained, is used by a patient suffering from Anaemia and oedema.

5. Suvarna- Ksiri, Syama- Trivrt – Operculina turpethum, Bhadra-daru and Nagara is triturated by adding 1 Anjali of cow's urine. The above mentioned drugs may also be boiled with milk. Intake of these potions causes downward movement (elimination) of Doshas (causing Pandu)

6. Alternatively, the patient [suffering from Pandu- Roga] should take a course (for 7 days) of Haritaki – Terminalia chebula along with cow's urine, and after the digestion of the recipe, he should take food with milk or sweetened meat soup and

7. The powder (bhasma) of iron is impregnated with cow's urine for 7 nights. The physician should administer this potion along with milk for the alleviation of Pandu- Roga (Anaemia). 63 1/3- 69]

Navayasa Churna

त्र्यूषण त्रिफला मुस्त विडङ्ग चित्रकाः समाः|
नवायोरजसो भागास्तच्चूर्णं क्षौद्र सर्पिषा||७०||
भक्षयेत् पाण्डु हृद्रोग कुष्ठार्शःकामलापहम्|
नवायसमिदं चूर्णं कृष्णात्रेयेण भाषितम्||७१||
इति नवायसचूर्णम्|

NavayasChuran:

1 part of each of the powders of

Sunthi – Zingiber officinale,

Pippali – Piper longum,

Maricha – Piper nigrum,

Haritaki – Terminalia chebula,

Bibhitaki – Terminalia bellerica,

Amalaki – Phyllanthus emblica,

Musta – Cyperus rotundus,

Vidanga – Embelia ribes and

Chitraka – Plumbago zeylanica and

9 parts of the powder (bhasma) of iron are mixed together.

Intake of this recipe along with honey and ghee cures

Pandu – Anaemia,

Hrud roga – heart diseases,

Kustha (skin diseases),

Arshas – Piles and

Kamala -Jaundice

This recipe propounded by Krsnatreya is called Navayasa- curna

Thus, ends the description of Navayasa- curna [70- 71]

Two Recipes of Mandura Vataka

गुड नागर मण्डूर तिलांशान्मानतः समान्|
पिप्पली द्विगुणां कुर्याद्गुटिकां पाण्डुरोगिणे||७२||
त्र्यूषणं त्रिफला मुस्तं विडङ्गं चव्य चित्रकौ|
दार्वीत्वइमाक्षिको धातुर्ग्रन्थिकं देवदारु च||७३||
एतान् द्विपलिकान्भागांश्चूर्णं कुर्यात् पृथक् पृथक्|

मण्डूरं द्विगुणं चूर्णाच्छुद्धमञ्जनसन्निभम्॥७४॥
गोमूत्रेऽष्टगुणे पक्त्वा तस्मिंस्तत् प्रक्षिपेततः।
उदुम्बर समान्कृत्वा वटकांस्तान् यथाग्नि ना॥७५॥
उपयुञ्जीत तक्रेण सात्म्यं जीर्णे च भोजनम्।
मण्डूर वटका ह्येते प्राणदाः पाण्डु रोगिणाम्॥७६॥
कुष्ठान्यजीर्णकं शोथमूरुस्तम्भं कफामयान्।
अर्शांसि कामलां मेहं प्लीहानं शमयन्ति च॥७७॥
इति मण्डूरवटकाः।

1 part of each of Jaggery, Sunthi – Zingiber officinale, Mandura and Taila 2 parts of Pippali – Piper longum is triturated [by adding water] and made into pills. This recipe is useful for patients suffering from Anaemia.

2 Palas of each of

Sunthi – Zingiber officinale

Pippali – Piper longum

Maricha – Piper nigrum

Haritaki – Terminalia chebula

Bibhitaka – Terminalia bellerica

Amalaka – Phyllanthus emblica

Musta – Cyperus rotundus

Vidanga – Embelia ribes

Chavya – Piper chaba

Chitraka – Plumbago zeylanica

Bark of devadaru – Cedrus deodara is made to powders separately.

The powder of 56 Palas of Mandura, which is dark in colour like collyrium is cooked by adding 8 times of cow's urine, and to this, the powders of the above mentioned drugs is added.

From out of this (Paste), Vatakas (large size Pills) of the shape of the fruit of Udumbara – Ficus racemosa are prepared.

This is taken by the patient in appropriate doses depending upon his Agni (powder of digestion and metabolism) along with butter-milk. After its digestion, the patient should takes wholesome food

These pills are called mandura-Vataka and these are the life givers for the patient suffering from Anaemia.

In addition, these pills cure

Kustha (skin diseases),

Ajirna – indigestion,

Shotha – oedema,

Uru-stambha (stiffening of the thighs),

Diseases caused by the aggravation of Kapha,

Arshas – piles,

Kamala – Jaundice,

Meha – urinary tract disorders, diabetes (obstinate urinary diseases including diabetes) and

Pliha – splenic diseases.

Thus ends the description of (2 types of) Manduravataka [72-77]

Tapyadi Yoga

ताप्याद्रिजतुरूप्यायोमलाः पञ्चपलाः पृथक्।
चित्रक त्रिफला व्योष विडङ्गैः पलिकैः सह॥७८॥
शर्कराष्टपलोन्मिश्राश्चूर्णिता मधुनाऽऽप्लुताः।
अभ्यस्यास्त्वक्षमात्रा हि जीर्णे हितमिताशिना॥७९॥
कुलत्थ काकमाच्यादिकपोतपरिहारिणा।८०।

5 palas of each of Tapya (svarna-Maksika), Silajatu, silver (bhasma or powder) and Mandura is added with (the powders of) 1 Pala of each of

Chitraka – Plumbago zeylanica

Haritaki – Terminalia chebula

Bhibhitaka – Terminalia bellerica

Amalaki – Phyllanthus emblica

Sunthi – Zingiber officinale

Pippali – Piper longum

Maricha – Piper nigrum and

Vidanga – Embelia ribes and

8 Palas of sugar

This recipe is taken habitually by the patient suffering from Pandu in the dose of 1 Karsha – 12 g along with an adequate quantity of honey.

After the digestion of this potion, the patient should take wholesome food in small quantities. He should avoid taking Kulattha (horse gram), Kakamachi – Solanum nigrum etc. and the meat of Kapota (pigeon). [78 ½ – 80]

Yogaraja

त्रिफलायास्त्रयो भागास्त्रयस्त्रिकटुकस्य च||८०||

भागश्चित्रकमूलस्य विडङ्गानां तथैव च|

पञ्चाश्मजतुनो भागास्तथा रूप्यमलस्य च||८१||

माक्षिकस्य च शुद्धस्य लौहस्य रजसस्तथा|

अष्टौ भागाः सितायाश्च तत्सर्वं सूक्ष्म चूर्णितम्||८२||

माक्षिकेणाप्लुतं स्थाप्यमायसे भाजने शुभे|

उदुम्बरसमां मात्रां ततः खादेद्यथाग्नि ना||८३||

दिने दिने प्रयुञ्जीत जीर्णं भोज्यं यथेप्सितम्|

वर्जयित्वा कुलत्थानि काकमाचीं कपोतकम्||८४||

योगराज इति ख्यातो योगोऽयममृतोपमः|

रसायनमिदं श्रेष्ठं सर्वरोगहरं शिवम्||८५||

पाण्डुरोगं विषं कासं यक्ष्माणं विषम ज्वरम्|

कुष्ठान्यजीर्णकं मेहं शोषं श्वासमरोचकम्||८६||

विशेषाद्धन्त्यपस्मारं कामलां गुदजानि च|

इति योगराजः|

1 part of each of

Haritaki – Terminalia chebula

Bibhitaka –Terminalia bellerica,

Amalaki – Phyllanthus emblica

Sunthi – Zingiber officinale

Pippali – Piper longum

Maricha – Piper nigrum

Root of Chitraka – Plumbago zeylanica and

Vidanga – Embelia ribes

5 parts of each of

Shilajatu,

Raupya Mala (silver rust),

Purified Maksika, and

Powder (Bhasma) of iron, and

8 parts of sugar is made into a fine powder.

This potion is mixed with an adequate quantity of honey and kept in a clam iron jar.

This recipe is taken by the patient in a quantity equal to a fruit of udumbara – Ficus racemosa according to his power of digestion every day.

After its digestion, he is given the desired food excluding kulattha, Kakamaci and meat of Kapota.

This ambrosia- like recipe is called Yogaraja.

It is an excellent rejuvenation recipe which cures all diseases and bestows auspiciousness.

It specially cures

Pandu – Anaemia,

Visham – poisoning,

Kasa – bronchitis,

Yakshma – tuberculosis,

VisamaJvara – fever (irregular fever),

Kustha – skin diseases),

Ajirna – indigestion,

Meha – obstinate urinary disorders including diabetes),

Kshya – consumption,

Shvasa – Asthma,

Aruchi – anorexia,

Apasmara – epilepsy,

Kamala – Jaundice and

Arshas – piles.

Thus ends the description of Yogaraja. [80 ½- 87½]

Shilajatu Vataka

कौटज त्रिफला निम्ब पटोलघन नागरैः||८७||

भावितानि दशाहानि रसैर्द्विर्वत्रिगुणानि वा|

शिलाजतुपलान्यष्टौ तावती सितशर्करा||८८||

त्वक्क्षीरी पिप्पली धात्री कर्कटाख्या पलोन्मिता|

निदिग्ध्याः फलमूलाभ्यां पलं युक्त्या त्रिगन्धकम्|||८९||

चूर्णितं मधुनः कुर्यात् त्रिपलेनाक्षिकान् गुडान्|

दाडिमाम्बुपयःपक्षिरसतोय सुरासवान्||९०||

तान् भक्षयित्वाऽनुपिबेन्निरन्नो भुक्त एव वा|

पाण्डु कुष्ठ ज्वर प्लीह तमकार्शो भगन्दरान्||९१||

पूतिहृच्छुक्रमूत्राग्निदोष शोषगरोदरान् |

कासासृग्दरपितासृक्शोथगुल्मगलामयान्||९२||

ते च सर्वव्रणान् हन्युः सर्वरोगहराः शिवाः|

इति शिलाजतुवटकाः|

8 Palas of Shilajatu is impregnated for 10, 20 or 30 days with the decoction of the fruit of Kutaja – , Haritaki , Bibhitaki , Amalaki , Nimba , Patola, Ghana, and Nagara.

To this Silajatu, 8 Palas of sugar, and the powder of 1 Pala of each of Tvak-Ksiri (Vamsa-Lochana), Pippali – Piper longum, Dhatri and Karkata- Srngi

½ Pala of each of the fruit and root of Nidigdhika and adequate quantity of the powder of tvak, Ela, and Patra is added by adding 3 Palas of honey to this powder, Vatakas or Gudas (large size pills) of 1 Aksha each is prepared.

Having taken these pills on empty stomach or after taking food, the patient is made to drink the juice of Dadima – punica granatum, milk, soup of the meat of birds, water, alcohol or Asava (medicated wine).

It cures

Pandu – Anaemia,

Kustha – skin diseases
Jwara – fever
Pliha – spleen disorders
Tamaka type of Asthma
Arshas – piles
Bhagandara – fistula-in-ano,
Puti – purified ulcers,
Hrut roga – heart diseases,
Shukra, mutra, agni dosha – diseases of semen, urine and agni (power of digestion),
Sosha – consumption,
Gara – poisoning,
Udara – obstinate abdominal diseases including ascites
Shvasa – bronchitis,
Asrgdara – Menorrhagia
Rakta-Pitta (a disease characterised by bleeding from different parts of the body),
Shotha — oedema,
Gulma – abdominal tumour, distension (phantom tumour),
Gala rogas – diseases of the throat, and all types of ulcer
It cures all types of diseases, and bestows auspiciousness.
Thus ends the description of Silajatu- Vataka. [87 ½ – 93½]

Punarnava Mandura
पुनर्नवा त्रिवृद्व्योषविडङ्गं दारु चित्रकम्||९३||
कुष्ठं हरिद्रे त्रिफला दन्ती चव्यं कलिङ्गकाः|
पिप्पली पिप्पलीमूलं मुस्तं चेति पलोन्मितम्||९४||
मण्डूरं द्विगुणं चूर्णाद्गोमूत्रे द्व्याढके पचेत्|
कोलवद्गुटिकाः कृत्वा तक्रेणालोड्य ना पिबेत्||९५||
ताः पाण्डुरोगान् प्लीहानमर्शांसि विषमज्वरम्|
श्वयथुं ग्रहणीदोषं हन्युः कुष्ठं क्रिमींस्तथा||९६||
इति पुनर्नवा मण्डूरम्|
The powder of 1 Pala each of
Punarnava – Boerhavia diffusa
Trivrt – Operculina turpethum
Sunthi – Zingiber officinale
Pippali – Piper longum
Maricha— Piper nigrum
Vidanga – Embelia ribes
Devadaru – Cedrus deodara
Chitraka – Plumbago zeylanica
Kustha – Sausserea lappa
Haridra – Curcuma longa
Daru- Haridra – Berberis aristata
Haritaki – Terminalia chebula
Bibhitaki – Terminalia bellerica
Amalaki – Phyllanthus emblica
Danti – Baliospermum montanum
Chavya – Piper chaba

Kalingaka

Pippali – Piper longum, Pippali Mula and

Musta – Cyperus rotundus and

40 Palas of Mandura (rest of iron) is cooked in 2 Adhakas of cow's urine. From out of this, Mandura cures

Pandu – Anemia,

Pliha – splenic disorders,

Arshas – piles,

Visama- Jvara (irregular fever),

Shotha – oedema

Grahani- Dosha – sprue syndrome

Kustha – skin diseases and parasitic infestation.

Thus, ends the description of Punarnava- Mandura. [93 ½- 96]

Darvyadi Leha

दार्वीत्वक् त्रिफला व्योषं विडङ्गमयसो रजः।

मधु सर्पिर्युतं लिह्यात् कामला पाण्डुरोगवान्॥९७॥

The powder of the

Bark of Daruharidra – Berberis aristata,

Haritaki, Bibhitaka, Amalaki

Sunthi – Zingiber officinale, Pippali – Piper longum, Maricha – Piper nigrum Vidanga and

Iron (Bhasma) is mixed with ghee and honey, and taken as linctus by the patients suffering from Jaundice & Anemia. [97]

Two Recipes

तुल्या अयोरजःपथ्या हरिद्राः क्षौद्र सर्पिषा।

चूर्णिताः कामली लिह्याद्गुडक्षौद्रेण वाऽभयाः॥९८॥

The patient suffering from Jaundice should take the powder of 1 part of each of iron (bhasma), Haridra along with honey and ghee. He may also take the linctus of the powder of Abhaya prepared by mixing with Jaggery and honey [98]

त्रिफला द्वे हरिद्रे च कटुरोहिण्ययोरजः।

चूर्णितं क्षौद्रसर्पिभर्यां स लेहः कामलापहः॥९९॥

Triphala

Haridra

Daruharidra

Katukurohini are powdered and mixed with honey. It is good for Jaundice.

Dhatryavaleha

द्विपलांशां तुगाक्षीरीं नागरं मधु यष्टिकाम्।

प्रास्थिकीं पिप्पलीं द्राक्षां शर्कराधैतुलां शुभाम्॥१००॥

धात्रीफलरसद्रोणे चूर्णितं लेहवत् पचेत्।

शीतं मधु प्रस्थयुतं लिह्यात् पाणितलं ततः॥१०१॥

हन्त्येष कामलां पित्तं पाण्डुं कासं हलीमकम्।

इति धात्र्यवलेहः।

The powder of 2 Palas of each of

Vamsa-lochana,

Sunthi and

Madhu-yasti

1 Prastha (768 g) of each

Pippali – Piper longum – long pepper and

Draksa – raisins – Vitis vinifera, and

½ a tula of crystal sugar is added with 1 drona of the juice of Amalaki- fruit – Phyllanthus emblica, and cooked till the whole thing becomes a linctus.

After it is cooled down, 1 Prastha of honey is added.

Intake of 1 Panitala of this linctus cures

Kamala – Jaundice,

Diseases caused by Pitta,

Pandu – Anaemia,

Kasa – bronchitis and

Halimaka (a type of Jaundice)

Thus, ends the description of Dhatryavaleha. [100 – 102½]

ManduraVataka (another recipe)

त्र्यूषणं त्रिफला चव्यं चित्रको देवदारु च||१०२||

विडङ्गान्यथ मुस्तं च वत्सकं चेति चूर्णयेत्|

मण्डूरतुल्यं तच्चूर्णं गोमूत्रेऽष्टगुणे पचेत्||१०३||

शनैः सिद्धास्तथा शीताः कार्याः कर्षसमा गुडाः|

यथाग्नि भक्षणीयास्ते प्लीह पाण्डवामयापहाः||१०४||

ग्रहण्यर्शोनुदश्चैव तक्रवाट्याशिनः स्मृताः|

इति मण्डूरवटकाः|

1 part of each of

Sunthi – Zingiber officinale

Pippali – Piper longum

Maricha – Piper nigrum

Haritaki – Terminalia chebula

Bibhitaka – Terminalia bellerica

Amalaki – Phyllanthus emblica

Chavya – Piper chaba

Chitraka – Plumbago zeylanica

Devadaru – Cedrus deodara

Vidanga – Embelia ribes

Musta – Cyperus rotundus and

Vatsaka (Kustaja) is made into a powder.

To this equal quantity (12 parts) of the Powder of Mandura (rust of iron) is added.

These powders are boiled by adding 8 times of cow's urine over mild fire. When the recipe becomes cool, pills of 1 Aksa each are ½ Tula of sugar is added it is then kept in a ghee-smeared earthen prepared and taken according to the power of digestion.

This cures:

Pliha – spleen diseases,

Pandu – Anaemia

Grahani (sprue syndrome) and

Arshas – piles.

While taking these pills, the patient should take butter- milk and Vatya (a preparation of roasted barley).

This ends the description of Mandura-vataka [102 ½- 105½]

Gaudarista

मञ्जिष्ठा रजनी द्राक्षा बलामूलान्ययोरजः||१०५||
लोध्रं चैतेषु गौडः स्यादरिष्टः पाण्डुरोगिणाम्|
इति गौडोऽरिष्टः|

Manjistha—Rubia cordifolia

Haridra – Curcuma longa

Draksa – Vitis vinifera

Roots of Bala – Sida cordifolia

Powder (bhasma) of iron and

Lodhra – Symplocos racemosa is (added with jaggery and) processed according to the method prescribed for Arista (a type of medicated wine).

This is called Gaudarista which is useful for the patients suffering from Anaemia [105 ½- 106½]

Thus ends the description of Gaudarista

Bijakarista:

बीजकात्षोडशपलं त्रिफलायाश्च विंशतिः||१०६||
द्राक्षायाः पञ्च लाक्षायाः सप्त द्रोणे जलस्य तत्|
साध्यं पादावशेषे तु पूतशेषे समावपेत्||१०७||
शर्करायास्तुलां प्रस्थं माक्षिकस्य च कार्षिकम्|
व्योषं व्याघ्रनखोशीरं क्रमुकं सैलवालुकम्||१०८||
मधुकं कुष्ठमित्येतच्चूर्णितं घृतभाजने|
यवेषु दशरात्रं तद्ग्रीष्मे दिवः शिशिरे स्थितम्||१०९||
पिबेतद्ग्रहणी पाण्डुरोगार्शःशोथ गुल्मनुत्|
मूत्रकृच्छ्राश्मरी मेह कामला सन्निपातजित्||११०||
बीजकारिष्ट इत्येष आत्रेयेण प्रकीर्तितः|
इति बीजकारिष्टः|

16 Palas of Bijaka (Asana)

20 of Triphala,

5 Palas of Draksha – Vitis vinifera and

7 Palas of Laksha is added with 1 Drona of water, and boiled till $1/4^{th}$ of water remains.

This water is then to be taken out by straining.

To this, 1 Tula of sugar and 1 Prastha of honey, and 1 Pala of the powder of each of

Sunthi – Zingiber officinale,

Pippali – Piper longum

Marica,

Vyaghra Nakha (a type of Nakhi),

Usira,

Karamuka,

Elavaluka,

Madhuka – Madhuca longifolia and

Kustha – Saussurea lappa is added.

The potion is stored in a jar smeared with ghee, and kept inside a heap of barley for 10 nights during summer, and for 20 nights in winter.

Intake of this potion cures

Grahani (sprue syndrome),

Pandu – Anaemia,

Arshas – piles,

Shotha – oedema,

Gulma (phantom tumour),

Mutra krcchra- dysuria, stone in urinary tract,

Meha – obstinate urinary disorders including diabetes

Kamala – jaundice and

Sannipata – diseases caused by the simultaneous vitiation of all the 3 Doshas

This is called bijakarista and it was propounded by Atreya. [106 ½ -111 ½]

Dhatryarista

धात्रीफल सहस्रे द्वे पीडयित्वा रसं तु तम्||१११||

क्षौद्राष्टांशेन संयुक्तं कृष्णार्धकुडवेन च|

शर्करार्धतुलोन्मिश्रं पक्षं स्निग्धघटे स्थितम्||११२||

प्रपिबेन्मात्रया प्रातर्जीर्णे हितमिताशनः|

कामला पाण्डु हृद्रोग वातासृग्विषमज्वरान्||११३||

कास हिक्कारुचि श्वासांश्चैषोऽरिष्टः प्रणाशयेत्|

इति धात्र्यरिष्टः|

1000 fruits of Amalaki are crushed and their juice is extracted.

To this, 1/8th the quantity of honey,

½ kudava of Pippali – Piper longum, and

½ Tula of sugar is added; it is then kept in a ghee-smeared earthen jar for 1 fortnight.

It is taken in the appropriate dose in the morning.

After the recipe is digested, the patient should take wholesome food in small quantities.

This Arista (medicated wine) cures

Kamala – jaundice,

Pandu – Anaemia,

Hrud roga – heart diseases,

Vata-rakta – gout,

Vishama jvara – irregular fever),

Kasa – bronchitis,

Hikka – hiccup,

Aruchi – aneroxia and

Shvasa – Asthma.

Thus ends the description of Dhatryrista [111 ½- 114 ½]

Drinks

स्थिरादिभिः श‍ृतं तोयं पानाहारे प्रशस्यते||११४||

पाण्डूनां, कामलार्तानां मृद्वीकामलकीरसः|११५|

Water boiled with the drugs belonging to the Sthiradi group (Salaparni, etc vide Sutrasthana 4:17) is useful for drinking, and for the preparation of food for the patient suffering from Anaemia.

For the patient of jaundice, the juice of Draksha – Vitis vinfera and Amalaki – Phyllanthus emblica is useful (as drink and for the preparation of food).

General line of treatment:

पाण्डुरोग प्रशान्त्यर्थमिति प्रोक्तं महर्षिणा||११५||

विकल्प्यमेतद्भिषजा पृथग्दोषबलं प्रति|

वातिके स्नेहभूयिष्ठं, पैतिके तिक्तशीतलम्||११६||

श्लैष्मिके कटुतिक्तोष्णं ,विमिश्रं सान्निपातिके|११७|

The above - mentioned recipes are described by the great sage (Punarvasu Atreya) for the cure of Pandu Roga (Anaemia).

The physician should make appropriate changes (Permutations and combinations) depending upon the strength of Doshas in the patient.

For Vatika type of Pandu the therapy is dominated by unctuous drugs (oil, ghee etc)

For the Paittika type of Pandu, it is dominated by bitter and cooling medicines.

For Kaphaja type of Pandu, the therapy is dominated by pungent, bitter and hot drugs.

For the Sannipatika type of Pandu all the above mentioned ingredients are combined. [115 ½- 117 ½]

Treatment of Mrid-Bhaksanaja- Pandu:

निपातयेच्छरीरातु मृत्तिकां भक्षितां भिषक्||११७||

युक्तिज्ञः शोधनैस्तीक्ष्णैः प्रसमीक्ष्य बलाबलम्|

शुद्धकायस्य सर्पींषि बलाधानानि योजयेत्||११८||

The physician, well versed in therapeutics, should give sharp (strong) elimination therapy, keeping in view the strength or otherwise of the patient, in order to remove the swallowed mud from his body.

After the body is cleansed, the patient is given different types of medicated ghee for the promotion of his strength. [117 ½- 118]

Vyoshadya –Ghruta

व्योषं बिल्वं हरिद्रे द्वे त्रिफला द्वे पुनर्नवे|

मुस्तान्ययोरजः पाठा विडङ्गं देवदारु च||११९||

वृश्चिकाली च भार्गी च सक्षीरैस्तैः समैर्घृतम्|

साधयित्वा पिबेद्युक्त्या नरो मृद्दोषपीडितः||१२०||

तद्वत् केशरयष्ट्याह्वपिप्पलीक्षारशाद्वलैः|

Ghee boiled with

Sunthi – Zingiber officinale

Pippali – Piper longum

Maricha – Piper nigrum

Bilva – Aegle marmelos

Haridra - Curcuma longa

Daru- Haridra – Berberis aristata

Haritaki – Terminalia chebula

Bibhitaka – Terminalia bellerica

Amalaki – Phyllanthus emblica

Sveta- Punarnava –

Rakta- Punarnava

Musta – Cyperus rotundus

Powder (bhasma) of Iron,

Patha – Cissampelos pariera

Vidanga – Embelia ribes

Deva-daru – Cedrus deodara

Vrscikali

Bhargi and

Milk is appropriately taken by the patient who suffers from Anaemia because of swallowing clay (mud)

Similarly, ghee boiled with

Kesara,

Yasti- Madhu – Liquorice

Pippali – Piper longum

Ksara – alkali preparation and

Sadvala (Durva – Cynodon dactylon (Linn.) is given to the patient suffering from Mrd- Bhaksanaja- Pandu. [119- ½ -121]

Recipe for Causing Aversion for Mud

मृद्भक्षणादातुरस्य लौल्यादविनिवर्तिनः||१२१||

द्वेष्यार्थं भावितां कामं दद्यात्तद्दोषनाशनैः|

विड्ङ्गैलातिविषया निम्बपत्रेण पाठया||१२२||

वार्ताकैः कटुरोहिण्या कौटजैर्मूर्वयाऽपि वा|१२३|

If the patient is unable to give up his clay-swallowing habits he is given clay impregnated with

Vidanga – Embelia ribes

Ela – Elettaria cardamomum

Ativisa – Aconitum heterophyllum

Neem-leaf – Azadirachta indica

Patha – Cissampelos pariera

Vartaka,

Katu-rohini – Picrorhiza kurroa

Kuthaja or

Murva – Marsedenia tenacissima with a view to creating aversion in him (for clay)

These drugs counteract the adverse effects of clay Swallowing. [121 ½- 123½]

Line of treatment of Mrud- Bhaksanaja- Pandu:

यथादोषं प्रकुर्वीत भैषज्यं पाण्डुरोगिणाम्||१२३||

क्रियाविशेष एषोऽस्य मतो हेतुविशेषतः|१२४|

Depending upon the Doshas aggravated, different types of treatment is given to the patient suffering from Mrd Bhaksanaja- pandu (Anaemia caused by clay swallowing).

However, because of the specific nature of the causative factor the type of Anaemia needs special type of treatment. [123 ½ – 124 ½]

Shakhasrita Kamala

तिलपिष्टनिभं यस्तु वर्चः सृजति कामली||१२४||

श्लेष्मणा रुद्धमार्गं तत् पित्तं कफहरैर्जयेत्|

रूक्ष शीत गुरु स्वादु व्यायामैर्वेगनिग्रहैः||१२५||

कफ सम्मूर्छितो वायुः स्थानात् पित्तं क्षिपेद्बली|

हारिद्र नेत्र मूत्र त्वक् श्वेत वर्चास्तदा नरः||१२६||

भवेत् साटोप विष्टम्भो गुरुणा हृदयेन च|

दौर्बल्याल्पाग्नि पार्श्वार्ति हिक्का श्वासारुचि ज्वरैः||१२७||

क्रमेणाल्पेऽनुसज्येत पित्ते शाखा समाश्रिते|१२८|

Shakhasrita Kamala

If a patient of jaundice voids stool having the colour of sesame paste – Tilapishtanibha Varchas, then it indicates the obstruction to the bile passage by Kapha.

Therefore, the Pitta (bile) of such a patient is eliminated by the administration of medicines which also balance Kapha.

Because of the excessive use of dry, cold and sweet ingredients, because of excessive exercise and because of the suppression of natural urges, Vata Dosha along with Kapha gets aggravated to cause displacement of Pitta.

Thus, the eyes, urine and skin of the patient become yellow in colour, and his stool becomes white in color.

In addition, the patient suffers from
Atopa (tympanitis),
Vistambha (constipation associated with flatulence) and
Heaviness in the cardiac region
Since the displaced Pitta gets located in the periphery (skin and Muscles), and there is reduction in the flow of Pitta (to the gastro-intestinal tract), the patient gradually suffers from weakness, Agnimandya (Suppression of the power of digestion), weakness, pain in the sides of the chest, hiccup, dyspnoea, anorexia and fever. [124 ½ – 128½]

Food for Sakhasrita- Kamala

बर्हितित्तिरि दक्षाणां रूक्षाम्लैः कटुकै रसैः||१२८||
शुष्कमूलक कौलत्थैर्यूषैश्चान्नानि भोजयेत्|
मातुलुङ्गरसं क्षौद्रपिप्पलीमरिचान्वितम्||१२९||
सनागरं पिबेत् पित्तं तथाऽस्यैति स्वमाशयम्|१३०|

The patient suffering from Shakhasrita- Kamala is given food along with the soup of the meat of peacock, partridge and cock sizzled with dry, sour and pungent articles, and vegetable soups of dry radish and Kulattha.
The patient is also given the juice of Matulunga – Citrus medica mixed with honey.
Pippali – Piper longum, Maricha – Piper nigrum and Sunthi – Zingiber officinale in order to bring the (diverged) Pitta to its own course [128 ½- 130½]

Duration of the treatment

कटु तीक्ष्णोष्ण लवणैर्भृशाम्लैश्चाप्युपक्रमः||१३०||
आपित्तरागाच्छकृतो वायोश्चाप्रशमाद्भवेत्|
स्वस्थानमागते पित्ते पुरीषे पित्तरञ्जिते||१३१||
निवृत्तोपद्रवस्य स्यात् पूर्वः कामलिको विधिः|१३२|

The treatment with pungent, sharp, hot, saline and extremely sour drugs is continued till the stool of the patient acquires the colour of pitta (yellow because of the presence of bile), and the vayu gets alleviated. When Pitta returns to its own habits (normal seat), and the stool starts getting coloured by Pitta (bile), and when the complications subside, the general treatment explained earlier for the treatment of Jaundice (kosthasrita Kamala) should be resumed. [130 ½ - 132½]

Halimaka Type of Jaundice

यदा तु पाण्डोर्वर्णः स्याद्धरित श्याव पीतकः||१३२||
बलोत्साह क्षयस्तन्द्रा मन्दाग्नित्वं मृदु ज्वरः|
स्त्रीष्वहर्षोऽङ्गमर्दश्च श्वासस्तृष्णाऽरुचिर्भ्रमः||१३३||
हलीमकं तदा तस्य विद्यादनिलपित्ततः|१३४|

If the colour of the patient suffering from Pandu (Anemia) because green, black or yellow, and he suffers from diminution of strength and enthusiasm, Tandra – Drowsiness, Agnimandya (Suppression of the power of digestion), Jwara – mild fever, lack of libido, malaise, Shvasa – dysponea, Trshuna – morbid thirst, Aruchi – anorexia and Bhrama – giddiness, the ailment is called Halimaka which is caused by the aggravation of Vayu and Pitta. [132 ½ – 134½]

Treatment of Halimaka

गुड़ूची स्वरस क्षीर साधितं माहिष घृतम्||१३४||
स पिबेत्त्रिवृतां स्निग्धो रसेनामलकस्य तु|
विरिक्तो मधुर प्रायं भजेत् पित्तानिलापहम्||१३५||
द्राक्षालेहं च पूर्वोक्तं सर्पीषि मधुराणि च|

यापनान् क्षीरबस्तींश्च शीलयेत्सानुवासनान्||१३६||
माद्वीकारिष्टयोगांश्च पिबेद्युक्त्याऽग्निवृद्धये|
कासिकं चाभयालेहं पिप्पलीं मधुकं बलाम्||१३७||
पयसा च प्रयुञ्जीत यथादोषं यथाबलम्|१३८|

The patient suffering from Halimaka should take the recipe prepared of the ghee from buffalo milk by adding the juice of Guduchi – Tinospora cordifolia and Milk.

After he is oleated, the patient should take Trivrt – Operculina turpethum mixed with the juice of Amalaki – Phyllanthus emblica which causes purgation. Thereafter, he should take (food and drinks) which are dominated by sweet taste and are alleviaters of pitta and Vayu.

He should take Draksavaleha described earlier. The recipe is described with the caption Dhatryavaleha and recipes of medicated ghee prepared by boiling with sweet medicines.

He should habitually resort to different types of Yapana- Basti (a type of medicated enema), Ksheera- Basthi and anuvasana- Basti (to be discussed in detail in Siddhi section).

He should also take different recipes of Arista (medicated wine) prepared of grape (Draksarista) for the promotion of the digestion Abhaya-leha (Agastya- haritaki) described in the chapter dealing with the treatment of Kasa or Bronchitis (wide Cikistsa 18: 57-62) may be taken by him.

Alternatively he may take Pippali – Piper longum, Madhuka – Madhuca longifolia and Bala—Abution indicum along with milk, depending upon the Doshas aggravated, and the strength of the patients. [134 ½- 138½]

Summary:
तत्र श्लोकौ-
पाण्डोः पञ्च विधस्योक्तं हेतु लक्षण भेषजम्||१३८||
कामला द्विविधा तेषां साध्यासाध्यत्वमेव च|
तेषां विकल्पो यश्चान्यो महा व्याधि हलीमकः|
तस्य चोक्तं समासेन व्यञ्जनं सचिकित्सितम्||१३९||

In this chapter, the following topics are described

1. 5 types of Pandu (Anemia) along with aetiology, signs and symptoms and treatment
2. 2 types of Kamala (Jaundice), and their curability as well as incurability
3. Different varieties (stages) of Kamala and
4. Halimaka which is a serious diseases along with its signs and symptoms, and treatment [138 ½- 139]

इत्यग्निवेशकृते तन्त्रेऽप्राप्ते दृढबल सम्पूरिते चिकित्सा स्थाने पाण्डुरोग चिकित्सितं नाम षोडशोऽध्यायः||१६||

Thus, ends the 16th chapter in Chikistha Sthana – treatment section, dealing with the treatment of Pandu Roga (Anemia) in the work of Agnivesha which was redacted by Charaka and supplemented by Dridhabala.

23

Chikitsasthana Chapter 17 Hikka Shwasa Chikitsitam

The 17th chapter of Charaka Samhita Chikitsasthana is called Hikka Shwasa Chikitsa. It deals with treatment for hiccups, asthma and respiratory disorders with difficulty in breathing.

Treatment of Hiccup and Asthma

अथातो हिक्का श्वास चिकित्सितं व्याख्यास्यामः||१||

इति ह स्माह भगवानात्रेयः||२||

Let us explore the chapter on the treatment of Hikka – hiccough (Hiccup) and Shvasa (asthma). Thus, said Lord Atreya [1-2]

Serious Nature of Hikka and Shvasa Roga:

वेदलोकार्थतत्त्वज्ञमात्रेयमृषिमुत्तमम्|

अपृच्छत् संशयं धीमानग्निवेशः कृताञ्जलिः||३||

य इमे द्विविधाः प्रोक्तास्त्रिदोषास्त्रिप्रकोपणाः|

रोगा नानात्मकास्तेषां कस्को भवति दुर्जयः||४||

अग्निवेशस्य तद्वाक्यं श्रुत्वा मतिमतां वरः|

उवाच परम प्रीतः परमार्थ विनिश्चयम्||५||

कामं प्राणहरा रोगा बहवो न तु ते तथा|

यथा श्वासश्च हिक्का च प्राणानाशु निकृन्ततः||६||

अन्यैरप्युपसृष्टस्य रोगैर्जन्तोः पृथग्विधैः|

अन्ते सञ्जायते हिक्का श्वासो वा तीव्रवेदनः||७||

Serious Nature of hiccups and dyspnoea related respiratory disorders:

Agnivesha, the learned disciple with folded hands, asked Lord Punarvasu Atreya, the illustrious sage proficient in spiritual and sane knowledge, the following questions:

All diseases that are caused by Tridosha imbalance can be classified into two, the ones that can be cured and the others which are incurable. Please elaborate on the incurable diseases.

After having heard this query of Agnivesha, Lord Punarvasu, the wisest among the learned, was immensely pleased and made a decisive statement –

"It is true that there are several diseases which can kill a patient. But none of these is as deadly as asthma and hiccup that can kill a patient instantaneously. Even if the patient has been ailing with several other types of diseases, ultimately, at the time of death, he would become a victim to hiccup and difficulty to breathing that are intensely painful". [3-7]

Pathogenesis of Hikka (hiccough) and Shvasa (respiratory disorders with difficulty in breathing):

कफ वातात्मकावेतौ पित्तस्थान समुद्भवौ|
हृदयस्य रसादीनां धातूनां चोपशोषणौ||८||
तस्मात् साधारणावेतौ मतौ परमदुर्जयौ|
मिथ्योपचरितौ क्रुद्धौ हत आशीविषाविव||९||

Origin: From site of Pitta

Caused by: The simultaneous aggravation of Kapha and Vata

Afflicts: The cardiac region (hrudaya) and all the 7 Dhatus (Rasa, Rakta etc)

Curability: Difficult to cure and have common pathogenesis.

If these two diseases are not properly treated at the right time or if the patient indulges in unwholesome regimen, these diseases being exacerbated become fatal like the deadly snake-venom [8-9]

Hikka and Shvasa Bheda, Nidana:

पृथक् पञ्चविधावेतौ निर्दिष्टौ रोग सङ्ग्रहे|
तयोः शृणु समुत्थानं लिङ्गं च सभिषग्जितम्||१०||
रजसा धूमवाताभ्यां शीत स्थानाम्बु सेवनात्|
व्यायामाद्ग्राम्यधर्माध्व रूक्षान्न विषमाशनात्||११||
आम प्रदोषादानाहाद्रौक्ष्यादत्यपतर्पणात्|
दौर्बल्यान्मर्मणो घाताद्द्वन्द्वाच्छुद्ध्यतियोगतः||१२||
अतीसार ज्वर च्छर्दि प्रतिश्याय क्षतक्षयात्|
रक्त पितादुदावर्तादिवसूच्यलसकादपि||१३||
पाण्डुरोगादिविषाच्चैव प्रवर्तेते गदाविमौ|
निष्पाव माष पिण्याक तिलतैल निषेवणात्||१४||
पिष्ट शालूक विष्टम्भि विदाहि गुरुभोजनात्|
जलजानूप पिशितदध्याम क्षीर सेवनात्||१५||
अभिष्यन्द्युपचाराच्च श्लेष्मलानां च सेवनात्|
कण्ठोरसः प्रतीघातादिवबन्धैश्च पृथग्विधैः||१६||

Types and causes of Hikka and Shwasa:

Each of these 2 diseases are described in the Roga- sangraha as of 5 types.

Aetiology, signs and symptoms, and treatment (of these diseases) are being described here after.

Etiological factors:

Both Hikka – hiccups and Shwasa – respiratory disorders with difficulty in breathing are influenced by aggravated Vata and Kapha Dosha. Hence, all diet and activities that cause an increase of these two Doshas may cause the said two diseases.

Causes for Hikka and Shwasa:

Rajasa Dhooma Vatabhyam – Exposure to dust, smoke and wind

Residing in a cold place and use of cold water

Exercise, sexual intercourse and long walk beyond one's capacity

Habitual intake of dry foods

Intake of food, deficient or excessive in quantity, and before or long after the meal time

Vitiation by Ama (product of improper digestion and metabolism)

Constipation associated with flatulence (Anaha)

Roukshyat – Dryness

Apatarpanaat – Fasting in excess

Weakness and injury to vital organs (Marmas)

Use of mutually contradictory ingredients

Shuddhi Atiyoga – Excessive administration of elimination therapies;

As a secondary affliction to Diarrhoea, fever, vomiting, Pratishyaya – coryza, phthisis, Depletion of body tissues, RaktaPitta (bleeding from different parts of the body), Udavarta (upward movement of the abdominal gases), Visuchika – Cholera, Alasaka (Intestinal torpor), Pandu (anemia) and poisoning.

Habitual intake of Nishpava – pigeon pea, black gram (masha), oil cake (Pinyaka) and excess consumption of sesame oil

Intake of Pastry (Pishta), Shaluka (Rhizome of lotus),

Vishtambhi – wind / gas forming ingredients,

Vidahi (ingredients which cause burning sensation in the abdomen and chest) and heavy food.

Intake of the meat of aquatic (Jalaja) and marshy animals (Anoopa) and birds (Pishita)

Intake of excess of curds and un-boiled milk (Ama Ksheera)

Intake of Abhisyandi (ingredients which cause obstruction to the channels of circulation)

Intake of kapha- aggravation ingredients

injury to throat and chest and

Different types of obstruction to the channels of circulation.[10-16]

Hikka Shwasa Samprapti: Pathogenesis

मारुतः प्राणवाहीनि स्रोतांस्याविश्य कुप्यति।

उरःस्थः कफमुद्धूय हिक्का श्वासान् करोति सः||१७||

घोरान् प्राणोपरोधाय प्राणिनां पञ्च पञ्च च|१८|

Pathogenesis of Hikka and Shvas:

Vata Dosha located in the chest after afflicting the channels carrying vital energy (pranavaha- srotas), gets aggravated and stimulates Kapha.

This leads to the causation of these 2 deadly diseases viz, hiccup and Shvas which are of 5types each and which may lead to the death of the patient. [17 ½- 18½]

Hikka and Swasa Poorvaroopa:

उभयोः पूर्वरूपाणि शृणु वक्ष्याम्यतः परम्||१८||

कण्ठोरसोर्गुरुत्वं च वदनस्य कषायता।

हिक्कानां पूर्वरूपाणि कुक्षेराटोप एव च||१९||

आनाहः पार्श्व शूलं च पीडनं हृदयस्य च।

प्राणस्य च विलोमत्वं श्वासानां पूर्वलक्षणम्||२०||

The premonitory signs and symptoms of hiccup are as follows:

Kanta uru gurutvam – Heaviness of the chest and throat

Vadanasya kashaya – Appearance of astringent taste in the mouth and

Kukshi aatopa – Distension in the pelvic region (Kuksi)

The premonitory signs and symptoms of asthma are as follows:

Anaha – Constipation with flatulence

Parshva shulam – Pain in the sides of the chest

Hridaya pidana – Pain in the cardiac region and

Pranasya vilomatvam - Reversal (vilomatva) of the respiratory functions (Prana). [18½ – 20]

Hikka Samprapti: Specific Pathogenesis of Hikka:

प्राणोदकान्नवाहीनि स्रोतांसि सकफोऽनिलः।

हिक्काः करोति संरुध्य तासां लिङ्गं पृथक् शृणु||२१||

Vata along with Kapha, having obstructed the

1. Pranavaha Srotas – channels carrying vital breath

2. Udakavaha Srotas – channels carrying watery elements and

3. Annavaha Srotas – Anna-Vaha- Srotas – channels carrying food, causes hiccup.

The signs and symptoms of various types of hiccups will be described hereafter. [21]

A. Mahahikka – Samprapti, Lakshana:

क्षीणमांस बल प्राण तेजसः सकफोऽनिलः।

गृहीत्वा सहसा कण्ठमुच्चैर्घोषवतीं भृशम्||२२||

करोति सततं हिक्कामेकद्विवत्रिगुणं तथा।

प्राणः स्रोतांसि मर्माणि संरुध्योष्माणमेव च||२३||

सञ्ज्ञां मुष्णाति गात्राणां स्तम्भं सञ्जनयत्यपि।

मार्गं चैवान्नपानानां रुणद्ध्युपहतस्मृतेः||२४||

साश्रुविप्लुत नेत्रस्य स्तब्ध शङ्खच्युतभ्रुवः।

सक्त जल्प प्रलापस्य निर्वृतिं नाधिगच्छतः||२५||

महामूला महावेगा महाशब्दा महाबला।

महाहिक्केति सा नृणां सद्यः प्राणहरा मता||२६||

इति महाहिक्का।

Pathogenesis, Signs and Symptoms of Maha- Hikka:

Vata in association with Kapha suddenly afflicts the throat of the patient who has depleted muscle tissue, strength, Elan Vitae (Prana) and lustre. It causes hiccups with exceedingly loud as well as resonant sound. This variety of hiccup is characterized by 1, 2 or 3 bouts at time, continuously.

The Prana-vayu obstructs the channels of circulation, vital parts (marma) as well as the heart of the patient. It makes the patient unconscious, and brings about stiffness of the body. This obstructs the channels of food and drinks.

He loses memory; his eyes become full of tears, his eyebrows become displaced because of the stiffness of the temple; he gets delirium accompanied by a choked voice; and he does not get any relief whatsoever. This disease is known as Maha- Hikka.

It is exceedingly deep- rooted (Maha- mula); its attack is enormous (maha- vega); it causes the patient to produce exceedingly loud sound (Maha- shabda) and its attacks are very strong (maha- bala). It may cause death of the patient instantaneously. Thus, ends the description of Maha- Hikka. [22-26]

B. Gambhira- Hikka

हिक्कते यः प्रवृद्धस्तु कृशो दीनमना नरः।

जर्जरेणोरसा कृच्छ्रं गम्भीरमनुनादयन्||२७||

सञ्जृम्भन् सङ्क्षिपंश्चैव तथाऽङ्गानि प्रसारयन्।

पार्श्वे चोभे समायम्य कूजन् स्तम्भरुगर्दितः||२८||

नाभेः पक्वाशयाद्वाऽपि हिक्का चास्योपजायते।

क्षोभयन्ती भृशं देहं नामयन्तीव ताम्यतः||२९||

रुणद्ध्युच्छ्वासमार्गं तु प्रनष्टबलचेतसः।

गम्भीरा नाम सा तस्य हिक्का प्राणान्तिकी मता||३०||

इति गम्भीरा हिक्का।

Gambheera Hikka

The patient is usually aged, emaciated and dispirited

He frequently hiccups, and produces deep, painful and resonant sounds with his afflicted chest

He yawns, contracts and expands his body

He raises both the sides of his chest making murmuring sound, afflicted with stiffness and pain

He gets hiccup from the umbilical and gastric regions with pain all over the body

His body bends and he gets shivering

His expiration is obstructed and

There is impairment of strength and consciousness
This type of Gambhira- Hikka may cause death. [27-30]

C. Vyapeta Hikka:

व्यपेता जायते हिक्का याऽन्नपाने चतुर्विधे।
आहारपरिणामान्ते भूयश्च लभते बलम्॥३१॥
प्रलाप वम्यतीसार तृष्णार्तस्य विचेतसः।
जृम्भिणो विप्लुताक्षस्य शुष्कास्यस्य विनामिनः॥३२॥
पर्याध्मातस्य हिक्का या जत्रुमूलादसन्तता।
सा व्यपेतेति विज्ञेया हिक्का प्राणोपरोधिनी॥३३॥
इति व्यपेता हिक्का।

C. Vyapeta Hikka: Vyapeta type of hiccup is produced during the course of the intake of 4 types of food.
It gets exceedingly aggravated after the digestion of food. Its signs and symptoms are.
Pralapa – Delirium, Vamya – Vomiting,
Atisara – Diarrhoea, Trushna – Morbid thirst
Jrumbha – Yawning,
Vipluta aksha – Tearful eyes,
Suskha asya – dryness of the mouth and Vinamata - contraction of the body and
Adhmana - Flatulence all around the body
Origin: From the base of the clavicle and the attack does not continue for a long time.
This type of Hikka – hiccough is called Vyapeta, and it is injurious to life. [31-33]

D. Kshudra Hikka – Minor hiccough

क्षुद्रवातो यदा कोष्ठाद्व्यायामपरिघट्टितः।
कण्ठे प्रपद्यते हिक्कां तदा क्षुद्रां करोति सः॥३४॥
अतिदुःखा न सा चोरःशिरो मर्म प्रबाधिनी।
न चोच्छ्वासान्नपानानां मार्गमावृत्य तिष्ठति॥३५॥
वृद्धिमायास्यतो याति भुक्तमात्रे च मार्दवम्।
यतः प्रवर्तते पूर्वं तत एव निवर्तते॥३६॥
हृदयं क्लोम कण्ठं च तालुकं च समाश्रिता।
मृद्वी सा क्षुद्र हिक्केति नृणां साध्या प्रकीर्तिता॥३७॥

D. Kshudra Hikka – Minor hiccup:
When the Vayu, which is slightly aggravated in the gastrointestinal region, is pushed up by physical exercise and arrives at the throat region, it causes Kshudra- Hikka (minor type of Hiccup).
It is not very painful. It does not exceedingly afflict the chest, head or vital organs (Marma). It also does not obstruct the channels of breath, food and drinks.
It gets aggravated during the course of exertion, and it becomes milder immediately after the meals.
It subsides immediately after its onset by implication, it does not continue for a long period.
It is located in the cardiac region, Kloman (Lungs / pancreas), throat and palate in a mild form.
This is called Ksudra- Hikka – hiccough, and it is curable. [34-37]

E. Annaja Hikka

सहसाऽत्यभ्यवह्रतैः पानान्नैः पीडितोऽनिलः।
ऊर्ध्वं प्रपद्यते कोष्ठान्मद्यैर्वाऽतिमदप्रदैः॥३८॥
तथाऽतिरोषभाष्याध्व हास्य भारातिवर्तनैः।
वायुः कोष्ठगतो धावन् पान भोज्य प्रपीडितः॥३९॥

उरःस्रोतः समाविश्य कुर्यादिधक्कां ततोऽन्नजाम्|
तथा शनैर सम्बन्धं क्षुवंश्चापि स हिक्कते||४०||
न मर्मबाधाजननी नेन्द्रियाणां प्रबाधिनी|
हिक्का पीते तथा भुक्ते शमं याति च साऽन्नजा||४१||
इत्यन्नजा हिक्का|

E. Annaja Hikka

Vata gets aggravated and moves upward in the Gastro intestinal tract because of the following:

Sudden intake of drinks and food in large quantity

Intake of excessively intoxicating alcohol and

Excessive anger, speech, long walk, laughter for a long time, and carrying heavy weight.

Being pressed by the drinks and food, this aggravated Vayu located in the Gastro- Intestinal tract quickly moves up to the channels in the chest and being located there, causes hiccup of Annaja type.

The Patient hiccups slowly and interruptions even while he sneezes. It does not cause any affliction of the vital spots (Marma) and sense organs. This type of hiccup gets alleviated by the intake of drinks and food. This is called Annaja Hikka – hiccough.

Thus, ends the description of Annaja- Hikka – hiccough. [38- 41]

Yamaka Hikka – hiccough

अति सञ्चित दोषस्य भक्त च्छेद कृशस्य च|
व्याधिभिः क्षीण देहस्य वृद्धस्यातिव्यवायिनः||४२||
आसां या सा समुत्पन्ना हिक्का हन्त्याशु जीवितम्|
यमिका च प्रलापार्ति तृष्णा मोह समन्विता||४३||
अक्षीणश्चाप्यदीनश्च स्थिर धात्विन्द्रियश्च यः|
तस्य साधयितुं शक्या यमिका हन्त्यतोऽन्यथा||४४||

Nidana: If the vitiated Doshas are accumulated in excess,

If there is weakness because of want of food,

If the body is emaciated on account of diseases,

If the patient is old, and

If a person over- indulges in sex,

He is liable to be afflicted by hiccups which can cause death instantaneously.

This is called Yamika- Hikka – hiccough.

Signs and Symptoms: It is associated with

Pralapa – delirium,

Arti – pain,

Trushna – morbid thirst and

Moha – unconsciousness

Curability:

Hikka is curable if –

The patient is not emaciated (no depletion of muscle tissues),

If he has not lost his will power (mental stamina) and

If Dhatus (tissue elements) and Indriyas (senses) are not impaired,

Otherwise, it is fatal. [42- 44]

Pathogenesis of Shvasaroga:

यदा स्रोतांसि संरुध्य मारुतः कफपूर्वकः|
विष्वग्व्रजति संरुद्धस्तदा श्वासान्करोति सः||४५||

Vata predominantly associated with Kapha obstructs the channels of circulation, and circulates all over the body, gets itself obstructed in the circulatory course. This aggravated Vayu causes Shvasa. [45]

A. Maha Shvasa

उद्धूयमानवातो यः शब्दवहुःखितो नरः।
उच्चैः श्वसिति संरुद्धो मत्तर्षभ इवानिशम्॥४६॥
प्रनष्ट ज्ञान विज्ञानस्तथा विभ्रान्त लोचनः।
विकृताक्ष्याननो बद्ध मूत्र वर्चा विशीर्ण वाक्॥४७॥
दीनः प्रश्वसितं चास्य दूरादिवज्ञायते भृशम्।
महाश्वासोपसृष्टः स क्षिप्रमेव विपद्यते॥४८॥
इति महाश्वासः।

A. Mahashwasa:

Because of the upward movement of aggravated Vayu, the patient takes deep breaths associated with loud sound continuously, like an intoxicated bull, on account of obstruction to the respiratory channel.

Signs and symptoms:

Loss of physical and mental senses;

His eyes (eyeballs) become bewildered;

His eyes and face become distorted;

Anaemia and constipation;

Voice becomes feeble;

Loses mental stamina, and

His deep inspiration becomes audible even from a distance.

Curability: The patient succumbs to death instantaneously.

Thus, ends the description of Maha Shvasa. [46-48]

B. Urdhva Shvasa

दीर्घ श्वसिति यस्तूर्ध्व न च प्रत्याहरत्यधः।
श्लेष्मावृत मुखस्रोताः क्रुद्ध गन्धवहार्दितः॥४९॥
ऊर्ध्व दृष्टि विपश्यंश्च विभ्रान्ताक्ष इतस्ततः।
प्रमुह्यन् वेदनार्तश्च शुष्कास्योऽरतिपीडितः॥५०॥
ऊर्ध्वश्वासे प्रकुपिते ह्यधःश्वासो निरुध्यते।
मुह्यतस्ताम्यतश्चोर्ध्व श्वासस्तस्यैव हन्त्यसून्॥५१॥
इत्यूर्ध्वश्वासः।

B. Urdhwa Shwasa – signs and symptoms:

Dirgha shvasam – Prolonged expiration and inability to have inspiration

Sleshma Aavruta mukha srotas – Adhesion of the mouth and (breathing) channels with Phlegm

Kruddha vata – Affliction with aggravated Vayu

Urdhva Drishti – Looking with the eye- balls moved upwards.

Vibhranta aksha – Bewildered eyes

Pramuhyan – Unconsciousness

Vedana aarta – Affliction with excessive pain

Shushka aasya – Dryness of the mouth and

Dislike for everything

When the upward moving breath (expiration) is aggravated, obstruction is caused to the downward moving breath (inspiration), because of which the patient becomes unconscious with tremors in his body.

The ailment having the above mentioned signs and symptoms is called Urdhva- Shvasa, and it causes death (of the patient)

Thus, ends the description of Urdhva Shvasa. [49- 51]

C. Chinna Shvasa

यस्तु श्वसिति विच्छिन्नं सर्वप्राणेन पीडितः।
न वा श्वसिति दुःखार्तो मर्म च्छेदरुगर्दितः॥५२॥
आनाह स्वेद मूर्च्छार्तो दह्यमानेन बस्तिना।
विप्लुताक्षः परिक्षीणः श्वसन् रक्तैकलोचनः॥५३॥
विचेताः परिशुष्कास्यो विवर्णः प्रलपन्नरः।
छिन्नश्वासेन विच्छिन्नः स शीघ्रं प्रजहात्यसून्॥५४॥
इति छिन्नश्वासः।

C. Chinna Shwasa

The signs and symptoms of Chinna- Shvasa are as follows:

Shvasiti vichinnam sarva pranena piditah – Interruption of stoppage of breath on account of affliction of all the channels carrying vital air (Prana-vayu)

Dukharta – Great distress

Marma chheda – Affliction with pain as if a vital organ (Marman) is injured'

Affliction with constipation associated with flatulence (Anaha), Sveda (Sweating) and Murchha (fainting)

Basti Daha – Burning sensation in the region of the urinary bladder

Excessive tears in the eyes

Excessive emaciation

Raktaika lochana – One of the eyes becomes red while the patient struggles for breath

Mental bewilderment

Pari shushha aasya – Dryness in the mouth

Vivarna and Pralapa – Discoloration of skin and delirium and

Looseness of the joints.

The patient afflicted with Chinna-Svasa, having the above mentioned signs and symptoms succumbs to death instantaneously.

Thus, ends the description of Chinna Shvasa.

D. Tamaka Shvasa

प्रतिलोमं यदा वायुः स्रोतांसि प्रतिपद्यते।
ग्रीवां शिरश्च सङ्गृह्य श्लेष्माणं समुदीर्य च॥५५॥
करोति पीनसं तेन रुद्धो घुर्घुरुकं तथा।
अतीव तीव्रवेगं च श्वासं प्राण प्रपीडकम्॥५६॥
प्रताम्यत्यतिवेगाच्च कासते सन्निरुध्यते।
प्रमोहं कासमानश्च स गच्छति मुहुर्मुहुः॥५७॥
श्लेष्मण्यमुच्यमाने तु भृशं भवति दुःखितः।
तस्यैव च विमोक्षान्ते मुहूर्तं लभते सुखम्॥५८॥
अथास्योद्ध्वंसते कण्ठः कृच्छ्राच्छक्नोति भाषितुम्।
न चापि निद्रां लभते शयानः श्वासपीडितः॥५९॥
पार्श्वे तस्यावगृह्णाति शयानस्य समीरणः।
आसीनो लभते सौख्यमुष्णं चैवाभिनन्दति॥६०॥
उच्छ्रिताक्षो ललाटेन स्विद्यता भृशमर्तिमान्।
विशुष्कास्यो मुहुः श्वासो मुहुश्चैवावधम्यते॥६१॥
मेघाम्बुशीतप्राग्वातैः श्लेष्मलैश्चाभिवर्धते।
स याप्यस्तमकश्वासः साध्यो वा स्यान्नवोत्थितः॥६२॥
इति तमकश्वासः।

D. Tamakashwasa

Vata moving in the reverse order (direction) pervades Pranavaha Srotas – channels of vital breath, afflicts the neck and head, and stimulates phlegm to cause rhinitis.

This vayu, thus obstructed, produces the following signs and symptoms:

Ghurghuraka (wheezing or murmuring sound)

Dyspnoea of exceeding deep velocity which is immensely injurious to life

Because of acute spasms, the patient gets tremors and coughs, and becomes motionless

Pramoham – He faints again and again while coughing

Since the phlegm does not come out, he becomes very restless;

He is relieved of restlessness for some time soon after the phlegm comes out

His throat is choked because of which he is unable to speak freely

Lack of sleep. While lying down for sleep, the difficulty in breathing increases because the sides of chest in that position get afflicted by Vayu. But he is relieved of this discomfort in sitting posture.

He develops a special liking for hot things.

His eyeballs become prominent (project outside)

Excess sweating in forehead and restlessness, dry mouth

Frequent outbursts of dyspnoea and

The attack gets aggravated when clouds appear in the sky, when he is exposed to water, humidity and cloud when the easterly wind blows, and when he resorts to Kapha- aggravating food and regimes.

This disease Tamaka Shvasa is curable in early stages and generally palliable. [55-62]

Pratamaka and santamaka Shvasa

ज्वर मूर्च्छापरीतस्य विद्यात् प्रतमकं तु तम्।

उदावर्त रजोऽजीर्ण क्लिन्न काय निरोधजः||६३||

तमसा वर्धतेऽत्यर्थं शीतैश्चाशु प्रशाम्यति।

मज्जतस्तमसीवाऽस्य विद्यात् सन्तमकं तु तम्||६४||

इति प्रतमक सन्तमक श्वासौ।

Pratamaka Shwasa:

If a patient suffering from Tamaka- Shvasa gets afflicted with fever and fainting, then the condition is called Pratamaka. This is caused by Udavarta – bloating (upward movement of Vayu in the abdomen), dust, indigestion, Humidity (Kleda) and suppression of the natural urges (Vega- nirodha) it gets aggravated in darkness (at night) and gets alleviated instantaneously by cooling regimens.

Santamaka Shwasa:

If such a patient feels as if he is submerged in darkness, then this condition is called Santamaka.

Thus, ends the description of Pratamaka and Santamaka types of Shvasa. [63-64]

E. Kshudra Shvasa

रूक्षायासोद्भवः कोष्ठे क्षुद्रो वात उदीरयन्।

क्षुद्रश्वासो न सोऽत्यर्थं दुःखेनाङ्ग प्रबाधकः||६५||

हिनस्ति न स गात्राणि न च दुःखो यथेतरे।

न च भोजनपानानां निरुणद्ध्युचितां गतिम्||६६||

नेन्द्रियाणां व्यथां नापि काञ्चिदापादयेदृजम्।

स साध्य उक्तो बलिनः सर्वे चाव्यक्त लक्षणाः||६७||

इति श्वासाः समुद्दिष्टा हिक्काश्चैव स्वलक्षणैः|६८|

E. Kshudra Shvasa

Vayu, mildly aggravated in the Kostha (gastrointestinal tract) on account of exertion and dry food and regimen, causes Kshudra- Shvasa (mild dyspnoea). It does not cause much discomfort in the body.

The body is not excessively afflicted thereby. It is not as painful as other forms of Shvasa (asthma). It does not obstruct the proper movement of food and drinks. It does not cause any pain or complication in the sense organs. This variety of dyspnoea is curable

All the other varieties of Shvasa (asthma) can also be cured if their signs and symptoms are not fully manifested and if the patient is strong (physically and mentally).

Thus, all the varieties of Shvasa (asthma) and Hikka – hiccough (hiccup) are explained along with their signs and symptoms. [65- 68½]

Prognosis

एषां प्राणहरा वर्ज्या घोरास्ते ह्याशुकारिणः||६८||

भेषजैः साध्ययाप्यांस्तु क्षिप्रं भिषगुपाचरेत्|

उपेक्षिता दहेयुर्हि शुष्कं कक्षमिवानलः||६९||

Patients suffering from the varieties of asthma which are fatal because of their serious nature (ghora) and because of their acuteness (Ashukarin) are not treated.

On the other hand, the curable and palliable varieties of asthma should be treated with due care by medicines without loss of any time. For if ignored (in the beginning) even they can cause death, like fire spreading and burning out dry grass [68 ½ – 69]

Chikitsa Sutra: Line of treatment:

कारण स्थान मूलैक्यादेकमेव चिकित्सितम्|

द्वयोरपि यथा दृष्टमृषिभिस्तन्निबोधत||७०||

हिक्का श्वासार्दितं स्निग्धैरादौ स्वेदैरुपाचरेत्|

आक्तं लवणतैलेन नाडीप्रस्तरसङ्करैः||७१||

तैरस्य ग्रथितः श्लेष्मा स्रोतःस्वभिविलीयते|

खानि मार्दवमायान्ति ततो वातानुलोमता||७२||

यथाऽद्रिकुञ्जेष्वर्काशुतप्तं विष्यन्दते हिमम्|

श्लेष्मा तप्तः स्थिरो देहे स्वेदैर्विष्यन्दते तथा||७३||

स्विन्नं ज्ञात्वा ततस्तूर्णं भोजयेत् स्निग्धमोदनम्|

मत्स्यानां शूकराणां वा रसैर्दध्युत्तरेण वा||७४||

ततः श्लेष्मणि संवृद्धे वमनं पाययेत् तम्|

पिप्पली सैन्धव क्षौद्रैर्युक्तं वाताविरोधि यत्||७५||

निर्हृते सुखमाप्नोति स कफे दुष्टविग्रहे|

स्रोतःसु च विशुद्धेषु चरत्यविहतोऽनिलः||७६||

Line of treatment

The sages, on the basis of their experience, have prescribed the same line of treatment for both hiccup and Shwasa. This is because of the similarity in causative factors, location of pathology, Doshas involved and similar pathogenesis. Now, the details of their line of treatment are explained.

The physician should treat the patient afflicted with hiccup and Asthma, in the beginning, with –

Snigdha Sweda – unctuous fomentation therapies like Nadi- Sveda, Prastara- Sveda, after anointing the body with oil, mixed with salt. This Snigdha Sweda dissolves knotted and granular Kapha. It makes sticky Kapha to detach from the respiratory channels (Pranavaha Srotas). It softens channels and causes normal movement of Vata Dosha by relieving obstruction.

Just like the snow accumulated on the peak melts when hot sun rays fall over it the kapha too which has been accumulated in the body gets melted / dissolved on account of the heat generated by sudation therapies.

After ascertaining that the patient is properly fomented, the patient should be given rice mixed with ghee, or soup of the fish or pork, followed by the cream of curd (Dadhi sara) to eat.

This causes aggravation (excitation, exacerbation) of Kapha Dosha. The patient is then given the emetic therapy, mixed with Pippali – long pepper, Saindhava – rock salt and honey. Care is taken that no Vata- aggravating ingredients are added to the recipe.

The patient gets relief after the vitiated Kapha is eliminated. When the channels of circulation are made clear (free from impediments) then Vayu moves in the channels at ease without any obstruction. [70-76]

Dhumapana – Smoking- therapy:

लीनश्चेद्दोषशेषः स्याद्धूमैस्तं निर्हरेद्बुधः|
हरिद्रां पत्रमेरण्डमूलं लाक्षां मनःशिलाम्||७७||
सदेवदारुवलं मांसीं पिष्ट्वा वर्तिं प्रकल्पयेत्|
तां घृताक्तां पिबेद्धूमं यवैर्वा घृतसंयुतैः||८७||
मधूच्छिष्टं सर्जरसं घृतं मल्लक सम्पुटे|
कृत्वा धूमं पिबेच्छृङ्गं बालं वा स्नायु वा गवाम्||७९||
स्योनाक वर्धमानानां नाडीं शुष्कां कुशस्य वा|
पद्मकं गुग्गुलं लोहं शल्लकीं वा घृताप्लुतम्||८०||

Dhumapana – Smoking- therapy:

In spite of Snehana, Swedana and Vamana treatments, if the residual Doshas still remains adhered to (inside) the channels, they are eliminated by the administration of Dhumapana (smoking therapy).

For this purpose, a Varti (cigarette or elongated pill) should be prepared with the paste of turmeric, Patra, castor root, Laksha – Laccifer lacca, Manahsila, Devadaru—Cedrus deodara, Ala (Haritala) and Jatamamsi. This cigarette (elongated pill) is smeared with ghee, and used for smoking. Alternatively, barley mixed with ghee can also be used for the smoking therapy.

Other recipes of smoking therapy which are also useful in these conditions are as follows:

Bee's wax and sarja- Rasa (Gum resin from the tree called Sarja) mixed with ghee is covered all around with arsenic (Malla) and kept inside two earthen plates. The fume which comes out of it by application of the heat by fire below is used for smoking.

Inside the above-mentioned Sarava- Samputa (two earthen plates), the horn, hair and sinew of cattle can be mixed with ghee and kept, surrounded by Malla. The fume which comes out by the application of the heat of fire can be used for this smoking

Padmaka, Guggulu, Aguru (Loha) and Sallaki may similarly be added with ghee, surrounded by Tala and kept inside the Sarava- Samputa. The fume which comes out of it by the application of heat below may be used in this smoking therapy.

The dried tender stems of Shyonaka – Oroxylum indicum, castor – Ricinus communis and Kusha grass – Desmostachya pinnata are used as a pipe to enable the patient to smoke the fume of the above-mentioned recipes placed inside the Sharava Samputa. [77-80]

Therapies to treat complications of Hikka and Shwasaroga:

स्वर क्षीणातिसारास्रृक्पित्त दाहानुबन्धजान्|
मधुर स्निग्ध शीताद्यैर्हिक्का श्वासानुपाचरेत्||८१||

If hiccup and asthma are associated with

Svara-Kshaya (thin voice or inability to speak),

Atisara – Diarrhoea,

Rakta Pitta (a disease characterised by bleeding from different parts of the body) and

Daha – burning sensation, then the patient is treated with ingredients which are sweet, unctuous, cooling etc. [81]

Patients Unsuitable for Fomentation Therapy:

न स्वेद्याः पित्तदाहार्ता रक्तस्वेदातिवर्तिनः|

क्षीणधातुबला रूक्षा गर्भिण्यश्चापि पित्तलाः||८२||

Patient afflicted with the following ailments are unsuitable for fomentation therapy

Daha – Burning sensation

Pitta roga – Diseases caused by Pitta

Ati rakta srava – Excessive bleeding

Ati sweda – Excessive sweating

Kshina dhatu bala – Feebleness of tissue element

Ruksha – Dryness in excess and

Garbhini – Pregnant woman and the patient who is of Pitta- Prakrti (Paittika constitution). [82]

Alternate Fomentation Therapy for Unsuitable Patients

कोष्णैः काममुरःकण्ठं स्नेहसेकैः सशर्करैः|

उत्कारिकोपनाहैश्च स्वेदयेन् मृदुभिः क्षणम्||८३||

तिलोमामाषगोधूमचूर्णैर्वातहरैः सह|

स्नेहैश्चोत्कारिका साम्लैः सक्षीरैर्वा कृता हिता||८४||

Depending upon the description of physician, such patients could be given mild fomentation therapy, for a moment, in their chest and neck by sprinkling luke-warm oil (Sneha) mixed with sugar and thereafter, by applying Upanaha with Utkarika (recipe for fomentation which is warm and which is in paste form).

Utkarika (poultice) prepared with the powders of Vayu- alleviating ingredients like Tila – Sesamum indicum, Uma – Linseed and black gram, mixed with oil, and cooked with sour drugs or milk is useful for this type of fomentation. [83-84]

Management of Complications

नव ज्वरामदोषेषु रूक्ष स्वेदं विलङ्घनम्|

समीक्ष्योल्लेखनं वाऽपि कारयेल्लवणाम्बुना||८५||

अतियोगोद्धतं वातं दृष्ट्वा वातहरै भिषक्|

रसाद्यैर्नाति शीतोष्णैरभ्यङ्गैश्च शमं नयेत्||८६||

उदावर्ते तथाऽऽध्माने मातुलुङ्गाम्लवेतसैः|

हिङ्गु पीलु बिडैश्चान्नं युक्तं स्यादनुलोमनम्||८७||

If the patient of hiccup and asthma suffers from fever (occurred recently) or Ama Dosha (ailments caused by Ama or uncooked products of food), then Rooksha Sweda (Dry type of fomentation) and fasting therapy – Langhana are administered.

After proper examination, such patients may also be given Vamana by administering saline water.

If Vata is increased due to excess Vamana treatment, then juice (decoction) of Vayu- alleviating herbs or massage with such ingredients as are neither very cold nor very hot (i.e., Luke warm) is administered.

If the patient suffers from

Udavarta – bloating (upward movement of Vayu) or

Adhmana (flatulence), then he is given food along with

Matulunga – Citrus medica,

Amla-Vetasa – Garcinia pedunculata

Hingu – Asafoetida

Pilu and

Bida salt

This type of food helps in the downward movement (Anulomana) of Vayu. [85-87]

Management of 4 Different Conditions of Patients

हिक्का श्वासामयी ह्येको बलवान् दुर्बलोऽपरः|

कफाधिकस्तथैवैको रूक्षो बह्वनिलोऽपरः||८८||
ककाधिके बलस्थे च वमनं सविरेचनम्|
कुर्यात् पथ्याशिने धूमलेहादिशमनं ततः||८९||
वातिकान् दुर्बलान् बालान् वृद्धांश्चानिलसूदनैः|
तर्पयेदेव शमनैः स्नेहयूषरसादिभिः||९०||

Patients suffering from hiccup and asthma are of 4 categories as follows:

Balavan – Strong

Durbala – weak

Kapha adhikyata -Kapha is Predominant

Vata adhikyata – Vata Dosha is predominant, and who are dry.

If Kapha is predominant and the patient has strength, then he is given wholesome food, Vamana and Virechana treatments, along with Dhumapana and Avaleha.

If Vata is aggravated, if the patient is weak, and if the patient is either an infant or old, then he or she is administered Vayu- alleviating medicines and nourishing recipes prepared of ghee (fat), Vegetable soup and meat soup. [88-99]

Contraindications for Panchakarma treatment:

अनुत्क्लिष्ट कफास्विन्न दुर्बलानां विशोधनात्|
वायुर्लब्धास्पदो मर्म संशोष्याश्च हरेदसून्||९१||
दृढान् बहुकफांस्तस्माद्रसैरानूपवारिजैः|
तृप्तान्विशोधयेत्स्विन्नान् बृंहयेदितरान् भिषक्||९२||
बर्हि तित्तिरि दक्षाश्च जाङ्गलाश्च मृगद्विजाः|
दशमूली रसे सिद्धाः कौलत्थे वा रसे हिताः||९३||

If Shodhan therapy is administered to a patient whose Kapha is not loosened, who is not administered fomentation therapy and who is weak, the aggravated Vayu gets lodged in the vital spots (marma) like heart etc. and causes dryness, leading to instantaneous death. Therefore, for a patient who is strong and who has aggravated Kapha, a wise physician should, first of all, administer fomentation therapy followed by the intake of soup of birds and animals living in marshy land (Anupa) and water (Varija).

This creates a sense of satisfaction (Trupti) when this is administered to such patients.

If, however, the patient has aggravated Vayu, and if he is weak, then nourishing therapy is administered.

For this purpose, the meat of peacock, Tittiri (partridge), cock, and birds and animals inhabiting arid zone boiled with the decoction of Dasha-Mula or the soup of Kulattha is useful. [91-93]

Soups and drinks for Hiccup and Asthma

निदिग्धिकां बिल्व मध्यं कर्कटाख्यां दुरालभाम्|
त्रिकण्टकं गुडूची च कुलत्थांश्च सचित्रकान्||९४||
जले पक्त्वा रसः पूतः पिप्पलीघृतभर्जितः|
सनागरः सलवणः स्याद्यूषो भोजने हितः||९५||
रास्नां बलां पञ्चमूलं ह्रस्वं मुद्गान् सचित्रकान्|
पक्त्वाऽम्भसि रसे तस्मिन् यूषः साध्यश्च पूर्ववत्||९६||
पल्लवान्मातुलुङ्गस्य निम्बस्य कुलकस्य च|
पक्त्वा मुद्गांश्च सव्योषान् क्षारयूषं विपाचयेत्||९७||
दत्त्वा सलवणं क्षारं शिग्रूणि मरिचानि च|
युक्त्या संसाधितो यूषो हिक्का श्वास विकारनुत्||९८||
कासमर्दकपत्राणां यूषः शोभाञ्जनस्य च|
शुष्कमूलकयूषश्च हिक्काश्वासनिवारणः||९९||
सदधि व्योष सर्पिष्को यूषो वार्ताकजो हितः|

Nidigdhika, the pulp of (unripe) bael, Karkata, Duralabha – Fagonia cretica Trikantaka – Tribulus, Guduchi – Tinospora cordifolia, horse gram and Chitraka – Plumbago zeylanica is boiled by adding water, and the liquid is filtered.

This liquid (decoction) is sizzled with Pippali – Piper nigrum and ghee. Intake of this soup, by adding the powder of ginger and salt during meals is useful (for curing asthma and hiccups).

Rasna – Alpinia galanga, Bala – country mallow, Salaparni – Desmodium gangeticum, Prisni Parni – Uraria picta, Kantakari – Solanum xantocarpum, Goksura – Tribulus terrestris, Mudga – green gram and Chitraka – Plumbago zeylanica is boiled by adding water and the decoction is prepared. Soup of this decoction is prepared as mentioned above and given to the patient (suffering from hiccup and asthma).

Tender leaves of Matulunga – Citrus medica, neem and Kulaka are mixed with Mudga – green gram and boiled by adding water. To this decoction, salt, Kshara, Shigru – Moringa oleifera and black pepper is cooked according to the prescribed appropriate quantity and the prescribed procedure. Intake of this alkaline soup (Ksara- Yusha) cures hiccup and Asthma.

The soup of the leaves of Kasamarda – Cassia occidentalis or Shobhanjana or dry- radish cures hiccup and Asthma.

Similarly, the soup of Vartaka prepared along with curd, ginger, long pepper and black pepper and ghee is useful (in curing hiccup and Asthma) [94½ - 100]

Diet and Yavagu for Hiccup and Asthma

शालि षष्टिक गोधूम यवान्नान्यनवानि च||१००||

हिङ्गु सौवर्चलाजाजी बिड पौष्कर चित्रकैः|

सिद्धा कर्कटशृङ्ग्या च यवागूः श्वास हिक्किनाम्||१०१||

दशमूली शटी रास्ना पिप्पलीमूल पौष्करैः|

शृङ्गी तामलकी भार्गी गुडूची नागराम्बुभिः||१०२||

यवागूं विधिना सिद्धां कषायं वा पिबेन्नरः|

कास हृद्ग्रहपार्श्वार्ति हिक्का श्वास प्रशान्तये||१०३||

पुष्कराह्व शटी व्योष मातुलुङ्गाम्लवेतसैः|

योजयेदन्नपानानि ससर्पिर्बिड हिङ्गुभिः||१०४||

The patient suffering from hiccup and Asthma should take food prepared of old Shali, Old Wheat or old barley.

The Yavagu (thick gruel) prepared by boiling with Hingu, Sauvarcala, Ajaji, Vida, Pauskara, Chitraka – Plumbago zeylanica and Karkata-Srngi – Rhus succedanea is useful for the patient suffering from hiccup and Asthma.

Intake of the Yavagu prepared with the decoction of Dashamula, Shati – Hedychium spicatum, Rasna – Alpinia galanga, Pippali- Mula – Piper nigrum, Puskaramula – Inula racemosa, Srngi, Tamalaki – Phyllanthus niruri, Bhargi, Guduchi – Tinospora cordifolia and nagara – Zingiber officinale is useful.

It is useful in

Kasa – cough / bronchitis,

Hrud roga -heart diseases,

Parshva shula – pain in the sides of the chest,

Hikka – hiccup and

Shvasa – asthma

Intake of the decoction alone of these drugs is also useful in the above-mentioned diseases.

Food and drinks of the patient suffering from hiccup and Asthma is given

Puskara (Puskara- Mula) – Inula racemosa

Shati – Hedychium spicatum

Sunthi—Zingiber officinale

Pippali – Piper longum

Maricha – Piper nigrum

Matulanga – Citrus medica and

Amlavetasa – Garcinia pedunculata along with Ghee, Vida and Hingu [½ 100- 104]

Drinks for Hiccup and Asthma

दशमूलस्य वा क्वाथमथवा देवदारुणः|
तृषितो मदिरां वाऽपि हिक्काश्वासी पिबेन्नरः||१०५||
पाठां मधुरसां रास्नां सरलं देवदारु च|
प्रक्षाल्य जर्जरीकृत्य सुरामण्डे निधापयेत्||१०६||
तं मन्दलवणं कृत्वा भिषक् प्रसृतसम्मितम्|
पाययेत्तु ततो हिक्का श्वासश्चैवोपशाम्यति||१०७||
हिङ्गु सौवर्चलं कोलं समङ्गां पिप्पलीं बलाम्|
मातुलुङ्गरसे पिष्टमारनालेन वा पिबेत्||१०८||
सौवर्चलं नागरं च भार्गीं द्विशर्करायुतम्|
उष्णाम्बुना पिबेदेतद्धिक्काश्वासविकारनुत्||१०९||
भार्गीनागरयोः कल्कं मरिचक्षारयोस्तथा|
पीतद्रुचित्रकास्फोतामूर्वाणां चाम्बुना पिबेत्||११०||
मधूलिका तुगाक्षीरी नागरं पिप्पली तथा|
उत्कारिका घृते सिद्धा श्वासे पित्तानुबन्धजे||१११||
श्वाविधं शशमांसं च शल्लकस्य च शोणितम्|
पिप्पलीघृत सिद्धानि श्वासे वातानुबन्धजे||११२||
सुवर्चलारसो दुग्धं घृतं त्रिकटुकान्वितम्|
शाल्योदनस्यानुपानं वातपित्तानुगे हितम्||११३||
शिरीषपुष्प स्वरसः सप्तपर्णस्य वा पुनः|
पिप्पलीमधुसंयुक्तः कफपित्तानुगे मतः||११४||
मधुकं पिप्पलीमूलं गुडो गोश्वशकृद्रसः|
घृतं क्षौद्रं कास श्वास हिक्काभिष्यन्दिनां शुभम्||११५||
खराश्वोष्ट्रवराहाणां मेषस्य च गजस्य च|
शकृद्रसं बहुकफे चैकैकं मधुना पिबेत्||११६||

If the patient suffering from hiccups and asthma is thirsty, then he should take (drink) the decoction of either Dasha-mula or Devadaru – Cedrus deodara. He may also drink Madira (a type of alcoholic drink).

The physician should wash and crush

Patha – Cyclea peltata,Madhurasa, Rasna – Alpinia galanga,

Sarala and Devadaru – Cedrus deodara and put these ingredients in Sura manda (a type of Alchoholic drink).

To this drink, a small quantity of salt is added and given to the patient to drink .The recipe so prepared cures hiccup and asthma.

Hingu, Sauvarcala, Kola, Samanga, Pippali – Piper longum and Bala – Abution indicum is made to a paste by triturating them with the juice of Matulunga –Citrus medica. This paste is mixed with Aranala (a type of sour drink). Intake of this drink cures hiccup and asthma.

Sauvarcala, Nagara – Zingiber officinale and Bhargi are added with double the quantity of sugar. Intake of this potion along with warm water cures hiccups and Asthma.

The paste of Bhargi or Maricha – Piper longum and Ksara (alkali preparation), or Pitadru, Chitraka – Plumbago zeylanica, Asphota and Murva – Marsedenia tenacissima is mixed with warm water and given as a drink (to the patient suffering from hiccup and Asthma).

Utkarika (a preparation in paste form) is prepared of Madhulika, Tuga-Ksiri, Nagara – Zingiber officinale and Pippali – Piper longum by cooking with ghee. Intake of this recipe is useful when Asthma is caused by the association (Anubandha) of Pitta.

The meat of (Svavit Sallaka) rabbit or the blood of Sallaka is cooked with Pippali Ghruta. This recipe is useful when asthma is caused by the association (Anubandha) of Vayu.

The juice prepared with Sauvarchala – black salt, milk or ghee is mixed with the powder of Trikatu (pepper, long pepper and ginger). Intake of this as post prandial drink (Anupana) after taking the boiled Shali- rice is useful for the patient suffering from Asthma caused by the association (Anubandha) of Vata and Pitta.

Intake of the Juice of the flower of Shirisha – Albizia lebbeck or Sapta Parna – Alstonia scholaris along with Pippali – Piper longum and honey is useful for the patient suffering from Asthma caused in association (Anubhandha) of Kapha and Pitta.

Intake of liquid prepared of Madhuka – Madhuca longifolia, Pippalimula – Piper longum, Jaggery, the juice of the dung of cow and horse, ghee and honey.

It is useful for the patient suffering from

Kasa – bronchitis,

Shvasa – Asthma,

Hikka – Hiccup and

Abhisyanda (name of one of the eye- diseases i.e. conjunctivitis; but in the present context, it refers to the obstruction of the channels of circulation by Ama)

If Kapha is aggravated in excess, the juice of the dungs of an ass, horse, camel, pig, sheep or elephant is given to the patient mixed with honey. [105-106]

Recipes of Linctus for Hiccup and Asthma

क्षारं चाप्यश्वगन्धाया लिह्यान्ना क्षौद्र सर्पिषा।
मयूरपादनालं वा शकलं शल्लकस्य वा||११७||
श्वाविज्जाण्डकचाषाणां रोमाणि कुररस्य वा।
शृङ्ग्येकद्विशफानां वा चर्मास्थीनि खुरांस्तथा||११८||
सर्वाण्येकैकशो वाऽपि दग्ध्वा क्षौद्रघृतान्वितम्।
चूर्ण लीढ्वा जयेत् कासं हिक्कां श्वासं च दारुणम्||११९||
एते हि कफसंरुद्धगतिप्राणप्रकोपजाः |
तस्मात्तन्मार्गशुद्ध्यर्थं देया लेहा न निष्कफे||१२०||

Intake of the Alkali- Preparation of Asvagandha – Withania somnifera along with honey and ghee, in linctus (Lehya) form is useful for the patients suffering from hiccup and asthma.

The stalk of Peacock feather, the quills of Sallaka, hair of Svavit, jandaka, Casa or Kurara, Skin, Bones and Hooves of horned animals, animals having one hoof or two hooves, all of these separately or together is reduced to ashes by burning.

Intake of these powders in the form of linctus by adding honey and ghee cures bronchitis, hiccup and serious types of asthma.

The above mentioned diseases (Viz, bronchitis, hiccup and asthma) are caused by aggravation of Prana- Vayu because of the obstruction to its path by Kapha. Therefore, to cleanse the channel (of Prana- vayu by alleviating Kapha), these recipes of linctus should be administered.

If however, Kapha is not involved in the causation of the diseases, then the above-mentioned recipes of linctus should be administered. [117- 120]

PanchaKarma Therapy – choice of Vamana and Virechana:

कासिने च्छर्दनं दद्यात् स्वरभङ्गे च बुद्धिमान्।
वातश्लेष्महरैर्युक्तं तमके तु विरेचनम्||१२१||
उदीर्यते भृशतरं मार्गरोधाद्वहज्जलम्।
यथा तथाऽनिलस्तस्य मार्गं नित्यं विशोधयेत्||१२२|| ·

If the patient suffering from hiccups and asthma gets afflicted with Kasa – bronchitis, Svara bheda – hoarseness of voice, then they are given emetic therapy by a wise physician.

Patients suffering from Tamaka Shwasa (Asthma) are given purgation therapy. – Tamake Tu Virechanam.

The ingredients for emetic and purgative therapies should have qualities to alleviate Vayu and Kapha.

If the flowing of a river is obstructed on its way, then the level of water rises further. Similarly, if the channels carrying mobile Vayu (in the chest) get obstructed, then the Vayu located at the point of obstruction gets very much aggravated. Therefore, the channels of Vayu should always be cleansed [by the elimination of obstructing Doshas]. [121-122]

Shatyadi Churna

शटी चोरक जीवन्ती त्वङ्मुस्तं पुष्कराह्वयम्|
सुरसं तामलक्येला पिप्पल्यगुरु नागरम्||१२३||
वालकं च समं चूर्णं कृत्वाऽष्टगुणशर्करम्|
सर्वथा तमके श्वासे हिक्कायां च प्रयोजयेत्||१२४||

Shati – Hedychium spicatum, Choraka, Jivanti- Leptadenia reticulata, Tvak, Musta – Cyperus rotundus, Puskaramula – Inula racemosa, Surasa, Tamalaki – Phyllanthus niruri, Ela – Elettaria cardamomum ,Pippali – Piper longum, Aguru – Aquilaria agallocha and Balaka is taken in equal quantities and made to a powder.

To this powder, 8 parts of sugar is added. This recipe is always administered to the patient suffering from Tamaka –Shvasa (Asthma) and hiccup. [123- 124]

Muktadi Churna

मुक्ता प्रवाल वैदूर्य शङ्ख स्फटिकमञ्जनम्|
ससारगन्धकाचार्कसूक्ष्मैलालवणद्वयम्||१२५||
ताम्रायोरजसी रूप्यं ससौगन्धिक सीसकम्|
जातीफलं शणाद्बीजमपामार्गस्य तण्डुलाः||१२६||
एषां पाणितलं चूर्णं तुल्यानां क्षौद्रसर्पिषा|
हिक्कां श्वासं च कासं च लीढमाशु नियच्छति||१२७||
अञ्जनातिमिरं काचं नीलिकां पुष्पकं तमः|
मल्यं कण्डूमभिष्यन्दमर्म चैव प्रणाशयेत्||१२८||
इति मुक्ताद्यं चूर्णम्|

Muktadya Churna

1 pani-tala of the powder of each of

Mukta – pearl

Pravala – coral

Vaidurya

Sankha – conch

Anjana,

Sasara-gandha (red variety of saindhava-Lavana),

Tamra-bhasma – calx of copper

Lauha- Bhasma – calx of Iron

Raupya- Bhasma,

Gandhaka,

Naga- Bhasma

Jatiphala – Myristica fragrans

Seeds of Sana and

Dehusked seeds of Apamarga – Achyranthes aspera are mixed with honey and ghee in equal quantities. Intake of this linctus instantaneously cures hiccup and asthma.

Application of this recipe in the form of collyrium cures

Timira,

Kaca,
Nikika,
Puspaka,
Tamas,
Malya,
Kandu,
Abhisyanda and Arma
Thus, ends the description of Muktadya-Churna [125- 128]

Recipes for Inhalation Therapy etc

शटी पुष्करमूलानां चूर्णमामलकस्य च|
मधुना संयुतं लेह्यं चूर्णं वा काललोहजम्||१२९||
सशर्करां तामलकीं द्राक्षां गोश्वशकृद्रसम्|
तुल्यं गुडं नागरं च प्राशयेन्नावयेत्तथा||१३०||
लशुनस्य पलाण्डोर्वा मूलं गृञ्जनकस्य वा|
नावयेच्चन्दनं वाऽपि नारीक्षीरेण संयुतम्||१३१||
सुखोष्णं घृतमण्डं वा सैन्धवेनावचूर्णितम्|
नावयेन्माक्षिकीं विष्ठामलक्तकरसेन वा||१३२||
नारीक्षीरेण सिद्धं वा सर्पिर्मधुरकैरपि|
पीतं नस्तो निषिक्तं वा सद्यो हिक्कां नियच्छति||१३३||
सकृदुष्णं सकृच्छीतं व्यत्यासादिद्धिक्किनां पयः|
पाने नस्तःक्रियायां वा शर्करा मधुसंयुतम्||१३४||

The powders of – Hedychium spicatum and Puskara- Mula – Inula racemosa or Amalaki – Phyllanthus emblica or Kala-loha is made to a linctus and taken by the patient suffering from hiccup and Asthma.

Tamalaki – Phyllanthus niruri, Draksa – Vitis vinifera and the juice of the dung of a cow and a horse mixed with sugar is given to the patient suffering from hiccup and Asthma.

It can be taken as linctus or to be used for the purpose of inhalation therapy. Similarly, Jaggery and ginger, taken in equal quantities can be used for the same purpose.

Mixed with the breast milk of a woman, garlic, onion, root of grnjanaka or Chandana – Santalum album can be administered as inhalation therapy to a patient suffering from hiccup and asthma.

Lukewarm ghrita Manda (scum of ghee) sprinkled with the powder of rock salt may similarly be used for inhalation therapy.

The stool of flies mixed with the juice of Alaktaka, or cooked by adding woman's breast milk or added with ghee medicated by boiling with drugs having sweet taste (belonging to Jivaniya group) can be given as a drink, or for inhalation therapy which instantaneously cures hiccup.

Alternately, hot and cool milk mixed with sugar and honey is administered as a drink or for inhalation therapy to the patient suffering from hiccup. [129-134]

Recipes for hiccup:

अधोभागैर्घृतं सिद्धं सद्यो हिक्कां नियच्छति|
पिप्पलीमधुयुक्तौ वा रसौ धात्री कपित्थयोः||१३५||
लाजा लाक्षा मधु द्राक्षा पिप्पल्यश्वशकृद्रसान्|
लिह्यात् कोल मधु द्राक्षा पिप्पली नागराणि वा||१३६||

Administration of the medicated ghee prepared by boiling purgative drugs instantaneously cures hiccup

Similarly, the linctus prepared of Laja, Laksa, Madhu, draksa – Vitis vinifera, Pippali – Piper longum and the juice of the dung of a horse, or of Kola, Madhu, Draksa, Pippali and Nagara – Zingiber officinale cures hiccup. [135-136]

Regimen to Avert Attacks of Hiccup

शीताम्बुसेकः सहसा त्रासो विस्मापनं भयम्|
क्रोध हर्ष प्रियोद्वेगा हिक्का प्रच्यावना मताः||१३७||

Subjecting the patient to sudden sprinkling of cold water, intimidation, distraction of memory and fear, and exposing him to anger, exhalation, love or anxiety averts the attack of hiccup. [137]

Avoiding the etiological factors

हिक्का श्वास विकाराणां निदानं यत् प्रकीर्तितम्|
वर्ज्यमारोग्यकामैस्तदिद्धिक्काश्वासविकारिभिः||१३८||

The etiological factors described to be responsible for the manifestation of hiccups and asthma should be kept away by the patients suffering from these diseases, if they want (to enjoy) good health. [138]

Administration of medicated Ghee

हिक्का श्वासानुबन्धा ये शुष्कोरःकण्ठतालुकाः|
प्रकृत्या रूक्ष देहाश्च सर्पिर्भिस्तानुपाचरेत्||१३९||

If the patient suffering from hiccup and asthma has the association (Anubandha) of Sushka uru, Kanta talu -dryness of the chest, throat and palate, and if he has dryness of the body by nature (Prakrti) then he is given recipes of medicated ghee. [139]

Dashamuladya Ghrita:

दशमूल रसे सर्पि र्दधिमण्डे च साधयेत्|
कृष्णा सौवर्चल क्षार वयःस्थाहिङ्गुचोरकैः||१४०||
कायस्थया च तत् पानादिद्धिक्काश्वासौ प्रणाशयेत्|१४१|

Intake of the ghee boiled by adding the decoction of

Dashamula – group of 10 roots

Dadhi manda (Mastu)

Krishna,

Sauvarcala,

Vayashtha (Brahmi) – Bacopa monnieri

Hingu

Choraka – Angelica glauca and

Kayastha (Surasa) cures Hiccup and asthma. [140- 141½]

Tejovatyadi Ghrta:

तेजोवत्यभया कुष्ठं पिप्पली कटुरोहिणी||१४१||
भूतीकं पौष्करं मूलं पलाशश्चित्रकः शटी|
सौवर्चलं तामलकी सैन्धवं बिल्व पेशिका||१४२||
तालीस पत्रं जीवन्ती वचा तैरक्षसम्मितैः|
हिङ्गु पादै घृतप्रस्थं पचेतोये चतुर्गुणे||१४३||
एतद्यथाबलं पीत्वा हिक्का श्वासौ जयेन्नरः|
शोथानिलार्शो ग्रहणी हृत्पार्श्वरुज एव च||१४४||
इति तेजोवत्यादिघृतम्|

1 Prastha of ghee is cooked by adding 4 Prastha of

Pippali – Piper longum

Katurohini – Picrorhiza kurroa

Bhutika

Pushkaramula – Inula racemosa

Palasha – Butea monosperma

Chitraka – Plumbago zeylanica

Shati – Hedychium spicatum

Sauvarcala – A kind of salt

Tamalaki – Phyllanthus niruri

Saindhava

Pulp of (unripe) Bilva – Aegle marmelos

Talisa-Patra,

Jivanti – Leptadenia reticulata and

Vacha – Acorus calamus and

1/4th Aksa of Hingu -asa foetida

Intake of this medicated ghee in a dose appropriate to the power of digestion cures

Hikka – hiccup,

Shvasa – asthma,

Shotha – oedema,

Vatika type of Arshas (piles),

Grahani – Malabsorption syndrome, Irritable Bowel Syndrome (sprue syndrome),

Hrud roga – heart- diseases and

Parshva pida – pain in the chest

Thus, ends the description of Tejovatyadi- ghrta. [141 ½- 144]

Manahsiladi- Ghrita

मनःशिला सर्ज रस लाक्षा रजनि पद्मकैः।

मञ्जिष्ठैलैश्च कर्षांशैः प्रस्थः सिद्धो घृतादि्धतः॥१४५॥

जीवनीयोपसिद्धं वा सक्षौद्रं लेहयेद्घृतम्।

त्र्यूषणं दाधिकं वाऽपि पिबेद्वासाघृतं तथा॥१४६॥

इति मनःशिलादिघृतम्।

1 Prastha of ghee is cooked by adding karsha of each of Manahsila

Sarjarasa, Rajani – turmeric, Padmaka – Prunus cerasoides, Manjistha – Rubia cordifolia and Ela

Intake of this medicated ghee is useful in hiccup and asthma.

Similarly, ghee cooked by adding drugs belonging to Jivaniya- group (vide Sutra 4: 9) is taken along with honey.

Patient suffering from hiccup and asthma may also take Tryusana- Ghrta (vide Cikitsa 18: 39-42), Dadhika- Ghrta (vide Hapusadi Ghrita in Cikitsa 5: 71- 73) and vasa- Ghrta (vide Cikitsa 5: 126- 127) along with honey] [145- 146]

Line of treatment in General

यत्किञ्चित् कफवातघ्नमुष्णं वातानुलोमनम्।

भेषजं पानमत्रं वा तदि्धतं श्वासहिक्किने॥१४७॥

वातकृद्वा कफहरं कफकृद्वाऽनिलापहम्।

कार्यं नैकान्तिकं ताभ्यां प्रायः श्रेयोऽनिलापहम्॥१४८॥

सर्वेषां बृंहणे ह्यल्पः शक्यश्च प्रायशो भवेत्।

नात्यर्थं शमनेऽपायो भृशोऽशक्यश्च कर्शने॥१४९॥

तस्माच्छुद्धानशुद्धांश्च शमनैर्बृंहणैरपि।

हिक्का श्वासार्दिताञ्जन्तून् प्रायः समुपाचरेत्॥१५०॥

Ingredients which cause alleviation of Vayu and Kapha, which are hot in potency, and which cause downward movement of Vayu, (vatanuloma) are useful as medicines, drinks and food preparations for the patients suffering from hiccup and asthma

The medicines and foods which increase vata but destroy kapha or those which increase kapha but destroy (alleviate) vata shall be used in the treatment of these conditions. But those medicines and foods which destroy / alleviate only vata or only kapha shall not be administered.

The patient suffering from hiccup and asthma can be given nourishing therapy (Bhrimhana) and its adverse effects will be minimal and curable.

Alleviation therapies (Shamana) for such patients are free from any adverse efforts. But the administration of depletion therapy (Karshana) is likely to produce serious adverse effects which are difficult to cure.

Therefore the patient suffering from hiccups and asthma should generally be treated with nourishing (bhrmana) or alleviating (Samana) therapy, irrespective of the fact whether he has undergone elimination therapy (Suddha) or not (Asuddha). [147-150]

To sum up

तत्र श्लोकः:-

दुर्जयत्वे समुत्पत्तौ क्रियैकत्वे च कारणम्|

लिङ्गं पथ्यं च हिक्कानां श्वासानां चेह दर्शितम्||१५१||

The following topics are discussed in this chapter:

The grounds responsible for making hiccup and asthma difficult of cure

The origin or pathogenesis of hiccup and asthma

The grounds for the identity of treatment of hiccup and asthma

The signs and symptoms of (different varieties of) hiccup and asthma and

The wholesome regimen to be administered for the cure of hiccup and asthma. [151]

इत्यग्निवेशकृते तन्त्रे चरक प्रतिसंस्कृतेऽप्राप्ते दृढबल सम्पूरिते चिकित्सास्थाने हिक्का श्वास चिकित्सितं नाम सप्तदशोऽध्यायः||१७||

Thus, ends the 17th chapter in Chikitsa-sthana, dealing with the treatment of Hikka and Shvasa in the work of Agnivesha, redacted by Charaka and supplemented by Dridhabala.

Easy Ayurveda Publications

All our book publications are available at
www.EasyAyurveda.com/Books

English Books:
Charaka Samhita Volume 1,2,3 and 4 - English Translation
Ashtanga Hrudayam Sutrasthanam - English Translation
Living Easy With Ayurveda
Easy Ayurveda Home Remedies
Tridosha Made Easy
Ayurveda Tarka

Hindi Books:
Ayurved Samadhan

Kannada Books:
Sugama Jivanakkagi Ayurveda
Ayurveda Santvana

Malayalam Books
Ayurveda Asvasam
Jeevitha Soukhyathinu Ayurvedam

All our book publications are available at
www.EasyAyurveda.com/Books